Lecture Notes in Computer Science 12908

Founding Editors

Gerhard Goos
Karlsruhe Institute of Technology, Karlsruhe, Germany
Juris Hartmanis
Cornell University, Ithaca, NY, USA

Editorial Board Members

Elisa Bertino
Purdue University, West Lafayette, IN, USA
Wen Gao
Peking University, Beijing, China
Bernhard Steffen
TU Dortmund University, Dortmund, Germany
Gerhard Woeginger
RWTH Aachen, Aachen, Germany
Moti Yung
Columbia University, New York, NY, USA

More information about this subseries at http://www.springer.com/series/7412

Marleen de Bruijne · Philippe C. Cattin ·
Stéphane Cotin · Nicolas Padoy ·
Stefanie Speidel · Yefeng Zheng ·
Caroline Essert (Eds.)

Medical Image Computing and Computer Assisted Intervention – MICCAI 2021

24th International Conference
Strasbourg, France, September 27 – October 1, 2021
Proceedings, Part VIII

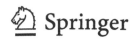 Springer

Editors
Marleen de Bruijne 🆔
Erasmus MC - University Medical Center
Rotterdam
Rotterdam, The Netherlands

University of Copenhagen
Copenhagen, Denmark

Stéphane Cotin 🆔
Inria Nancy Grand Est
Villers-lès-Nancy, France

Stefanie Speidel 🆔
National Center for Tumor Diseases
(NCT/UCC)
Dresden, Germany

Caroline Essert 🆔
ICube, Université de Strasbourg, CNRS
Strasbourg, France

Philippe C. Cattin 🆔
University of Basel
Allschwil, Switzerland

Nicolas Padoy 🆔
ICube, Université de Strasbourg, CNRS
Strasbourg, France

Yefeng Zheng 🆔
Tencent Jarvis Lab
Shenzhen, China

ISSN 0302-9743   ISSN 1611-3349   (electronic)
Lecture Notes in Computer Science
ISBN 978-3-030-87236-6   ISBN 978-3-030-87237-3   (eBook)
https://doi.org/10.1007/978-3-030-87237-3

LNCS Sublibrary: SL6 – Image Processing, Computer Vision, Pattern Recognition, and Graphics

This Springer imprint is published by the registered company Springer Nature Switzerland AG
The registered company address is: Gewerbestrasse 11, 6330 Cham, Switzerland

Preface

The 24th edition of the International Conference on Medical Image Computing and Computer Assisted Intervention (MICCAI 2021) has for the second time been placed under the shadow of COVID-19. Complicated situations due to the pandemic and multiple lockdowns have affected our lives during the past year, sometimes perturbing the researchers work, but also motivating an extraordinary dedication from many of our colleagues, and significant scientific advances in the fight against the virus. After another difficult year, most of us were hoping to be able to travel and finally meet in person at MICCAI 2021, which was supposed to be held in Strasbourg, France. Unfortunately, due to the uncertainty of the global situation, MICCAI 2021 had to be moved again to a virtual event that was held over five days from September 27 to October 1, 2021. Taking advantage of the experience gained last year and of the fast-evolving platforms, the organizers of MICCAI 2021 redesigned the schedule and the format. To offer the attendees both a strong scientific content and an engaging experience, two virtual platforms were used: Pathable for the oral and plenary sessions and SpatialChat for lively poster sessions, industrial booths, and networking events in the form of interactive group video chats.

These proceedings of MICCAI 2021 showcase all 531 papers that were presented at the main conference, organized into eight volumes in the Lecture Notes in Computer Science (LNCS) series as follows:

- Part I, LNCS Volume 12901: Image Segmentation
- Part II, LNCS Volume 12902: Machine Learning 1
- Part III, LNCS Volume 12903: Machine Learning 2
- Part IV, LNCS Volume 12904: Image Registration and Computer Assisted Intervention
- Part V, LNCS Volume 12905: Computer Aided Diagnosis
- Part VI, LNCS Volume 12906: Image Reconstruction and Cardiovascular Imaging
- Part VII, LNCS Volume 12907: Clinical Applications
- Part VIII, LNCS Volume 12908: Microscopic, Ophthalmic, and Ultrasound Imaging

These papers were selected after a thorough double-blind peer review process. We followed the example set by past MICCAI meetings, using Microsoft's Conference Managing Toolkit (CMT) for paper submission and peer reviews, with support from the Toronto Paper Matching System (TPMS), to partially automate paper assignment to area chairs and reviewers, and from iThenticate to detect possible cases of plagiarism.

Following a broad call to the community we received 270 applications to become an area chair for MICCAI 2021. From this group, the program chairs selected a total of 96 area chairs, aiming for diversity — MIC versus CAI, gender, geographical region, and a mix of experienced and new area chairs. Reviewers were recruited also via an open call for volunteers from the community (288 applications, of which 149 were selected by the program chairs) as well as by re-inviting past reviewers, leading to a total of 1340 registered reviewers.

We received 1630 full paper submissions after an original 2667 intentions to submit. Four papers were rejected without review because of concerns of (self-)plagiarism and dual submission and one additional paper was rejected for not adhering to the MICCAI page restrictions; two further cases of dual submission were discovered and rejected during the review process. Five papers were withdrawn by the authors during review and after acceptance.

The review process kicked off with a reviewer tutorial and an area chair meeting to discuss the review process, criteria for MICCAI acceptance, how to write a good (meta-)review, and expectations for reviewers and area chairs. Each area chair was assigned 16–18 manuscripts for which they suggested potential reviewers using TPMS scores, self-declared research area(s), and the area chair's knowledge of the reviewers' expertise in relation to the paper, while conflicts of interest were automatically avoided by CMT. Reviewers were invited to bid for the papers for which they had been suggested by an area chair or which were close to their expertise according to TPMS. Final reviewer allocations via CMT took account of reviewer bidding, prioritization of area chairs, and TPMS scores, leading to on average four reviews performed per person by a total of 1217 reviewers.

Following the initial double-blind review phase, area chairs provided a meta-review summarizing key points of reviews and a recommendation for each paper. The program chairs then evaluated the reviews and their scores, along with the recommendation from the area chairs, to directly accept 208 papers (13%) and reject 793 papers (49%); the remainder of the papers were sent for rebuttal by the authors. During the rebuttal phase, two additional area chairs were assigned to each paper. The three area chairs then independently ranked their papers, wrote meta-reviews, and voted to accept or reject the paper, based on the reviews, rebuttal, and manuscript. The program chairs checked all meta-reviews, and in some cases where the difference between rankings was high or comments were conflicting, they also assessed the original reviews, rebuttal, and submission. In all other cases a majority voting scheme was used to make the final decision. This process resulted in the acceptance of a further 325 papers for an overall acceptance rate of 33%.

Acceptance rates were the same between medical image computing (MIC) and computer assisted interventions (CAI) papers, and slightly lower where authors classified their paper as both MIC and CAI. Distribution of the geographical region of the first author as indicated in the optional demographic survey was similar among submitted and accepted papers.

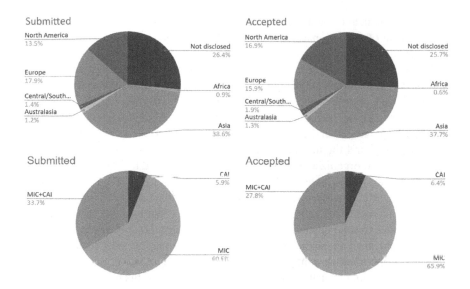

New this year, was the requirement to fill out a reproducibility checklist when submitting an intention to submit to MICCAI, in order to stimulate authors to think about what aspects of their method and experiments they should include to allow others to reproduce their results. Papers that included an anonymous code repository and/or indicated that the code would be made available were more likely to be accepted. From all accepted papers, 273 (51%) included a link to a code repository with the camera-ready submission.

Another novelty this year is that we decided to make the reviews, meta-reviews, and author responses for accepted papers available on the website. We hope the community will find this a useful resource.

The outstanding program of MICCAI 2021 was enriched by four exceptional keynote talks given by Alyson McGregor, Richard Satava, Fei-Fei Li, and Pierre Jannin, on hot topics such as gender bias in medical research, clinical translation to industry, intelligent medicine, and sustainable research. This year, as in previous years, high-quality satellite events completed the program of the main conference: 28 workshops, 23 challenges, and 14 tutorials; without forgetting the increasingly successful plenary events, such as the Women in MICCAI (WiM) meeting, the MICCAI Student Board (MSB) events, the 2nd Startup Village, the MICCAI-RSNA panel, and the first "Reinforcing Inclusiveness & diverSity and Empowering MICCAI" (or RISE-MICCAI) event.

MICCAI 2021 has also seen the first edition of CLINICCAI, the clinical day of MICCAI. Organized by Nicolas Padoy and Lee Swanstrom, this new event will hopefully help bring the scientific and clinical communities closer together, and foster collaborations and interaction. A common keynote connected the two events. We hope this effort will be pursued in the next editions.

We would like to thank everyone who has contributed to making MICCAI 2021 a success. First of all, we sincerely thank the authors, area chairs, reviewers, and session chairs for their dedication and for offering the participants and readers of these proceedings content of exceptional quality. Special thanks go to our fantastic submission platform manager Kitty Wong, who has been a tremendous help in the entire process from reviewer and area chair selection, paper submission, and the review process to the preparation of these proceedings. We also thank our very efficient team of satellite events chairs and coordinators, led by Cristian Linte and Matthieu Chabanas: the workshop chairs, Amber Simpson, Denis Fortun, Marta Kersten-Oertel, and Sandrine Voros; the challenges chairs, Annika Reinke, Spyridon Bakas, Nicolas Passat, and Ingerid Reinersten; and the tutorial chairs, Sonia Pujol and Vincent Noblet, as well as all the satellite event organizers for the valuable content added to MICCAI. Our special thanks also go to John Baxter and his team who worked hard on setting up and populating the virtual platforms, to Alejandro Granados for his valuable help and efficient communication on social media, and to Shelley Wallace and Anna Van Vliet for marketing and communication. We are also very grateful to Anirban Mukhopadhay for his management of the sponsorship, and of course many thanks to the numerous sponsors who supported the conference, often with continuous engagement over many years. This year again, our thanks go to Marius Linguraru and his team who supervised a range of actions to help, and promote, career development, among which were the mentorship program and the Startup Village. And last but not least, our wholehearted thanks go to Mehmet and the wonderful team at Dekon Congress and Tourism for their great professionalism and reactivity in the management of all logistical aspects of the event.

Finally, we thank the MICCAI society and the Board of Directors for their support throughout the years, starting with the first discussions about bringing MICCAI to Strasbourg in 2017.

We look forward to seeing you at MICCAI 2022.

September 2021

Marleen de Bruijne
Philippe Cattin
Stéphane Cotin
Nicolas Padoy
Stefanie Speidel
Yefeng Zheng
Caroline Essert

Organization

General Chair

Caroline Essert — Université de Strasbourg, CNRS, ICube, France

Program Chairs

Marleen de Bruijne — Erasmus MC Rotterdam, The Netherlands, and University of Copenhagen, Denmark
Philippe C. Cattin — University of Basel, Switzerland
Stéphane Cotin — Inria, France
Nicolas Padoy — Université de Strasbourg, CNRS, ICube, IHU, France
Stefanie Speidel — National Center for Tumor Diseases, Dresden, Germany
Yefeng Zheng — Tencent Jarvis Lab, China

Satellite Events Coordinators

Cristian Linte — Rochester Institute of Technology, USA
Matthieu Chabanas — Université Grenoble Alpes, France

Workshop Team

Amber Simpson — Queen's University, Canada
Denis Fortun — Université de Strasbourg, CNRS, ICube, France
Marta Kersten-Oertel — Concordia University, Canada
Sandrine Voros — TIMC-IMAG, INSERM, France

Challenges Team

Annika Reinke — German Cancer Research Center, Germany
Spyridon Bakas — University of Pennsylvania, USA
Nicolas Passat — Université de Reims Champagne-Ardenne, France
Ingerid Reinersten — SINTEF, NTNU, Norway

Tutorial Team

Vincent Noblet — Université de Strasbourg, CNRS, ICube, France
Sonia Pujol — Harvard Medical School, Brigham and Women's Hospital, USA

Clinical Day Chairs

Nicolas Padoy   Université de Strasbourg, CNRS, ICube, IHU, France
Lee Swanström   IHU Strasbourg, France

Sponsorship Chairs

Anirban Mukhopadhyay   Technische Universität Darmstadt, Germany
Yanwu Xu   Baidu Inc., China

Young Investigators and Early Career Development Program Chairs

Marius Linguraru   Children's National Institute, USA
Antonio Porras   Children's National Institute, USA
Daniel Racoceanu   Sorbonne Université/Brain Institute, France
Nicola Rieke   NVIDIA, Germany
Renee Yao   NVIDIA, USA

Social Media Chairs

Alejandro Granados   King's College London, UK
   Martinez
Shuwei Xing   Robarts Research Institute, Canada
Maxence Boels   King's College London, UK

Green Team

Pierre Jannin   INSERM, Université de Rennes 1, France
Étienne Baudrier   Université de Strasbourg, CNRS, ICube, France

Student Board Liaison

Éléonore Dufresne   Université de Strasbourg, CNRS, ICube, France
Étienne Le Quentrec   Université de Strasbourg, CNRS, ICube, France
Vinkle Srivastav   Université de Strasbourg, CNRS, ICube, France

Submission Platform Manager

Kitty Wong   The MICCAI Society, Canada

Virtual Platform Manager

John Baxter   INSERM, Université de Rennes 1, France

Program Committee

Ehsan Adeli	Stanford University, USA
Iman Aganj	Massachusetts General Hospital, Harvard Medical School, USA
Pablo Arbelaez	Universidad de los Andes, Colombia
John Ashburner	University College London, UK
Meritxell Bach Cuadra	University of Lausanne, Switzerland
Sophia Bano	University College London, UK
Adrien Bartoli	Université Clermont Auvergne, France
Christian Baumgartner	ETH Zürich, Switzerland
Hrvoje Bogunovic	Medical University of Vienna, Austria
Weidong Cai	University of Sydney, Australia
Gustavo Carneiro	University of Adelaide, Australia
Chao Chen	Stony Brook University, USA
Elvis Chen	Robarts Research Institute, Canada
Hao Chen	Hong Kong University of Science and Technology, Hong Kong SAR
Albert Chung	Hong Kong University of Science and Technology, Hong Kong SAR
Adrian Dalca	Massachusetts Institute of Technology, USA
Adrien Depeursinge	HES-SO Valais-Wallis, Switzerland
Jose Dolz	ÉTS Montréal, Canada
Ruogu Fang	University of Florida, USA
Dagan Feng	University of Sydney, Australia
Huazhu Fu	Inception Institute of Artificial Intelligence, United Arab Emirates
Mingchen Gao	University at Buffalo, The State University of New York, USA
Guido Gerig	New York University, USA
Orcun Goksel	Uppsala University, Sweden
Alberto Gomez	King's College London, UK
Ilker Hacihaliloglu	Rutgers University, USA
Adam Harrison	PAII Inc., USA
Mattias Heinrich	University of Lübeck, Germany
Yi Hong	Shanghai Jiao Tong University, China
Yipeng Hu	University College London, UK
Junzhou Huang	University of Texas at Arlington, USA
Xiaolei Huang	The Pennsylvania State University, USA
Jana Hutter	King's College London, UK
Madhura Ingalhalikar	Symbiosis Center for Medical Image Analysis, India
Shantanu Joshi	University of California, Los Angeles, USA
Samuel Kadoury	Polytechnique Montréal, Canada
Fahmi Khalifa	Mansoura University, Egypt
Hosung Kim	University of Southern California, USA
Minjeong Kim	University of North Carolina at Greensboro, USA

Ender Konukoglu	ETH Zürich, Switzerland
Bennett Landman	Vanderbilt University, USA
Ignacio Larrabide	CONICET, Argentina
Baiying Lei	Shenzhen University, China
Gang Li	University of North Carolina at Chapel Hill, USA
Mingxia Liu	University of North Carolina at Chapel Hill, USA
Herve Lombaert	ÉTS Montréal, Canada, and Inria, France
Marco Lorenzi	Inria, France
Le Lu	PAII Inc., USA
Xiongbiao Luo	Xiamen University, China
Dwarikanath Mahapatra	Inception Institute of Artificial Intelligence, United Arab Emirates
Andreas Maier	FAU Erlangen-Nuremberg, Germany
Erik Meijering	University of New South Wales, Australia
Hien Nguyen	University of Houston, USA
Marc Niethammer	University of North Carolina at Chapel Hill, USA
Tingying Peng	Technische Universität München, Germany
Caroline Petitjean	Université de Rouen, France
Dzung Pham	Henry M. Jackson Foundation, USA
Hedyeh Rafii-Tari	Auris Health Inc, USA
Islem Rekik	Istanbul Technical University, Turkey
Nicola Rieke	NVIDIA, Germany
Su Ruan	Laboratoire LITIS, France
Thomas Schultz	University of Bonn, Germany
Sharmishtaa Seshamani	Allen Institute, USA
Yonggang Shi	University of Southern California, USA
Darko Stern	Technical University of Graz, Austria
Carole Sudre	King's College London, UK
Heung-Il Suk	Korea University, South Korea
Jian Sun	Xi'an Jiaotong University, China
Raphael Sznitman	University of Bern, Switzerland
Amir Tahmasebi	Enlitic, USA
Qian Tao	Delft University of Technology, The Netherlands
Tolga Tasdizen	University of Utah, USA
Martin Urschler	University of Auckland, New Zealand
Archana Venkataraman	Johns Hopkins University, USA
Guotai Wang	University of Electronic Science and Technology of China, China
Hongzhi Wang	IBM Almaden Research Center, USA
Hua Wang	Colorado School of Mines, USA
Qian Wang	Shanghai Jiao Tong University, China
Yalin Wang	Arizona State University, USA
Fuyong Xing	University of Colorado Denver, USA
Daguang Xu	NVIDIA, USA
Yanwu Xu	Baidu, China
Ziyue Xu	NVIDIA, USA

Zhong Xue	Shanghai United Imaging Intelligence, China
Xin Yang	Huazhong University of Science and Technology, China
Jianhua Yao	National Institutes of Health, USA
Zhaozheng Yin	Stony Brook University, USA
Yixuan Yuan	City University of Hong Kong, Hong Kong SAR
Liang Zhan	University of Pittsburgh, USA
Tuo Zhang	Northwestern Polytechnical University, China
Yitian Zhao	Chinese Academy of Sciences, China
Luping Zhou	University of Sydney, Australia
S. Kevin Zhou	Chinese Academy of Sciences, China
Dajiang Zhu	University of Texas at Arlington, USA
Xiahai Zhuang	Fudan University, China
Maria A. Zuluaga	EURECOM, France

Reviewers

Alaa Eldin Abdelaal
Khalid Abdul Jabbar
Purang Abolmaesumi
Mazdak Abulnaga
Maryam Afzali
Priya Aggarwal
Ola Ahmad
Sahar Ahmad
Euijoon Ahn
Alireza Akhondi-Asl
Saad Ullah Akram
Dawood Al Chanti
Daniel Alexander
Sharib Ali
Lejla Alic
Omar Al-Kadi
Maximilian Allan
Pierre Ambrosini
Sameer Antani
Michela Antonelli
Jacob Antunes
Syed Anwar
Ignacio Arganda-Carreras
Mohammad Ali Armin
Md Ashikuzzaman
Mehdi Astaraki
Angélica Atehortúa
Gowtham Atluri

Chloé Audigier
Kamran Avanaki
Angelica Aviles-Rivero
Suyash Awate
Dogu Baran Aydogan
Qinle Ba
Morteza Babaie
Hyeon-Min Bae
Woong Bae
Junjie Bai
Wenjia Bai
Ujjwal Baid
Spyridon Bakas
Yaël Balbastre
Marcin Balicki
Fabian Balsiger
Abhirup Banerjee
Sreya Banerjee
Shunxing Bao
Adrian Barbu
Sumana Basu
Mathilde Bateson
Deepti Bathula
John Baxter
Bahareh Behboodi
Delaram Behnami
Mikhail Belyaev
Aicha BenTaieb

Camilo Bermudez
Gabriel Bernardino
Hadrien Bertrand
Alaa Bessadok
Michael Beyeler
Indrani Bhattacharya
Chetan Bhole
Lei Bi
Gui-Bin Bian
Ryoma Bise
Stefano B. Blumberg
Ester Bonmati
Bhushan Borotikar
Jiri Borovec
Ilaria Boscolo Galazzo
Alexandre Bousse
Nicolas Boutry
Behzad Bozorgtabar
Nathaniel Braman
Nadia Brancati
Katharina Breininger
Christopher Bridge
Esther Bron
Rupert Brooks
Qirong Bu
Duc Toan Bui
Ninon Burgos
Nikolay Burlutskiy
Hendrik Burwinkel
Russell Butler
Michał Byra
Ryan Cabeen
Mariano Cabezas
Hongmin Cai
Jinzheng Cai
Yunliang Cai
Sema Candemir
Bing Cao
Qing Cao
Shilei Cao
Tian Cao
Weiguo Cao
Aaron Carass
M. Jorge Cardoso
Adrià Casamitjana
Matthieu Chabanas

Ahmad Chaddad
Jayasree Chakraborty
Sylvie Chambon
Yi Hao Chan
Ming-Ching Chang
Peng Chang
Violeta Chang
Sudhanya Chatterjee
Christos Chatzichristos
Antong Chen
Chang Chen
Cheng Chen
Dongdong Chen
Geng Chen
Hanbo Chen
Jianan Chen
Jianxu Chen
Jie Chen
Junxiang Chen
Lei Chen
Li Chen
Liangjun Chen
Min Chen
Pingjun Chen
Qiang Chen
Shuai Chen
Tianhua Chen
Tingting Chen
Xi Chen
Xiaoran Chen
Xin Chen
Xuejin Chen
Yuhua Chen
Yukun Chen
Zhaolin Chen
Zhineng Chen
Zhixiang Chen
Erkang Cheng
Jun Cheng
Li Cheng
Yuan Cheng
Farida Cheriet
Minqi Chong
Jaegul Choo
Aritra Chowdhury
Gary Christensen

Daan Christiaens
Stergios Christodoulidis
Ai Wern Chung
Pietro Antonio Cicalese
Özgün Çiçek
Celia Cintas
Matthew Clarkson
Jaume Coll-Font
Toby Collins
Olivier Commowick
Pierre-Henri Conze
Timothy Cootes
Luca Corinzia
Teresa Correia
Hadrien Courtecuisse
Jeffrey Craley
Hui Cui
Jianan Cui
Zhiming Cui
Kathleen Curran
Claire Cury
Tobias Czempiel
Vedrana Dahl
Haixing Dai
Rafat Damseh
Bilel Daoud
Neda Davoudi
Laura Daza
Sandro De Zanet
Charles Delahunt
Yang Deng
Cem Deniz
Felix Denzinger
Hrishikesh Deshpande
Christian Desrosiers
Blake Dewey
Neel Dey
Raunak Dey
Jwala Dhamala
Yashin Dicente Cid
Li Ding
Xinghao Ding
Zhipeng Ding
Konstantin Dmitriev
Ines Domingues
Liang Dong

Mengjin Dong
Nanqing Dong
Reuben Dorent
Sven Dorkenwald
Qi Dou
Simon Drouin
Niharika D'Souza
Lei Du
Hongyi Duanmu
Nicolas Duchateau
James Duncan
Luc Duong
Nicha Dvornek
Dmitry V. Dylov
Oleh Dzyubachyk
Roy Eagleson
Mehran Ebrahimi
Jan Egger
Alma Eguizabal
Gudmundur Einarsson
Ahmed Elazab
Mohammed S. M. Elbaz
Shireen Elhabian
Mohammed Elmogy
Amr Elsawy
Ahmed Eltanboly
Sandy Engelhardt
Ertunc Erdil
Marius Erdt
Floris Ernst
Boris Escalante-Ramírez
Maria Escobar
Mohammad Eslami
Nazila Esmaeili
Marco Esposito
Oscar Esteban
Théo Estienne
Ivan Ezhov
Deng-Ping Fan
Jingfan Fan
Xin Fan
Yonghui Fan
Xi Fang
Zhenghan Fang
Aly Farag
Mohsen Farzi

Lina Felsner
Jun Feng
Ruibin Feng
Xinyang Feng
Yuan Feng
Aaron Fenster
Aasa Feragen
Henrique Fernandes
Enzo Ferrante
Jean Feydy
Lukas Fischer
Peter Fischer
Antonio Foncubierta-Rodríguez
Germain Forestier
Nils Daniel Forkert
Jean-Rassaire Fouefack
Moti Freiman
Wolfgang Freysinger
Xueyang Fu
Yunguan Fu
Wolfgang Fuhl
Isabel Funke
Philipp Fürnstahl
Pedro Furtado
Ryo Furukawa
Jin Kyu Gahm
Laurent Gajny
Adrian Galdran
Yu Gan
Melanie Ganz
Cong Gao
Dongxu Gao
Linlin Gao
Siyuan Gao
Yixin Gao
Yue Gao
Zhifan Gao
Alfonso Gastelum-Strozzi
Srishti Gautam
Bao Ge
Rongjun Ge
Zongyuan Ge
Sairam Geethanath
Shiv Gehlot
Nils Gessert
Olivier Gevaert

Sandesh Ghimire
Ali Gholipour
Sayan Ghosal
Andrea Giovannini
Gabriel Girard
Ben Glocker
Arnold Gomez
Mingming Gong
Cristina González
German Gonzalez
Sharath Gopal
Karthik Gopinath
Pietro Gori
Michael Götz
Shuiping Gou
Maged Goubran
Sobhan Goudarzi
Dushyant Goyal
Mark Graham
Bertrand Granado
Alejandro Granados
Vicente Grau
Lin Gu
Shi Gu
Xianfeng Gu
Yun Gu
Zaiwang Gu
Hao Guan
Ricardo Guerrero
Houssem-Eddine Gueziri
Dazhou Guo
Hengtao Guo
Jixiang Guo
Pengfei Guo
Xiaoqing Guo
Yi Guo
Yulan Guo
Yuyu Guo
Krati Gupta
Vikash Gupta
Praveen Gurunath Bharathi
Boris Gutman
Prashnna Gyawali
Stathis Hadjidemetriou
Mohammad Hamghalam
Hu Han

Liang Han
Xiaoguang Han
Xu Han
Zhi Han
Zhongyi Han
Jonny Hancox
Xiaoke Hao
Nandinee Haq
Ali Hatamizadeh
Charles Hatt
Andreas Hauptmann
Mohammad Havaei
Kelei He
Nanjun He
Tiancheng He
Xuming He
Yuting He
Nicholas Heller
Alessa Hering
Monica Hernandez
Carlos Hernandez-Matas
Kilian Hett
Jacob Hinkle
David Ho
Nico Hoffmann
Matthew Holden
Sungmin Hong
Yoonmi Hong
Antal Horváth
Md Belayat Hossain
Benjamin Hou
William Hsu
Tai-Chiu Hsung
Kai Hu
Shi Hu
Shunbo Hu
Wenxing Hu
Xiaoling Hu
Xiaowei Hu
Yan Hu
Zhenhong Hu
Heng Huang
Qiaoying Huang
Yi-Jie Huang
Yixing Huang
Yongxiang Huang

Yue Huang
Yufang Huang
Arnaud Huaulmé
Henkjan Huisman
Yuankai Huo
Andreas Husch
Mohammad Hussain
Raabid Hussain
Sarfaraz Hussein
Khoi Huynh
Seong Jae Hwang
Emmanuel Iarussi
Kay Igwe
Abdullah-Al-Zubaer Imran
Ismail Irmakci
Mobarakol Islam
Mohammad Shafkat Islam
Vamsi Ithapu
Koichi Ito
Hayato Itoh
Oleksandra Ivashchenko
Yuji Iwahori
Shruti Jadon
Mohammad Jafari
Mostafa Jahanifar
Amir Jamaludin
Mirek Janatka
Won-Dong Jang
Uditha Jarayathne
Ronnachai Jaroensri
Golara Javadi
Rohit Jena
Rachid Jennane
Todd Jensen
Won-Ki Jeong
Yuanfeng Ji
Zhanghexuan Ji
Haozhe Jia
Jue Jiang
Tingting Jiang
Xiang Jiang
Jianbo Jiao
Zhicheng Jiao
Amelia Jiménez-Sánchez
Dakai Jin
Yueming Jin

Bin Jing
Anand Joshi
Yohan Jun
Kyu-Hwan Jung
Alain Jungo
Manjunath K N
Ali Kafaei Zad Tehrani
Bernhard Kainz
John Kalafut
Michael C. Kampffmeyer
Qingbo Kang
Po-Yu Kao
Neerav Karani
Turkay Kart
Satyananda Kashyap
Amin Katouzian
Alexander Katzmann
Prabhjot Kaur
Erwan Kerrien
Hoel Kervadec
Ashkan Khakzar
Nadieh Khalili
Siavash Khallaghi
Farzad Khalvati
Bishesh Khanal
Pulkit Khandelwal
Maksim Kholiavchenko
Naji Khosravan
Seyed Mostafa Kia
Daeseung Kim
Hak Gu Kim
Hyo-Eun Kim
Jae-Hun Kim
Jaeil Kim
Jinman Kim
Mansu Kim
Namkug Kim
Seong Tae Kim
Won Hwa Kim
Andrew King
Atilla Kiraly
Yoshiro Kitamura
Tobias Klinder
Bin Kong
Jun Kong
Tomasz Konopczynski

Bongjin Koo
Ivica Kopriva
Kivanc Kose
Mateusz Kozinski
Anna Kreshuk
Anithapriya Krishnan
Pavitra Krishnaswamy
Egor Krivov
Frithjof Kruggel
Alexander Krull
Elizabeth Krupinski
Serife Kucur
David Kügler
Hugo Kuijf
Abhay Kumar
Ashnil Kumar
Kuldeep Kumar
Nitin Kumar
Holger Kunze
Tahsin Kurc
Anvar Kurmukov
Yoshihiro Kuroda
Jin Tae Kwak
Yongchan Kwon
Francesco La Rosa
Aymen Laadhari
Dmitrii Lachinov
Alain Lalande
Tryphon Lambrou
Carole Lartizien
Bianca Lassen-Schmidt
Ngan Le
Leo Lebrat
Christian Ledig
Eung-Joo Lee
Hyekyoung Lee
Jong-Hwan Lee
Matthew Lee
Sangmin Lee
Soochahn Lee
Étienne Léger
Stefan Leger
Andreas Leibetseder
Rogers Jeffrey Leo John
Juan Leon
Bo Li

Chongyi Li
Fuhai Li
Hongming Li
Hongwei Li
Jian Li
Jianning Li
Jiayun Li
Junhua Li
Kang Li
Mengzhang Li
Ming Li
Qing Li
Shaohua Li
Shuyu Li
Weijian Li
Weikai Li
Wenqi Li
Wenyuan Li
Xiang Li
Xiaomeng Li
Xiaoxiao Li
Xin Li
Xiuli Li
Yang Li
Yi Li
Yuexiang Li
Zeju Li
Zhang Li
Zhiyuan Li
Zhjin Li
Gongbo Liang
Jianming Liang
Libin Liang
Yuan Liang
Haofu Liao
Ruizhi Liao
Wei Liao
Xiangyun Liao
Roxane Licandro
Gilbert Lim
Baihan Lin
Hongxiang Lin
Jianyu Lin
Yi Lin
Claudia Lindner
Geert Litjens

Bin Liu
Chi Liu
Daochang Liu
Dong Liu
Dongnan Liu
Feng Liu
Hangfan Liu
Hong Liu
Huafeng Liu
Jianfei Liu
Jingya Liu
Kai Liu
Kefei Liu
Lihao Liu
Mengting Liu
Peng Liu
Qin Liu
Quande Liu
Shengfeng Liu
Shenghua Liu
Shuangjun Liu
Sidong Liu
Siqi Liu
Tianrui Liu
Xiao Liu
Xinyang Liu
Xinyu Liu
Yan Liu
Yikang Liu
Yong Liu
Yuan Liu
Yue Liu
Yuhang Liu
Andrea Loddo
Nicolas Loménie
Daniel Lopes
Bin Lou
Jian Lou
Nicolas Loy Rodas
Donghuan Lu
Huanxiang Lu
Weijia Lu
Xiankai Lu
Yongyi Lu
Yueh-Hsun Lu
Yuhang Lu

Imanol Luengo
Jie Luo
Jiebo Luo
Luyang Luo
Ma Luo
Bin Lv
Jinglei Lv
Junyan Lyu
Qing Lyu
Yuanyuan Lyu
Andy J. Ma
Chunwei Ma
Da Ma
Hua Ma
Kai Ma
Lei Ma
Anderson Maciel
Amirreza Mahbod
S. Sara Mahdavi
Mohammed Mahmoud
Saïd Mahmoudi
Klaus H. Maier-Hein
Bilal Malik
Ilja Manakov
Matteo Mancini
Tommaso Mansi
Yunxiang Mao
Brett Marinelli
Pablo Márquez Neila
Carsten Marr
Yassine Marrakchi
Fabio Martinez
Andre Mastmeyer
Tejas Sudharshan Mathai
Dimitrios Mavroeidis
Jamie McClelland
Pau Medrano-Gracia
Raghav Mehta
Sachin Mehta
Raphael Meier
Qier Meng
Qingjie Meng
Yanda Meng
Martin Menten
Odyssée Merveille
Islem Mhiri

Liang Mi
Stijn Michielse
Abhishek Midya
Fausto Milletari
Hyun-Seok Min
Zhe Min
Tadashi Miyamoto
Sara Moccia
Hassan Mohy-ud-Din
Tony C. W. Mok
Rafael Molina
Mehdi Moradi
Rodrigo Moreno
Kensaku Mori
Lia Morra
Linda Moy
Mohammad Hamed Mozaffari
Sovanlal Mukherjee
Anirban Mukhopadhyay
Henning Müller
Balamurali Murugesan
Cosmas Mwikirize
Andriy Myronenko
Saad Nadeem
Vishwesh Nath
Rodrigo Nava
Fernando Navarro
Amin Nejatbakhsh
Dong Ni
Hannes Nickisch
Dong Nie
Jingxin Nie
Aditya Nigam
Lipeng Ning
Xia Ning
Tianye Niu
Jack Noble
Vincent Noblet
Alexey Novikov
Jorge Novo
Mohammad Obeid
Masahiro Oda
Benjamin Odry
Steffen Oeltze-Jafra
Hugo Oliveira
Sara Oliveira

Arnau Oliver
Emanuele Olivetti
Jimena Olveres
John Onofrey
Felipe Orihuela-Espina
José Orlando
Marcos Ortega
Yoshito Otake
Sebastian Otálora
Cheng Ouyang
Jiahong Ouyang
Xi Ouyang
Michal Ozery-Flato
Danielle Pace
Krittin Pachtrachai
J. Blas Pagador
Akshay Pai
Viswanath Pamulakanty Sudarshan
Jin Pan
Yongsheng Pan
Pankaj Pandey
Prashant Pandey
Egor Panfilov
Shumao Pang
Joao Papa
Constantin Pape
Bartlomiej Papiez
Hyunjin Park
Jongchan Park
Sanghyun Park
Seung-Jong Park
Seyoun Park
Magdalini Paschali
Diego Patiño Cortés
Angshuman Paul
Christian Payer
Yuru Pei
Chengtao Peng
Yige Peng
Antonio Pepe
Oscar Perdomo
Sérgio Pereira
Jose-Antonio Pérez-Carrasco
Fernando Pérez-García
Jorge Perez-Gonzalez
Skand Peri

Matthias Perkonigg
Mehran Pesteie
Jorg Peters
Jens Petersen
Kersten Petersen
Renzo Phellan Aro
Ashish Phophalia
Tomasz Pieciak
Antonio Pinheiro
Pramod Pisharady
Kilian Pohl
Sebastian Pölsterl
Iulia A. Popescu
Alison Pouch
Prateek Prasanna
Raphael Prevost
Juan Prieto
Sergi Pujades
Elodie Puybareau
Esther Puyol-Antón
Haikun Qi
Huan Qi
Buyue Qian
Yan Qiang
Yuchuan Qiao
Chen Qin
Wenjian Qin
Yulei Qin
Wu Qiu
Hui Qu
Liangqiong Qu
Kha Gia Quach
Prashanth R.
Pradeep Reddy Raamana
Mehdi Rahim
Jagath Rajapakse
Kashif Rajpoot
Jhonata Ramos
Lingyan Ran
Hatem Rashwan
Daniele Ravì
Keerthi Sravan Ravi
Nishant Ravikumar
Harish RaviPrakash
Samuel Remedios
Yinhao Ren

Yudan Ren
Mauricio Reyes
Constantino Reyes-Aldasoro
Jonas Richiardi
David Richmond
Anne-Marie Rickmann
Leticia Rittner
Dominik Rivoir
Emma Robinson
Jessica Rodgers
Rafael Rodrigues
Robert Rohling
Michal Rosen-Zvi
Lukasz Roszkowiak
Karsten Roth
José Rouco
Daniel Rueckert
Jaime S. Cardoso
Mohammad Sabokrou
Ario Sadafi
Monjoy Saha
Pramit Saha
Dushyant Sahoo
Pranjal Sahu
Maria Sainz de Cea
Olivier Salvado
Robin Sandkuehler
Gianmarco Santini
Duygu Sarikaya
Imari Sato
Olivier Saut
Dustin Scheinost
Nico Scherf
Markus Schirmer
Alexander Schlaefer
Jerome Schmid
Julia Schnabel
Klaus Schoeffmann
Andreas Schuh
Ernst Schwartz
Christina Schwarz-Gsaxner
Michaël Sdika
Suman Sedai
Anjany Sekuboyina
Raghavendra Selvan
Sourya Sengupta

Youngho Seo
Lama Seoud
Ana Sequeira
Maxime Sermesant
Carmen Serrano
Muhammad Shaban
Ahmed Shaffie
Sobhan Shafiei
Mohammad Abuzar Shaikh
Reuben Shamir
Shayan Shams
Hongming Shan
Harshita Sharma
Gregory Sharp
Mohamed Shehata
Haocheng Shen
Li Shen
Liyue Shen
Mali Shen
Yiqing Shen
Yiqiu Shen
Zhengyang Shen
Kuangyu Shi
Luyao Shi
Xiaoshuang Shi
Xueying Shi
Yemin Shi
Yiyu Shi
Yonghong Shi
Jitae Shin
Boris Shirokikh
Suprosanna Shit
Suzanne Shontz
Yucheng Shu
Alberto Signoroni
Wilson Silva
Margarida Silveira
Matthew Sinclair
Rohit Singla
Sumedha Singla
Ayushi Sinha
Kevin Smith
Rajath Soans
Ahmed Soliman
Stefan Sommer
Yang Song

Youyi Song
Aristeidis Sotiras
Arcot Sowmya
Rachel Sparks
William Speier
Ziga Spiclin
Dominik Spinczyk
Jon Sporring
Chetan Srinidhi
Anuroop Sriram
Vinkle Srivastav
Lawrence Staib
Marius Staring
Johannes Stegmaier
Joshua Stough
Robin Strand
Martin Styner
Hai Su
Yun-Hsuan Su
Vaishnavi Subramanian
Gérard Subsol
Yao Sui
Avan Suinesiaputra
Jeremias Sulam
Shipra Suman
Li Sun
Wenqing Sun
Chiranjib Sur
Yannick Suter
Tanveer Syeda-Mahmood
Fatemeh Taheri Dezaki
Roger Tam
José Tamez-Peña
Chaowei Tan
Hao Tang
Thomas Tang
Yucheng Tang
Zihao Tang
Mickael Tardy
Giacomo Tarroni
Jonas Teuwen
Paul Thienphrapa
Stephen Thompson
Jiang Tian
Yu Tian
Yun Tian

Aleksei Tiulpin
Hamid Tizhoosh
Matthew Toews
Oguzhan Topsakal
Antonio Torteya
Sylvie Treuillet
Jocelyne Troccaz
Roger Trullo
Chialing Tsai
Sudhakar Tummala
Verena Uslar
Hristina Uzunova
Régis Vaillant
Maria Vakalopoulou
Jeya Maria Jose Valanarasu
Tom van Sonsbeek
Gijs van Tulder
Marta Varela
Thomas Varsavsky
Francisco Vasconcelos
Liset Vazquez Romaguera
S. Swaroop Vedula
Sanketh Vedula
Harini Veeraraghavan
Miguel Vega
Gonzalo Vegas Sanchez-Ferrero
Anant Vemuri
Gopalkrishna Veni
Mitko Veta
Thomas Vetter
Pedro Vieira
Juan Pedro Vigueras Guillén
Barbara Villarini
Satish Viswanath
Athanasios Vlontzos
Wolf-Dieter Vogl
Bo Wang
Cheng Wang
Chengjia Wang
Chunliang Wang
Clinton Wang
Congcong Wang
Dadong Wang
Dongang Wang
Haifeng Wang
Hongyu Wang

Hu Wang
Huan Wang
Kun Wang
Li Wang
Liansheng Wang
Linwei Wang
Manning Wang
Renzhen Wang
Ruixuan Wang
Sheng Wang
Shujun Wang
Shuo Wang
Tianchen Wang
Tongxin Wang
Wenzhe Wang
Xi Wang
Xiaosong Wang
Yan Wang
Yaping Wang
Yi Wang
Yirui Wang
Zeyi Wang
Zhangyang Wang
Zihao Wang
Zuhui Wang
Simon Warfield
Jonathan Weber
Jürgen Weese
Dong Wei
Donglai Wei
Dongming Wei
Martin Weigert
Wolfgang Wein
Michael Wels
Cédric Wemmert
Junhao Wen
Travis Williams
Matthias Wilms
Stefan Winzeck
James Wiskin
Adam Wittek
Marek Wodzinski
Jelmer Wolterink
Ken C. L. Wong
Chongruo Wu
Guoqing Wu

Ji Wu
Jian Wu
Jie Ying Wu
Pengxiang Wu
Xiyin Wu
Ye Wu
Yicheng Wu
Yifan Wu
Tobias Wuerfl
Pengcheng Xi
James Xia
Siyu Xia
Wenfeng Xia
Yingda Xia
Yong Xia
Lei Xiang
Deqiang Xiao
Li Xiao
Yiming Xiao
Hongtao Xie
Lingxi Xie
Long Xie
Weidi Xie
Yiting Xie
Yutong Xie
Xiaohan Xing
Chang Xu
Chenchu Xu
Hongming Xu
Kele Xu
Min Xu
Rui Xu
Xiaowei Xu
Xuanang Xu
Yongchao Xu
Zhenghua Xu
Zhoubing Xu
Kai Xuan
Cheng Xue
Jie Xue
Wufeng Xue
Yuan Xue
Faridah Yahya
Ke Yan
Yuguang Yan
Zhennan Yan

Changchun Yang
Chao-Han Huck Yang
Dong Yang
Erkun Yang
Fan Yang
Ge Yang
Guang Yang
Guanyu Yang
Heran Yang
Hongxu Yang
Huijuan Yang
Jiancheng Yang
Jie Yang
Junlin Yang
Lin Yang
Peng Yang
Xin Yang
Yan Yang
Yujiu Yang
Dongren Yao
Jiawen Yao
Li Yao
Qingsong Yao
Chuyang Ye
Dong Hye Ye
Menglong Ye
Xujiong Ye
Jingru Yi
Jirong Yi
Xin Yi
Youngjin Yoo
Chenyu You
Haichao Yu
Hanchao Yu
Lequan Yu
Qi Yu
Yang Yu
Pengyu Yuan
Fatemeh Zabihollahy
Ghada Zamzmi
Marco Zenati
Guodong Zeng
Rui Zeng
Oliver Zettinig
Zhiwei Zhai
Chaoyi Zhang

Daoqiang Zhang
Fan Zhang
Guangming Zhang
Hang Zhang
Huahong Zhang
Jianpeng Zhang
Jiong Zhang
Jun Zhang
Lei Zhang
Lichi Zhang
Lin Zhang
Ling Zhang
Lu Zhang
Miaomiao Zhang
Ning Zhang
Qiang Zhang
Rongzhao Zhang
Ru-Yuan Zhang
Shihao Zhang
Shu Zhang
Tong Zhang
Wei Zhang
Weiwei Zhang
Wen Zhang
Wenlu Zhang
Xin Zhang
Ya Zhang
Yanbo Zhang
Yanfu Zhang
Yi Zhang
Yishuo Zhang
Yong Zhang
Yongqin Zhang
You Zhang
Youshan Zhang
Yu Zhang
Yue Zhang
Yueyi Zhang
Yulun Zhang
Yunyan Zhang
Yuyao Zhang
Can Zhao
Changchen Zhao
Chongyue Zhao
Fenqiang Zhao
Gangming Zhao

He Zhao
Jun Zhao
Li Zhao
Qingyu Zhao
Rongchang Zhao
Shen Zhao
Shijie Zhao
Tengda Zhao
Tianyi Zhao
Wei Zhao
Xuandong Zhao
Yiyuan Zhao
Yuan-Xing Zhao
Yue Zhao
Zixu Zhao
Ziyuan Zhao
Xingjian Zhen
Guoyan Zheng
Hao Zheng
Jiannan Zheng
Kang Zheng
Shenhai Zheng
Yalin Zheng
Yinqiang Zheng
Yushan Zheng
Jia-Xing Zhong
Zichun Zhong

Bo Zhou
Haoyin Zhou
Hong-Yu Zhou
Kang Zhou
Sanping Zhou
Sihang Zhou
Tao Zhou
Xiao-Yun Zhou
Yanning Zhou
Yuyin Zhou
Zongwei Zhou
Dongxiao Zhu
Hancan Zhu
Lei Zhu
Qikui Zhu
Xinliang Zhu
Yuemin Zhu
Zhe Zhu
Zhuotun Zhu
Aneeq Zia
Veronika Zimmer
David Zimmerer
Lilla Zöllei
Yukai Zou
Lianrui Zuo
Gerald Zwettler
Reyer Zwiggelaar

Outstanding Reviewers

Neel Dey   New York University, USA
Monica Hernandez   University of Zaragoza, Spain
Ivica Kopriva   Rudjer Boskovich Institute, Croatia
Sebastian Otálora   University of Applied Sciences and Arts Western
                         Switzerland, Switzerland
Danielle Pace   Massachusetts General Hospital, USA
Sérgio Pereira   Lunit Inc., South Korea
David Richmond   IBM Watson Health, USA
Rohit Singla   University of British Columbia, Canada
Yan Wang   Sichuan University, China

Honorable Mentions (Reviewers)

Mazdak Abulnaga	Massachusetts Institute of Technology, USA
Pierre Ambrosini	Erasmus University Medical Center, The Netherlands
Hyeon-Min Bae	Korea Advanced Institute of Science and Technology, South Korea
Mikhail Belyaev	Skolkovo Institute of Science and Technology, Russia
Bhushan Borotikar	Symbiosis International University, India
Katharina Breininger	Friedrich-Alexander-Universität Erlangen-Nürnberg, Germany
Ninon Burgos	CNRS, Paris Brain Institute, France
Mariano Cabezas	The University of Sydney, Australia
Aaron Carass	Johns Hopkins University, USA
Pierre-Henri Conze	IMT Atlantique, France
Christian Desrosiers	École de technologie supérieure, Canada
Reuben Dorent	King's College London, UK
Nicha Dvornek	Yale University, USA
Dmitry V. Dylov	Skolkovo Institute of Science and Technology, Russia
Marius Erdt	Fraunhofer Singapore, Singapore
Ruibin Feng	Stanford University, USA
Enzo Ferrante	CONICET/Universidad Nacional del Litoral, Argentina
Antonio Foncubierta-Rodríguez	IBM Research, Switzerland
Isabel Funke	National Center for Tumor Diseases Dresden, Germany
Adrian Galdran	University of Bournemouth, UK
Ben Glocker	Imperial College London, UK
Cristina González	Universidad de los Andes, Colombia
Maged Goubran	Sunnybrook Research Institute, Canada
Sobhan Goudarzi	Concordia University, Canada
Vicente Grau	University of Oxford, UK
Andreas Hauptmann	University of Oulu, Finland
Nico Hoffmann	Technische Universität Dresden, Germany
Sungmin Hong	Massachusetts General Hospital, Harvard Medical School, USA
Won-Dong Jang	Harvard University, USA
Zhanghexuan Ji	University at Buffalo, SUNY, USA
Neerav Karani	ETH Zurich, Switzerland
Alexander Katzmann	Siemens Healthineers, Germany
Erwan Kerrien	Inria, France
Anitha Priya Krishnan	Genentech, USA
Tahsin Kurc	Stony Brook University, USA
Francesco La Rosa	École polytechnique fédérale de Lausanne, Switzerland
Dmitrii Lachinov	Medical University of Vienna, Austria
Mengzhang Li	Peking University, China
Gilbert Lim	National University of Singapore, Singapore
Dongnan Liu	University of Sydney, Australia

Bin Lou	Siemens Healthineers, USA
Kai Ma	Tencent, China
Klaus H. Maier-Hein	German Cancer Research Center (DKFZ), Germany
Raphael Meier	University Hospital Bern, Switzerland
Tony C. W. Mok	Hong Kong University of Science and Technology, Hong Kong SAR
Lia Morra	Politecnico di Torino, Italy
Cosmas Mwikirize	Rutgers University, USA
Felipe Orihuela-Espina	Instituto Nacional de Astrofísica, Óptica y Electrónica, Mexico
Egor Panfilov	University of Oulu, Finland
Christian Payer	Graz University of Technology, Austria
Sebastian Pölsterl	Ludwig-Maximilians Universität, Germany
José Rouco	University of A Coruña, Spain
Daniel Rueckert	Imperial College London, UK
Julia Schnabel	King's College London, UK
Christina Schwarz-Gsaxner	Graz University of Technology, Austria
Boris Shirokikh	Skolkovo Institute of Science and Technology, Russia
Yang Song	University of New South Wales, Australia
Gérard Subsol	Université de Montpellier, France
Tanveer Syeda-Mahmood	IBM Research, USA
Mickael Tardy	Hera-MI, France
Paul Thienphrapa	Atlas5D, USA
Gijs van Tulder	Radboud University, The Netherlands
Tongxin Wang	Indiana University, USA
Yirui Wang	PAII Inc., USA
Jelmer Wolterink	University of Twente, The Netherlands
Lei Xiang	Subtle Medical Inc., USA
Fatemeh Zabihollahy	Johns Hopkins University, USA
Wei Zhang	University of Georgia, USA
Ya Zhang	Shanghai Jiao Tong University, China
Qingyu Zhao	Stanford University, China
Yushan Zheng	Beihang University, China

Mentorship Program (Mentors)

Shadi Albarqouni	Helmholtz AI, Helmholtz Center Munich, Germany
Hao Chen	Hong Kong University of Science and Technology, Hong Kong SAR
Nadim Daher	NVIDIA, France
Marleen de Bruijne	Erasmus MC/University of Copenhagen, The Netherlands
Qi Dou	The Chinese University of Hong Kong, Hong Kong SAR
Gabor Fichtinger	Queen's University, Canada
Jonny Hancox	NVIDIA, UK

Nobuhiko Hata	Harvard Medical School, USA
Sharon Xiaolei Huang	Pennsylvania State University, USA
Jana Hutter	King's College London, UK
Dakai Jin	PAII Inc., China
Samuel Kadoury	Polytechnique Montréal, Canada
Minjeong Kim	University of North Carolina at Greensboro, USA
Hans Lamecker	1000shapes GmbH, Germany
Andrea Lara	Galileo University, Guatemala
Ngan Le	University of Arkansas, USA
Baiying Lei	Shenzhen University, China
Karim Lekadir	Universitat de Barcelona, Spain
Marius George Linguraru	Children's National Health System/George Washington University, USA
Herve Lombaert	ETS Montreal, Canada
Marco Lorenzi	Inria, France
Le Lu	PAII Inc., China
Xiongbiao Luo	Xiamen University, China
Dzung Pham	Henry M. Jackson Foundation/Uniformed Services University/National Institutes of Health/Johns Hopkins University, USA
Josien Pluim	Eindhoven University of Technology/University Medical Center Utrecht, The Netherlands
Antonio Porras	University of Colorado Anschutz Medical Campus/Children's Hospital Colorado, USA
Islem Rekik	Istanbul Technical University, Turkey
Nicola Rieke	NVIDIA, Germany
Julia Schnabel	TU Munich/Helmholtz Center Munich, Germany, and King's College London, UK
Debdoot Sheet	Indian Institute of Technology Kharagpur, India
Pallavi Tiwari	Case Western Reserve University, USA
Jocelyne Troccaz	CNRS, TIMC, Grenoble Alpes University, France
Sandrine Voros	TIMC-IMAG, INSERM, France
Linwei Wang	Rochester Institute of Technology, USA
Yalin Wang	Arizona State University, USA
Zhong Xue	United Imaging Intelligence Co. Ltd, USA
Renee Yao	NVIDIA, USA
Mohammad Yaqub	Mohamed Bin Zayed University of Artificial Intelligence, United Arab Emirates, and University of Oxford, UK
S. Kevin Zhou	University of Science and Technology of China, China
Lilla Zollei	Massachusetts General Hospital, Harvard Medical School, USA
Maria A. Zuluaga	EURECOM, France

Contents – Part VIII

Computational (Integrative) Pathology

Modalities - Microscopy

Modalities - Histopathology

Modalities - Ultrasound

Clinical Applications - Ophthalmology

Relational Subsets Knowledge Distillation for Long-Tailed Retinal Diseases Recognition

Lie Ju[1,2], Xin Wang[1], Lin Wang[1,3], Tongliang Liu[4], Xin Zhao[1],
Tom Drummond[2], Dwarikanath Mahapatra[5], and Zongyuan Ge[1,2(✉)]

[1] Airdoc LLC, Beijing, China
julie@airdoc.com
[2] Monash Medical AI Group, Monash University, Melbourne, Australia
zongyuan.ge@monash.edu
[3] Harbin Engineering University, Harbin, China
[4] The University of Sydney, Sydney, Australia
[5] Inception Institute of Artificial Intelligence, Abu Dhabi, UAE
https.//mmai.group

Abstract. In the real world, medical datasets often exhibit a long-tailed data distribution (i.e., a few classes occupy most of the data, while most classes have rarely few samples), which results in a challenging imbalance learning scenario. For example, there are estimated more than 40 different kinds of retinal diseases with variable morbidity, however with more than 30+ conditions are very rare from the global patient cohorts, which results in a typical long-tailed learning problem for deep learning-based screening models. In this study, we propose class subset learning by dividing the long-tailed data into multiple class subsets according to prior knowledge, such as regions and phenotype information. It enforces the model to focus on learning the subset-specific knowledge. More specifically, there are some relational classes that reside in the fixed retinal regions, or some common pathological features are observed in both the majority and minority conditions. With those subsets learnt teacher models, then we are able to distil the multiple teacher models into a unified model with weighted knowledge distillation loss. The proposed framework proved to be effective for the long-tailed retinal diseases recognition task. The experimental results on two different datasets demonstrate that our method is flexible and can be easily plugged into many other state-of-the-art techniques with significant improvements.

Keywords: Retinal diseases recognition · Long-tailed learning · Knowledge distillation · Deep learning

Electronic supplementary material The online version of this chapter (https://doi.org/10.1007/978-3-030-87237-3_1) contains supplementary material, which is available to authorized users.

M. de Bruijne et al. (Eds.): MICCAI 2021, LNCS 12908, pp. 3–12, 2021.
https://doi.org/10.1007/978-3-030-87237-3_1

1   Introduction

Recent studies have demonstrated successful applications of deep learning-based models for retinal disease screening such as diabetic retinopathy (DR) and glaucoma [2,4,8]. However, diseases and lesions that occurred less frequently in the training set may not perform well in real clinical test settings due to the algorithm fails to generalize those pathologies. Recently released datasets [7,11] collected more than **40** different kinds of fundus diseases that may appear in clinical screening. As Fig. 1 shows, this dataset shows a typical long-tailed distribution attribute, whose ratio of majority class (head) to minority class (tail) exceeds 100, indicating a serious class-imbalance issue. This is not uncommon in many medical image datasets. Besides, some samples may contain more than a single retinal disease label (label co-occurrence), leading to a multi-label challenge.

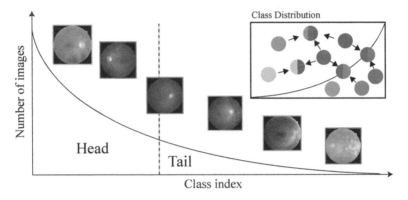

Fig. 1. The retinal disease distribution from [7] exhibits a prominent long-tailed attribute. Label co-occurrence is also a common observation among head, medium and tailed classes (shown in color dots in the class distribution window). (Color figure online)

Most of the existing algorithms to tackle imbalanced long-tailed datasets use either re-sampling [12] or re-weighting [6] strategy. However, since there is label co-occurrence between each class (e.g., macular edema is often accompanied by splenic vein occlusion), the repetitive sampling for those associated instances introduces inner-class imbalance. Recently, Wang et al. proposed a multi-task deep learning framework [13] which can identify 36 kinds of retinal diseases. The data imbalanced is partially solved by bringing all diseases into subsets with regional location information. However, it requires extra annotations for the optic disc and macula's location in the first stage. Xiang et al. learned to divide the original samples into multiple class subsets and train several models on those subsets since they often yield better performances than their jointly-trained counterpart [15]. However, the multi-label challenge is not discussed and can not be decoupled directly.

Inspired by the observation that the model trained from less imbalanced class subsets performs better than that trained from the full long-tailed data [15], we leverage the prior knowledge of retinal diseases and divide the original long-tailed

Table 1. Region-based subsets and corresponding lesions/diseases.

Region	Lesions/Diseases
Optic disc	Glaucoma, retinal myelinated nerve fiber, etc.
Macula	Epiretinal membrane, drusen, macular hole, hypo-pigmentation, etc.
Vessels	Arterionevous crossing phenomenon, perivascular sheathing, etc.
Global	Hemorrhage, pigmentation, hard exudates, soft exudates, etc.

classes into **relational** subsets. For instance, some diseases (glaucoma, etc.) only occur around the optic disc, while others (epiretinal membrane, macular hole, etc.) only affect the macular area, so we can divide those classes into subsets based on pathology region. Besides, some diseases may share similar semantics (hypertension, splenic vein occlusion and DR can all cause hemorrhages) in the pathology features. Based on this cognitive law of retinal diseases, we enforce those correlated categories/diseases to be in the same class subset. This article proposes three different rules for class subsets partition, which are **Shot-based**, **Region-based** and **Feature-based**. From those subsets, then we train the 'teacher' models accordingly to 'enforce' the model to focus on learning the specific information or features from those class subsets. With all teacher models trained, we later distill the knowledge of several 'teacher' models into one unified 'student' model with an extra weighted knowledge distillation loss, which also contributes to decouple the label co-occurrence in a multi-label setting (Table 1).

The contributions are summarized as follows: (1) We propose to train the retinal diseases classification model from relational subsets to tackle the long-tailed class distribution problem. (2) We leverage the prior knowledge and design three different class partition rules for the relational subsets generation and propose to distill the knowledge from multiple teacher models into a unified model with dynamic weights. (3) We conduct comprehensive experiments on two medical datasets *Lesion-10* and *Disease-48* with different tail length. The experimental results demonstrate that our proposed method improves the recognition performance of up to 48 kinds of retinal diseases. Our method can be easily combined with many other state-of-the-art techniques with significant improvements.

2   Methods

The overview of our proposed framework is shown in Fig. 2. In the first stage, we divide the original samples into several subsets under the constraint of different rules and train the individual teacher models. In the second stage, we train the unified student model with the knowledge being transferred from the teacher models with a weighted knowledge distillation loss. We show some examples of the regions/lesions in Fig. 2 for a better understanding of our methods.

2.1   Relational Subsets Generation

Formally, given the original long-tailed samples $S_{original}$, we divide them into several subsets $\{S^1_{[i_1,...,i_{o-1}]}, S^2_{[i_o,...i_p]}, ..., S^k_{[i_{p+1},...,i_n]}\}$, where k denotes the subset

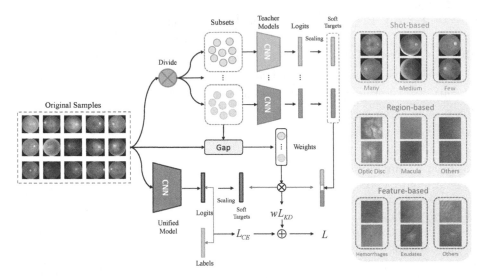

Fig. 2. The overview of our proposed framework. In the first stage, we divide the original long-tailed samples into multiple subsets under the relational class constraint and train separate teacher models. In the second stage, we train a unified student model using a weighted knowledge distillation loss on the trained teacher models' parameters.

ID and i_o denotes the o_{th} class ID in the sorted all n classes. There are two main advantages: **(1)** subsets can help reduce the label co-occurrence in a multi-label setting. More specifically, for $S_{original}$ with N_{all} instances. We randomly select some instances, which belong to class i or j. So we have the sampling probability $p_i = \frac{N_i}{N_{all}}$, $p_j = \frac{N_j}{N_{all}}$, and $p_i \gg p_j$. Less label co-occurrence helps to have $p_j \to p_i$ as close as possible. **(2)** learning from class subsets reduces the length of tail classes and makes the class distribution towards a more balanced state. We thus have proposed the following three rules for class subsets generation:

Shot-based. Inspired by [15], we divide the long-tailed samples into class-subsets according to their sampling probability, which is equivalent to the number of shots: many, medium and few. Hence, those subsets are all in a relatively less-imbalanced state than that of the original sample distribution, and the learning process involves less interference between the majority and the minority.

Region-based. Here, we divide the lesions/diseases which are frequently appeared in the specific regions into the same subsets, as Table 2 shows. We leverage this kind of prior knowledge to have the model enforced to focus on the local area in an unsupervised manner. We extracted the locations of lesions in *Lesion-10* dataset and drew heatmaps for various categories to verify our hypothesis, which is shown in Fig. 3.

Feature-based. Many diseases share similar pathological features. For example, hypertension and DR both manifest phenotypes such as fundus hemorrhage. Therefore, we divide the diseases which share similar semantics into the same class-subsets, and those common features can be shared and learned between the

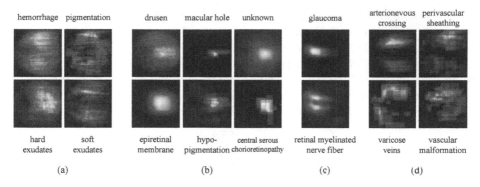

Fig. 3. The heatmap of the locations of various medical signs (lesions) tended to appear frequently in one region: (a) global fundus areas; (b) macula; (c) optic disc; (d) vessels.

majority and minority. This subset divide rule can also help to improve the model to distinguish the fine-grained local features such as drusen and exudates [3].

2.2 Multiple Weighted Knowledge Distillation

We pre-train the teacher models $[M_{s_1}, ..., M_{s_k}]$ on generated subsets. Each teacher model tends to learn specific information under less imbalanced cardinality class samples. For example, Coat's disease, congenital retinoschisis, retina vasculitis and uveitis are the main etiological factors in non-traumatic vitreous hemorrhage (a relational subset). Training from such subsets remains the locality preserving characteristic and utilizes the common feature shared between majority and minority class while the within-class distance in the representation space is minimized. After all the teacher models being trained, the obtained logits are used for training the unified student model with KD technique. Formally, for the subset S^j and its i_{th} class, we have the calibrated soft targets q_i and $\hat{q}_i$ with respect to the logits z_i and $\hat{z}_i$ from teacher models and unified model:

$$q_i = \frac{\exp(z_i/T)}{\sum_{0,1} \exp(z_i/T)}, \; \hat{q}_i = \frac{\exp(\hat{z}_i/T)}{\sum_{0,1} \exp(\hat{z}_i/T)}, \tag{1}$$

where T is the hyper-parameter. Then the knowledge distillation loss for M_{s_i} is given by:

$$L_{KD_i} = KL(\hat{q}_i|q_i) = \sum_{0,1} \hat{q}_i \cdot \ln\frac{\hat{q}_i}{q_i}, \tag{2}$$

where $KL(\cdot)$ is the Kullback-Leibler divergence loss. Since we obtain the KD loss from multiple teacher models $L_{RS-KD} = [L_{KD_1}, ..., L_{KD_n}]$ for n sorted classes. So we need to find a way to aggregate them for joint optimizing under one unified model. The most intuitive way is to summing up however may lead to unsatisfactory performance. For instance, NPDRI and NPDRIII both belong to the same subset (medium/hemorrhage-related), and the former has more samples for training, but the semantic information of the latter is more obvious and easier to be learnt by the model, which results in the difference in the performance. In this way, since the performance of some tailed classes of the student model is the same as that of the teacher model, it is unfair to distill all subsets at the same rate and weight. Hence, we expect the teacher models to produce positive and dynamic guidance for the unified model. Here, we compute the performance gap between the teacher and student model as the weights for the KD loss:

$$w_i = \begin{cases} 1.0 & \text{if } \delta Acc_{M_S^i} \geq Acc_{M_{U,c}^i} \\ \dfrac{Acc_{M_S^i} - Acc_{M_{U,c}^i}}{Acc_{M_S^i} \cdot (1-\delta)} & \text{if } \delta Acc_{M_S^i} < Acc_{M_{U,c}^i} \end{cases} \quad (3)$$

where c denotes the c_{th} epoch for the i_{th} class when training the unified model and its performance $Acc_{M_{U,c}^i}$. $Acc_{M_S^i}$ is the performance of teacher model which is a fixed value. The w will be updated after every epoch. δ is set for controlling the KD decaying schedule. The final loss we aim to optimize becomes:

$$L = L_{BCE} + \sum_i w_i L_{KD_i} \quad (4)$$

where L_{BCE} calculates the original outputs of the softmax and its corresponding ground-truth in the unified model with respect to the fed long-tailed samples.

3 Experiments

3.1 Experimental Settings

We use ResNet-50 [5] pre-trained on ImageNet as our backbone. The input size of the network is 256×256. We apply Adam to optimize the model. The learning rate starts at 1×10^{-4} and reduces ten-fold when there is no drop on validation loss till 1×10^{-7} with the patience of 5. δ is set as 0.6. We use the mean average precision (mAP) as the evaluation metric and all the results are evaluated on test set based on 4-fold cross-validation with a total of 100 epochs. All experiments are implemented with Pytorch and $8 \times$ GTX 1080Ti GPUs.

3.2 Data Collections and Annotations

We conduct our experiments on two datasets *Lesion-10* and *Disease-48* with different tail length. The evaluated datasets consist of two parts: re-labeled public dataset and private dataset from hospitals. We follow [7] and select 10 kinds of lesions and 48 kinds of diseases as our target task. In the ophthalmology field, the occurred lesions always determine the diagnostic results of the specific diseases. Both datasets contain multi-label annotations and the statistics are shown in Table 2. For instance, more than 22,000 images have 2+ kinds of diseases in the *Disease-48*. The dataset is divided for training: validating: testing = 7: 1: 2. To verify the idea of our proposed region-based subsets training, we also labeled the locations of lesions (bounding box) for *Lesion-10* dataset. We will make the test dataset publicly available to the community for future study and benchmark.

3.3   Quantitative Evaluation

Table 3 shows the long-tailed classification results on *Lesion-10* and *Disease-48*. We consider the following baseline method families: (a) ERM model; (b) re-sampling [12]; (c) re-weighting; (d) focal loss [9]; (e) other state-of-the-art methods such as OLTR [10]. Results in the middle section show that our proposed methods have greatly improved the ERM model with at most 3.29% mAP, and are also competitive or even better than results comparing with other state-of-the-art methods. For those two datasets, our method gives a sharp rise in mAP to the tail classes with 15.18% mAP and 7.78% mAP, respectively. We find that the feature-based relational subsets learning claims the best performance on the *Lesion-10* dataset, and the shot-based relational subsets learning outperforms the other two rules on the *Disease-48* dataset that has a longer tail length.

Table 2. The statistics (number) of multi-label datasets.

Multi-label	Lesion-10	Disease-48
1	5929	27368
2	1569	29766
3	321	17102
3+	52	5574
Sum	7871	79810

As we declare that our framework has the plug-and-play feature for most frameworks, we validate it with the combination of ours (best baseline out of three rules is chosen for each dataset. e.g., feature-based for *Lesion-10*) and other state-of-the-art methods. As shown in Table 3, for *Lesion-10*, LDAM [1] and focal loss [9] are further improved by 0.94% and 1.38% mAP. However, DB Loss and OLTR drop by 1.48% and 0.20%. We further evaluate our methods on the *Disease-48*, and all methods obtain significant improvements, including DB Loss and OLTR.

3.4   Ablation Study

Visualization of the Label Co-Occurrence. Table 3 indicates that the regular re-sampling technique does not benefit head and medium classes with performance decrease due to the label co-occurrence. As discussed in Sect. 2, the relational subsets are in a relatively more balanced state by decoupling the original class labels. Here, we showcase shot-based subsets learning for the *Lesion-10* dataset in Fig. 4. We mainly consider the local co-occurrence labels between classes in the same relational subset with specific semantic information. Then we leverage weighted KD to reduce the risk of regarding the out-of-subsets classes (e.g. classes with label co-occurrence but not included in subsets) as outliers.

Table 3. Long-tailed classification results (mAP) on Lesion-10 and Disease-48.

Datasets	Lesion-10				Disease-48			
Methods	Head	Medium	Tail	Total	Head	Medium	Tail	Total
ERM Model	86.84	69.13	27.01	60.99	62.80	46.87	18.60	42.76
RS [12]	81.42	65.97	32.99	60.13	55.57	37.55	23.99	39.04
RW	83.42	68.10	37.74	63.00	63.41	**47.76**	20.87	44.01
Focal Loss [9]	86.84	68.67	39.60	65.04	62.03	47.12	22.66	43.94
OLTR [10]	87.55	**70.41**	26.99	61.65	60.41	45.24	22.45	42.70
LDAM [1]	86.90	69.09	30.68	62.22	61.00	46.90	26.73	44.88
DB Loss [14]	88.01	69.24	39.77	65.67	63.19	46.61	25.99	45.26
Ours (shot-based)	86.87	67.93	34.31	63.04	**64.17**	47.02	26.38	45.85
Ours (region-based)	87.22	69.35	35.61	64.06	64.15	46.99	25.33	45.49
Ours (feature-based)	85.42	65.24	42.19	64.28	62.42	46.67	21.08	43.39
Ours + DB Loss [14]	84.15	69.99	38.44	64.19	62.94	46.97	**27.82**	**45.91**
Ours + OLTR [10]	85.73	68.44	30.17	61.45	61.78	45.22	23.98	43.66
Ours + LDAM [1]	84.88	67.04	37.56	63.16	61.01	47.31	27.00	45.11
Ours + Focal Loss [9]	**86.97**	69.75	**42.55**	**66.42**	63.44	47.03	25.65	45.37

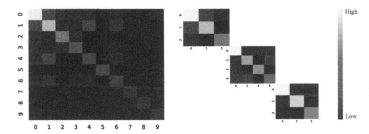

Fig. 4. Left: original distribution. Right: subsets distribution.

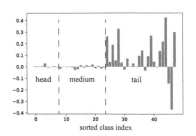

Fig. 5. The per-class mAP increments between ERM model and ours on Disease-48 dataset.

Table 4. Ablation study results on Lesion-10.

Methods	Head	Medium	Tail	Total
ERM Model	**86.84**	**69.13**	27.01	60.99
KD (T = 3)	86.08	67.09	32.59	61.92
KD (T = 10)	86.59	66.82	36.07	63.16
KD (T = 20)	85.76	68.54	30.20	61.55
Weighted	85.42	65.24	**42.19**	**64.28**

The Effectiveness of Each Component. In order to test how each factor contributes to our model performance, we conduct further ablation studies on various method components. Results are shown in Table 4. Firstly, we assess the sensitivity of knowledge distillation (KD) and how different temperature scaling hyper-parameters affect the model's performance. It can be seen that the KD can only obtain marginal improvements with a low (T = 3) or high temperature (T = 20) value due to the trade-off between CE loss and KD loss. We also show the per-class mAP increments between ERM model and our proposed method on the *Disease-48* dataset in Fig. 5. With the weighted KD Loss, the model has a better detection rate on the tail classes with little performance trade-off on the head and medium classes, which results in an overall gain in performance.

4   Conclusion

In this work, we present relational subsets knowledge distillation for long-tailed retinal diseases recognition. We leverage the prior knowledge of retinal diseases such as the regions information, phenotype information and distribution information among all classes, to divide the original long-tailed classes into multiple relational subsets and train teacher models on them respectively to learn a more effective representation. Then we transfer the teacher models into a unified model with the knowledge distillation. Our experiments evaluated on *Lesion-10* and *Disease-48* demonstrate our method can greatly improve the diagnostic result for retinal diseases under the challenging long-tail distribution setting.

References

1. Cao, K., Wei, C., Gaidon, A., Arechiga, N., Ma, T.: Learning imbalanced datasets with label-distribution-aware margin loss. arXiv preprint arXiv:1906.07413 (2019)
2. Fu, H., et al.: Disc-aware ensemble network for glaucoma screening from fundus image. IEEE Trans. Med. Imaging **37**(11), 2493–2501 (2018)
3. Ge, Z., McCool, C., Sanderson, C., Corke, P.: Subset feature learning for fine-grained category classification. In: Proceedings of the IEEE Conference on Computer Vision and Pattern Recognition Workshops, pp. 46–52 (2015)
4. Gulshan, V., et al.: Development and validation of a deep learning algorithm for detection of diabetic retinopathy in retinal fundus photographs. JAMA **316**(22), 2402–2410 (2016)
5. He, K., Zhang, X., Ren, S., Sun, J.: Deep residual learning for image recognition. In: Proceedings of the IEEE Conference on Computer Vision and Pattern Recognition, pp. 770–778 (2016)
6. Huang, C., Li, Y., Loy, C.C., Tang, X.: Learning deep representation for imbalanced classification. In: Proceedings of the IEEE Conference on Computer Vision and Pattern Recognition, pp. 5375–5384 (2016)
7. Ju, L., et al.: Improving medical image classification with label noise using dual-uncertainty estimation. arXiv preprint arXiv:2103.00528 (2021)
8. Ju, L., et al.: Synergic adversarial label learning for grading retinal diseases via knowledge distillation and multi-task learning. IEEE J. Biomed. Health Inform. (2021)

9. Lin, T.Y., Goyal, P., Girshick, R., He, K., Dollár, P.: Focal loss for dense object detection. In: Proceedings of the IEEE International Conference on Computer Vision, pp. 2980–2988 (2017)
10. Liu, Z., Miao, Z., Zhan, X., Wang, J., Gong, B., Yu, S.X.: Large-scale long-tailed recognition in an open world. In: Proceedings of the IEEE/CVF Conference on Computer Vision and Pattern Recognition, pp. 2537–2546 (2019)
11. Quellec, G., Lamard, M., Conze, P.H., Massin, P., Cochener, B.: Automatic detection of rare pathologies in fundus photographs using few-shot learning. Med. Image Anal. **61**, 101660 (2020)
12. Shen, L., Lin, Z., Huang, Q.: Relay backpropagation for effective learning of deep convolutional neural networks. In: Leibe B., Matas J., Sebe N., Welling M. (eds) Computer Vision, vol. 9911, pp. 467–482. Springer, Heidelberg (2016). https://doi.org/10.1007/978-3-319-46478-7_29
13. Wang, X., Ju, L., Zhao, X., Ge, Z.: Retinal abnormalities recognition using regional multitask learning. In: Shen, D., et al. (eds) Medical Image Computing and Computer Assisted Intervention, vol. 11764, pp. 30–38. Springer, Cham (2019). https://doi.org/10.1007/978-3-030-32239-7_4
14. Wu, T., Huang, Q., Liu, Z., Wang, Y., Lin, D.: Distribution-balanced loss for multi-label classification in long-tailed datasets. In: Vedaldi, A., Bischof, H., Brox, T., Frahm, J.M. (eds) Computer Vision, vol. 12349, pp. 162–178. Springer, Cham (2020).https://doi.org/10.1007/978-3-030-58548-8_10
15. Xiang, L., Ding, G., Han, J.: Learning from multiple experts: self-paced knowledge distillation for long-tailed classification. In: Vedaldi, A., Bischof, H., Brox, T., Frahm, J.M., (eds) Computer Vision, vol. 12350, pp. 247–263. Springer, Cham (2020). https://doi.org/10.1007/978-3-030-58558-7_15

Cross-Domain Depth Estimation Network for 3D Vessel Reconstruction in OCT Angiography

Shuai Yu[1,6], Yonghuai Liu[2], Jiong Zhang[3], Jianyang Xie[1], Yalin Zheng[4], Jiang Liu[5], and Yitian Zhao[1(✉)]

[1] Cixi Institute of Biomedical Engineering, Ningbo Institute of Materials Technology and Engineering, Chinese Academy of Sciences, Ningbo, China
`yitian.zhao@nimte.ac.cn`
[2] Department of Computer Science, Edge Hill University, Ormskirk, UK
[3] Keck School of Medicine, University of Southern California, Los Angeles, USA
[4] Department of Eye and Vision Science, University of Liverpool, Liverpool, UK
[5] Department of Computer Science and Engineering, Southern University of Science and Technology, Shenzhen, China
[6] University of Chinese Academy of Sciences, Beijing, China

Abstract. Optical Coherence Tomography Angiography (OCTA) has been widely used by ophthalmologists for decision-making due to its superiority in providing caplillary details. Many of the OCTA imaging devices used in clinic provide high-quality 2D *en face* representations, while their 3D data quality are largely limited by low signal-to-noise ratio and strong projection artifacts, which restrict the performance of depth-resolved 3D analysis. In this paper, we propose a novel 2D-to-3D vessel reconstruction framework based on the 2D *en face* OCTA images. This framework takes advantage of the detailed 2D OCTA depth map for prediction and thus does not rely on any 3D volumetric data. Based on the data with available vessel depth labels, we first introduce a network with structure constraint blocks to estimate the depth map of blood vessels in other cross-domain *en face* OCTA data with unavailable labels. Afterwards, a depth adversarial adaptation module is proposed for better unsupervised cross-domain training, since images captured using different devices may suffer from varying image contrast and noise levels. Finally, vessels are reconstructed in 3D space by utilizing the estimated depth map and 2D vascular information. Experimental results demonstrate the effectiveness of our method and its potential to guide subsequent vascular analysis in 3D domain.

Keywords: OCTA · Domain adaptation · 3D vessel reconstruction

1 Introduction

Optical Coherence Tomography Angiography (OCTA) is a novel 3D imaging technique that has the ability to acquire rich blood flow details at capillary-level,

M. de Bruijne et al. (Eds.): MICCAI 2021, LNCS 12908, pp. 13–23, 2021.
https://doi.org/10.1007/978-3-030-87237-3_2

as shown in Fig. 1 (a). OCTA is non-invasive and does not expose patients with side effects such as nausea or anaphylaxis compared with fluorescein angiography (FA). As a result, this budding technology has shown considerable potential in the diagnosis of various eye-related diseases [1].

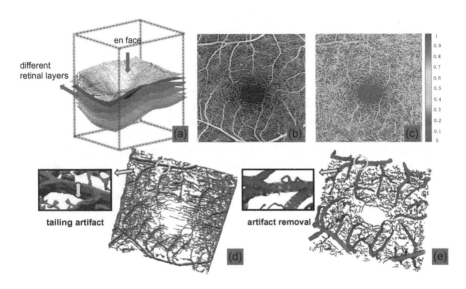

Fig. 1. Illustration of (a) an example 3D OCTA volume. (b) 2D *en face* angiogram. (c) Color encoded depth map of (b). (d) Vessel 3D reconstruction by an existing method [2], and (e) reconstruction result by our method.

Recently, several works have been conducted to study retinal blood vasculatures in OCTA images. Hwang *et al.* [3] used a quantification method to analyze the correlation between OCTA features and DR. Arrigo *et al.* [4] applied OCTA images for the detection of the choroidal neovascularization area. Xie *et al.* [5] classified the retinal vessels into artery and vein from OCTA *en face* images. Some studies [6–8] have developed automatic methods for vessel segmentation. However, all the above-mentioned works are only performed on 2D *en face* angiograms (Fig. 1 (b)), and the 3D spatial information of the vessels are not utilized. 3D analysis and visualization of blood vessels can provide additional spatial information and are very useful for observing vascular changes [2,9,10]. Zhang *et al.* [2] built a 3D microvascular shape modeling framework based on the original volume of OCTA. Although this work provides an effective vascular analysis framework, it still suffers from projection artifacts as shown in Fig. 1 (d), and requires direct processing of 3D data. 3D vessel reconstruction from an OCTA volume faces several challenges: limited data quality, complex topological structures, and high computational demand. On the other hand, it is not always straightforward to have the required 3D volumetric data in real application. For example, some public datasets such as ROSE [8] does not provide 3D data which makes it impossible to achieve 3D reconstruction of vessels through volumetric data-based methods. In addition, some OCTA devices, e.g., Heidelberg OCT2 has difficulty exporting 3D data due to restriction from manufacture. To this end, 3D vessel reconstruction from 2D *en face* image is desirable.

With the development of OCTA imaging technology, the dedicated depth-resolved information becomes available in current devices such as the CIRRUS HD-OCT 5000 System (Carl Zeiss Meditec Inc., USA), which is equipped with an *AngioPlex^{TM}* OCT Angiography software with an additional color-coded *en face* OCTA image (i.e., *depth map* in this study) as shown in Fig. 1 (c). The depth map is intrinsically a combination of the retinal layers shown in Fig. 1 (a), whose pixel intensity score is the distance from the imaging sensor to each spatial position in the retinal structure [11]. The blue color indicates that the vessels are further away to the sensor, and red implies the vessels are closer.

In this work, we propose a framework to reconstruct the 3D structure of blood vessels from 2D OCTA images, while 3D data is utilized for verification. It is worth noting that our previous work [12] aims for preliminary 3D retinal vessel reconstruction by only exploring the data from a single domain (i.e., the Cirrus HD-OCT device), which is not an ideal framework with good generalization ability. However, it is important to set up a unified framework that can work well on microvascular data from a variety of imaging domains, in particular to those devices which do not provide a depth map. The previous work [12] introduced a supervised depth prediction network with MSE loss. However, in this work, we specifically designed a new domain-adaptive method with unsupervised training strategies, to predict a vessel depth map solely based on input 2D en face OCTA images from multi-domains (i.e., multiple OCTA devices). Therefore, we introduce a depth adversarial adaptation module to narrow the domain discrepancies, and further employ adversarial loss which gives better performance instead of using MSE loss in our new domain-adaptive framework. For validation, we choose Zeiss Cirrus HD-OCT data as the source domain, and the data acquired from Optovue RTVue XR Avanti device (without a machine-provided depth map) as the target domain for cross-domain prediction and validation. It is also worth noting that while achieving reconstruction accuracy equal to that of the existing state-of-the-art (SOTA) method, our method can also avoid the interference of projection artifact as illustrated in Fig. 1 (e), and is not limited by data domains.

2   Proposed Method

We will detail our 3D vessel reconstruction method in this section, and it mainly consists of two steps: depth map prediction and 3D reconstruction.

2.1   Cross-Domain Depth Estimation Network

Network Architecture: In view of the excellent performance of the U-shaped network [13] in biomedical images, we apply it as the backbone. However, direct skipping connections between encoder and decoder in [13] will transmit redundant information. In our depth prediction task, the accuracy of spatial depth of blood vessels is primarily factor for the subsequent reconstruction. To this end, we employ a structure branch to manage only vessel-related information by means of our previously designed SCB [12] and local supervision.

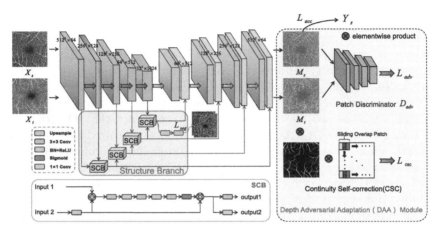

Fig. 2. Architecture of our cross-domain depth map estimation network. It comprises of our previous introduced structure constraint blocks (SCB) [12] and the Depth Adversarial Adaptation (DAA) Module.

As illustrated in Fig. 2, SCB is enforced after each encoder block and connected to the corresponding decoder block. Let e_t ($t \in 2, ..., 5$) denotes the output of t_{th} encoder block, and $s_{\tilde{t}}$ denotes the corresponding intermediate representations of the structure branch. Firstly, the concatenate e_t and $s_{\tilde{t}}$ followed by convolution, batch normalization and nonlinear activation layers is employed to estimate an attention map a_{t-1}. Then an element-wise product is applied between e_t and a_{t-1} to acquire a weighted map. It is worth noting that upsampling is utilized on e_t before concatenation, so as to make sure that e_t and $s_{\tilde{t}}$ have the same size. In practice, the region with more blood vessel can be treated as an attention map a_{t-1}. The *output2* in Fig. 2 is the filtered feature maps by SCB, and are cascaded with the feature maps of corresponding decoder so as to provide optimized structure-related information. The final output of the SCB is subject to upsampling and convolution operations to finally yield the prediction of vessel depth map.

To optimize the capability for domain adaptation, a DAA module is then attached to narrow the domain discrepancies. Typically, the source and target domain are denoted as S and T, respectively. The input images from S are denoted as $\mathcal{X}_s \in \mathbb{R}^{C \times H \times W}$ while those from T are denoted as $\mathcal{X}_t \in \mathbb{R}^{C \times H \times W}$, where C is the channel dimension, H and W are spatial dimensions. $\mathcal{M}_s$ and $\mathcal{M}_t$ represent the predictions of S and T, while $\mathcal{Y}_s$ denotes the label of the source image. We first feed $\mathcal{M}_s$ and $\mathcal{M}_t$ into the patch discriminator D_{adv} for adversarial training, so as to make the distribution of $\mathcal{M}_t$ closer to that of $\mathcal{M}_s$. In addition, we make full use of the prior knowledge of vascular continuity and employ continuity self-correction (CSC) to obtain final outputs.

CSC first multiplies $\mathcal{M}_t$, and its segmented image includes a pixel by pixel depth map $\mathcal{M}_{\tilde{t}}$ in effective vessel areas. As an ordered topology, in fact the depths of adjacent blood vessels are continuous in physical space. Based on this important prior knowledge, we then use a sliding overlapping patch to traverse $\mathcal{M}_{\tilde{t}}$. In each infinitesimal patch size, we minimize the variance of the depth of blood vessels so that the continuity of vascular depth can be guaranteed, and the outliers can be corrected. The overlapping part is set to make adjacent blood vessels in the same vascular tree continuous in depth.

Loss Functions: In this work, the loss function consists of four parts $\mathcal{L}_{seg}$, $\mathcal{L}_{acc}$, $\mathcal{L}_{adv}$ and $\mathcal{L}_{continuity}$, to be defined below. We first use the cross-entropy (CE) loss $\mathcal{L}_{seg}$ on the predicted segmentation maps $pred_{seg}$:

$$\mathcal{L}_{seg} = \mathcal{L}_{CE}(pred_{seg\_s}, gt_{seg\_s}) + \mathcal{L}_{CE}(pred_{seg\_t}, gt_{seg\_t}), \tag{1}$$

where $gt_{seg\_s} \in \mathbb{R}^{C \times H \times W}$ and $gt_{seg\_t} \in \mathbb{R}^{C \times H \times W}$ denote the groundtruths of the source and target domain, respectively. In order to improve the prediction performance at both pixel- and overall structure- level, we merge MSE and SSIM [14] loss as $\mathcal{L}_{acc}$ between $\mathcal{M}_s$ and $\mathcal{Y}_s$:

$$\mathcal{L}_{acc} = \mathcal{L}_{MSE}(\mathcal{M}_s, \mathcal{Y}_s) + \mathcal{L}_{SSIM}(\mathcal{M}_s, \mathcal{Y}_s). \tag{2}$$

For the adversarial training, we use the adversarial loss $\mathcal{L}_{adv}$ as:

$$\mathcal{L}_{adv} = \min_G \max_D \mathbb{E}[log D(\mathcal{M}_s)] + \mathbb{E}[log(1 - D(G(\mathcal{X}_t)))], \tag{3}$$

where G is the generator (i.e. $G(\mathcal{X}_t) = \mathcal{M}_t$) and D is the patch discriminator D_{adv}. $\mathcal{L}_{adv}$ is designed to train the network and to deceive D_{adv} by maximizing the probability of T being considered as S.

Additionally, a continuity self-correction loss $\mathcal{L}_{csc}$ is defined to ensure the continuity of the depth of adjacent blood vessels:

$$\mathcal{L}_{csc} = \mathcal{V}ar[\sum_i Patch(i)], \tag{4}$$

in which $\mathcal{V}ar[\cdot]$ denotes the variance of input $\cdot$ and $Patch(i)$ denotes the i_{th} sliding patch of $\mathcal{M}_{\tilde{t}}$ (the patch size is set to 8×8 and the sliding step is 4 in this paper). The final loss function $\mathcal{L}_{total}$ of the proposed method is thus:

$$\mathcal{L}_{total} = \lambda_1 \mathcal{L}_{acc} + \lambda_2 \mathcal{L}_{seg} + \lambda_3 \mathcal{L}_{adv} + \lambda_4 \mathcal{L}_{csc}, \tag{5}$$

where λ_1, λ_2, λ_3 and λ_4 are empirically set in this paper to 100, 7, 1 and 1, respectively.

2.2   3D Vessel Reconstruction via Depth Map

The 3D reconstruction of blood vessels can be regarded as a mapping problem from 2D to 3D with the availability of 2D segmented vessels and depth maps. In this step, we remove artifacts in OCTA, so that the final reconstructed surface can be used for subsequent 3D feature extraction and analysis.

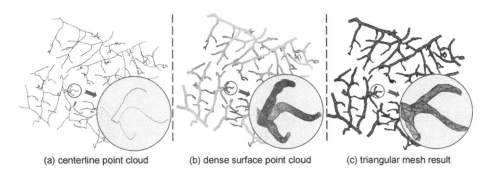

(a) centerline point cloud   (b) dense surface point cloud   (c) triangular mesh result

Fig. 3. Illustration of vascular reconstruction from point cloud to mesh surface.

3D Centerline Point Cloud Extraction: Given an OCTA segmentation image, the vessel centerlines as well as diameters can be extracted using the skeletonization method [15], and the vessel bifurcation may be detected by locating the pixels with more than two neighbours, i.e., intersection points. All the bifurcation and crossover region are then removed from the skeleton map, so as to yield a separated vessel map. The depth of each centerline point depends on the corresponding position of its depth map and is shifted downward by a distance of radius of vessel. Therefore, a 3D point cloud comprising the centerline points is obtained, as shown in Fig. 3 (a), where adjacent segments are connected based on the topology consistency using bilinear interpolation.

Vessel Surface Reconstruction: Using the previously obtained centerline point cloud, a center-to-surface method is employed to convert centerline to surface. Taking each center point as the centroid of a circle and the line between two adjacent points as the normal vector, a circle is then generated with a predefined radius.

Next, we obtain sampling points at equal intervals for each circle, and traverse all segments to obtain a dense surface point cloud, as shown in Fig. 3 (b). Furthermore, a constrained Poisson-disk sampling [16] was employed to optimize the surface so as to obtain a point cloud uniformly, Finally, a Ball-pivoting algorithm [17] is utilized to generate the final 3D triangular mesh, as shown in Fig. 3 (c).

3   Experiments

We validate the performance of the proposed method in terms of depth map prediction and 3D retinal vessel reconstruction.

3.1   Datasets and Evaluation Metrics

Datasets: Two OCTA datasets each containing 80 pairs of images were obtained from a CIRRUS HD-OCT 5000 system (Carl Zeiss Meditec Inc., USA) and an RTVue XR Avanti system (Optovue, Fremont Inc., USA). The former was selected as the source domain as it is associated with depth maps, the latter was selected as the target domain. The scan area was $3\,\text{mm} \times 3\,\text{mm} \times 2\,\text{mm}$ centered on the fovea.

56 of 80 images in the source domain were used for training, and the rest for testing. 56 of 80 images in the target domain were used for training, and the rest for validation. Note that a SOTA vessel segmentation model which is particularly designed for OCTA image, OCTA-Net [8], was used to detect blood vessels from the training set, and an image analysis expert further refined the obtained vessel maps as the ground truth, i.e., gt_{seg_s} in Eq. (1). The target domain data include the corresponding segmentation annotations, i.e., gt_{seg_t} in Eq. (1).

The method utilized in [2] was employed to obtain a 3D vessel segmentation result from the raw 3D volume. A centerline point cloud was obtained by taking the upper surface of the vessel as the depth, and moving downward with a distance of the corresponding radius. Finally, the aforementioned method was applied to obtain the surface as the ground truth. For comparison purposes, the ground truth point cloud was mapped to the same spatial depth range (0–255) as that reconstructed via the predicted depth map in the target domain.

Metrics: A total of five metrics were utilized to verify the performance of the proposed method in both the source and target domains. For the source domain, the accuracy (ACC) metric δ [18] was used to validate the predicted depth map with its ground truth: $\delta = max(\frac{D_i}{D_i^*}, \frac{D_i^*}{D_i}) < T$, where D_i and D_i^* are the obtained depth and the corresponding depth of the i-th pixel of the ground truth, respectively. Following [19], a threshold $T = 1.25$ was used in this metric. The Absolute Relative Difference (ARD) and Root Mean Squared Error (RMSE), two most commonly-used metrics in evaluating monocular image depth estimation, were also used in this work. For the target domain, Chamfer Distance (CD) [20] and Hausdorff Distance (HD) [21] were utilized to measure the similarity between two sets of pointclouds.

3.2   Experimental Results

The experiments were carried out on PyTorch library with a single NVIDIA GPU GeForce GTX 2080Ti. The learning rate was set to 0.0001, the number of training

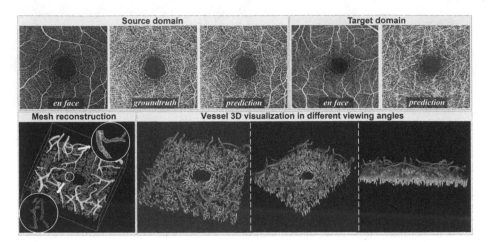

Fig. 4. Illustrative results of depth prediction in terms of source and target domain images, and 3D vessel reconstruction.

Table 1. Comparison of the proposed method with the state-of-the-art methods.

Methods	Source domain			Target domain	
	ACC	ARD	RMSE	CD	HD
Eigen *et al.* [22]	0.596	0.310	0.343	5.266	6.913
Laina *et al.* [19]	0.925	0.138	0.213	3.452	6.874
Chen *et al.* [23]	0.973	0.114	0.138	2.921	5.147
Yu *et al.* [12]	0.971	0.058	0.107	2.624	3.502
Tzeng *et al.* [24]	0.795	0.241	0.293	1.892	4.730
Yue *et al.* [25]	0.983	0.056	0.098	1.549	**4.088**
Li *et al.* [26]	0.971	0.125	0.187	1.463	4.279
Proposed method	**0.984**	**0.049**	**0.096**	**1.375**	4.107

iterations was 200 epochs and the batch size was set to one. All training images were rescaled to 512×512 and random rotation of $[-10,10]$ degrees as well as random horizontal/vertical flipping were employed for data augmentation. The mean values across all testing images are reported.

Figure 1(d–e) illustrate the 3D vessel reconstruction results by method [2] and the proposed method, where we can observe the projection artifact along big vessels. This problem has been certainly addressed based our method, and thus it will be more helpful to ophthalmologists of retinal diseases diagnosis and treatment. More visual results may be found in bottom row of Fig. 4. To further verify the superiority of our method, the following comparative and ablation studies were also carried out.

Comparison with Previous Methods: Table 1 reports the performances of the proposed method compared with SOTA depth predicting methods [12, 19, 22, 23] and the most commonly-used domain adaptation algorithms [24–26]. For the source domain, it may be observed clearly that the proposed method is capable of obtaining a depth map similar to the ground truth as shown in top row of Fig. 4: this is confirmed by ACC, ARD and RMSE in Table 1. For the target domain, both CD and HD show the similarity between the reconstructed point cloud and corresponding ground truth. Overall, the proposed method outperforms the previous methods in terms of almost all the metrics by significant margins for both depth prediction and domain adaptation.

Table 2. Ablation study of the proposed method.

SCB	D_{adv}	CSC	CD	HD
			3.413	6.610
	✓		1.897	4.662
✓	✓		1.764	4.575
✓	✓	✓	**1.375**	**4.107**

Ablation Study: To understand the roles of different components in the proposed method, an ablation study is performed. Table 2 summarizes the results of the proposed method with different combinations of components. D_{adv} significantly decreases the value of CD from 3.413 to 1.897, and HD from 6.610 to 4.662. The addition of SCB and CSC, separately and in combination, also effectively improves the network capacity. A combination of the SCB, D_d and CSC provides significant improvements, which confirms that the proposed method produces the best results.

4 Conclusion

In conclusion, a novel method for the 3D reconstruction of vessels in OCTA images via depth map estimation is proposed, which is suitable for OCTA images obtained from a variety of devices. The remarkable significance of this work is that it successfully demonstrates the effective use of 2D OCTA *en face* angiograms alone for 3D vessel reconstruction, and that it is applicable to images in two different data domains. Moreover, it effectively solves the projection artifact problem. The high evaluation performance demonstrates the effectiveness of our method both qualitatively and quantitatively. It reveals considerable potential to exploring the subsequent vessel analysis in 3D space, and to assist clinical research in the future.

Acknowledgment. This work was supported in part by the Zhejiang Provincial Natural Science Foundation of China (LZ19F010001), in part by the Youth Innovation Promotion Association CAS (2021298), in part by the Ningbo 2025 S&T Megaprojects (2019B10033 and 2019B1006).

References

1. Kashani, A.H., et al.: Optical coherence tomography angiography: a comprehensive review of current methods and clinical applications. Prog. Retinal Eye Res. **60**, 66–100 (2017)
2. Zhang, J., et al.: 3D shape modeling and analysis of retinal microvasculature in oct-angiography images. IEEE Trans. Med. Imaging **39**(5), 1335–1346 (2019)
3. Hwang, T.S., et al.: Automated quantification of capillary nonperfusion using optical coherence tomography angiography in diabetic retinopathy. JAMA Ophthalmol. **134**(4), 367–373 (2016)
4. Arrigo, A., et al.: Advanced optical coherence tomography angiography analysis of age-related macular degeneration complicated by onset of unilateral choroidal neovascularization. Am. J. Ophthalmol. **195**, 233–242 (2018)
5. Xie, J., et al.: Classification of retinal vessels into artery-vein in oct angiography guided by fundus images. In: Martel, A.L., et al. (eds.) Medical Image Computing and Computer Assisted Intervention. LNCS, vol. 12266, pp. 117–127. Springer, Cham (2020). https://doi.org/10.1007/978-3-030-59725-2_12
6. Eladawi, N., et al.: Automatic blood vessels segmentation based on different retinal maps from OCTA scans. Comput. Biol. Med. **89**, 150–161 (2017)
7. Mou, L., et al.: CS-Net: channel and spatial attention network for curvilinear structure segmentation. In: Shen, D., et al. (eds.) Medical Image Computing and Computer Assisted Intervention. LNCS, vol. 11764, pp. 721–730. Springer, Heidelberg (2019)
8. Ma, Y., et al.: Rose: a retinal oct-angiography vessel segmentation dataset and new model. IEEE Trans. Med. Imaging **40**(3), 928–939 (2021)
9. Zhao, Y., et al.: Automatic 2-D/3-D vessel enhancement in multiple modality images using a weighted symmetry filter. IEEE Trans. Med. Imaging **37**(2), 438–450 (2017)
10. Sarabi, M.S., et al.: 3D retinal vessel density mapping with oct-angiography. IEEE J. Biomed. Health Inform. **24**(12), 3466–3479 (2020)
11. Majcher, C., Johnson, S.L.: Imaging motion: a review of oct-a: this new, noninvasive technology is giving us a more detailed view of the retinal vasculature than ever. Rev. Optom. **154**(3), 36–44 (2017)
12. Yu, S., et al.: 3D vessel reconstruction in oct-angiography via depth map estimation. In: 2021 IEEE 18th International Symposium on Biomedical Imaging (ISBI), pp. 1609–1613. IEEE (2021)
13. Ronneberger, O., Fischer, P., Brox, T.: U-Net: Convolutional networks for biomedical image segmentation. In: Navab, N., Hornegger, J., Wells, W., Frangi, A. (eds.) Medical Image Computing and Computer-Assisted Intervention. LNCS, vol. 9351, pp. 234–241. Springer, Cham (2015)
14. Wang, Z., et al.: Image quality assessment: from error visibility to structural similarity. IEEE Trans. Image Process. **13**(4), 600–612 (2004)
15. Bankhead, P., et al.: Fast retinal vessel detection and measurement using wavelets and edge location refinement. PloS ONE **7**(3), e32435 (2012)
16. Corsini, M., Cignoni, P., Scopigno, R.: Efficient and flexible sampling with blue noise properties of triangular meshes. IEEE Trans. Vis. Comput. Graph. **18**(6), 914–924 (2012)
17. Bernardini, F., et al.: The ball-pivoting algorithm for surface reconstruction. IEEE Trans. Vis. Comput. Graph. **5**(4), 349–359 (1999)

18. Ladicky, L., Shi, J., Pollefeys, M.: Pulling things out of perspective. In: IEEE Conference on Computer Vision and Pattern Recognition, pp. 89–96 (2014)
19. Laina, I., et al.: Deeper depth prediction with fully convolutional residual networks. In: International Conference on 3D Vision (3DV), pp. 239–248. IEEE (2016)
20. Borgefors, G.: Distance transformations in digital images. Comput. Vis. Graph. Image Process. **34**(3), 344–371 (1986)
21. Huttenlocher, D.P., et al.: Comparing images using the Hausdorff distance. IEEE Trans. Pattern Anal. Mach. Intell. **15**(9), 850–863 (1993)
22. Eigen, D., Fergus, R.: Predicting depth, surface normals and semantic labels with a common multi-scale convolutional architecture. In: IEEE International Conference on Computer Vision, pp. 2650–2658 (2015)
23. Chen, W., Fu, Z., Yang, D., Deng, J.: Single-image depth perception in the wild. In: International Conference and Workshop on Neural Information Processing Systems (2016)
24. Tzeng, E., et al.: Adversarial discriminative domain adaptation. In: IEEE Conference on Computer Vision and Pattern Recognition, pp. 7167–7176 (2017)
25. Yue, X., et al.: Domain randomization and pyramid consistency: simulation-to-real generalization without accessing target domain data. In: IEEE/CVF International Conference on Computer Vision, pp. 2100–2110 (2019)
26. Li, S., et al.: Domain conditioned adaptation network. In: AAAI Conference on Artificial Intelligence, vol. 34, pp. 11386–11393 (2020)

Distinguishing Differences Matters: Focal Contrastive Network for Peripheral Anterior Synechiae Recognition

Yifan Yang[1,2], Huihui Fang[3], Qing Du[1], Fei Li[4], Xiulan Zhang[4], Mingkui Tan[1,2,5(✉)], and Yanwu Xu[3(✉)]

[1] South China University of Technology, Guangzhou, China
mingkuitan@scut.edu.cn
[2] Pazhou Lab, Guangzhou, China
[3] Intelligent Healthcare Unit, Baidu, Beijing, China
ywxu@ieee.org
[4] State Key Laboratory of Ophthalmology, Zhongshan Ophthalmic Center,
Sun Yat-sen University, Guangzhou, China
[5] Key Laboratory of Big Data and Intelligent Robot, Ministry of Education, Guangzhou, China

Abstract. We address the problem of Peripheral Anterior Synechiae (PAS) recognition, which aids clinicians in better understanding the progression of the type of irreversible angle-closure glaucoma. Clinical identification of PAS requires indentation gonioscopy, which is patient-contacting and time-consuming. Thus, we aim to design an automatic deep-learning-based method for PAS recognition based on non-contacting anterior segment optical coherence tomography (AS-OCT). However, modeling structural differences between tissues, which is the key for clinical PAS recognition, is especially challenging for deep learning methods. Moreover, the class imbalance issue and the tiny region of interest (ROI) hinder the learning process. To address these issues, we propose a novel Focal Contrastive Network (FC-Net), which contains a Focal Contrastive Module (FCM) and a Focal Contrastive (FC) loss to model the structural differences of tissues, and facilitate the learning of hard samples and minor class. Meanwhile, to weaken the impact of irrelevant structure, we introduce a zoom-in head to localize the tiny ROI. Extensive experiments on two AS-OCT datasets show that our proposed FC-Net yields 2.3%–8% gains on the PAS recognition performance regarding AUC, compared with the baseline models using different backbones. The code is available at https://github.com/YifYang993/FC-Net.

Keywords: PAS recognition · Contrastive loss · AS-OCT · Glaucoma

1 Introduction

Peripheral Anterior Synechiae (PAS), an eye condition in which the iris adheres to the cornea, causes closure of the anterior chamber angle [1,2] and further increases the risk of angle-closure glaucoma [3]. Clinically, experts identify PAS by measuring whether

---

Y. Yang, H. Fang and Q. Du—Authors contributed equally.

© Springer Nature Switzerland AG 2021
M. de Bruijne et al. (Eds.): MICCAI 2021, LNCS 12908, pp. 24–33, 2021.
https://doi.org/10.1007/978-3-030-87237-3_3

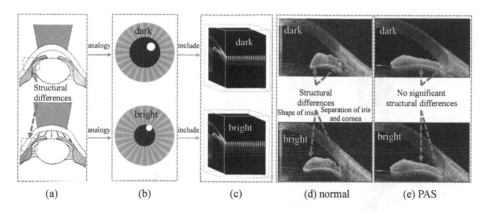

(a)   (b)   (c)   (d) normal   (e) PAS

Fig. 1. A description of the motivation for the proposed FC-Net. (a) The structural differences (the dashed boxes) of the eye observed by indentation gonioscopy [9], (b) the eye in different light conditions, (c) the paired AS-OCT sequence, (d) the normal case with the existence of structural differences, (e) the PAS case without a significant structural difference. (Color figure online)

the adhesion between iris and cornea could be disrupted (*i.e.,* structural differences, as shown in Fig. 1(a)) using indentation gonioscopy [4]. However, this diagnostic approach is patient-contacting. Anterior segment optical coherence tomography (AS-OCT), with the characteristics of easy-to-perform and non-contact, has become a critical tool to evaluate the anterior segment of an eye [5]. Thus, we seek to design an AS-OCT based algorithm to detect the PAS automatically.

Currently, there are a few deep-learning-based research endeavors pertaining to AS-OCT based automatic recognition of PAS, whereas several attempts have been made to recognize glaucoma related disease. Fu *et al.* combined clinical parameters and multi-scale features to improve the accuracy of a angle-closure screening method [6]. Hao *et al.* proposed a coarse-to-fine method to localize anterior chamber angle regions and then classified them into primary open-angle glaucoma (POAG), primary angle-closure suspect (PACS) and primary angle-closure glaucoma (PACG) [7]. Recently, Hao *et al.* proposed a novel MSDA block and multi-loss function to classify AS-OCT images into POAG, PACG and synechiae [8]. Although these deep learning methods can improve the performance of automatic recognition of glaucoma related diseases, they lack information regarding the structural differences of an eye (see Figs. 1(a), 1(d) and 1(e)), which is critical in identifying PAS in clinic [3]. Moreover, these methods ignore the class imbalance problem, which is unavoidable due to the difficulty in collecting positive data (*e.g.,* In the two AS-OCT datasets used in the experiment, the PAS samples accounted for 7.5% and 30.4%, respectively).

In view of the shortcomings of the above methods, we propose a novel framework to recognize PAS by considering distinguishing the structural differences of an eye, which requires a paired data representing conditions during indentation gonioscopy and a strategy to measure the differences between the paired data. Inspired by the diagnostic processes of doctors, PAS is identified if the adhesion of iris and cornea cannot be separated using indentation gonioscopy [4]. We introduce a medical prior [3], which states that the structural differences of the eye observed by indentation gonioscopy (Fig. 1 (a))

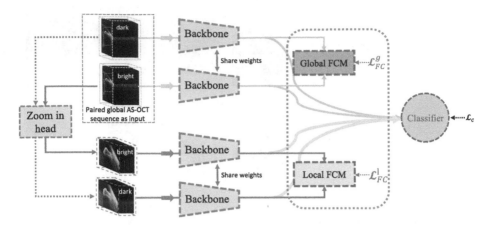

Fig. 2. Our proposed framework takes paired AS-OCT sequence under bright and dark conditions as input. The zoom-in head crops the discriminative area. Differences of the paired AS-OCT sequence are distinguished by means of the focal contrastive module in global and local views.

is analogized to the structural difference of an eye in different light conditions (Fig. 1 (b)), which can be observed from the paired AS-OCT sequence (Fig. 1 (c)). In normal cases, bright conditions cause pupillary constriction, which results in separation of iris and cornea (see the red dashed boxes in Fig. 1 (d)). For patients with PAS, the adhesion of iris and cornea prevents the separation (Fig. 1 (e)).

To distinguish the differences between the paired AS-OCT sequence for PAS recognition, we design a Focal Contrastive Network (FC-Net) with a focal contrastive (FC) loss. The network consists of two modules including a zoom-in head module and a Focal Contrastive Module (FCM). The zoom-in head module is designed to address the difficulty in capturing the tiny region, where the iris and cornea intersect. The main idea of FCM is to distinguish differences of features from two light conditions, and to guide the network to focus on hard samples and minor class by the designed FC loss. The major contributions of this paper are threefold. (1) We introduce a medical prior of clinical PAS recognition to the deep-learning-based method, and experimentally demonstrate that this medical prior knowledge can enhance the performances. (2) We design a novel focal contrastive module with a focal contrastive loss, which can distinguish the differences between the paired AS-OCT images, as well as alleviate the class imbalance problem and focus on the hard samples. (3) Our proposed FC-Net can be implemented with different backbones, and the promising experimental results show that the FC-Net has strong generalizability and can be applied to 3D data such as video or CT volume for difference measurement.

2   Methodology

Dividing an eye into 12 paired sectors (Fig. 3 (a1)–(a2)), a paired sectors (*e.g.*, 2–3 o'clock, shown as the yellow fan area) of the eye under dark and bright conditions is represented by a paired AS-OCT sequence, *i.e.*, 2×21 AS-OCT images (Fig. 1 (c)) [2]. We aim to classify the 12 paired sectors of an eye into normal or PAS, respectively.

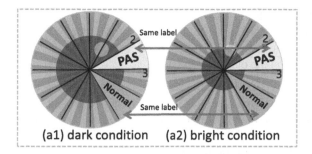

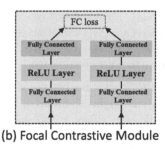

Fig. 3. (a1–a2) Illustration of the paired sectors of an eye in different light conditions. Colored paired sectors shares same label and is represented by paired AS-OCT sequence. (b) Overview of the focal contrastive module (FCM). (Color figure online)

The pipeline of our FC-Net is illustrated in Fig. 2 given a paired AS-OCT sequence $\{\mathcal{X}_d, \mathcal{X}_b\}$ that represents a paired sectors of an eye from different light conditions. First, a zoom-in head module is implemented to extract the discriminative area by cropping $\{\mathcal{X}_d, \mathcal{X}_b\}$ into local version $\{\mathcal{X}_d^l, \mathcal{X}_b^l\}$. After the dual stream backbone, the learned features $\{\mathcal{H}_d, \mathcal{H}_b\}$, and $\{\mathcal{H}_d^l, \mathcal{H}_b^l\}$ are sent to the focal contrastive module(FCM) to distinguish the differences between two light conditions ($C(\mathcal{H}_d, \mathcal{H}_b) \rightarrow \mathcal{L}_{FC}^g, C(\mathcal{H}_d^l, \mathcal{H}_b^l) \rightarrow \mathcal{L}_{FC}^l$), generating corresponding global focal contrastive (FC) loss $\mathcal{L}_{FC}^g$ and local FC loss $\mathcal{L}_{FC}^l$ which measure the difference between the paired AS-OCT sequence in global and local views. Note that the FC loss in FCM introduces two factors to guide the contrastive module to focus on hard samples and minor class simultaneously. Finally, the supervised information of FC loss ($\mathcal{L}_{FC}^l$ and $\mathcal{L}_{FC}^g$) and classification loss ($\mathcal{L}_c$) is fused by the decay learning strategy, which iteratively decreases the weight of FC loss. The overall training procedure of PAS recognition aims to minimize the following objective function:

$$\mathcal{L}_{all} = \mathcal{L}_c + decay(\mathcal{L}_{FC}), \ \mathcal{L}_{FC} = \mathcal{L}_{FC}^g + \mu\mathcal{L}_{FC}^l \tag{1}$$

where *decay* is our proposed decay learning strategy to balance between $\mathcal{L}_c$ and $\mathcal{L}_{FC}$, and μ is a given ratio between local FC loss and global FC loss. The details of our FC-Net are illustrated as follows.

2.1 Focal Contrastive Neural Network

The focal contrastive network (FC-Net) contains a zoom-in head module for cropping the AS-OCT sequence, a dual-stream backbone for learning representation of the paired AS-OCT sequence and a focal contrastive module for measuring the differences between the dark and bright conditions.

Zoom-in head: Clinically, PAS is identified by the adhesion of iris and cornea [4], yet the adhesion region is tiny comparing with an eye. Hence, we introduce a localization method termed the zoom-in head to crop the tiny ROI of the AS-OCT sequence, based on an observation that the horizontal centerline of the ROI is close to the horizontal line with max sum of pixels. Consider a matrix X representing an image, the zoom-in head module traverses each row of X to search the row with the largest sum of pixels (*i.e.,* $\max_i\{\sum_j X_{ij}\}$), then we set the row as the horizontal centerline of the ROI. With the centerline, we crop X at a fixed size to obtain the ROI. The original and the cropped sequence are simultaneously learned by the dual-stream backbone.

Dual Stream Backbone: Motivated by an observation that the AS-OCT sequence in different light conditions differ on both global scale (*e.g.,* change in lens size) and local scale (*i.e.,* adhesion and separation of the conjunction of iris and cornea), we design a dual-stream neural network that includes global and local information of the paired data. The backbone aims to extract features of the sequence from multiple levels in the two light conditions. Specifically, the global and local sequence ($\mathcal{X}_d$ and $\mathcal{X}_d^l$) captured in the dark condition are fed into a global dark stream (*i.e.,* $\mathcal{X}_d \rightarrow \mathcal{H}_d$) and a local dark stream (*i.e.,* $\mathcal{X}_d^l \rightarrow \mathcal{H}_d^l$), and their counterparts ($\mathcal{X}_b$ and $\mathcal{X}_b^l$) work in the same manner. Note that the backbones of the same scale share weights to benefit from the corresponding representation learning and to reduce computational complexity.

Focal Contrastive Module: Modeling the difference between the dark and bright sequence is the core procedure for PAS recognition, which is achieved by our proposed FCM, as shown in Fig. 3 (b). Taking the global branch as an example, the feature vectors $\mathcal{H}_d^g$, $\mathcal{H}_b^g$ are fed into FCM to generate representation vectors of corresponding AS-OCT sequence (*i.e.,* $\mathcal{C}_d$, and $\mathcal{C}_b$). Then, the difference, *i.e.,* Euclidean distance d between $\mathcal{C}_d$ and $\mathcal{C}_b$, is selected by the mining strategy in [10] and then measured by the FC loss.

2.2   Designed Loss Function

Focal Contrastive Loss: The novel FC loss is designed to measure the difference of the paired AS-OCT sequence and to alleviate the class imbalance problem. Inspired by contrastive loss [11] and focal loss [12], the FC loss is designed as follows.

$$\mathcal{L}_{FC} = \frac{S}{m} \sum_{i=1}^{m} \left\{ \alpha^{\mathcal{P}} \sum_{y_i=1} \beta_i^{\mathcal{P}} d_i^2 + \alpha^{\mathcal{N}} \sum_{y_i=0} \beta_i^{\mathcal{N}} \left([M - d_i]_+\right)^2 \right\} \qquad (2)$$

where m denotes the number of training samples, S is a scale factor that determines the largest scale of the FC loss, and M is a fixed margin for similarity separation, which is set as 2 following [11]. d is the Euclidean distance that measures similarity between a data pair (*e.g.,* paired AS-OCT sequence from different light conditions). β and α are a focal factor and a balance factor following the focal loss style. β is formulated as:

$$\beta^{\mathcal{P}} = [\text{sigmoid}\,(d)]^2, \ \beta^{\mathcal{N}} = [1 - \text{sigmoid}\,(d)]^2 \qquad (3)$$

where $\mathcal{P}$ and $\mathcal{N}$ denote PAS and normal samples(*i.e.,* similar pairs and dissimilar pairs).

   β measures the amount of information that a data pair contains. Starting from scaling non-negative value d to range $[0.5, 1)$ by a sigmoid function, we then measure the information of each pair according to how far the distance d is from the expected distance by Eq. 3 (*e.g.,* the expected distance of a pair is near 1, thus a hard dissimilar pair with a close distance contains much information). We specify a property of the focal factor. When a similar pair is a hard one and leads to sigmoid(d) near 1, the corresponding $\beta^{\mathcal{P}}$ approaches 1. In this way, the loss for the hard similar pair is up-weighted.

Table 1. The statistics of AS-I and AS-II. Note that a sample in the table denotes a paired sequence (Fig. 1 (c)) consisting of 2×21 AS-OCT images, except for the last column, which represents the number of eyes.

Dataset	Set	Category		#Total	#Eye
		#Normal	#PAS		
AS-I	Train	212	64	276	23
	Test	202	62	264	22
AS-II	Train	2109	159	2268	189
	Test	2099	157	2256	188

α balances the impact of the similar and dissimilar pairs. Since class imbalance problem leads the training to be dominated by the dissimilar pairs, we design $\alpha^{\mathcal{P}}$ and $\alpha^{\mathcal{N}}$ subject to $\alpha^{\mathcal{P}} + \alpha^{\mathcal{N}} = 1$. Specifically, for a normal pair that occupies the majority, $\alpha^{\mathcal{N}}$ is set to less than 0.5 and hence down-weights the impact of the major class.

Decay Learning Strategy: To use the information obtained from the structural differences, we design a decay learning strategy to fuse the above FC loss and a classification loss. In our network, the α-balanced focal loss [12–14] is used as the classification loss. Specifically, recall that the overall loss is formulated as in Eq. 1, where *decay* controls the impact of FC loss. We down-weight the ratio of FC loss by:

$$decay = 1 - \left(\frac{T}{T_{\max}} \right) \tag{4}$$

where T denotes the current training epoch, and $T_{\max}$ denotes the total epochs. During the training procedure, the decay learning strategy aims to first learn an embedding by distinguishing the difference via the FC loss and then gradually focus on the classification by making use of the difference. Thus, in our designed decay strategy, as $T \rightarrow T_{max}$, *decay* goes to 0 and the impact of FC loss is down-weighted.

3 Experimental Results

Datasets: Our experiments utilize AS-I and AS-II, which are captured from 377 eyes using a CASIA II machine and from 45 eyes using a CASIA I machine, respectively. Each eye is collected in bright and dark conditions to obtain bright and dark volumes, and contains 2×128 AS-OCT images with 800×1876 pixels in AS-II, with 800×1000 in AS-I. Differences between the AS-OCT images in these two datasets lie in noise, iris and crystalline lens, which lead to variation in prediction performance. Following [15], we crop 128 images of an AS-OCT volume into 256 left/right images. Then, 256 images are divided into 12 AS-OCT sequence, each of which denotes a sector of an eye under dark or bright light condition. The statistics of the category distribution, as well as the data distribution in training and testing processes, are shown in Table 1. Note that we carefully checked the datasets to ensure that there was no patient overlap between the training and testing sets.

Table 2. Performance comparison based on two datasets. The suffix "*-FC" represents FC-Net with "*" as the backbone, "*-B(D)" denotes methods taking bright(dark) sequence as input only, and "*-C" indicates baselines concatenating features extracted from paired AS-OCT sequence.

Method	AS-I		AS-II	
	AUC	F1	AUC	F1
SMA-Net-D [8]	0.8675	0.6400	0.9271	0.4013
SMA-Net-B [8]	0.8521	0.5856	0.9024	0.5086
S3D-D [16]	0.8084	0.5492	0.8581	0.3402
S3D-B [16]	0.8204	0.5665	0.8532	0.3303
S3D-FC(ours)	**0.8986**	**0.6853**	**0.9381**	**0.5428**
I3D-D [17]	0.8713	0.6345	0.9360	0.4945
I3D-B [17]	0.8403	0.6341	0.9340	0.5056
I3D-FC(Ours)	**0.8986**	**0.6906**	**0.9599**	**0.5646**
NL I3D-D [18]	0.8907	0.6667	0.9082	0.4103
NL I3D-B [18]	0.8897	0.6212	0.9162	0.3657
NL I3D-C(Ours)	0.9016	**0.6667**	0.9359	0.4217
NL I3D-FC(Ours)	**0.9342**	0.6526	**0.9401**	**0.4778**

Implementation Details: We implement FC-Net via Pytorch. During training, we use an SGD optimizer with learning rate $= 10^{-3}$ and weight decay $= 10^{-4}$ on NVIDIA TITAN X GPU. The learning rate is decayed by 0.01 at the 120-th and 160-th epochs. We implement the decay learning strategy to trade off between classification loss ($\mathcal{L}_C$) and FC loss ($\mathcal{L}_{FC}$). For the trade-off parameters, we set $\mu = 0.5$, $M = 2$, and $\alpha = 0.25$ on all datasets, and set $S = 16$ and $S = 24$ for AS-I and AS-II, respectively.

Baselines: We compare our FC-Net with 4 3D deep learning models: S3D [16], I3D [17], NL I3D [18], and SMA-Net [8]. For fair comparisons, we evaluate each model on both dark and bright AS-OCT sequence, which are termed as "*-D" and "*-B". In addition, "*-C" denotes a variation of our proposed method that simply concatenates features of dark and bright sequence, while our proposed method "*-FC" considers the difference between both AS-OCT sequence. Note that "*" denotes different backbones.

Metrics: We use AUC and F_1-score as the metrics. Both metrics are robust with respect to the class imbalance problem. The AUC shows desirable properties in the binary classification task [19], and the F_1-score can trade off between precision and recall [20].

3.1 Overall Performance

Table 2 shows the PAS recognition results of different methods under different light conditions for two datasets. Specifically, on AS-II, when using the AS-OCT sequence captured only in dark or bright condition, the best performance of the methods with SMA-Net, S3D, I3D and NL I3D as backbones is the $AUC = 0.9360$ obtained by the I3D-D method. When adding FCM to I3D, the corresponding performance is improved by 2.39%. Similarly, on AS-I, using the proposed FCM, the PAS recognition performance is increased by 4.35% over the NL I3D-D method, which exhibits the best performance among the methods when using only one light condition. Besides, as illustrated

Table 3. Ablation studies performed on AS-I and AS-II in terms of AUC, where ZIH means zoom-in head, FCM indicates the focal contrastive module with FC loss, and DSL denotes decay learning strategy.

Component			Dataset	
ZIH	FCM	DLS	AS-I	AS-II
			0.8395	0.8784
✓			0.9003	0.9425
✓	✓		0.9177	0.9540
✓	✓	✓	**0.9342**	**0.9599**

Table 4. Effect of α in FC loss on the performance of NL I3D-FC in terms of AUC (on AS-I).

$\alpha^{\mathcal{N}}, \alpha^{\mathcal{P}}$	0.25, 0.75	0.5, 0.5	0.75, 0.25
AUC	**0.9342**	0.9107	0.8753

in the table, our proposed FC-Net can be added to different backbones, and outperforms the one stream counterpart by 2.3%–8% in terms of AUC. Such results demonstrate the superiority as well as the generalizability of our FC-Net. Thus, these experimental results show that distinguishing the differences between dark and bright sequence with our proposed FCM and FC loss boosts the performance of PAS recognition.

To verify the effect of only adding AS-OCT sequence of two illumination conditions, we use the NL I3D backbone to extract the features of the paired sequence and concatenate them (NL I3D-C) for PAS recognition. From Table 2, NL I3D-C achieves 2.77% and 1.97% gains compared with NL I3D-D and NL I3D-B in terms of AUC on AS-II, respectively. A similar conclusion can be drawn from AS-I, which demonstrates the effectiveness of the clinical prior, i.e., the differences of an eye observed by clinical indentation gonioscopy are analogized to the difference of a paired AS-OCT sequence captured under dark and bright conditions.

3.2 Ablation Studies and Parameter Discussion

In this section, we discuss the ablation studies (Table 3) and the selection of α (Table 4). We choose I3D as the backbone for AS-II, and NL I3D is set as the backbone for AS-I. In Table 3, the method in the first line simply concatenates the features of the AS-OCT sequence from different light conditions. The table demonstrates that the model with the zoom-in head module (ZIH) achieves 6.41% and 6.08% gains regarding AUC on AS-II and AS-I compared with that without ZIH, since ZIH can introduce the discriminative information by cropping the AS-OCT sequence. Based on ZIH, the focal contrastive module with FC loss (FCM) further increases AUC by 1.15% and 1.74% on AS-II and AS-I respectively, by modeling the structural differences of tissues. Moreover, the decay learning strategy (DLS) also boosts the model performance owint to its characteristic of gradually down-weighting FC loss that focuses on modeling structural differences instead of classification. In addition, we introduce parameter α in FC loss to re-weight the minority class. To further evaluate the impact of α, we discuss its sensitivity at different values while retaining other parameter settings. According to Table 4, when we reduce $\alpha^{\mathcal{N}}$ from 0.75 to 0.25, the minor class in Eq. 2 is up-weighted and the re-weighting procedure leads to improvement of the experimental results.

4   Conclusion

In this paper, we demonstrated that the paired AS-OCT sequence captured from dark and bright conditions can provide fruitful information for PAS recognition. Additionally, we proposed a FC-Net to model the difference of the paired data, which contains an FCM and an FC loss to distinguish the difference of tissues accompanied by up-weighting hard samples and minor class, and a zoom-in head to crop the discriminative area of the AS-OCT sequence. Our FC-Net outperforms the state-of-the-art methods on both AS-II and AS-I. The ablation study shows that the modules designed in this paper are meaningful and effective. Moreover, the proposed FCM with the FC loss can be applied to more tasks aiming at identification of differences between paired 3D data such as video and CT volume, which we leave to our future work.

Acknowledgements. This work was partially supported by Key Realm R&D Program of Guangzhou (202007030007), National Natural Science Foundation of China (NSFC) 62072190, Program for Guangdong Introducing Innovative and Enterpreneurial Teams 2017ZT07X183, Fundamental Research Funds for the Central Universities D2191240, Guangdong Natural Science Foundation Doctoral Research Project (2018A030310365), International Cooperation open Project of State Key Laboratory of Subtropical Building Science, South China University of Technology (2019ZA02).

References

1. Foster, P.J., Aung, T., et al.: Defining "occludable" angles in population surveys: drainage angle width, peripheral anterior synechiae, and glaucomatous optic neuropathy in East Asian people. Brit. J. Ophthalmol. **88**(4), 486–490 (2004)
2. Lee, J.Y., Kim, Y.Y., Jung, H.R.: Distribution and characteristics of peripheral anterior synechiae in primary angle-closure glaucoma. Korean J. Ophthalmol. **20**(2), 104–108 (2006)
3. Lai, I., Mak, H., Lai, G., Yu, M., Lam, D.S., Leung, C.: Anterior chamber angle imaging with swept-source optical coherence tomography: measuring peripheral anterior synechia in glaucoma. Ophthalmology **120**(6), 1144–1149 (2013)
4. Forbes, M.: Gonioscopy with corneal indentation: a method for distinguishing between appositional closure and synechial closure. Arch. Ophthalmol. **76**(4), 488–492 (1966)
5. Ang, M., Baskaran, M., et al.: Anterior segment optical coherence tomography. Prog. Retinal Eye Res. **66**, 132–156 (2018)
6. Fu, H., Xu, Y., et al.: Multi-context deep network for angle-closure glaucoma screening in anterior segment OCT. In: Frangi, A., Schnabel, J., Davatzikos, C., Alberola-Lopez, C., Fichtinger, G. (eds) Medical Image Computing and Computer Assisted Intervention, vol. 11071, pp. 356–363. Springer, Cham (2018). https://doi.org/10.1007/978-3-030-00934-2_40
7. Hao, H., Zhao, Y., Fu, H., Shang, Q., Li, F., Zhang, X., Liu, J.: Anterior chamber angles classification in anterior segment oct images via multi-scale regions convolutional neural networks. In: International Conference of the IEEE Engineering in Medicine and Biology Society, pp. 849–852 (2019)

8. Hao, H.: Open-appositional-synechial anterior chamber angle classification in AS-OCT sequences. In: Martel, A.L., et al. (eds) Medical Image Computing and Computer Assisted Intervention, vol. 12265, pp. pp. 715–724. Springer, Cham (2020). https://doi.org/10.1007/978-3-030-59722-1_69

9. Friedman, D.S., He, M.: Anterior chamber angle assessment techniques. Surv. Ophthalmol. **53**(3), 250–273 (2008)

10. Wang, X., Han, X., Huang,W., Dong, D., Scott, M.R.: Multi-similarity loss with general pair weighting for deep metric learning. In: Proceedings of the IEEE Conference on Computer Vision and Pattern Recognition, pp. 5022–5030 (2019)

11. Hadsell, R., Chopra, S., LeCun, Y.: Dimensionality reduction by learning an invariant mapping. In: IEEE Computer Society Conference on Computer Vision and Pattern Recognition, vol. 2, pp. 1735–1742 (2006)

12. Lin, T.Y., Goyal, P., Girshick, R., He, K., Dollar, P.: Focal loss for dense object detection. IEEE Trans. Pattern Anal. Mach. Intell. **42**(2), 318–327 (2020)

13. Zhang, Y., Wei, Y., et al.: Collaborative unsupervised domain adaptation for medical image diagnosis. IEEE Trans. Image Process. **29**, 7834–7844 (2020)

14. Zhang, Y., Chen, H., et al.: From whole slide imaging to microscopy: deep microscopy adaptation network for histopathology cancer image classification. In: Shen, D., et al. (eds) Medical Image Computing and Computer Assisted Intervention, vol. 11764, pp. 360–368. Springer, Cham (2019). https://doi.org/10.1007/978-3-030-32239-7_40

15. Fu, H., Xu, Y., et al.: Segmentation and quantification for angle-closure glaucoma assessment in anterior segment OCT. IEEE Trans. Med. Imaging **36**, 1930–1938 (2017)

16. Xie, S., Sun, C., Huang, J., Tu, Z., Murphy, K.: Rethinking spatiotemporal feature learning: speed-accuracy trade-offs in video classification. In: The European Conference on Computer Vision, pp. 318–335 (2018)

17. Carreira, J., Zisserman, A.: Quo vadis, action recognition? A new model and the kinetics dataset. In: IEEE Conference on Computer Vision and Pattern Recognition, pp. 4724–4733 (2017)

18. Wang, X., Girshick, R., Gupta, A., He, K.: Non-local neural networks. In: IEEE Computer Society Conference on Computer Vision and Pattern Recognition, pp. 7794–7803 (2018)

19. Bradley, A.P.: The use of the area under the ROC curve in the evaluation of machine learning algorithms. Pattern Recogn. **30**(7), 1145–1159 (1997)

20. Powers, D.: Evaluation: from precision, recall and F-factor to ROC, informedness, markedness and correlation. Mach. Learn. Technol. 2 (2008)

RV-GAN: Segmenting Retinal Vascular Structure in Fundus Photographs Using a Novel Multi-scale Generative Adversarial Network

Sharif Amit Kamran[1]([✉]), Khondker Fariha Hossain[1], Alireza Tavakkoli[1], Stewart Lee Zuckerbrod[2], Kenton M. Sanders[3], and Salah A. Baker[3]

[1] Department of Computer Science and Engineering, University of Nevada, Reno, NV, USA
skamran@nevada.unr.edu
[2] Houston Eye Associates, Houston, TX, USA
[3] School of Medicine, University of Nevada, Reno, NV, USA

Abstract. High fidelity segmentation of both macro and microvascular structure of the retina plays a pivotal role in determining degenerative retinal diseases, yet it is a difficult problem. Due to successive resolution loss in the encoding phase combined with the inability to recover this lost information in the decoding phase, autoencoding based segmentation approaches are limited in their ability to extract retinal microvascular structure. We propose RV-GAN, a new multi-scale generative architecture for accurate retinal vessel segmentation to alleviate this. The proposed architecture uses two generators and two multi-scale autoencoding discriminators for better microvessel localization and segmentation. In order to avoid the loss of fidelity suffered by traditional GAN-based segmentation systems, we introduce a novel weighted feature matching loss. This new loss incorporates and prioritizes features from the discriminator's decoder over the encoder. Doing so combined with the fact that the discriminator's decoder attempts to determine real or fake images at the pixel level better preserves macro and microvascular structure. By combining reconstruction and weighted feature matching loss, the proposed architecture achieves an area under the curve (AUC) of 0.9887, 0.9914, and 0.9887 in pixel-wise segmentation of retinal vasculature from three publicly available datasets, namely DRIVE, CHASE-DB1, and STARE, respectively. Additionally, RV-GAN outperforms other architectures in two additional relevant metrics, mean intersection-over-union (Mean-IOU) and structural similarity measure (SSIM).

Keywords: Retinal vessel segmentation · Generative networks · Medical imaging · Opthalmology · Retinal fundus

1 Introduction

The fundoscopic exam is a procedure that provides necessary information to diagnose different retinal degenerative diseases such as Diabetic Retinopathy, Macular Edema, Cytomegalovirus Retinitis [27]. A highly accurate system is required to segment retinal

Electronic supplementary material The online version of this chapter (https://doi.org/10.1007/978-3-030-87237-3_4) contains supplementary material, which is available to authorized users.

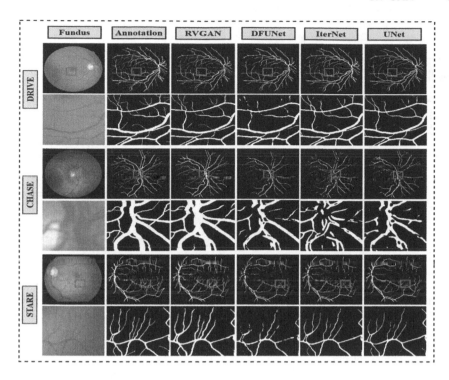

Fig. 1. RV-GAN segments vessel with better precision than other architectures. The 1st row is the whole image, while 2nd row is specific zoomed-in area of the image. The Red bounded box signifies the zoomed-in region. Here, the confidence score is, $t > 0.5$. The row contains DRIVE, CHASE-DB1 and STARE data-set. Whereas the column contains fundus images, ground-truths and segmentation maps for RV-GAN, DFUNet, IterNet and UNet. (Color figure online)

vessels and find abnormalities in the retinal subspace to diagnose these vascular diseases. Many image processing and machine learning-based approaches for retinal vessel segmentation have so far been proposed [7,13,23,26]. However, such methods fail to precisely pixel-wise segment blood vessels due to insufficient illumination and periodic noises. Attributes like this present in the subspace can create false-positive segmentation [7]. In recent times, UNet based deep learning architectures have become very popular for retinal vessel segmentation. UNet consists of an encoder to capture context information and a decoder for enabling precise localization [24]. Many derivative works based on UNet have been proposed, such as Dense-UNet, Deformable UNet [10], Iter-Net [16] etc. These models were able to achieve quite good results for macro vessel segmentation. However, these architectures fail when segmenting microvessels with higher certainty. One reason is successive resolution loss in the encoder, and failure to capture those features in the decoder results in inferior microvessel segmentation. Recent GAN-based architecture [21,32] tries to address this by incorporating discriminative features from adversarial examples while training. However, the discriminator being an encoder [9], only trains on patches of images rather than pixels, affecting the true-positive-rate of the model. We need an architecture that can retain discriminative manifold features

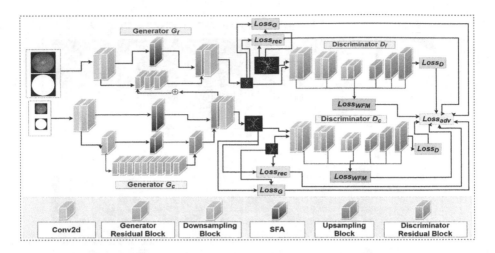

Fig. 2. RV-GAN consisting of Coarse and Fine generators G_f, G_c and discriminators D_f, D_c. The generators incorporates reconstruction loss, $Loss_{rec}$ and Hinge loss $Loss_G$. Whereas the discriminators uses weighted feature matching loss, $Loss_{wfm}$ and Hinge loss $Loss_D$. All of these losses are multiplied by weight multiplier and then added in the final adversarial loss, $Loss_{adv}$. The generators consists of Downsampling, Upsampling, SFA and its distinct residual blocks. On the other hand, the discriminators consists of Downsampling, Upsampling and counterpart residual blocks.

and segment microvessels on pixel-level with higher confidence. Confidence signifies the probability distribution function of the segmented pixel falling under vessel or background. By taking all of these into account, we propose Retinal-Vessel GAN, consisting of coarse and fine generators and multi-scale autoencoder-based discriminators for producing highly accurate segmentation of blood vessel with strong confidence score. Additionally, we come up with a new weighted feature matching loss with inner and outer weights. And we combine it with reconstruction and hinge loss for adversarial training of our architecture. From Fig. 1, it is apparent that our architecture produces a segmentation map with a high confidence score.

2   Proposed Methodology

2.1   Multi-scale Generators

Pairing multi-scale coarse and fine generators produces high-quality domain-specific retinal image synthesis, as observed in recent generative networks, such as Fundus2Angio [12], V-GAN [27] and [29]. Inspired by this, we also adopt this feature in our architecture by using two generators (G_{fine} and G_{coarse}), as visualized in Fig. 2. The generator G_{fine} synthesizes fine-grained vessel segmentation images by extracting local features such as micro branches, connections, blockages, etc. In contrast, the generator G_{coarse} tries to learn and conserve global information, such as the structures of the maco branches, while producing less detailed microvessel segmentation. The detailed structure of these generators is illustrated in Fig. 2.

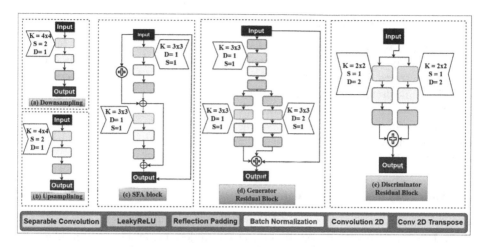

Fig. 3. Proposed Downsampling, Upsampling, Spatial Feature Aggregation block, Generator and Discriminator Residual blocks. Here, K=Kernel size, S=Stride, D=Dilation.

2.2 Residual Downsampling and Upsampling Blocks

Our generators and discriminators consist of both downsampling and upsampling blocks to get the desired feature maps and output. The downsampling block comprises of a convolution layer, a batch-norm layer and a Leaky-ReLU activation function consecutively and is illustrated in Fig. 3(a). Contrarily, the decoder block consists of a transposed convolution layer, batch-norm, and Leaky-ReLU activation layer successively and can be visualized in Fig. 3(b).

2.3 Distinct Identity Blocks for Generator & Discriminator

For spatial and depth feature propagation, residual identity blocks have become go-to building blocks for image style transfer, image inpainting, and image segmentation tasks [3,4,22,25,30]. Vanilla convolution layers are both computationally inefficient and fail to retain accurate spatial and depth information, as opposed to separable convolution [5]. Separable convolution comprises of a depth-wise convolution and a point-wise convolution successively. As a result, it extracts and preserves depth and spatial features while forward propagating the network. Recent advancement in retinal image classification has shown that combining separable convolutional layers with dilation allows for more robust feature extraction [11]. We design two unique residual identity blocks, for our generators and discriminators, as illustrated in Fig. 3(d) & Fig. 3(e).

2.4 Spatial Feature Aggregation

In this section, we discuss our proposed spatial feature aggregation (SFA) block, as illustrated in Fig. 3(c). We use spatial feature aggregation block for combining spatial and depth features from the bottom layers of the network with the top layers of the network, as illustrated in Fig. 2. The rationale behind employing the SFA block is to extract and retain spatial and depth information, that is otherwise lost in deep networks. Consequently, these features can be combined with the learned features of the deeper layers of the network to get an accurate approximation, as observed in similar GAN architectures [2, 33].

2.5 Auto-Encoder as Discriminators

For better pixel-wise segmentation, we need an architecture that can extract both global and local features from the image. To mitigate this underlying problem, we need a deep and dense architecture with lots of computable parameters. It, in turn, might lead to overfitting or vanishing gradient while training the model. To address this issue, rather than having a single dense segmentation architecture, we adopt light-weight discriminators as autoencoders. Additionally, we use multi-scale discriminators for both our coarse and fine generators, as previously proposed in [15, 30]. The arrangement consists of two discriminators with variable sized input and can help with the overall adversarial training. We define two discriminators as D_f and D_c as illustrated in Fig. 2.

2.6 Proposed Weighted Feature Matching Loss

Feature matching loss [30] was incorporated by extracting features from discriminators to do semantic segmentation. The feature-matching loss is given in Eq. 1 As the authors used Patch-GAN as a discriminator, it only contains an encoding module. By contrast, our work involves finding pixel-wise segmentation of retinal vessel and background and thus requires an additional decoder. By successive downsampling and upsampling, we lose essential spatial information and features; that is why we need to give weightage to different components in the overall architecture. We propose a new weighted feature matching loss, as given in Eq. 2 that combines elements from both encoder and decoder and prioritizes particular features to overcome this. For our case, we experiment and see that giving more weightage to decoder feature map results in better vessel segmentation.

$$\mathcal{L}_{fm}(G, D_{enc}) = \mathbb{E}_{x,y} \frac{1}{N} \sum_{i=1}^{k} \|D_{enc}^i(x, y) - D_{enc}^i(x, G(x))\| \tag{1}$$

$$\mathcal{L}_{wfm}(G, D_n) = \mathbb{E}_{x,y} \frac{1}{N} \sum_{i=1}^{k} \lambda_{enc}^i \|D_{enc}^i(x, y) - D_{enc}^i(x, G(x))\| + \lambda_{dec}^i \|D_{dec}^i(x, y)$$
$$- D_{dec}^i(x, G(x))\| \tag{2}$$

Equation 1 is calculated by taking only the features from the downsampling blocks of the discriminator's encoder, D_{enc}^i. Contrarily, the proposed Eq. 2 takes features from both the downsampling and upsampling blocks of the discriminator's encoder, D^i_{enc} and decoder, D^i_{dec}. We insert the real x, y and the synthesized $x, G(x)$, image & segmentation map pairs consecutively. The N signifies the number of features. Here, λ_{enc} and λ_{dec} is the inner weight multiplier for each of the extracted feature maps. The weight values are between $[0, 1]$, and the total sum of the weight is 1, and we use a higher weight value for the decoder feature maps than the encoder feature maps.

2.7 Weighted Objective and Adversarial Loss

For adversarial training, we use Hinge-Loss [18,33] as given in Eq. 3 and Eq. 4. Conclusively, all the fundus images and their corresponding segmentation map pairs are normalized, to $[-1, 1]$. As a result, it broadens the difference between the pixel intensities of the real and synthesized segmentation maps. In Eq. 5, we multiply $\mathcal{L}_{adv}(G)$ with λ_{adv} as weight multiplier. Next, we add $\mathcal{L}_{adv}(D)$ with the output of the multiplication.

$$\mathcal{L}_{adv}(D) = \mathbb{E}_{x,y}\big[\min(0, -1 + D(x, y))\big] - \mathbb{E}_x\big[\min(0, -1 - D(x, G(x)))\big] \quad (3)$$

$$\mathcal{L}_{adv}(G) = -\mathbb{E}_{x,y}\big[(D(G(x), y))\big] \quad (4)$$

$$\mathcal{L}_{adv}(G, D) = \mathcal{L}_{adv}(D) + \lambda_{adv}(\mathcal{L}_{adv}(G)) \quad (5)$$

In Eq. 4 and Eq. 5, we first train the discriminators on the real fundus, x and real segmentation map, y. After that, we train with the real fundus, x, and synthesized segmentation map, $G(x)$. We begin by batch-wise training the discriminators D_f, and D_c for a couple of iterations on the training data. Following that, we train the G_c while keeping the weights of the discriminators frozen. In a similar fashion, we train G_f on a batch training image while keeping weights of all the discriminators frozen.

The generators also incorporate the reconstruction loss (Mean Squared Error) as shown in Eq. 6. By utilizing the loss we ensure the synthesized images contain more realistic microvessel, arteries, and vascular structure.

$$\mathcal{L}_{rec}(G) = \mathbb{E}_{x,y}\|G(x) - y\|^2 \quad (6)$$

By incorporating Eqs. 2, 5 and 6, we can formulate our final objective function as given in Eq. 7.

$$\min_{G_f, G_c} \big(\max_{D_f, D_c} (\mathcal{L}_{adv}(G_f, G_c, D_f, D_c)) +$$
$$\lambda_{rec}[\mathcal{L}_{rec}(G_f, G_c)] + \lambda_{wfm}[\mathcal{L}_{wfm}(G_f, G_c, D_f, D_c)]\big) \quad (7)$$

Here, λ_{adv}, λ_{rec}, and λ_{wfm} implies different weights, that is multiplied with their respective losses. The loss weighting decides which architecture to prioritize while training. For our system, more weights are given to the $\mathcal{L}_{adv}(G)$, $\mathcal{L}_{rec}$, $\mathcal{L}_{wfm}$, and thus we select bigger λ values for those.

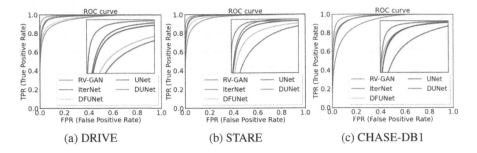

Fig. 4. ROC Curves on (a) DRIVE (b) STARE (c) CHASE-DB1.

3 Experiments

3.1 Dataset

For benchmarking, we use three retinal segmentation datasets, namely, DRIVE [28], CHASE-DB1 [20], and STARE [8]. The images are respectively in $.tif(565 \times 584)$, $.jpg(999 \times 960)$, and $.ppm(700 \times 605)$. We train three different RV-GAN networks with each of these datasets using 5-fold cross-validation. We use overlapping image patches with a stride of 32 and an image size of 128×128 for training and validation. So we end up having 4320 for STARE, 15120 for CHASE-DB1, and 4200 for DRIVE from 20, 20, and 16 images. DRIVE dataset comes with official FoV masks for the test images. For CHASE-DB1 and STARE dataset, we also generate FoV masks similar to Li et al. [16]. For testing, overlapping image patches with a stride of 3 were extracted and averaged by taking 20, 8 and 4 images from DRIVE, CHASE-DB1, and STARE.

3.2 Hyper-parameter Initialization

For adversarial training, we used hinge loss [18,33]. We picked $\lambda_{enc} = 0.4$ (Eq. 1), $\lambda_{dec} = 0.6$ (Eq. 2), $\lambda_{adv} = 10$ (Eq. 5), $\lambda_{rec} = 10$ (Eq. 6) and $\lambda_{wfm} = 10$ (Eq. 7). We used Adam optimizer [14], with learning rate $\alpha = 0.0002$, $\beta_1 = 0.5$ and $\beta_2 = 0.999$. We train with mini-batches with batch size, $b = 24$ for 100 epochs in three stages using Tensorflow. It took between 24–48 h to train our model on NVIDIA P100 GPU depending on data-set. Because DRIVE and STARE have lower number of patches compared to CHASE-DB1, it takes less amount to train. The inference time is 0.025 second per image. The code repository is provided in this link.

3.3 Threshold vs. Confidence Score

Confidence score signifies the per-pixel probability density value of the segmentation map. U-Net-derived models incorporate binary cross-entropy loss with a threshold of 0.5 to predict if the pixel is a vessel or background. So a pixel, predicted with a 0.5001 probability, will be classified as a vessel. As a result, the model suffers from Type I error or a high false-positive rate (FPR). In contrast, we use the generators to produce realistic

Table 1. Performance comparison on DRIVE [28], CHASE-DB1 [20], & STARE [8].

Dataset	Method	Year	F1 Score	Sensitivity	Specificity	Accuracy	AUC-ROC	Mean-IOU	SSIM
DRIVE	UNet [10]	2018	0.8174	0.7822	0.9808	0.9555	0.9752	0.9635	0.8868
	Residual UNet [1]	2018	0.8149	0.7726	0.9820	0.9553	0.9779	–	–
	Recurrent UNet [1]	2018	0.8155	0.7751	0.9816	0.9556	0.9782	–	–
	R2UNet [1]	2018	0.8171	0.7792	0.9813	0.9556	0.9784	–	–
	DFUNet [10]	2019	0.8190	0.7863	0.9805	0.9558	0.9778	0.9605	0.8789
	IterNet [16]	2019	0.8205	0.7735	0.9838	0.9573	0.9816	0.9692	0.9008
	SUD-GAN [32]	2020	–	0.8340	0.9820	0.9560	0.9786	–	–
	M-GAN [21]	2020	0.8324	**0.8346**	0.9836	0.9706	0.9868	–	–
	RV-GAN (Ours)	2021	**0.8690**	0.7927	**0.9969**	**0.9790**	**0.9887**	**0.9762**	**0.9237**
CHASE-DB1	UNet [10]	2018	0.7993	0.7841	0.9823	0.9643	0.9812	0.9536	0.9029
	DenseBlock-UNet [17]	2018	0.8006	0.8178	0.9775	0.9631	0.9826	0.9454	0.8867
	DFUNet [10]	2019	0.8001	0.7859	0.9822	0.9644	0.9834	0.9609	0.9175
	IterNet [16]	2019	0.8073	0.7970	0.9823	0.9655	0.9851	0.9584	0.9123
	M-GAN [21]	2020	0.8110	0.8234	**0.9938**	**0.9736**	0.9859	–	–
	RV-GAN (Ours)	2021	**0.8957**	**0.8199**	0.9806	0.9697	**0.9914**	**0.9705**	**0.9266**
STARE	UNet [10]	2018	0.7595	0.6681	0.9915	0.9639	0.9710	0.9744	0.9271
	DenseBlock-UNet [17]	2018	0.7691	0.6807	0.9916	0.9651	0.9755	0.9604	0.9034
	DFUNet [10]	2019	0.7629	0.6810	0.9903	0.9639	0.9758	0.9701	0.9169
	IterNet [16]	2019	0.8146	0.7715	0.9886	0.9701	0.9881	0.9752	0.9219
	SUD-GAN [32]	2020	–	0.8334	0.9897	0.9663	0.9734	–	–
	M-GAN [21]	2020	**0.8370**	0.8234	**0.9938**	**0.9876**	0.9873	–	–
	RV-GAN (Ours)	2021	0.8323	**0.8356**	0.9864	0.9754	**0.9887**	**0.9754**	**0.9292**

segmentation maps and utilize the weighted feature matching loss to combine inherent manifold information to predict real and fake pixels with higher certainty. Consequently, we can see in Fig. 4 that our model's Receiver Operating (ROC) curves for three datasets are relatively better than other previous methods due to a high confidence score.

3.4 Quantitative Bench-Marking

We compared our architecture with some best performing ones, including UNet [10], DenseBlock-UNet [17], Deform-UNet [10] and IterNet [16] as illustrated in Fig. 1. We trained and evaluated the first three architectures using their publicly available source code by ourselves on the three datasets. For testing, we only use the generators, G_f and G_c for synthesizing retinal segmentation maps. First, we generate the feature vector from G_c by feeding the resized Fundus and FOV mask. After that, we use the original Fundus, FOV mask, and the feature vector from G_c to generate the fine segmentation map using G_f. For IterNet, the pre-trained weight was provided, so we used that to get the inference result. Next, we do a comparative analysis with existing retinal vessel segmentation architectures, which includes both UNet and GAN based models. The prediction results for DRIVE, CHASE-DB1 and STARE are provided in Table 1. We report traditional metrics such as F1-score, Sensitivity, Specificity, Accuracy, and AUC-ROC. Additionally, we use two other metrics for predicting accurate segmentation and structural similarity of the retinal vessels, namely Mean-IOU (Jaccard Similarity Coefficient) and Structural Similarity Index [31]. We chose Mean-IOU because its the gold standard for measuring segmentation results for many Semantic Segmentation Challenges such as Pascal-VOC2012 [6], MS-COCO [19]. Contrarily, SSIM is a standard metric for evaluating GANs for image-to-image translation tasks. As illustrated in all the tables, our model outperforms both UNet derived architectures and recent GAN based models in terms of AUC-ROC, Mean-IOU, and SSIM, the three main metrics for this task. M-GAN achieves better Specificity and Accuracy in CHASE-DB1 and STARE. However, higher Specificity means better background pixel segmentation (True Negative), which is less essential than having better retinal vessel segmentation (True Positive). We want both, better Sensitivity and AUC-ROC, which equates to having a higher confidence score. In Fig. 4 we can see that our True positive Rate is always better than other architectures for all three data-set. We couldn't report SSIM and Mean-IOU for some of the architectures as source codes and pre-trained, weights weren't provided.

4   Conclusion

In this paper, we proposed a new multi-scale generative architecture called RV-GAN. By combining our novel featuring matching loss, the architecture synthesizes precise venular structure segmentation with high confidence scores for two relevant metrics. As a result, we can efficiently employ this architecture in various applications of ophthalmology. The model is best suited for analyzing retinal degenerative diseases and monitoring future prognosis. We hope to extend this work to other data modalities.

Acknowledgments. This material is based upon work supported by the National Aeronautics and Space Administration under Grant No. 80NSSC20K1831 issued through the Human Research Program (Human Exploration and Operations Mission Directorate).

References

1. Alom, M.Z., Hasan, M., Yakopcic, C., Taha, T.M., Asari, V.K.: Recurrent residual convolutional neural network based on U-Net (R2U-Net) for medical image segmentation. arXiv preprint arXiv:1802.06955 (2018)
2. Chen, X., Xu, C., Yang, X., Tao, D.: Attention-GAN for object transfiguration in wild images. In: Proceedings of the European Conference on Computer Vision, pp. 164–180 (2018)
3. Choi, Y., Choi, M., Kim, M., Ha, J.W., Kim, S., Choo, J.: StarGAN: unified generative adversarial networks for multi-domain image-to-image translation. In: Proceedings of the IEEE Conference on Computer Vision and Pattern Recognition, pp. 8789–8797 (2018)
4. Choi, Y., Uh, Y., Yoo, J., Ha, J.W.: StarGAN V2: diverse image synthesis for multiple domains. In: Proceedings of the IEEE/CVF Conference on Computer Vision and Pattern Recognition, pp. 8188–8197 (2020)
5. Chollet, F.: Xception: deep learning with depthwise separable convolutions. In: Proceedings of the IEEE Conference on Computer Vision and Pattern Recognition, pp. 1251–1258 (2017)
6. Everingham, M., Eslami, S.A., Van Gool, L., Williams, C.K., Winn, J., Zisserman, A.: The pascal visual object classes challenge: a retrospective. Int. J. Comput. Vis. **111**(1), 98–136 (2015). https://doi.org/10.1007/s11263-014-0733-5
7. Fraz, M.M., Remagnino, P., Hoppe, A., Uyyanonvara, B., Rudnicka, A.R., Owen, C.G., Barman, S.A.: Blood vessel segmentation methodologies in retinal images-a survey. Comput. Methods Progr. Biomed. **108**(1), 407–433 (2012)

8. Hoover, A., Kouznetsova, V., Goldbaum, M.: Locating blood vessels in retinal images by piecewise threshold probing of a matched filter response. IEEE Trans. Med. Imaging **19**(3), 203–210 (2000)

9. Isola, P., Zhu, J.Y., Zhou, T., Efros, A.A.: Image-to-image translation with conditional adversarial networks. In: Proceedings of the IEEE Conference on Computer Vision and Pattern Recognition, pp. 1125–1134 (2017)

10. Jin, Q., Meng, Z., Pham, T.D., Chen, Q., Wei, L., Su, R.: DUNet: a deformable network for retinal vessel segmentation. Knowl.-Based Syst. **178**, 149–162 (2019)

11. Kamran, S.A., Saha, S., Sabbir, A.S., Tavakkoli, A.: Optic-Net: a novel convolutional neural network for diagnosis of retinal diseases from optical tomography images. In: 2019 18th IEEE International Conference on Machine Learning And Applications (ICMLA), pp. 964–971 (2019)

12. Kamran, S.A., Hossain, K.F., Tavakkoli, A., Zuckerbrod, S., Baker, S.A., Sanders, K.M.: Fundus2Angio: a conditional GAN architecture for generating fluorescein angiography images from retinal fundus photography. In: Bebis, G., et al. (eds) Advances in Visual Computing, vol. 12510, pp. 125–138. Springer, Heidelberg (2020). https://doi.org/10.1007/978-3-030-64559-5_10

13. Kamran, S.A., Tavakkoli, A., Zuckerbrod, S.L.: Improving robustness using joint attention network for detecting retinal degeneration from optical coherence tomography images. arXiv preprint arXiv:2005.08094 (2020)

14. Kingma, D.P., Ba, J.: Adam: a method for stochastic optimization. arXiv preprint arXiv:1412.6980 (2014)

15. Li, C., Wand, M.: Precomputed real-time texture synthesis with Markovian generative adversarial networks. In: Leibe, B., Matas, J., Sebe, N., Welling, M. (eds) Computer Vision, vol. 9907, pp. 702–716. Springer, Heidelberg (2016). https://doi.org/10.1007/978-3-319-46487-9_43

16. Li, L., Verma, M., Nakashima, Y., Nagahara, H., Kawasaki, R.: IterNet: retinal image segmentation utilizing structural redundancy in vessel networks. In: The IEEE Winter Conference on Applications of Computer Vision, pp. 3656–3665 (2020)

17. Li, X., Chen, H., Qi, X., Dou, Q., Fu, C.W., Heng, P.A.: H-DenseUNet: hybrid densely connected UNet for liver and tumor segmentation from CT volumes. IEEE Trans. Med. Imaging **37**(12), 2663–2674 (2018)

18. Lim, J.H., Ye, J.C.: Geometric GAN. arXiv preprint arXiv:1705.02894 (2017)

19. Lin, T.Y., et al.: Microsoft COCO: common objects in context. In: Fleet, D., Pajdla, T., Schiele, B., Tuytelaars, T. (eds) Computer Vision, vol. 8693, pp. 740–755. Springer, Cham (2014). https://doi.org/10.1007/978-3-319-10602-1_48

20. Owen, C.G., et al.: Measuring retinal vessel tortuosity in 10-year-old children: validation of the computer-assisted image analysis of the retina (CAIAR) program. Investigat. Ophthalmol. Vis. Sci. **50**(5), 2004–2010 (2009)

21. Park, K.B., Choi, S.H., Lee, J.Y.: M-GAN: retinal blood vessel segmentation by balancing losses through stacked deep fully convolutional networks. IEEE Access **8**, 146308–146322 (2020)

22. Park, T., Liu, M.Y., Wang, T.C., Zhu, J.Y.: Semantic image synthesis with spatially-adaptive normalization. In: Proceedings of the IEEE Conference on Computer Vision and Pattern Recognition, pp. 2337–2346 (2019)

23. Ricci, E., Perfetti, R.: Retinal blood vessel segmentation using line operators and support vector classification. IEEE Trans. Med. Imaging **26**(10), 1357–1365 (2007)

24. Ronneberger, O., Fischer, P., Brox, T.: U-Net: convolutional networks for biomedical image segmentation. In: Navab, N., Hornegger, J., Wells, W., Frangi, A. (eds) Medical Image Computing and Computer-Assisted Intervention, vol. 9351, pp. 234–241. Springer, Cham (2015).https://doi.org/10.1007/978-3-319-24574-4_28

25. Shaham, T.R., Dekel, T., Michaeli, T.: SinGAN: learning a generative model from a single natural image. In: Proceedings of the IEEE International Conference on Computer Vision, pp. 4570–4580 (2019)
26. Soares, J.V., Leandro, J.J., Cesar, R.M., Jelinek, H.F., Cree, M.J.: Retinal vessel segmentation using the 2-D Gabor wavelet and supervised classification. IEEE Trans. Med. Imaging **25**(9), 1214–1222 (2006)
27. Son, J., Park, S.J., Jung, K.H.: Retinal vessel segmentation in fundoscopic images with generative adversarial networks. arXiv preprint arXiv:1706.09318 (2017)
28. Staal, J., Abràmoff, M.D., Niemeijer, M., Viergever, M.A., Van Ginneken, B.: Ridge-based vessel segmentation in color images of the retina. IEEE Trans. Med. Imaging **23**(4), 501–509 (2004)
29. Tavakkoli, A., Kamran, S.A., Hossain, K.F., Zuckerbrod, S.L.: A novel deep learning conditional generative adversarial network for producing angiography images from retinal fundus photographs. Sci. Rep. **10**(1), 1–15 (2020)
30. Wang, T.C., Liu, M.Y., Zhu, J.Y., Tao, A., Kautz, J., Catanzaro, B.: High-resolution image synthesis and semantic manipulation with conditional GANs. In: Proceedings of the IEEE Conference on Computer Vision and Pattern Recognition, pp. 8798–8807 (2018)
31. Wang, Z., Bovik, A.C., Sheikh, H.R., Simoncelli, E.P.: Image quality assessment: from error visibility to structural similarity. IEEE Trans. Image Process. **13**(4), 600–612 (2004)
32. Yang, T., Wu, T., Li, L., Zhu, C.: SUD-GAN: deep convolution generative adversarial network combined with short connection and dense block for retinal vessel segmentation. J. Digit. Imaging 1–12 (2020). https://doi.org/10.1007/s10278-020-00339-9
33. Zhang, H., Goodfellow, I., Metaxas, D., Odena, A.: Self-attention generative adversarial networks. In: International Conference on Machine Learning, pp. 7354–7363 (2019)

MIL-VT: Multiple Instance Learning Enhanced Vision Transformer for Fundus Image Classification

Shuang Yu[1], Kai Ma[1(✉)], Qi Bi[1], Cheng Bian[1], Munan Ning[1], Nanjun He[1], Yuexiang Li[1], Hanruo Liu[2], and Yefeng Zheng[1]

[1] Tencent Jarvis Lab, Tencent, Shenzhen, China
kylekma@tencent.com
[2] Beijing Tongren Hospital, Capital Medical University, Beijing, China

Abstract. With the advancement and prevailing success of Transformer models in the natural language processing (NLP) field, an increasing number of research works have explored the applicability of Transformer for various vision tasks and reported superior performance compared with convolutional neural networks (CNNs). However, as the proper training of Transformer generally requires an extremely large quantity of data, it has rarely been explored for the medical imaging tasks. In this paper, we attempt to adopt the Vision Transformer for the retinal disease classification tasks, by pre-training the Transformer model on a large fundus image database and then fine-tuning on downstream retinal disease classification tasks. In addition, to fully exploit the feature representations extracted by individual image patches, we propose a multiple instance learning (MIL) based 'MIL head', which can be conveniently attached to the Vision Transformer in a plug-and-play manner and effectively enhances the model performance for the downstream fundus image classification tasks. The proposed MIL-VT framework achieves superior performance over CNN models on two publicly available datasets when being trained and tested under the same setup. The implementation code and pre-trained weights are released for public access (Code link: https://github.com/greentreeys/MIL-VT).

Keywords: Vision Transformer · Multiple instance learning · Fundus image · Deep learning

1 Introduction

Transformer models have been widely used for natural language processing (NLP) related tasks and demonstrated superior performance [4,15]. Different from convolutional neural networks (CNNs) that focus on the local receptive field at each convolution layer, the essence of Transformer networks is the self-attention mechanism, which enables the global or long-range interactions among all the embedded entries for the prediction task [8,15]. Recently, Transformer

© Springer Nature Switzerland AG 2021
M. de Bruijne et al. (Eds.): MICCAI 2021, LNCS 12908, pp. 45–54, 2021.
https://doi.org/10.1007/978-3-030-87237-3_5

networks have attracted a great amount of interest and attention from the computer vision field, and have been successfully adapted to various vision tasks [3,5,14,16,17,19]. For instance, Carion et al. [3] proposed a hybrid Transformer framework DETR for object detection by combining CNNs with Transformer architecture, which eliminated the necessity of complex framework design of the detection networks. Zhu et al. [19] further extended the work of DETR by introducing a deformable attention module to process the feature maps and achieved better performance with faster convergence speed.

Very recently, Dosovitskiy et al. [5] explored the possibility of using pure Transformer based structure, named as Vision Transformer (ViT), for image classification, which eliminated all the convolutional layers from the network architecture. However, as the ViT architecture does not assume any prior knowledge about the image content, it requires an extremely large dataset for pre-training, and only then it can perform well on downstream classification tasks via fine-tuning [5,8]. To alleviate the ViT model's heavy reliance on data quantity, Touvron et al. [14] proposed a data-efficient image Transformer (DeiT) to utilize a CNN model as the teacher and distillate knowledge to the Transformer based student model via a distillation token, which achieved better performance than EfficientNet when trained and tested on the mid-sized ImageNet dataset. However, for medical image classification tasks, due to the high cost associated with data collection and annotation, generally, the image quantity is often limited and is far less than the quantity of natural images [18]. Thus, it remains an open problem whether Transformer based classification models trained on medical images with limited quantity can achieve comparable performance to that of CNNs.

From another aspect, for pure Transformer based classification models like ViT [5], a unique learnable classification token is appended at the beginning of the input patch series, whose state at the output of the Transformer encoder is taken as the exclusive image representation and used for the image classification. However, all the embedded features from individual patches, which may contain important complementary information to that of the class token, are neglected and does not contribute to the final classification. Therefore, we raise a second problem whether the feature representation of individual patches can be helpful for improving the classification performance.

In this paper, we aim to address the above mentioned two problems, by adopting Vision Transformer to the medical image classification task and making full utilization of the feature representations from individual patches. Two major contributions are achieved with this paper. Firstly, the applicability of Transformer models is explored for the retinal disease classification with fundus images, which, to the best of our knowledge, is the first attempt of using Vision Transformer for medical image classification tasks. We pre-train the Transformer model with a large fundus database, which substantively improves the model performance when fine-tuned on downstream retinal disease classification tasks. Secondly, we enhance the performance of Vision Transformer model by introducing a multiple instance learning head ('MIL head') to fully exploit the features

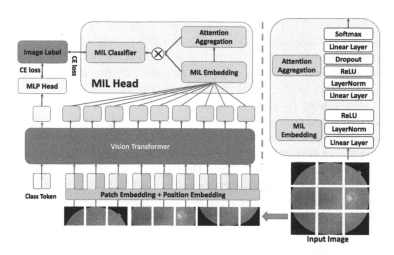

Fig. 1. Framework of the proposed multiple instance learning enhanced Vision Transformer (MIL-VT).

extracted from individual patches, which can be easily attached to existing Vision Transformer in a plug-and-play manner and effectively improves the model performance. Last but not least, the implementation code and pre-trained weights are released for public access, so as to promote further research of Vision Transformer for fundus image related tasks.

2   Method

Figure 1 shows the overall framework of the proposed Multiple Instance Learning enhanced Vision Transformer network (MIL-VT). Different from ViT [5] where only the feature representations from the class token are utilized for classification, we propose a novel 'MIL head' to fully utilize the features extracted by individual image patches. The proposed 'MIL head' is based on the multiple instance learning paradigm and can be conveniently attached to existing Vision Transformer structures in a plug-and-play manner to enhance the model performance.

2.1   Vision Transformer

The structure of Vision Transformer used in this research is the same to that of ViT [5], which is a pure Transformer based architecture without any convolutional layers. The classic Transformer structure is initially designed for NLP tasks, which takes embeddings of characters or words as input, instead of an image. To prepare the fundus image data compatible for the Vision Transformer format, the input image $X \in \mathbb{R}^{H \times W \times C}$ (where H, W, and C denote the image height, width, and color channel number, respectively) is divided into individual patches with size of $P \times P$, where P is set as 16 in this research following the optimal experimental setup as that of [5]. Then we can obtain $N = HW/P^2$ patches from one single image. The patches are further flattened into 1D format and then get embedded via a linear layer into D dimensions, which is the compatible data format for the Transformer networks.

Since the patch embedding contains no information regarding the spatial position of individual patches, thus position embedding is necessary to encode the position information. For ViT [5], the position embedding is encoded as a learnable 1D vector and added to the patch embedding to obtain the final embedding of individual patches. Apart from the embedding of individual patches, a unique learnable class token with corresponding position embedding is appended at the beginning of the embedding series, which serves as the global feature representation for the full image. For DeiT [14], an extra learnable distillation token is appended before the image patch series to learn the another global feature representation by the supervision of a CNN teacher model.

Until now, the original fundus image is processed in a format that is suitable for Vision Transformer with the dimension of $B \times (N + 1) \times D$, where B is the batch size, N is the patch number from one single image and D is the embedding dimension. The processed data is further fed into the Transformer encoder, which consists of repeated Transformer blocks. More specifically, each block is composed of the multi-head attention (MHA) and feed forward network (FFN), with layer normalization and residual operations via skip connection before and after the MHA and FFN, respectively.

2.2   Multiple Instance Learning

For the ViT structure, only the feature representations corresponding to the class token are fed to a multi-layer perceptron (MLP head) for the final classification of the image. Meanwhile, features extracted from individual patches are discarded and fail to contribute towards the final classification. However, the individual patches may contain important complementary information that is neglected or not fully expressed by the feature representation of the class token, especially concerning that pathologies of retinal disease may distribute at different positions [9] and thus the contribution of different patches may vary. In MIL scheme, it regards an image as a bag, which consists of a set of instances either in the format of pixels or image patches. The bag-instance relationship presented in MIL highly resembles that of the image-patch relationship in the Vision Transformer. Thus, in this paper, we propose to introduce the classic MIL formulation [7,12] to the Vision Transformer structures so as to fully utilize the features from individual patches.

To realize this objective, our adoption of MIL scheme into ViT network involves three steps, that is, 1) building a lower-dimension embedding for ViT features from individual patches, 2) an aggregation function to obtain the bag representation, and 3) a bag-level classifier to obtain the final bag-level probabilities, respectively.

Low-dimensional Embedding. Assume the bag-instance relationship in individual images is denoted as $X = \{x_1, x_2, \cdots, x_N\}$. After processing by the Transformer blocks, an instance (image patch) x_i is encoded into a feature vector v_i with the dimension of D, i.e., $v_i = \mathbb{T}(x_i)$. The obtained feature vector v_i is transferred to a lower-dimension embedding, by using a linear layer followed by layer normalization and ReLU activation. This embedding procedure can be denoted as:

$$h_i = max(Norm(W^T v_i), 0), \quad h_i \in \mathcal{H}, \mathcal{H} = \mathbb{R}^M,$$

$$Norm(x) = \frac{x - E(x)}{Var(x) + \epsilon} * \gamma + \beta, \tag{1}$$

where M is the dimension of the embedding $\mathcal{H}$; $W \in \mathbb{R}^{D \times M}$ represents the weight of the projection operation by the linear layer; γ and β denote the learnable parameter of the layer normalization operation.

Attention Aggregation Function. As different image patches contribute differently to the bag, to fully exploit the contribution of all the patches while distinguishing their difference, an attention module with two linear layers is utilized in our framework to extract the spatial weight matrix for the instance embedding. To further normalize the hidden features and prevent potential overfitting, layer normalization, ReLU activation and dropout layers are inserted between the two linear layers, as illustrated in Fig. 1. This process can be presented as:

$$\alpha_i = softmax(W_2^T max(Norm(W_1 h_i^T), 0)), \tag{2}$$

where $W_1 \in \mathbb{R}^{L \times M}$ and $W_2 \in \mathbb{R}^{L \times 1}$ are the parameters of the two linear layers. The *softmax* denotes the Softmax function so as to ensure that the weight for all the instances sums up to 1.

Then, our aggregation function assigns the above attention weights to the instance embeddings to highlight the different contribution of different instances and to provide a feasible approach of end-to-end training. It works as:

$$\mathcal{R} = \sum_{i=1}^{N} \alpha_i h_i. \tag{3}$$

Bag-level Classifier. The aggregated bag representation $\mathcal{R}$ is further fed into a linear classifier to obtain the final bag-level probability, presented as

$$p = w^T \mathcal{R}, \tag{4}$$

where p is the final prediction probability; $w \in \mathbb{R}^{L \times C}$ denotes the parameter of the bag-level classifier and C is the number of categories.

To summarize, the classic MIL formulation is packed and modularized in our entire framework, which we term as 'MIL head' in Fig. 1. The proposed 'MIL head' can be conveniently attached to the Vision Transformer structure in a plug-and-play manner and takes full utilization of the feature representation from individual patches.

2.3   Framework Pre-training and Fine-Tuning

In order to enhance the performance of Vision Transformer specifically for fundus images, a large fundus image classification database is utilized in this research for the pre-training of the Transformer structure. Note that when training the Transformer structure, the model parameters are initialized using the pre-trained weight from ImageNet, so as to fully exploit the learned inductive bias for vision tasks and speed up the training process.

After pre-training, the proposed MIL-VT structure is then fine-tuned on the downstream disease classification tasks with fundus images. The Transformer structure can deal with an arbitrary number of input patches, but the position embedding needs to be interpolated to handle a longer or shorter patch series resulted by a different image size to the pre-training size. For the training of the downstream model, both 'MLP head' and 'MIL head' receive supervision from the classification label, with the cross entropy loss function:

$$L(y, y', y'') = -\lambda \sum_{i=1}^{C} y_i log(y_i') - (1 - \lambda) \sum_{i=1}^{C} y_i log(y_i''), \tag{5}$$

where y denotes the ground-truth label; y' and y'' denote the prediction of 'MLP head' and 'MIL head', respectively; C denotes the number of categories for the downstream task; and λ is the hyper-parameter that controls the relative weight between the two heads and empirically set as 0.5. At inference stage, the outputs of the two heads are weight-averaged by λ to obtain the final prediction.

3   Experiments

For the pre-training of the Vision Transformer structure, a large fundus image dataset is collected and graded from a tele-opthalmology platform, which contains a total of 345,271 fundus images. Five common retinal conditions are labeled, including normal (208,733), diabetic retinopathy (DR, 38,284), age-related macular degeneration (21,962), glaucoma (24,082), and cataract (67,230). Multiple retinal diseases may appear on the same fundus image concurrently and thus the pre-training is set as a multi-label classification problem with the binary cross-entropy loss function. We randomly split 95% of the dataset for training and the rest 5% for validation. All fundus images are resized to the dimension of 384 × 384 for pre-training. The model parameters are initialized using the ImageNet pre-trained weights [5] to speed up the convergence.

For the downstream tasks, two publicly available benchmark databases are utilized to evaluate the effectiveness of the proposed MIL-VT framework, including the APTOS 2019 Blindness Detection (APTOS2019) [1] and 2020 Retinal Fundus Multi-disease Image Dataset (RFMiD2020) [2]. The APTOS2019 contains a total of 3,662 fundus images for DR grading, with five label categories ranging for 0 to 4, representing the DR severity. The RFMiD2020 dataset contains 1,900 images, with binary disease label being provided: 0 for normal images and 1 for image with pathologies. For both datasets, images are split into 5 folds for cross validation and resized to the dimension of 512×512 before being fed into the network.

All experiments are performed on a GPU cluster with four NVIDIA Tesla P40 GPUs and each with 24 GB of memory. The Adam optimizer is adopted to optimize the model parameter with a batch size of 16 and maximum training epochs of 30. The initial learning rate is set as 2×10^{-4} and halved every 2000 iterations. Data augmentation strategies, including random cropping, rotation, horizontal flipping and color jitting, are utilized during the training procedure, so as to increase the diversity of the training data.

3.1 Ablation Studies

Ablation studies have been performed to evaluate the performance boosted by further pre-training on a large fundus dataset, compared with original pre-training from ImageNet. In addition, the efficacy of the proposed MIL-VT structure by introducing the 'MIL head' is also evaluated. We adopt the ViT-Small structure with embedding dimension of 384, multi-head number of 6, and 12 stacked Transformer blocks as the backbone for the experiments. The ablation studies are performed on both APTOS2019 and RFMiD2020 datasets. For the APTOS2019, as a multi-class classification problem, we utilize evaluation metrics of accuracy, area under the curve (AUC), weighted F1 and weighted Kappa. For the RFMiD2020, as it contains only two classes of either disease or normal, evaluation metrics of AUC, accuracy, F1, recall and precision are used.

As listed in Table 1 and Table 2, the further pre-training with the fundus database has improved the performance of Vision Transformer dramatically under all metrics for both APTOS2019 and RFMiD2020. Specifically, for the APTOS2019, the F1 and Kappa metrics of DR grading are improved by 2.3% and 2.1%, respectively. Meanwhile, for the RFMiD2020, the AUC is increased by 1.5% and F1 score is increased by 1.4%, with the pre-training from the fundus dataset.

More importantly, by introducing the 'MIL head' on top of the existing 'MLP head' in the classic Vision Transformer, the model performance is further improved. For the DR grading of APTOS2019, F1 and Kappa scores are improved by 1.5% and 0.9%, respectively. Meanwhile, for RFMiD2020, by adding the 'MIL head' on top of the ViT structure, the AUC and F1 are further improved by 1.4% and 1.8%, arriving at the final performance with AUC of 95.9% and F1 of 94.4%. The experimental results indicate that the proposed 'MIL-head' can take advantage of the feature representations of individual patches and effectively enhance the model performance of the existing Vision Transformer.

3.2 Comparison to State-of-the-art Methods

We compare the proposed MIL-VT framework with other research works for DR grading, including the typical CNN model ResNet34 [6] (with and without fundus pre-training) and the proposed method. Apart from this, we also compared

Table 1. The ablation study results of MIL-VT on APTOS2019 (%).

Model	Combination		DR Grading			
	Pre-train	MIL	AUC	Acc	F1	Kappa
VT (ImageNet)			96.7	82.3	81.5	89.0
VT (Fundus)	✓		97.5	84.6	83.8	91.1
MIL-VT (Fundus)	✓	✓	**97.9**	**85.5**	**85.3**	**92.0**

Table 2. The ablation study results of MIL-VT on RFMiD2020 (%).

Model	Combination		Disease Classification				
	Pre-train	MIL	AUC	Acc	F1	Recall	Precision
VT (ImageNet)			93.0	86.5	91.2	89.1	93.4
VT (Fundus)	✓		94.5	88.5	92.6	90.4	94.8
MIL-VT (Fundus)	✓	✓	**95.9**	**91.1**	**94.4**	**93.7**	**95.0**

Table 3. Comparison with state-of-the-art methods on APTOS2019 (%).

Method	AUC	Acc	F1	Kappa
ResNet34 (ImageNet)	96.5	82.9	82.4	88.8
ResNet34 (Fundus)	97.0	85.0	84.7	90.2
DLI [13]	–	82.5	80.3	89.5
CANet [10]	–	83.2	81.3	90.0
GREEN-ResNet50 [11]	–	84.4	83.6	90.8
GREEN-SE-ResNext50 [11]	–	**85.7**	85.2	91.2
MIL-VT (Proposed)	**97.9**	85.5	**85.3**	**92.0**

Table 4. Comparison with state-of-the-art methods on RFMiD2020 (%).

Method	AUC	Acc	F1	Recall	Precision
ResNet34 (ImageNet)	93.5	87.8	92.6	92.4	92.1
ResNet34 (Fundus)	94.7	89.1	93.0	91.4	94.5
MIL-VT (Proposed)	**95.9**	**91.1**	**94.4**	**93.7**	**95.0**

with recent publications on DR gradings for the APTOS2019 dataset. As listed in Table 3, the weighted F1 and Kappa score of the proposed MIL-VT surpass that of GREEN [11], which is specifically designed for DR grading with a strong backbone and is the current state-of-the-art method for APTOS2019. In addition, the performance of the proposed MIL-VT also surpasses that of ResNet34, when being trained and tested under the same pre-training setup. Similarly, for the performance comparison of RFMiD2020 as listed on Table 4, the proposed MIL-VT also surpasses that of ResNet34, indicating that Transformer structures under proper pre-training can achieve better performance than CNNs.

4   Conclusion

In this paper, the applicability of Vision Transformer was explored for the retinal disease classification task, which, with proper pre-training on a large fundus database, achieved superior performance to that of CNN under the same pre-training setup. In addition, we proposed the MIL-VT framework based on multiple instance learning scheme with a novel 'MIL head' to fully exploit the feature representations extracted from individual patches, which were usually neglected by Vision Transformer. The proposed 'MIL head' could be easily attached to existing Vision Transformer structures via a plug-and-play manner and effectively improved the model performance. When being tested on the fundus image classification datasets of APTOS2019 and RFMiD2020, the proposed MIL-VT achieved the state-of-the-art performance compared with ResNet and other comparison methods in literature.

Acknowledgment. This work was funded by Key-Area Research and Development Program of Guangdong Province, China (No. 2018B010111001), and Scientific and Technical Innovation 2030 - 'New Generation Artificial Intelligence' Project (No.2020AAA0104100).

References

1. APTOS 2019 blindness detection (2019). https://www.kaggle.com/c/aptos2019-blindness-detection/
2. Retinal image analysis for multi-disease detection challenge (2020). https://riadd.grand-challenge.org/
3. Carion, N., Massa, F., Synnaeve, G., Usunier, N., Kirillov, A., Zagoruyko, S.: End-to-end object detection with transformers. In: Vedaldi, A., Bischof, H., Brox, T., Frahm, J.M., (eds) Computer Vision, vol. 12346, pp. 213–229. Springer, Cham (2020). https://doi.org/10.1007/978-3-030-58452-8_13
4. Devlin, J., Chang, M.W., Lee, K., Toutanova, K.: BERT: pre-training of deep bidirectional transformers for language understanding. In: Proceedings of the 2019 Conference of the North American Chapter of the Association for Computational Linguistics: Human Language Technologies, vol. 1 (Long and Short Papers), pp. 4171–4186. Association for Computational Linguistics (2019)
5. Dosovitskiy, A., et al.: An image is worth 16x16 words: transformers for image recognition at scale. arXiv preprint arXiv:2010.11929 (2020)
6. He, K., Zhang, X., Ren, S., Sun, J.: Deep residual learning for image recognition. In: Proceedings of the IEEE Conference on Computer Vision and Pattern Recognition, pp. 770–778 (2016)
7. Ilse, M., Tomczak, J., Welling, M.: Attention-based deep multiple instance learning. In: International Conference on Machine Learning, pp. 2127–2136. PMLR (2018)
8. Khan, S., Naseer, M., Hayat, M., Zamir, S.W., Khan, F.S., Shah, M.: Transformers in vision: a survey. arXiv preprint arXiv:2101.01169 (2021)
9. Li, T., et al.: Applications of deep learning in fundus images: a review. Med. Image Anal. **69**, 101971 (2021)
10. Li, X., Hu, X., Yu, L., Zhu, L., Fu, C.W., Heng, P.A.: CANet: cross-disease attention network for joint diabetic retinopathy and diabetic macular edema grading. IEEE Trans. Med. Imaging **39**(5), 1483–1493 (2019)

11. Liu, S., Gong, L., Ma, K., Zheng, Y.: GREEN: a graph residual re-ranking network for grading diabetic retinopathy. In: Martel, A.L., et al. (eds) Medical Image Computing and Computer Assisted Intervention, vol. 12265, pp. 585–594. Springer, Cham (2020). https://doi.org/10.1007/978-3-030-59722-1_56
12. Peng, T., Wang, X., Xiang, B., Liu, W.: Multiple instance detection network with online instance classifier refinement. In: IEEE Conference on Computer Vision and Pattern Recognition (2017)
13. Rakhlin, A.: Diabetic retinopathy detection through integration of deep learning classification framework. bioRxiv p. 225508 (2018)
14. Touvron, H., Cord, M., Douze, M., Massa, F., Sablayrolles, A., Jégou, H.: Training data-efficient image transformers and distillation through attention. arXiv preprint arXiv:2012.12877 (2020)
15. Vaswani, A., et al.: Attention is all you need. In: Advances in Neural Information Processing Systems, pp. 5998–6008 (2017)
16. Yang, F., Yang, H., Fu, J., Lu, H., Guo, B.: Learning texture transformer network for image super-resolution. In: Proceedings of the IEEE/CVF Conference on Computer Vision and Pattern Recognition, pp. 5791–5800 (2020)
17. Yuan, L., et al.: Tokens-to-token ViT: Training vision transformers from scratch on ImageNet. arXiv preprint arXiv:2101.11986 (2021)
18. Zhou, S.K., et al.: A review of deep learning in medical imaging: image traits, technology trends, case studies with progress highlights, and future promises. arXiv preprint arXiv:2008.09104 (2020)
19. Zhu, X., Su, W., Lu, L., Li, B., Wang, X., Dai, J.: Deformable DETR: deformable transformers for end-to-end object detection. arXiv preprint arXiv:2010.04159 (2020)

Local-Global Dual Perception Based Deep Multiple Instance Learning for Retinal Disease Classification

Qi Bi[1], Shuang Yu[1], Wei Ji[1], Cheng Bian[1], Lijun Gong[1], Hanruo Liu[2], Kai Ma[1(✉)], and Yefeng Zheng[1]

[1] Tencent Jarvis Lab, Tencent, Shenzhen, China
kylekma@tencent.com
[2] Beijing Tongren Hospital, Capital Medical University, Beijing, China

Abstract. With the rapidly growing number of people affected by various retinal diseases, there is a strong clinical interest for fully automatic and accurate retinal disease recognition. The unique characteristics of how retinal diseases are manifested on the fundus images pose a major challenge for automatic recognition. In order to tackle the challenges, we propose a local-global dual perception (LGDP) based deep multiple instance learning (MIL) framework that integrates the instance contribution from both local scale and global scale. The major components of the proposed framework include a local pyramid perception module (LPPM) that emphasizes the key instances from the local scale, and a global perception module (GPM) that provides a spatial weight distribution from a global scale. Extensive experiments on three major retinal disease benchmarks demonstrate that the proposed framework outperforms many state-of-the-art deep MIL methods, especially for recognizing the pathological images. Last but not least, the proposed deep MIL framework can be conveniently embedded into any convolutional backbones via a plug-and-play manner and effectively boost the performance.

Keywords: Retina disease classification · Multiple instance learning · Deep learning · Interpretability

1 Introduction

The number of people with visual impairment and blindness is growing rapidly, resulted from the global issue of population aging and growth [1]. Among various retinal diseases, diabetic retinopathy (DR), glaucoma and age-related macular degeneration (AMD) are reported to be the top three leading causes for moderate to severe vision loss [2,3]. By year 2040, it is estimated that approximately 200 million people will suffer from DR, 111 million potential patients with glaucoma and 288 million people with AMD worldwide [2,4–6]. Thus, early screening and timely treatment is critical to prevent disease progression and potential

Electronic supplementary material The online version of this chapter (https://doi.org/10.1007/978-3-030-87237-3_6) contains supplementary material, which is available to authorized users.

vision loss [2]. In order to reduce manpower cost and make up for the shortage of ophthalmologists and specialists, fully automatic retinal disease screening approaches based on deep learning techniques have been actively investigated in recent years, for instance, [7,8] for DR recognition, [9,10] for glaucoma detection, [11,12] for AMD detection.

Although deep learning approaches have boosted the performance of image recognition significantly [13–16], some unique characteristics of fundus images make it challenging to accurately identify the diseases.

1) Low Contrast Between Tiny and Subtle Pathological Regions and Fundus Background: The pathological regions of retinal disease, also termed as *Region of Interest (RoIs)* in general, are often small in sizes, as well as having a relatively low contrast with the fundus background, especially for diseases in the early stage. Current convolutional neural networks (CNNs) tend to preserve primary global semantic features [13,14], and thus confront challenges in perceiving such low-contrast and small-sized RoIs [17].

2) Scattered Distribution of Pathological Regions: For natural images, foreground objects are often easy to distinguish because of the relatively large object size and the nearly centric distribution due to the photographer's awareness [18]. In contrast, the pathological regions in fundus images are often scattered over the entire retina. This characteristic also poses another challenge for the CNNs to identify the retinal diseases.

Different from general image classification models that predict the target label based on the image directly, multiple instance learning (MIL) regards an image as a bag which consists of a series of instances (i.e., pixels or patches) [19–21]. In the MIL scheme, although the bag category is determined by instances, there are no specific individual instance labels, thus making it critical to automatically infer the importance of each instance.

Although recently some efforts have been made to adopt MIL into current deep learning frameworks [17,22,23], the above characteristics of fundus images are still challenging for current deep MIL approaches to precisely perceive these pathological RoIs, which are often relatively small and occupy a small portion of the whole image, especially for diseases in the early stage. Therefore, in the paper, we are motivated to tackle the above challenges in recognizing retinal diseases by developing a deep MIL framework which can investigate the influence of individual instances from both local scale and global scale, so as to better suit the specific characteristics of how various retinal diseases are manifested in the fundus image. Four major contributions are achieved with this paper:

- We propose a standardized deep MIL scheme for retinal disease recognition, which can be conveniently adapted to any CNN backbones in a plug-and-play manner and substantively boost the performance by a large margin.
- We propose a local-global dual perception based MIL module. To the best of our knowledge, it is the first MIL aggregator that simultaneously integrates the instance contribution from both the local scale and global scale to determine the bag label.

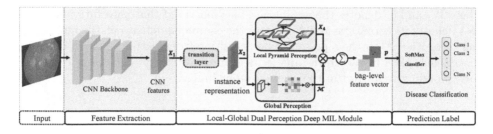

Fig. 1. Our proposed framework for funds image disease recognition.

- We propose a local pyramid instance selection strategy in mining the key instances relevant to the bag label from the local perspective with the utilization of sliding windows.
- Extensive experiments on three major retinal disease benchmarks have demonstrated the effectiveness of the proposed MIL module. In addition, its generalization capability has been validated on multiple backbones.

2   Methodology

Figure 1 demonstrates the proposed framework for the retinal disease recognition task. The feature maps, extracted by a CNN backbone from the original input image, are converted into the instance representations via a transition layer inside the proposed deep MIL framework. Then, our local pyramid perception module (LPPM) selects the key instances under different local scales, so as to increase the importance of locally prominent instances. At the same time, allowing for the scattered distribution of the RoIs, our global perception module (GPM) measures the importance of each instance from the view of the entire image. Finally, the local instance representation and the global instance weights are fused to generate the bag score.

Notably, the proposed local-global dual perception (LGDP) based deep MIL module can conveniently transform current CNNs into the MIL scheme by replacing the global average pooling and fully connected layers in current CNNs. This effort is significantly beneficial as the fully connected layers are parameter costing and are the most potential components to cause over-fitting [13,14].

2.1   Instance Representation Transition

As demonstrated in Fig. 1, after extracting convolutional features X_1 via a CNN backbone, a transitional layer with 1×1 convolution kernels is utilized to obtain the instance representation X_2. Here, the output channel number of the transitional layer equals to the number of bag categories N, and thus enabling the direct generation of bag scores from the instance scores under the instance space paradigm. The process can be represented as:

$$X_2 = W_1^{(1 \times 1, N)} X_1 + b_1^{(1 \times 1, N)}, \tag{1}$$

where W_1 and b_1 denotes the weight and bias matrix of this convolutional layer, 1×1 denotes its kernel size and N denotes the channel number, i.e., the number of bag categories. After the representation transition from feature space to instance space, each pixel in the down-sampled feature map is regarded as an instance, corresponding to an RoI in the original input image.

2.2   Local Pyramid Perception Module (LPPM)

For retinal diseases, the subtle pathological RoIs are generally small-size and have relatively low contrast to the background, thus it is challenging to select the key instances that contribute to the bag score, especially when using the traditional MIL aggregators such as mean or max pooling. Distinguishing these key instances from a variety of local scales helps to fully mine the minor differences between the RoIs and the fundus background. Thus, we develop a local pyramid perception module (LPPM) to fulfill this goal.

Figure 2 illustrates how the LPPM module works. To be specific, given a k-channel sliding window G with the size of $w \times w$, each of the k channels corresponds to a pyramid layer of the LPPM. Then, the operation of G is defined as follows. For the lth layer ($l = 1, 2, ..., k$), the feature responses of the top-l max instances in the local window of this channel G_l are preserved and other instance responses are set zero for suppression. Bear in mind that here the instance representation X_2 is still organized as a set of stacked feature maps and each pixel in X_2 corresponds to an instance.

This k-channel sampling window G slides on the instance representation X_2 with the stride of one. Then, the output of the lth layer $X_{3,l}$ is calculated as

$$X_{3,l} = X_2 \star G_l, \tag{2}$$

where the '$\star$' operation denotes applying G_l on X_2 via the sliding operation. Note that, by using k pyramid layers, the top-l max in the same sampling window will be repeatedly selected for $(k - l + 1)$ times, which will further emphasize the importance of the prominent instances.

The final output of our LPPM X_4 is the sum and normalization of the output of all the k pyramid layers, which can be presented as:

$$X_4 = softmax(\sum_{l=1}^{k} X_{3,l}), \tag{3}$$

where $softmax$ denotes the softmax normalization function among different classes, helping to strengthen the inter-class difference of individual instances meanwhile normalize the feature distribution into $[0, 1]$. Empirically, we set $k = 5$ and $w = 3$ in our deep MIL module.

2.3   Global Perception Module (GPM)

Apart from the local scale, it is also very important to inspect the relative importance of instances from a global perspective while taking their overall contribution to the disease recognition into account. To this end, we design a global perception module (GPM), working as a parallel branch combined with the above mentioned LPPM, so as to better calibrate the contribution of individual instances from both local and global perspectives simultaneously.

The evaluation of these instances from the global view is straight-forward. The instance representation X_2 is fed into a 1×1 convolutional layer with single channel output, with weights W_2 and bias b_2. In this way, a spatial weight distribution matrix $\mathcal{M}$ is generated via:

$$\mathcal{M} = softmax(relu(W_2X_2 + b_2)), \tag{4}$$

where $relu$ denotes the ReLU activation function. This spatial weight distribution matrix $\mathcal{M}$ helps to better describe the relative importance of individual instance on the entire feature map scale.

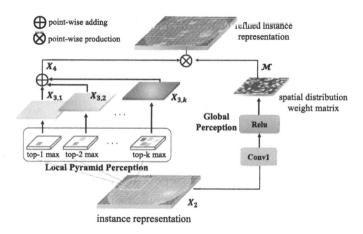

Fig. 2. Illustration of our local-global dual perception based deep multiple instance learning module.

2.4   Local-Global Perception Fusion

In order to take advantage of the information from both the local and global scales to generate the bag score distribution p, our MIL aggregator $g(\cdot)$ fuses the refined instance representation X_3 from the local scale and the spatial weight distribution $\mathcal{M}$ from the global scale via:

$$p = g(\mathcal{M}, X_4) = \sum_{i,j} \mathcal{M}_{i,j} X_{4,(i,j)}. \tag{5}$$

Note that the bag score distribution p has the same channel number as the total category number N, each of which presents the score of a certain bag category. Then, p is fed into a *softmax* activation function to obtain the final probability of each category, and optimized with a commonly utilized cross entropy loss.

3   Experiments and Analysis

Dataset: The proposed deep MIL framework is validated on APTOS [24], LAG [25] and a private AMD dataset respectively, corresponding to the top three major retinal diseases of DR, glaucoma and AMD. APTOS contains 1,857 DR images and 1,805 non-DR images [24]. LAG contains 1,710 glaucoma images and 3,140 non-glaucoma images [25]. The AMD private dataset obtained from a regional hospital contains 2,678 AMD images and 2,978 non-AMD images.

Evaluation Metric: Precision, recall, overall accuracy and F1-score are utilized to evaluate the performance of our approach and other SOTA approaches. Here, recall and precision mainly evaluate the model's capability to retrieve the disease images and the fraction of the correctly recognized disease images among all the retrieved images. Overall accuracy and F1-score evaluate how the model distinguishes samples across all the categories. Following the same data split protocol in [24, 25], five-fold cross validation is performed.

Table 1. Ablation study of our proposed approach (Metrics presented in %).

Dataset	Module			Evaluation metric			
	ResNet	GPM	LPPM	Precision	Recall	F1-score	Accuracy
APOTS	✓			98.33	91.64	94.87	95.04
	✓	✓		98.64	96.80	97.72	97.74
	✓		✓	98.14	96.50	97.31	97.33
	✓	✓	✓	**98.90**	**99.46**	**99.18**	**99.18**
LAG	✓			**98.69**	87.92	92.99	93.38
	✓	✓		98.02	94.74	96.35	96.41
	✓		✓	97.84	93.57	95.65	95.75
	✓	✓	✓	98.39	**97.08**	**97.73**	**97.74**
AMD	✓			98.12	91.36	94.62	94.80
	✓	✓		96.66	97.25	96.95	96.94
	✓		✓	95.49	97.80	96.63	96.59
	✓	✓	✓	**98.32**	**98.09**	**98.20**	**98.20**

3.1   Ablation Studies

The proposed local-global dual perception (LGDP) based deep MIL approach consists of a ResNet-50 backbone, a local pyramid perception module (LPPM) and a global perception module (GPM). All the four experiment results from the ablation study are listed in Table 1. It is clearly observed that:

1) The proposed approach (ResNet+LPPM+GPM) achieves the best performance on all the three benchmarks. Deep MIL with a single local perception or global perception module also outperforms the baseline. Its effectiveness can be explained that our approach is capable of both perceiving locally low contrast

Table 2. Comparison between state-of-the-art methods and our proposed approach.

Dataset	Method	Evaluation metrics (%)			
		Precision	Recall	F1-Score	Accuracy
APTOS	Max pooling	97.20	96.27	96.73	96.75
	Mean pooling	95.48	99.45	97.43	97.36
	GA-MIL	97.43	96.99	97.21	97.22
	CSA-MIL	97.33	98.39	97.86	97.85
	MS-MIL	97.12	97.14	97.13	97.13
	Ours	**98.90**	**99.46**	**99.18**	**99.18**
LAG	Max pooling	97.73	88.96	93.14	93.45
	Mean pooling	97.44	90.94	94.08	94.27
	GA-MIL	96.81	96.78	96.80	96.80
	CSA-MIL	96.30	95.32	95.81	95.83
	MS-MIL	98.12	92.69	95.33	95.46
	Ours	**98.39**	**97.08**	**97.73**	**97.74**
AMD	Max pooling	96.86	92.02	94.38	94.52
	Mean pooling	97.33	93.30	95.27	95.37
	GA-MIL	98.11	91.39	94.63	94.81
	CSA-MIL	97.18	93.56	95.33	95.42
	MS-MIL	97.13	94.04	95.56	95.63
	Ours	**98.32**	**98.09**	**98.20**	**98.20**

and small-sized pathologies and capturing scattered pathologies globally. Several representative visualizations of the instance response heatmaps in Fig. 3 clearly indicates that the pathological regions are well captured and perceived by the proposed modules and result in a stronger instance response.

2) The improvement of *recall* is most prominent among all the evaluation metrics. To be more specific, the proposed framework (ResNet+LPPM+GPM) boosts the recall by 7.82%, 4.74% and 6.73% for APTOS, LAG and AMD, respectively, when compared with the baseline performance. Clinically, for the retinal disease screening task, a higher *recall* is very important, so as not to miss the potential patients.

Moreover, Table 3 lists the performance of the proposed deep MIL module on the LAG benchmark when being embedded into VGG-16 [13], ResNet-50 [27] and Inception [14] backbone. In all three cases, a significant boost is witnessed in terms of the *recall, F1-score* and *overall accuracy*, indicating the effectiveness of the proposed module across different backbones.

Table 3. Generalization ability of our LGDP MIL on different CNN backbones on the LAG benchmark (Metrics presented in %).

	Precision	Recall	F1-score	Accuracy
VGG	**98.77**	76.61	86.29	87.83
VGG+LGDP	94.26	**91.52**	**92.87**	**92.97**
ResNet	**98.69**	87.92	92.99	93.38
ResNet+LGDP	98.39	**97.08**	**97.73**	**97.74**
Inception	96.47	87.13	91.57	91.97
Inception+LGDP	**97.25**	**95.91**	**96.58**	**96.60**

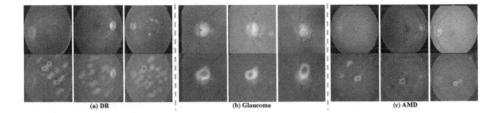

Fig. 3. Visualization of instance response for major retinal diseases; (a): diabetic retinopathy (DR); (b): glaucoma; (c): age-related macular degeneration (AMD).

3.2 Comparison with SOTA Methods

Since this paper focuses on integrating MIL paradigm into existing CNN backbones for the retinal disease recognition, we mainly compare our deep MIL module with other state-of-the-art (SOTA) deep MIL methods, including: mean pooling (Mean), max pooling (Max) [26], gated attention (GA-MIL) [17], channel-spatial attention (CSA-MIL) [22] and multi-scale (MS-MIL) [23] deep MIL modules. In order to compare with the proposed module under the same criteria, the SOTA methods are also embedded into the same backbone with the same parameter settings as mentioned above.

The comparison experiments on three benchmarks are listed in Table 2. It is obvious that the proposed LGDP module significantly outperforms the other SOTA deep MIL modules for all the three benchmarks across four evaluation metrics, especially for *recall*. On top of the SOTA methods, our proposed LGDP module integrates the instance contributions from both local scale and global scale, and thus is able to achieve superior performance. In contrast, the other three recently-developed SOTA deep MIL modules (GA-MIL, CSA-MIL and MS-MIL) only emphasize the key instances from a global perspective.

4 Conclusion

We proposed a local-global dual perception deep MIL module for retinal disease recognition, which can be conveniently embedded into any CNN backbones in an end-to-end trainable manner. Instance responses from both local and global scales are considered and integrated, so as to better tackle the challenge of how various pathologies are presented on the retinal image. Extensive experiments on three benchmarks validated that the proposed module could effectively boost the recognition performance. Moreover, experiments on different backbone networks further validated its effectiveness and generalization capability.

Acknowledgment. This work was funded by Key-Area Research and Development Program of Guangdong Province, China (No. 2018B010111001), and Scientific and Technical Innovation 2030 - 'New Generation Artificial Intelligence' Project (No.2020AAA0104100).

References

1. Bourne, R., et al.: Magnitude, temporal trends, and projections of the global prevalence of blindness and distance and near vision impairment: a systematic review and meta-analysis. Lancet Glob. Health **5**(9), e888–e897 (2017)
2. Ting, D., et al.: Deep learning in ophthalmology: the technical and clinical considerations. Prog. Retinal Eye Res. **72**, 100759 (2019)
3. Abràmoff, M., Garvin, M., Sonka, M.: Retinal imaging and image analysis. IEEE Rev. Biomed. Eng. **3**, 169–208 (2010)
4. Yau, J., et al.: Global prevalence and major risk factors of diabetic retinopathy. Diab. Care **35**(3), 556–564 (2012)
5. Tham, Y., Li, X., Wong, T., Quigley, H., Aung, T., Cheng, C.: Global prevalence of glaucoma and projections of glaucoma burden through 2040: a systematic review and meta-analysis. Ophthalmology **121**(11), 2081–2090 (2014)
6. Wong, W., et al.: Global prevalence of age-related macular degeneration and disease burden projection for 2020 and 2040: a systematic review and meta-analysis. Lancet Glob. Health **2**(2), e106–e116 (2014)
7. Gulshan, V., et al.: Development and validation of a deep learning algorithm for detection of diabetic retinopathy in retinal fundus photographs. J. Am. Med. Assoc. **316**(22), 2402–2410 (2016)
8. Ting, D., et al.: Development and validation of a deep learning system for diabetic retinopathy and related eye diseases using retinal images from multiethnic populations with diabetes. J. Am. Med. Assoc. **318**(22), 2211–2223 (2017)
9. Phene, S., et al.: Deep learning and glaucoma specialists: the relative importance of optic disc features to predict glaucoma referral in fundus photographs. Ophthalmology **126**(12), 1627–1639 (2019)
10. Liu, H., et al.: Development and validation of a deep learning system to detect glaucomatous optic neuropathy using fundus photographs. JAMA Ophthalmol. **137**(12), 1353–1360 (2019)
11. Burlina, P., Joshi, N., Pekala, M., Pacheco, K., Freund, D., Bressler, N.: Automated grading of age-related macular degeneration from color fundus images using deep convolutional neural networks. JAMA Ophthalmol. **135**(11), 1170–1176 (2017)
12. Grassmann, F., et al.: A deep learning algorithm for prediction of age-related eye disease study severity scale for age-related macular degeneration from color fundus photography. Ophthalmology **125**(6), 1410–1420 (2018)
13. Simonyan, K., Zisserman, A.: Very deep convolutional networks for large-scale image recognition. In: International Conference on Learning Representation (2015)

14. Szegedy, C., et al.: Going deeper with convolutions. In: IEEE Conference on Computer Vision and Pattern Recognition, pp. 1–9 (2015)
15. Zhang, M., Li, J., Ji, W., Piao, Y., Lu, H.: Memory-oriented decoder for light field salient object detection. In: Advances in Neural Information Processing Systems, pp. 898–908 (2019)
16. Ji, W., et al.: Learning calibrated medical image segmentation via multi-rater agreement modeling. In: IEEE Conference on Computer Vision and Pattern Recognition, pp. 12341–12351 (2021)
17. Ilse, M., Tomczak, J., Welling, M.: Attention-based deep multiple instance learning. In: International Conference on Machine Learning, vol. 80, pp. 2127–2136 (2018)
18. Oliva, A., Torralba, A.: Modeling the shape of the scene: a holistic representation of the spatial envelope. Int. J. Comput. Vision **42**, 145–175 (2001)
19. Dietterich, T., Lathrop, R., Lozano-Pérez, T.: Solving the multiple instance problem with axis-parallel rectangles. Artif. Intell. **89**(1), 31–71 (1997)
20. Zhang, M., Zhou, Z.: Improve multi-instance neural networks through feature selection. Neural Process. Lett. **19**(1), 1–10 (2004)
21. Andrews, S., Tsochantaridis, I., Hofmann, T.: Support vector machines for multiple-instance learning. In: Advances in Neural Information Processing Systems (2003)
22. Bi, Q., Qin, K., Zhang, H., Li, Z., Xu, K., Xia, G.: A multiple-instance densely-connected ConvNet for aerial scene classification. IEEE Trans. Image Process. **29**, 4911–4926 (2020)
23. Li, S., et al.: Multi-instance multi-scale CNN for medical image classification. In: Shen, D., et al. (eds.) MICCAI 2019. LNCS, vol. 11767, pp. 531–539. Springer, Cham (2019). https://doi.org/10.1007/978-3-030-32251-9_58
24. APTOS 2019 Blindness Detection (2019). https://www.kaggle.com/c/aptos2019-blindness-detection/data
25. Li, L., Xu, M., Wang, X., Jiang, L., Liu, H.: Attention based glaucoma detection: a large-scale database and CNN model. In: IEEE Conference on Computer Vision and Pattern Recognition, pp. 10571–10580 (2019)
26. Wang, X., Yan, Y., Peng, T., Xiang, B., Liu, W.: Revisiting multiple instance neural networks. Pattern Recogn. **74**, 15–24 (2016)
27. He, K., Zhang, X., Ren, S., Sun, J.: Deep residual learning for image recognition. In: IEEE Conference on Computer Vision and Pattern Recognition, pp. 770–778 (2016)

BSDA-Net: A Boundary Shape and Distance Aware Joint Learning Framework for Segmenting and Classifying OCTA Images

Li Lin[1,2], Zhonghua Wang[1], Jiewei Wu[1,2], Yijin Huang[1], Junyan Lyu[1], Pujin Cheng[1], Jiong Wu[3], and Xiaoying Tang[1]([✉])

[1] Department of Electrical and Electronic Engineering,
Southern University of Science and Technology, Shenzhen, China
tangxy@sustech.edu.cn
[2] SEIT, Sun Yat-Sen University, Guangzhou, China
[3] School of Computer and Electrical Engineering,
Hunan University of Arts and Science, Hunan, China

Abstract. Optical coherence tomography angiography (OCTA) is a novel non-invasive imaging technique that allows visualizations of vasculature and foveal avascular zone (FAZ) across retinal layers. Clinical researches suggest that the morphology and contour irregularity of FAZ are important biomarkers of various ocular pathologies. Therefore, precise segmentation of FAZ has great clinical interest. Also, there is no existing research reporting that FAZ features can improve the performance of deep diagnostic classification networks. In this paper, we propose a novel multi-level boundary shape and distance aware joint learning framework, named BSDA-Net, for FAZ segmentation and diagnostic classification from OCTA images. Two auxiliary branches, namely boundary heatmap regression and signed distance map reconstruction branches, are constructed in addition to the segmentation branch to improve the segmentation performance, resulting in more accurate FAZ contours and fewer outliers. Moreover, both low-level and high-level features from the aforementioned three branches, including shape, size, boundary, and signed directional distance map of FAZ, are fused hierarchically with features from the diagnostic classifier. Through extensive experiments, the proposed BSDA-Net is found to yield state-of-the-art segmentation and classification results on the OCTA-500, OCTAGON, and FAZID datasets.

Keywords: Boundary shape and distance · FAZ · Segmentation · Classification · OCTA · Joint learning

---

L. Lin and Z. Wang—Contributed equally to this work.

Electronic supplementary material The online version of this chapter (https://doi.org/10.1007/978-3-030-87237-3_7) contains supplementary material, which is available to authorized users.

© Springer Nature Switzerland AG 2021
M. de Bruijne et al. (Eds.): MICCAI 2021, LNCS 12908, pp. 65–75, 2021.
https://doi.org/10.1007/978-3-030-87237-3_7

1   Introduction

Optical coherence tomography angiography (OCTA) is an emerging non-invasive ophthalmological imaging technique with an ability to generate high-resolution volumetric images of retinal vasculature. It has been increasingly recognized as an invaluable imaging technique to visualize retinal vessels and foveal avascular zone (FAZ) [19]. OCTA *en face* maps are produced by projection over regions of selective depths, and can be basically divided into superficial images and deep ones with different fields of view (FOVs), e.g., $3\,mm \times 3\,mm$ and $6\,mm \times 6\,mm$, obtained from different scan modes. The former mode has a higher scan resolution than the latter one, and thus the FAZ and capillaries are depicted more clearly. In contrast, the latter mode covers a broader area and has a greater ability in detecting pathological features such as microaneurysms and non-perfusion [6,13]. Many retinal biomarkers are extracted from the OCTA *en face* maps (hereinafter collectively referred to as OCTA images), given that the flattened retinal structures in OCTA images are more informative and convenient for oph-thalmologists to examine [14]. Existing evidence suggests that the morphology and contour irregularity of FAZ are highly relevant to various ocular pathologies such as diabetic retinopathy (DR), age-related macular degeneration (AMD), and so on [17,23,31]. For instance, patients with high myopia typically have reduced FAZ areas, whereas macular ischemia caused by diabetes have enlarged FAZ areas [4,21]. As such, precise FAZ segmentation is of great clinical signifi-cance. Moreover, OCTA as a new modality shows its potential in computer-aided eye disease and eye-related systemic disease diagnoses [19].

In the past few years, several automatic FAZ segmentation algorithms have been proposed, which can be mainly divided into two categories. The first cate-gory is unsupervised methods, typically including statistical segmentation meth-ods and mathematical morphology methods. For instance, Haddouche et al. [9] employed a Markov random fields based method to detect FAZ. Pipelines based on combinations of morphology processing methods and transformation meth-ods also yielded reasonable results [7,18,24]. The past few years have witnessed a rapid development of the second category of methods, the deep learning based methods, which achieved overwhelming performance in almost all computer vision fields. Several works based on UNet [22] and its variants for FAZ seg-mentation have been reported [8,14–16]. Despite their progress, these methods still have limitations, such as imprecise boundaries due to inferior image quality, confusing FAZ with interfering structures, generating inevitable outliers when there exists erroneous layer projection, and failing to segment low contrast FAZ from its surrounding region. Some representative images are shown on the left panel of Figs. 1 and 2. The main reason for these problems is that UNet based methods typically lack the ability to learn sufficiently strong prior knowledge via single task/loss constraint on small medical image datasets. As for OCTA-based automatic diagnostic classification, only a few papers have reported their attempts. For example, Minhaj et al. designed several hand-crafted features such as vessel tortuosity and FAZ area, and employed support vector machine for clas-sification and staging [2]. Deep ImageNet-pretrained networks have also been proposed for classifying small-sampled OCTA datasets [3,12]. However, these methods are still very preliminary given most of them only utilized pretrained models followed by fine-tuning OCTA images from the specific study of interest, and there is still room for improvement. Meanwhile, there is no research showing that explicit or implicit FAZ-related features can be effectively and interpretably utilized in deep classification networks.

In such context, we propose a novel hierarchical and multi-level boundary shape and distance aware joint learning framework for FAZ segmentation and eye-related disease classification utilizing OCTA images. Two auxiliary branches, namely boundary heatmap regression and signed distance map (SDM) reconstruction branches, are constructed in addition to the segmentation branch following a shared encoder to improve the segmentation performance. Also, both low-level and high-level features from the aforementioned three branches, including shape, boundary, and signed directional distance map of FAZ, are fused hierarchically with features from the diagnostic classifier.

The main contributions of this paper are four-fold: (1) We present the first joint learning framework, named BSDA-Net, for FAZ segmentation and multi-disease (e.g. DR, AMD, diabetes and myopia) classification from OCTA images. (2) We propose boundary heatmap regression and SDM reconstruction auxiliary tasks, which can effectively improve the performance of FAZ segmentation in both joint learning and single-task learning settings. (3) Via hierarchically fusing features from decoders of the three segmentation-related tasks and the classifier, we demonstrate the effectiveness of FAZ features in guiding and boosting deep classification networks interpretably. (4) We validate the effectiveness of our method on three publicly-accessible OCTA datasets, and our approach achieves state-of-the-art (SOTA) performance in both tasks, establishing new baselines for the community. We make our code available at https://github.com/llmir/MultitaskOCTA.

2   Methodology

The proposed joint learning framework of BSDA-Net is shown in Fig. 1, which is composed of a multi-branch segmentation network (segmentor) and a classifier. Each component will be described detailedly in the following subsections.

2.1   Segmentation Network

As illustrated in Fig. 1, the segmentor in BSDA-Net adopts the widely employed encoder-decoder architecture, which is composed of a shared encoder E and three different decoders, namely a segmentation branch S, a soft boundary regression branch B, and a SDM reconstruction branch D.

BSDA-Net is a general framework, and any segmentation network with an encoder-decoder architecture, such as UNet [22], UNet++ [32], PSPNet [30], and DeepLabv3+ [5], can fit in. In this paper, we employ an adapted UNet structure with ResNeSt50 being the encoder for illustration [29]. The three decoders have the same structure, and features from the penultimate layer of branch B are concatenated to features from the corresponding layer of branch S for better contour perception and preservation. Each decoder module comprises nearest

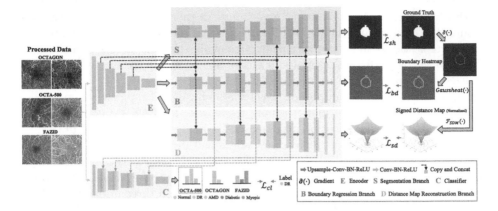

Fig. 1. Schematic representation of the architecture of our proposed framework.

upsampling with a scale factor of 2, followed by two layers of 3 × 3 filters, batch normalization (BN), and ReLU. In our setting, three small decoders are adopted, with the initial number of feature maps being 256 and getting halved after every upsampling layer. Under small dataset conditions, the edge region of a predicted mask may be inaccurate and has a high probability of being over or under segmented. Also, interfering structures and erroneous layer projection in OCTA images typically lead to outliers. We therefore propose a novel multi-task combination by constructing two auxiliary tasks to reconstruct edges and SDM, which provide the encoder with more topological priors both explicitly and implicitly and make them collaborate with the primary segmentation task to obtain a more accurate target segmentation mask.

Given a target FAZ and a point x in the OCTA image, the SDM of the ground truth G is formulated as

$$G_{sd} = \mathcal{F}_{SDM}(\partial G) = \begin{cases} -\inf_{y \in \partial G} \|x - y\|_2, & x \in G_{in} \\ 0, & x \in \partial G \\ \inf_{y \in \partial G} \|x - y\|_2, & x \in G_{out} \end{cases} \tag{1}$$

where $\|x - y\|_2$, ∂G, G_{in}, and G_{out} respectively denote the Euclidean distance between pixels x and y, the boundary, the inside and outside of the FAZ. Compared to the fixed distance map (DM) suggested in [14] which may produce wrong guidance and fail when the foveal center deviates from the image center and the normal DM which only calculates distance of either foreground or background [26,27], SDM has two main advantages. It considers the distance transformation information of both foreground and background, which also characterizes the diameter of FAZ and the fovea position. Moreover, since the target area is typically smaller than the background, through respectively normalizing the distance inside and outside FAZ to $[-1, 0]$ and $[0, 1]$, SDM naturally imposes more weights on the interior region and is beneficial for solving the class imbalance issue. As for the boundary regression branch, considering the subjectivity in manual annotations, we generate a Gaussian kernel matrix $\mathcal{G}(\cdot)$ centered at each point c_n on the boundary ∂G and construct a soft label heatmap in the form of *Heatsum* and treat it as a regression task using mean squared error (MSE) loss instead of treating it as a single pixel boundary segmentation problem:

$$\mathcal{G}(c_n) = \frac{1}{2\pi\sigma^2} e^{-\|x-c_n\|_2^2/2\sigma^2}, \tag{2}$$

$$Heatsum(\mathcal{G}(c_1), \mathcal{G}(c_2)) = 1 - (1 - \mathcal{G}(c_1)) \circ (1 - \mathcal{G}(c_2)), \tag{3}$$

$$G_{bd} = Guussheat(\partial G) = Heatsum(\mathcal{G}(c_1), \mathcal{G}(c_2), ..., \mathcal{G}(c_n)), \forall c_n \in \partial G, \tag{4}$$

where $\circ$ denotes the Hadamard product. Also, G_{bd} is normalized to $[0, 1]$ with values less than 0.001 set to be 0 before normalization. For the segmentation branch S, we use Dice loss to evaluate the pixel-wise agreement between the prediction and the ground truth. Therefore, with trade-off parameters λ_1, λ_2, λ_3, the total objective function of the segmentation model is defined as

$$
\begin{aligned}
\mathcal{L}_{seg} &= \lambda_1 \mathcal{L}_{sh} + \lambda_2 \mathcal{L}_{bd} + \lambda_3 \mathcal{L}_{sd} \\
&= \lambda_1 \mathcal{L}_{dice}(\mathcal{S}(p_i^s), G) + \lambda_2 \mathcal{L}_{mse}(p_i^b, G_{bd}^n) + \lambda_3 \mathcal{L}_{mse}(p_i^d, G_{sd}^n),
\end{aligned}
\tag{5}
$$

where p_i^s, p_i^b, and p_i^d respectively denote the predictions from branches S, B, and D given an input image i, and $\mathcal{S}$ represents the Sigmoid function. G_{bd}^n and G_{sd}^n are the normalized G_{bd} and G_{sd}.

2.2 Classification Network and Joint Learning Strategy

In the training phase, the segmentor is first trained via the aforementioned tasks, while the classifier C is initially frozen to avoid instability caused by inaccurate features from the segmentation network. We set a starting flag τ when the segmentation network almost converges to start joint learning. During joint learning, the multi-level features reconstructed by branches S, B, and D are sufficiently percepted by the unfrozen classifier in a hierarchical and interpretable way. For each feature concatenation, randomly initialized 1×1 convolutions are adopted for dimensionality reduction. Being consistent with the encoder E, we use ResNeSt50 partially (expect the above convolutions) initialized with weights pretrained on ImageNet as the classifier and employ the standard Cross-Entropy loss as $\mathcal{L}_{cl}$. So the final loss of BSDA-Net is defined as (with coefficient λ_0 to balance the two loss terms):

$$
\mathcal{L}_{joint} = \begin{cases} \mathcal{L}_{seg}, & \text{epoch} \leqslant \tau \\ \mathcal{L}_{seg} + \lambda_0 \mathcal{L}_{cl}, & \text{epoch} > \tau \end{cases}. \tag{6}
$$

3 Experiments and Results

Dataset and Preprocessing. We evaluate our proposed BSDA-Net framework on three recently released OCTA datasets: OCTA-500, OCTAGON, and

Foveal Avascular Zone Image Database (FAZID), the details of which are listed in Table 1. In OCTA-500, we only use data from three categories (normal, DR, and AMD) each with a sample size greater than 20. For OCTAGON, the two categories are normal and DR, and FAZID includes normal, diabetic, and myopic. For each dataset, to enlarge the sample size and to better evaluate the classification performance, we unify and combine images with different spatial resolutions via resizing and center cropping. The final category distributions within the three datasets are listed in Tables A1 to A3 (in appendix). We adopt data augmentation methods that will not change the spatial resolution and FAZ shape, including random rotation, flipping, contrast adjustment, adding Gaussian noise, and random blurring.

Table 1. Details and preprocessing of the three datasets utilized in our experiments.

Dataset	OCTA-500 [14,15]		OCTAGON [7]		FAZID [1]
FOV [mm]	3×3	6×6	3×3	6×6	6×6
Original resolution [px]	304×304	400×400	320×320		420×420
Retinal depth	Superficial		Both superficial and deep		superficial
Number	195	169	108	105	304
Preprocessing	Resize	Crop + resize	Resize	Crop	Crop
Processed size [px]	192×192		160×160		224×224

Implementation Details. All compared models and the proposed BSDA-Net framework are implemented with Pytorch using NVIDIA Tesla A100 GPUs. We adopt ResNeSt50 as the encoder of both the segmentation network and the classifier in this work. We use the Adam optimizer with a learning rate of 1 $\times 10^{-4}$ with no learning rate policy for the segmentation network and another separate Adam optimizer with a learning rate of 2×10^{-5} for the classifier. Empirically, we set the starting point of the joint learning τ as 20 and train the network for a total of 200 epochs. Trade-off coefficients λ_0, λ_1, λ_2, λ_3, and σ for soft contour are respectively set to be 1, 3, 1, 1, and 2. For internal validation, we split each dataset into 70%, 20%, and 10% for training, testing, and validation. Five-fold cross-validation is used for fair comparison in all settings.

Evaluation of FAZ Segmentation. All methods are evaluated using four metrics, i.e., Dice[%], Jaccard[%], Average Symmetric Surface Distance (ASD[px]), and 95% Hausdorff Distance (95HD[px]) [11]. Table 2 tabulates the segmentation results on the three OCTA datasets. We compare BSDA-Net with the baseline ResNeSt-UNet (based on our implementation) and several ablation models (to verify the impact of each auxiliary task), as well as several SOTA segmentation models, e.g., Deeplabv3+, PSPNet for natural image segmentation and UNet, UNet++ for medical image segmentation. By compared with the sixth row, the seventh and eighth rows in Table 2 indicate that the soft boundary regression constraint and the SDM reconstruction are effective in enhancing the FAZ segmentation performance in terms of every evaluation metric for all three datasets. The last two rows of that table indicate that when jointly learning classification and segmentation, though subsequent results identify the effectiveness of such joint learning strategy for boosting the classification performance, BSDA-Net may not achieve the best segmentation results. In other words, the joint learning framework slightly sacrifices the segmentation performance (without significant difference in any metric of any dataset, p-value > 0.05), with a reward of a much greater degree of improvement in the classification performance, as we will show later. Results shown in the penultimate row of Table 2 can be treated as the upper bound of our FAZ segmentation. Figure 2 displays representative segmentation results of the proposed method and four compared models. We also present two sets of intermediate outputs from BSDA-Net, which clearly show the effectiveness of the regressed soft boundary in assessing model's uncertainty and the reconstructed SDM in extracting fovea.

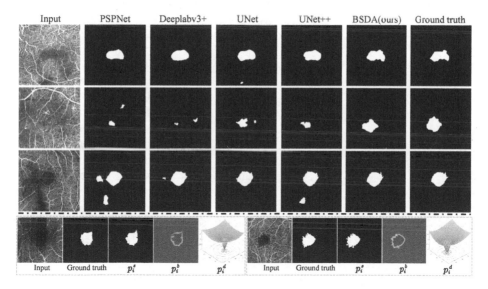

Fig. 2. Visualization results. The upper panel displays segmentation predictions of compared models and the proposed BSDA-Net. The bottom panel shows representative segmentation predictions p_x^s, regressed soft boundary p_x^b, and reconstructed SDM p_x^d. Zoom-in for details.

Evaluation of OCTA Classification. As for classification, accuracy and Cohen's kappa are adopted to evaluate all models. The compared methods include VGG16 (employed in previously proposed OCTA classification works), ResNet50, ResNeXt50, and the SOTA ResNeSt50 (with and without ImageNet pretrained). Moreover, we compare with the YNet [20] of a shared-encoder structure for joint classification and segmentation (based on our reimplementation using ResNeSt50 as the encoder), and the ablation structure without branches B and D. The quantitative results are shown in Table 3, which demonstrates

Table 2. Quantitative evaluations of different networks for FAZ segmentation. Joint learning slightly sacrifices the segmentation performance with no significant difference in any metric.

Method	OCTA-500				OCTAGON				FAZID			
	Dice↑	Jaccard↑	95HD↓	ASD↓	Dice↑	Jaccard↑	95HD↓	ASD↓	Dice↑	Jaccard↑	95HD↓	ASD↓
UNet [22] (w BN)	94.51 ± 6.71	90.16 ± 9.23	5.35 ± 9.67	1.02 ± 1.81	87.71 ± 7.09	78.73 ± 9.95	7.63 ± 12.93	2.28 ± 3.01	89.29 ± 8.09	81.40 ± 10.53	7.65 ± 11.48	2.34 ± 2.60
UNet++ [32]	94.71 ± 6.61	90.53 ± 9.42	5.33 ± 8.61	0.99 ± 1.81	87.86 ± 6.75	78.94 ± 9.90	6.35 ± 9.58	2.05 ± 2.33	88.73 ± 7.94	80.51 ± 10.95	8.26 ± 11.92	2.50 ± 2.81
PSPNet [30]	91.48 ± 6.89	84.87 ± 9.29	6.91 ± 11.01	1.63 ± 2.07	86.87 ± 6.69	77.34 ± 9.49	6.89 ± 10.92	2.18 ± 1.98	87.58 ± 9.40	78.91 ± 12.17	10.04 ± 16.94	2.96 ± 3.57
DeepLabv3+ [5]	92.35 ± 7.33	86.44 ± 9.71	6.06 ± 7.01	1.34 ± 1.49	87.28 ± 6.82	78.00 ± 9.50	6.65 ± 10.39	2.17 ± 2.38	88.22 ± 8.98	79.82 ± 11.57	8.02 ± 13.57	2.74 ± 4.12
Baseline (E + S)	95.24 ± 7.00	91.49 ± 9.05	4.52 ± 7.20	0.89 ± 2.25	87.73 ± 7.82	78.84 ± 10.24	6.95 ± 11.61	2.19 ± 2.81	89.89 ± 7.16	82.27 ± 10.02	7.05 ± 10.36	2.20 ± 2.57
BSDA (w/o D, C)	95.90 ± 4.20	92.40 ± 6.71	4.37 ± 7.26	0.76 ± 1.48	88.30 ± 6.32	79.56 ± 9.04	6.23 ± 9.81	2.00 ± 2.02	90.77 ± 5.87	83.57 ± 8.63	6.52 ± 10.15	1.98 ± 2.31
BSDA (w/o B, C)	95.84 ± 4.40	92.30 ± 6.92	4.08 ± 5.81	0.72 ± 1.20	88.14 ± 6.45	79.31 ± 9.10	5.94 ± 9.63	1.97 ± 2.18	90.60 ± 7.12	83.43 ± 9.57	6.19 ± 7.42	1.90 ± 2.26
BSDA (w/o C)	**96.21** ± 3.78	**92.92** ± 6.14	**3.61** ± 5.68	**0.63** ± 1.23	**88.64** ± 8.66	**80.00** ± 5.89	**5.43** ± 6.86	**1.80** ± 1.26	**91.03** ± 5.13	**83.91** ± 7.92	5.85 ± 6.05	**1.81** ± **1.23**
BSDA (ours)	96.07 ± 4.28	92.72 ± 6.82	3.90 ± 6.03	0.68 ± 1.28	88.37 ± 6.03	79.64 ± 8.75	5.79 ± 8.95	1.92v ± 1.96	90.98 ± 5.19	83.84 ± 8.03	**5.67** ± **5.53**	1.82 ± 1.23

Table 3. Classification performance of all methods on the three OCTA datasets.

Method	Pretrained (ImageNet)	OCTA-500		OCTAGON		FAZID	
		Acc	Kappa	Acc	Kappa	Acc	Kappa
VGG16 [3,12,25]	–	84.62	64.23	95.31	89.36	66.78	49.35
	✓	86.53	72.40	96.24	91.55	70.72	55.63
ResNet50 [10]	–	81.59	60.01	90.61	78.23	70.72	55.68
	✓	89.84	77.88	**97.65**	**94.58**	74.67	61.70
ResNeXt50 [28]	–	82.97	62.16	87.79	71.92	70.72	55.78
	✓	90.11	78.38	96.24	91.29	72.37	58.10
ResNeSt50 [29]	–	89.01	76.62	95.77	90.32	**75.00**	**62.08**
	✓	**90.93**	**80.32**	96.71	92.53	**75.00**	**62.08**
YNet (ResNeSt50)[20]	✓	91.76	82.21	96.71	92.53	74.34	61.24
BSDA (w/o B, D)	✓	92.03	82.67	97.65	94.58	78.62	67.81
BSDA (ours)	✓	**94.23**	**87.68**	**99.53**	**98.92**	**82.57**	**73.67**

that our model achieves the best performance and identifies the effectiveness of FAZ features and the proposed hierarchical feature perception strategy in boosting deep classification networks. Comparing results listed in the last two rows of Table 3, there is no doubt that our proposed joint learning strategy benefits the classification significantly, with only a very mild decrease in the segmentation performance (Table 2). In addition, we display detailed classification reports, including the precision, recall, F1-score of each disease and the macro avg, weight avg of each dataset, in Tables A1 to A3 (from our appendix) for the three datasets. These results establish new SOTA classification baselines for OCTA images. Across all three datasets, BSDA-Net is found to yield the best classification results on DR. Even in FAZID, samples misclassified in the diabetic category are mainly diabetic non-retinopathy samples. The classification performance on myopia in the FAZID dataset is relatively inferior (79.68%), which partially agrees with existing evidence that FAZ features are relatively indistinguishable in low-moderate myopia [1,4].

4 Conclusion

This paper presents a novel hierarchical and multi-level boundary shape and distance aware joint learning (BSDA-Net) framework for FAZ segmentation and diagnostic classification. Specifically, by constructing a boundary heatmap regression branch and a SDM reconstruction branch, we essentially propose a soft contour and directional signed distance aware segmentation loss, which is found to predict more accurate FAZ boundaries and suppress outliers. We also design a hierarchical and interpretable joint learning strategy to fuse FAZ features with those from the classifier. Extensive experiments on three publicly-accessible OCTA datasets show that our BSDA-Net achieves significantly better performance than SOTA methods on both segmentation and classification. Collectively, our results demonstrate the potential of OCTA for automated ophthalmological and systemic disease assessments and the effectiveness of FAZ features in boosting deep learning classifiers' performance.

References

1. Agarwal, A., Balaji, J., Raman, R., Lakshminarayanan, V.: The Foveal avascular zone image database (FAZID). In: Applications of Digital Image Processing XLIII, vol. 11510, pp. 1151027. International Society for Optics and Photonics (2020)
2. Alam, M., Le, D., Lim, J., Chan, R., Yao, X.: Supervised machine learning based multi-task artificial intelligence classification of retinopathies. J. Clin. Med. **8**(6), 872 (2019)
3. Andreeva, R., Fontanella, A., Giarratano, Y., Bernabeu, M.: DR detection using optical coherence tomography angiography (OCTA): a transfer learning approach with robustness analysis. In: Fu, H., Garvin, M.K., MacGillivray, T., Xu, Y., Zheng, Y. (eds.) International Workshop on Ophthalmic Medical Image Analysis, vol. 12069, pp. 11–20. Springer, Cham (2020). https://doi.org/10.1007/978-3-030-63419-3_2
4. Balaji, J., Agarwal, A., Raman, R., Lakshminarayanan, V.: Comparison of foveal avascular zone in diabetic retinopathy, high myopia, and normal fundus images. In: Ophthalmic Technologies XXX, vol. 11218, pp. 1121810. International Society for Optics and Photonics (2020)
5. Chen, L., Zhu, Y., Papandreou, G., Schroff, F., Adam, H.: Encoder-decoder with Atrous separable convolution for semantic image segmentation. In: Ferrari, V., Hebert, M., Sminchisescu, C., Weiss, Y. (eds.) Proceedings of the European Conference on Computer Vision (ECCV). LNCS, vol. 11211, pp. 801–818 (2018)
6. De Carlo, T., Romano, A., Waheed, N., Duker, J.: A review of optical coherence tomography angiography (OCTA). Int. J. Retin. Vitr. **1**(1), 5 (2015)
7. Díaz, M., Novo, J., Cutrín, P., Gómez-Ulla, F., Penedo, M., Ortega, M.: Automatic segmentation of the Foveal avascular zone in ophthalmological OCT-A images. PLoS One **14**(2), e0212364 (2019)

8. Guo, M., Zhao, M., Cheong, A., Dai, H., Lam, A., Zhou, Y.: Automatic quantification of superficial foveal avascular zone in optical coherence tomography angiography implemented with deep learning. Vis. Comput. Ind. Biomed. Art **2**(1), 1–9 (2019)

9. Haddouche, A., Adel, M., Rasigni, M., Conrath, J., Bourennane, S.: Detection of the foveal avascular zone on retinal angiograms using Markov random fields. Digital Sig. Process. **20**(1), 149–154 (2010)

10. He, K., Zhang, X., Ren, S., Sun, J.: Deep residual learning for image recognition. In: Proceedings of the IEEE Conference on Computer Vision and Pattern Recognition, pp. 770–778 (2016)

11. Heimann, T., et al.: Comparison and evaluation of methods for liver segmentation from CT datasets. IEEE Trans. Med. Imag. **28**(8), 1251–1265 (2009)

12. Le, D., et al.: Transfer learning for automated OCTA detection of diabetic retinopathy. Transl. Vis. Sci. Technol. **9**(2), 35 (2020)

13. Leitgeb, R.: En face optical coherence tomography: a technology review. Biomed. Opt. Express **10**(5), 2177–2201 (2019)

14. Li, M., et al.: Image projection network: 3D to 2D image segmentation in octa images. IEEE Trans. Med. Imag. **39**(11), 3343–3354 (2020)

15. Li, M., et al.: IPN-V2 and OCTA-500: methodology and dataset for retinal image segmentation. arXiv preprint arXiv:2012.07261 (2020)

16. Li, M., Wang, Y., Ji, Z., Fan, W., Yuan, S., Chen, Q.: Fast and robust fovea detection framework for OCT images based on Foveal avascular zone segmentation. OSA Continuum **3**(3), 528–541 (2020)

17. Linderman, R., Salmon, A., Strampe, M., Russillo, M., Khan, J., Carroll, J.: Assessing the accuracy of Foveal avascular zone measurements using optical coherence tomography angiography: segmentation and scaling. Transl. Vis. Sci. Technol. **6**(3), 16 (2017)

18. Lu, Y., et al.: Evaluation of automatically quantified foveal avascular zone metrics for diagnosis of diabetic retinopathy using optical coherence tomography angiography. Investig. Ophthalmol. Vis. Sci. **59**(6), 2212–2221 (2018)

19. Ma, Y., et al.: ROSE: a retinal OCT-angiography vessel segmentation dataset and new model. IEEE Trans. Med. Imag. (2020, in Press)

20. Mehta, S., et al.: Y-Net: joint segmentation and classification for diagnosis of breast biopsy images. In: In: Frangi, A., Schnabel, J., Davatzikos, C., Alberola-López, C., Fichtinger, G. (eds.) MICCAI 2018. MICCAI 2018. LNCS, vol. 11071, pp. 893–901. Springer, Cham (2018). https://doi.org/10.1007/978-3-030-00934-2_99

21. Ometto, G., Montesano, G., Chakravarthy, U., Kee, F., Hogg, R., Crabb, D.: Fast 3-dimensional estimation of the foveal avascular zone from OCTA. arXiv preprint arXiv:2012.09945 (2020)

22. Ronneberger, O., Fischer, P., Brox, T.: U-Net: convolutional networks for biomedical image segmentation. In: Maier-Hein, G.E.B., Fritzsche, K., Deserno, G.E.B., Lehmann, T., Handels, H., Tolxdorff, T. (eds.) International Conference on Medical Image Computing and Computer-Assisted Intervention, pp. 234–241. Springer, Cham (2015). https://doi.org/10.1007/978-3-319-24574-4_28

23. Salles, M., Kvanta, A., Amrén, U., Epstein, D.: Optical coherence tomography angiography in central retinal vein occlusion: correlation between the foveal avascular zone and visual acuity. Investig. Ophthalmol. Vis. Sci. **57**(9), OCT242–OCT246 (2016)

24. Silva, A., et al.: Segmentation of Foveal avascular zone of the retina based on morphological alternating sequential filtering. In: Proceedings of the IEEE 28th International Symposium on Computer-Based Medical Systems, pp. 38–43 (2015)

25. Simonyan, K., Zisserman, A.: Very deep convolutional networks for large-scale image recognition. arXiv preprint arXiv:1409.1556 (2014)
26. Tan, C., et al.: Deep multi-task and task-specific feature learning network for robust shape preserved organ segmentation. In: IEEE International Symposium on Biomedical Imaging, pp. 1221–1224 (2018)
27. Wijnen, K., et al.: Automated Lesion detection by regressing intensity-based distance with a neural network. In: Shen, D., et al. (eds.) MICCAI 2019. LNCS, pp. 234–242. Springer, Cham (2019). https://doi.org/10.1007/978-3-030-32251-9_26
28. Xie, S., Girshick, R., Dollár, P., Tu, Z., He, K.: Aggregated residual transformations for deep neural networks. In: Proceedings of the IEEE Conference on Computer Vision and Pattern Recognition, pp. 1492–1500 (2017)
29. Zhang, H., et al.: ResNeSt: split-attention networks. arXiv preprint arXiv:2004.08955 (2020)
30. Zhao, H., Shi, J., Qi, X., Wang, X., Jia, J.: Pyramid scene parsing network. In: Proceedings of the IEEE Conference on Computer Vision and Pattern Recognition, pp. 2881–2890 (2017)
31. Zheng, Y., Gandhi, J., Stangos, A., Campa, C., Broadbent, D., Harding, S.: Automated segmentation of foveal avascular zone in Fundus Fluorescein angiography. Investig. Ophthalmol. Vis. Sci. **51**(7), 3653–3659 (2010)
32. Zhou, Z., Siddiquee, M., Tajbakhsh, N., Liang, J.: UNet++: redesigning skip connections to exploit multiscale features in image segmentation. IEEE Trans. Med. Imag. **39**(6), 1856–1867 (2019)

LensID: A CNN-RNN-Based Framework Towards Lens Irregularity Detection in Cataract Surgery Videos

Negin Ghamsarian[1(✉)], Mario Taschwer[1], Doris Putzgruber-Adamitsch[2], Stephanie Sarny[2], Yosuf El-Shabrawi[2], and Klaus Schoeffmann[1]

[1] Department of Information Technology, Alpen-Adria-Universität Klagenfurt, Klagenfurt, Austria
{negin,mt,ks}@itec.aau.at
[2] Department of Ophthalmology, Klinikum Klagenfurt, Klagenfurt, Austria
{doris.putzgruber-adamitsch,stephanie.sarny, Yosuf.El-Shabrawi}@kabeg.at

Abstract. A critical complication after cataract surgery is the dislocation of the lens implant leading to vision deterioration and eye trauma. In order to reduce the risk of this complication, it is vital to discover the risk factors during the surgery. However, studying the relationship between lens dislocation and its suspicious risk factors using numerous videos is a time-extensive procedure. Hence, the surgeons demand an automatic approach to enable a larger-scale and, accordingly, more reliable study. In this paper, we propose a novel framework as the major step towards lens irregularity detection. In particular, we propose (I) an end-to-end recurrent neural network to recognize the lens-implantation phase and (II) a novel semantic segmentation network to segment the lens and pupil after the implantation phase. The phase recognition results reveal the effectiveness of the proposed surgical phase recognition approach. Moreover, the segmentation results confirm the proposed segmentation network's effectiveness compared to state-of-the-art rival approaches.

Keywords: Semantic segmentation · Surgical phase recognition · Cataract surgery

1 Introduction

Cataract refers to the eye's natural lens, having become cloudy and causing vision deterioration. Cataract surgery is the procedure of restoring clear eye vision via cataract removal followed by artificial lens implantation. This operation is conducted with the aid of a binocular microscope providing a 3D magnified and illuminated image of the eye. The camera mounted on the microscope records and stores the whole surgery for postoperative objectives.

This work was funded by the FWF Austrian Science Fund under grant P 31486-N31.

Electronic supplementary material The online version of this chapter (https://doi.org/10.1007/978-3-030-87237-3_8) contains supplementary material, which is available to authorized users.

© Springer Nature Switzerland AG 2021
M. de Bruijne et al. (Eds.): MICCAI 2021, LNCS 12908, pp. 76–86, 2021.
https://doi.org/10.1007/978-3-030-87237-3_8

Over several years, there have been numerous advances in surgical techniques, tools, and instruments in ophthalmic surgeries. Such advances resulted in decreasing the risk of severe intraoperative and postoperative complications. Still, there are many ongoing research efforts to prevent the current implications during and after surgery. A critical issue in cataract surgery that has not yet been addressed is intraocular lens (IOL) dislocation. This complication leads to various human sight issues such as vision blur, double vision, or vision inference as observing the lens implant edges. Intraocular inflammation, corneal edema, and retinal detachment are some other consequences of lens relocation. Since patient monitoring after the surgery or discharge is not always possible, the surgeons seek ways to diagnose evidence of potential irregularities that can be investigated during the surgery.

Recent studies show that particular intraocular lens characteristics can contribute to lens dislocation after the surgery [15]. Moreover, the expert surgeons argue that there can be a direct relationship between the overall time of lens unfolding and the risk of lens relocation after the surgery. Some surgeons also hypothesize that severe lens instability during the surgery is a symptom of lens relocation. To discover the potential correlations between lens relocation and its possibly contributing factors, surgeons require a tool for systematic feature extraction. Indeed, an automatic approach is required for (i) detecting the lens implantation phase to determine the starting time for lens statistics' computation and (ii) segmenting the lens and pupil to compute the lens statistics over time. The irregularity-related statistics can afterward be extracted by tracking the lens's relative size (normalized by the pupil's size) and relative movements (by calibrating the pupil). Due to the dearth of computing power in the operation rooms, automatic phase detection and lens/pupil segmentation on the fly is not currently achievable. Alternatively, this analysis can be performed in a post hoc manner using recorded cataract surgery videos. The contributions of this paper are:

1. We propose a novel CNN-RNN-based framework for evaluating lens unfolding delay and lens instability in cataract surgery videos.
2. We propose and evaluate a recurrent convolutional neural network architecture to detect the "implantation phase" in cataract surgery videos.
3. We further propose a novel semantic segmentation network architecture termed as *AdaptNet*[1], that can considerably improve the segmentation performance for the intraocular lens (and pupil) compared to ten rival state-of-the-art approaches.
4. We introduce three datasets for phase recognition, pupil segmentation, and lens segmentation that are publicly released with this paper to support reproducibility and allow further investigations for lens irregularity detection[2].

2   Related Work

Since this work involves *phase recognition* and *semantic segmentation*, we briefly review the state-of-the-art approaches related to the mentioned subjects.

Phase recognition in surgical videos has experienced three stages of development. In the first stage, hand-engineered features such as color, shape, and instrument

---

[1] The PyTorch implementation of AdaptNet is publicly available at https://github.com/Negin-Ghamsarian/AdaptNet-MICCAI2021.

[2] http://ftp.itec.aau.at/datasets/ovid/LensID/.

presence information [14,19,21] are exploited as the input to classical machine learning approaches. Using Conditional Random Fields (CRF), Random Forests, and Hidden Markov Models (HMM), the corresponding phase of each feature vector is classified [19,21,23]. Because of pruning to suboptimal results, the classical approaches are replaced with convolutional neural networks in the second stage [22]. To improve the classification accuracy by taking advantage of the temporal information, the third generation of phase recognition approaches adopt LSTM [11] or GRU [4] or bidirectional recurrent layers [9,13,27].

Since semantic segmentation plays a prominent role in medical image analysis, considerable attention has been devoted to this subject in recent years. Specifically, U-Net [20], which takes advantage of skip connections between symmetric layers in encoder and decoder, demonstrated pioneering results in medical image segmentation. Many approaches based on U-Net are proposed to improve its segmentation accuracy or address its weaknesses [7,10,12,24,26]. UNet++ [26] ensembles varying-depth U-Nets to deal with network depth optimization. CPFNet [7] adopts a scale-aware module by fusing the output feature maps of atrous convolutions [2] with different dilation rates. MultiResUNet [12] fuses the feature maps coming from sequential convolutions as an effective alternative to convolutional layers with large filters and atrous convolutions. Many other attention modules are proposed to boost segmentation accuracy for different medically-relevant content such as surgical instruments [16–18], liver lesion [3], and general medical image segmentation [10].

3   Methodology

Figure 1 demonstrates the block diagram of *LensID* and the network architecture of the phase recognition and segmentation steps. As the first step towards lens irregularity

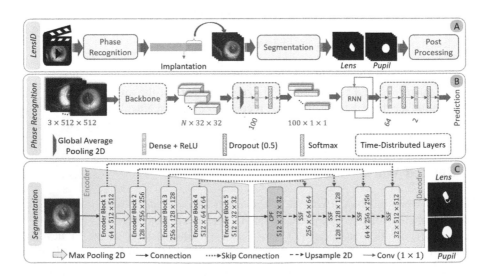

Fig. 1. The block diagram of *LensID* and the architecture of *Phase Recognition* and *Semantic Segmentation* networks.

detection, we adopt a recurrent convolutional network (Fig. 1-B) to detect the lens implantation phase (the temporal segment in which the lens implantation instrument is visible). We start segmenting the artificial lens and pupil exactly after the lens implantation phase using the proposed semantic segmentation network (Fig. 1-C). The pupil and lens segmentation results undergo some post-processing approaches to compute lens instability and lens unfolding delay. More precisely, we draw the smallest convex polygon surrounding pupil's and lens' masks using binary morphological operations. For lens instability, we use the normalized distance between the lens and pupil centers. For lens unfolding, we track the lens' area over time, considering its relative position.

Phase Recognition. As shown in Fig. 1-B, we use a pre-trained backbone followed by global average pooling to obtain a feature vector per each input frame. These features undergo a sequence of Dense, Dropout, and ReLU layers to extract higher-order semantic features. A recurrent layer with five units is then employed to improve the feature representation by taking advantage of temporal dependencies. These features are then fed into a sequence of layers to finally output the predicted class for each input frame.

Lens and Pupil Segmentation. In cataract surgery, a folded artificial lens is implanted inside the eye. The lens is transparent and inherits the pupil's color after implantation. Moreover, it is usually being unfolded very fast (sometimes with the help of an instrument). The transparency and unpredictable formation of this object, as well as occlusion, defocus blur, and motion blur [8], make lens segmentation and tracking more challenging. Hence, we require a semantic segmentation network that can be adapted to the changes in the artificial lens's shape and scale. We adopt a U-Net-based encoder-decoder architecture for the proposed semantic segmentation network termed as AdaptNet. AdaptNet consists of three main components: encoder, *cascade pooling fusion (CPF)* module, and *shape/scale-adaptive feature fusion (SSF)* module. We use the VGG16 network as the encoder network. The encoder's output feature map is fed into the CPF module to enhance the feature representation using pyramid features. This feature map is then fed into a sequence of SSF modules, which decode low-resolution semantic features.

As shown in Fig. 2, the CPF module applies a sequence of three average pooling layers (with a stride of two pixels) followed by a global average pooling layer to the input features. The obtained feature maps are upsampled to the original size of the input and concatenated together with the input feature map in a depth-wise manner. Each group of five channels in the generated feature map undergoes a distinct convolution for intra-channel feature refinement (which is performed using a convolutional layer with C groups). Besides, the upsampled features are mapped into a smaller channel space while extracting higher-order semantic features using convolutional layers with shared weights. The obtained features are concatenated with the intra-channel refined features and undergo a convolutional layer for inter-channel feature refinement.

The *SSF* module starts with concatenating the upsampled semantic feature map with the fine-grained feature map coming from the encoder. The concatenated feature map is fed into a sequence of convolutional, layer normalization, and ReLU layers for feature enhancement and dimensionality reduction. The resulting features are fed into the *scale-adaptive block*, which aims to fuse the features coming from cascade convolutional blocks. This succession of convolutional layers with small filter sizes

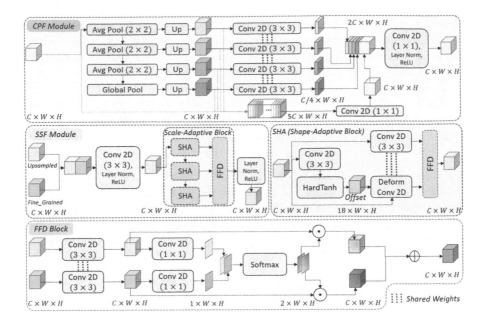

Fig. 2. The detailed architecture of the *CPF* and *SFF* modules of AdaptNet.

can factorize the large and computationally expensive receptive fields [12]. Moreover, the fusion of these successive feature maps can play the role of scale-awareness for the network. The *shape-adaptive (SHA) block* is responsible for fusing the resulting feature maps of deformable and structured convolutions. At first, a convolutional layer followed by a hard tangent hyperbolic function is employed to produce the offsets for the deformable convolutional layer [5]. The input features are also fed into a regular convolutional layer that shares the weights with the deformable layer for structured-feature extraction. These features are then fused to induce the awareness of shape and deformation to the network.

The *feature fusion decision (FFD)* block inspired by CPFNet [7] accounts for determining the importance of each input feature map in improving semantic features. Figure 2 shows the *FFD Block* in the case of two input branches. At first, shared convolutional layers are applied to the input feature maps to extract the shared semantic features. The resulting feature maps undergo shared pixel-wise convolutions to produce the pixel-wise attention maps. The concatenated attention maps are fed into a softmax activation layer for normalization. The obtained features are used as pixel-wise weights of the shared-semantic feature maps. The shape/scale adaptive features are computed as the sum of pixel-wise multiplications ($\odot$) between the normalized attention maps and their corresponding semantic feature maps.

4   Experimental Setup

We use three datasets for this study: (i) a large dataset containing the annotations for the lens implantation phase versus the rest of phases from 100 videos of cataract surgery, (ii) a dataset containing the lens segmentation of 401 frames from 27 videos (292 images from 21 videos for training, and 109 images from six videos for testing), and (iii) a dataset containing the pupil segmentation of 189 frames from 16 videos (141 frames from 13 videos for training, and 48 frames from three videos for testing). Regarding the phase recognition dataset, since lens implantation is a very short phase (around four seconds) compared to the whole surgery (seven minutes on average), creating a balanced dataset that can cover the entire content of videos from the "Rest" class is quite challenging. Hence, we propose a video clip generator that can provide diverse training sequences for the recurrent neural network by employing stochastic functions. At first, 12 three-second video clips with overlapping frames are extracted from the implantation phase of each cataract surgery video. Besides, the video segments before and after the implantation phase are divided into eight and four video clips, respectively (these clips have different lengths depending on the length of the input video). Accordingly, we have a balanced dataset containing 2040 video clips from 85 videos for training and 360 video clips from the other 15 videos for testing. For each training example, the video generator uses a stochastic variable to randomly select a three-second clip from the input clip. We divide this clip into N sub-clips, and N stochastic variables are used to randomly select one frame per sub-clip (in our experiments, N is set to five to reduce computational complexity and avoid network overfitting).

For phase recognition, all networks are trained for 20 epochs. The initial learning rate for these networks is set to 0.0002 and 0.0004 for the networks with VGG19 and Resnet50 backbones, respectively, and halved after ten epochs. Since the segmentation networks used for evaluations have different depths, backbones, and the number of trainable parameters, all networks are trained with three different initial learning rates ($lr_0 \in \{0.0005, 0.001, 0.002\}$). For each network, the results with the highest Dice coefficient are listed. All segmentation networks are trained for 30 epochs, and the learning rate is decreased by a factor of 0.8 in every other epoch. To prevent overfitting and improve generalization performance, we have used motion blur, Gaussian blur, random contrast, random brightness, shift, scale, and rotation for data augmentation. The backbones of all networks evaluated for phase recognition and lens/pupil semantic segmentation are initialized with ImageNet [6] weights. The size of input images to all networks is set to $512 \times 512 \times 3$. The loss function for the phase recognition network is set to *Binary Cross Entropy*. For the semantic segmentation task, we adopt a loss function consisting of categorical cross entropy and logarithm of soft Dice coefficient as follows (in Eq. (1), *CE* stands for *Cross Entropy*, and $\mathcal{X}_{Pred}$ and $\mathcal{X}_{True}$ denote the predicted and ground-truth segmentation images, respectively. Besides, we use a Dice smoothing factor equal to 1, and set $\lambda = 0.8$ in our experiments):

$$\mathcal{L} = \lambda \times CE(\mathcal{X}_{Pred}, \mathcal{X}_{True}) - (1 - \lambda) \times \log_2 Dice(\mathcal{X}_{Pred}, \mathcal{X}_{True}) \qquad (1)$$

To evaluate the performance of phase recognition networks, we use *Precision*, *Recall*, *F1-Score*, and *Accuracy*, which are the common classification metrics. The semantic segmentation performance is evaluated using *Dice coefficient* and *Intersection over Union (IoU)*. We compare the segmentation accuracy of the proposed approach (Adapt-Net) with ten state-of-the-art approaches including UNet++ (and UNet++/DS) [26], MultiResUNet [12], CPFNet [7], dU-Net [24], CE-Net [10], FEDNet [3], PSPNet [25], SegNet [1], and U-Net [20]. It should be mentioned that the rival approaches employ different backbone networks, loss functions (cross entropy or cross entropy log Dice), and upsampling methods (bilinear, transposed convolution, pixel-shuffling, or max unpooling).

5   Experimental Results and Discussion

Table 1 compares the classification reports of the proposed architecture for phase recognition considering two different backbone networks and four different recurrent layers. Thanks to the large training set and taking advantage of recurrent layers, all networks have shown superior performance in classifying the implantation phase versus other phases. However, the LSTM and bidirectional LSTM (BiLSTM) layers have shown better performance compared to GRU and BiGRU layers, respectively. Surprisingly, the network with a VGG19 backbone and BiLSTM layer has achieved 100% accuracy in classifying the test clips extracted from the videos which are not used during training. Figure 3 compares the segmentation results (mean and standard deviation of IoU and Dice coefficient) of AdaptNet and ten rival state-of-the-art approaches. Overall, it can be perceived that AdaptNet, UNet++, UNet++/DS, and FEDNet have achieved the top four segmentation results. However, AdaptNet has achieved the highest mean IoU and Dice coefficient compared to the rival approaches. In particular, the proposed approach achieves 3.48% improvement in mean IoU and 2.22% improvement in mean Dice for lens segmentation compared to the best rival approach (UNet++). Moreover, the smaller standard deviation of IoU (10.56% vs. 12.34%) and Dice (8.56% vs. 9.65%) for AdaptNet compared to UNet++ confirms the reliability and effectiveness of the proposed architecture. For pupil segmentation, AdaptNet shows subtle improvement over the best rival approach (UNet++) regarding mean IoU and Dice while showing significant improvement regarding the standard deviation of IoU (1.91 vs. 4.05). Table 2 provides an ablation study of AdaptNet. We have listed the Dice and IoU percentage with two different learning rates by gradually adding the proposed modules and blocks (for lens segmentation). It can be perceived from the results that regardless of the learning

Table 1. Phase recognition results of the end-to-end recurrent convolutional networks.

RNN	Backbone: VGG19				Backbone: ResNet50			
	Precision	Recall	F1-Score	Accuracy	Precision	Recall	F1-Score	Accuracy
GRU	0.97	0.96	0.96	0.96	0.9	0.94	0.94	0.94
LSTM	0.98	0.98	0.98	0.98	0.96	0.96	0.96	0.96
BiGRU	0.97	0.96	0.96	0.96	0.95	0.95	0.95	0.95
BiLSTM	**1.00**	**1.00**	**1.00**	**1.00**	**0.98**	**0.98**	**0.98**	**0.98**

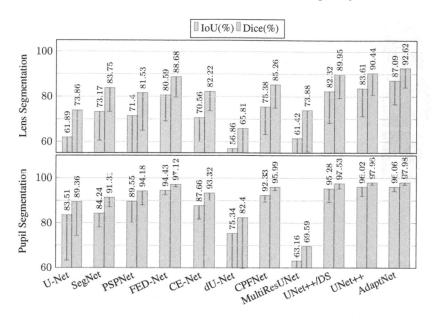

Fig. 3. Quantitative comparison of segmentation results for the proposed approach (AdaptNet) and rival approaches.

Table 2. Impact of different modules on the segmentation results of AdaptNet.

Components				lr = 0.001		lr = 0.002	
Baseline	SSF	SHA	CPF	IoU(%)	Dice(%)	IoU(%)	Dice(%)
✓	✗	✗	✗	82.79	89.94	84.33	90.90
✓	✓	✗	✗	83.54	90.33	84.99	91.22
✓	✓	✓	✗	84.76	91.12	86.34	92.17
✓	✓	✓	✓	**85.03**	**91.28**	**87.09**	**92.62**

rate, each distinctive module and block has a positive impact on segmentation performance. We cannot test the FFD block separately since it is bound with the SSF module.

Figure 4 shows the post-processed lens segments (pink) and pupil segments (cyan) from a representative video in different time slots (a), the relative lens area over time (b), and relative lens movements over time (c). Due to lens instability, a part of the lens is sometimes placed behind the iris, as shown in the segmentation results in the 35th second. Accordingly, the visible area of the lens can change independently of the unfolding state. Hence, the relative position of the lens should also be taken into account for lens unfolding delay computations. As can be perceived, the visible area of the lens is near maximum at 20 s after the implantation phase, and the lens is located nearly at the center of the pupil at this time. Therefore, the lens unfolding delay is 20 s in this case. However, the lens is quite unstable until 70 s after implantation.

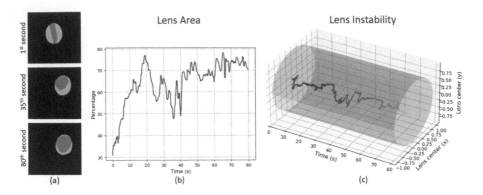

Fig. 4. The lens statistics for one representative cataract surgery video.

6   Conclusion

Lens irregularity detection is a highly relevant problem in ophthalmology, which can play a prominent role in predicting and preventing lens relocation after surgery. This paper focuses on two significant steps towards lens irregularity detection: (i) "lens implantation phase" detection and (ii) lens/pupil segmentation. We propose an end-to-end recurrent convolutional network to detect the lens implantation phase. Moreover, we propose a novel semantic segmentation network termed as AdaptNet. The proposed approach can deal with severe deformations and scale variations in the intraocular lens by adaptively fusing sequential and parallel feature maps. Experimental results reveal the effectiveness of the proposed phase recognition and semantic segmentation networks.

References

1. Badrinarayanan, V., Kendall, A., Cipolla, R.: SegNet: a deep convolutional encoder-decoder architecture for image segmentation. IEEE Trans. Pattern Anal. Mach. Intell. **39**(12), 2481–2495 (2017). https://doi.org/10.1109/TPAMI.2016.2644615
2. Chen, L., Papandreou, G., Kokkinos, I., Murphy, K., Yuille, A.L.: DeepLab: semantic image segmentation with deep convolutional nets, atrous convolution, and fully connected CRFs. IEEE Trans. Pattern Anal. Mach. Intell. **40**(4), 834–848 (2018). https://doi.org/10.1109/TPAMI.2017.2699184
3. Chen, X., Zhang, R., Yan, P.: Feature fusion encoder decoder network for automatic liver lesion segmentation. In: 2019 IEEE 16th International Symposium on Biomedical Imaging (ISBI 2019), pp. 430–433 (2019). https://doi.org/10.1109/ISBI.2019.8759555
4. Cho, K., van Merrienboer, B., Gülçehre, Ç., Bougares, F., Schwenk, H., Bengio, Y.: Learning phrase representations using RNN encoder-decoder for statistical machine translation. CoRR abs/1406.1078 (2014). http://arxiv.org/abs/1406.1078
5. Dai, J., Qi, H., Xiong, Y., Li, Y., Zhang, G., Hu, H., Wei, Y.: Deformable convolutional networks. In: 2017 IEEE International Conference on Computer Vision (ICCV), pp. 764–773 (2017). https://doi.org/10.1109/ICCV.2017.89
6. Deng, J., Dong, W., Socher, R., Li, L.J., Li, K., Fei-Fei, L.: ImageNet: a large-scale hierarchical image database. In: CVPR 2009 (2009)

7. Feng, S., et al.: CPFNet: context pyramid fusion network for medical image segmentation. IEEE Trans. Med. Imag. **39**(10), 3008–3018 (2020). https://doi.org/10.1109/TMI.2020.2983721

8. Ghamsarian, N., Taschwer, M., Schoeffmann, K.: Deblurring cataract surgery videos using a multi-scale deconvolutional neural network. In: 2020 IEEE 17th International Symposium on Biomedical Imaging (ISBI), pp. 872–876 (2020)

9. Ghamsarian, N., Taschwer, M., Putzgruber-Adamitsch, D., Sarny, S., Schoeffmann, K.: Relevance detection in cataract surgery videos by spatio- temporal action localization. In: 2020 25th International Conference on Pattern Recognition (ICPR), pp. 10720–10727 (2021). https://doi.org/10.1109/ICPR48806.2021.9412525

10. Gu, Z., et al.: CE-NET: context encoder network for 2D medical image segmentation. IEEE Trans. Med. Imag. **38**(10), 2281–2292 (2019). https://doi.org/10.1109/TMI.2019.2903562

11. Hochreiter, S., Schmidhuber, J.: Long short-term memory. Neural Comput. **9**(8), 1735–1780 (1997). https://doi.org/10.1162/neco.1997.9.8.1735

12. Ibtehaz, N., Rahman, M.S.: MultiResUNet : rethinking the U-Net architecture for multimodal biomedical image segmentation. Neural Netw. **121**, 74–87 (2020). https://doi.org/10.1016/j.neunet.2019.08.025, https://www.sciencedirect.com/science/article/pii/S0893608019302503

13. Jin, Y., Dou, Q., Chen, H., Yu, L., Qin, J., Fu, C., Heng, P.: SV-RCNet: workflow recognition from surgical videos using recurrent convolutional network. IEEE Trans. Med. Imag. **37**(5), 1114–1126 (2018). https://doi.org/10.1109/TMI.2017.2787657, https://ieeexplore.ieee.org/document/8240734

14. Lalys, F., Riffaud, L., Bouget, D., Jannin, P.: A framework for the recognition of high-level surgical tasks from video images for cataract surgeries. IEEE Trans. Biomed. Eng. **59**(4), 966–976 (2012). https://doi.org/10.1109/TBME.2011.2181168

15. Mayer-Xanthaki, C.F., et al.: Impact of intraocular lens characteristics on intraocular lens dislocation after cataract surgery. Br. J. Ophthalmol. (2020). https://doi.org/10.1136/bjophthalmol-2020-317124, https://bjo.bmj.com/content/early/2020/09/18/bjophthalmol-2020-317124

16. Ni, Z.L., Bian, G.B., Wang, G.A., Zhou, X.H., Hou, Z.G., Chen, H.B., Xie, X.L.: Pyramid attention aggregation network for semantic segmentation of surgical instruments. In: Proceedings of the AAAI Conference on Artificial Intelligence, vol. 34, no. 07, pp. 11782–11790 (2020). https://doi.org/10.1609/aaai.v34i07.6850, https://ojs.aaai.org/index.php/AAAI/article/view/6850

17. Ni, Z.L., et al.: BarNet: bilinear attention network with adaptive receptive fields for surgical instrument segmentation. In: Bessiere, C. (ed.) Proceedings of the Twenty-Ninth International Joint Conference on Artificial Intelligence, IJCAI 2020, pp. 832–838. International Joint Conferences on Artificial Intelligence Organization (2020). https://doi.org/10.24963/ijcai.2020/116

18. Ni, Z.L., et al.: RAUNet: residual attention U-Net for semantic segmentation of cataract surgical instruments. In: Gedeon, T., Wong, K.W., Lee, M. (eds.) Neural Information Processing, pp. 139–149. Springer International Publishing, Cham (2019). https://doi.org/10.1007/978-3-030-36711-4_13

19. Quellec, G., Lamard, M., Cochener, B., Cazuguel, G.: Real-time segmentation and recognition of surgical tasks in cataract surgery videos. IEEE Trans. Med. Imag. **33**, 2352–2360 (2014). https://doi.org/10.1109/TMI.2014.2340473

20. Ronneberger, O., Fischer, P., Brox, T.: U-Net: convolutional networks for biomedical image segmentation. In: Navab, N., Hornegger, J., Wells, W.M., Frangi, A.F. (eds.) MICCAI 2015. LNCS, vol. 9351, pp. 234–241. Springer, Cham (2015). https://doi.org/10.1007/978-3-319-24574-4_28

21. Stauder, R., et al.: Random forests for phase detection in surgical workflow analysis. In: Stoyanov, D., Collins, D.L., Sakuma, I., Abolmaesumi, P., Jannin, P. (eds.) Information Processing in Computer-Assisted Interventions, vol. 8498, pp. 148–157. Springer, Cham (2014). https://doi.org/10.1007/978-3-319-07521-1_16

22. Twinanda, A.P., Shehata, S., Mutter, D., Marescaux, J., de Mathelin, M., Padoy, N.: EndoNet: a deep architecture for recognition tasks on laparoscopic videos. IEEE Trans. Med. Imag. **36**(1), 86–97 (2017). https://doi.org/10.1109/TMI.2016.2593957, https://ieeexplore.ieee.org/abstract/document/7519080

23. Zappella, L., Béjar, B., Hager, G., Vidal, R.: Surgical gesture classification from video and kinematic data. Med. Image Anal. **17**(7), 732–745 (2013). https://doi.org/10.1016/j.media.2013.04.007, http://www.sciencedirect.com/science/article/pii/S1361841513000522, special Issue on the 2012 Conference on Medical Image Computing and Computer Assisted Intervention

24. Zhang, M., Li, X., Xu, M., Li, Q.: Automated semantic segmentation of red blood cells for sickle cell disease. IEEE J. Biomed. Health Inform. **24**(11), 3095–3102 (2020). https://doi.org/10.1109/JBHI.2020.3000484

25. Zhao, H., Shi, J., Qi, X., Wang, X., Jia, J.: Pyramid scene parsing network. In: Proceedings of the IEEE Conference on Computer Vision and Pattern Recognition (CVPR) (2017)

26. Zhou, Z., Siddiquee, M.M.R., Tajbakhsh, N., Liang, J.: UNET++: redesigning skip connections to exploit multiscale features in image segmentation. IEEE Trans. Med. Imag. **39**(6), 1856–1867 (2020). https://doi.org/10.1109/TMI.2019.2959609

27. Zisimopoulos, O., et al.: DeepPhase: surgical phase recognition in CATARACTS videos. CoRR abs/1807.10565 (2018). http://arxiv.org/abs/1807.10565

I-SECRET: Importance-Guided Fundus Image Enhancement via Semi-supervised Contrastive Constraining

Pujin Cheng[1], Li Lin[1,2], Yijin Huang[1], Junyan Lyu[1], and Xiaoying Tang[1(✉)]

[1] Department of Electrical and Electronic Engineering, Southern University of Science and Technology, Shenzhen, China
tangxy@sustech.edu.cn
[2] School of Electronics and Information Technology, Sun Yat-sen University, Guangzhou, China

Abstract. Fundus image quality is crucial for screening various ophthalmic diseases. In this paper, we proposed and validated a novel fundus image enhancement method, named importance-guided semi-supervised contrastive constraining (I-SECRET). Specifically, our semi-supervised framework consists of an unsupervised component, a supervised component, and an importance estimation component. The unsupervised part makes use of a large publicly-available dataset of unpaired high-quality and low-quality images via contrastive constraining, whereas the supervised part utilizes paired images through degrading pre-selected high-quality images. The importance estimation provides a pixel-wise importance map to guide both unsupervised and supervised learning. Extensive experiments on both authentic and synthetic data identify the superiority of our proposed method over existing state-of-the-art ones, both quantitatively and qualitatively.

Keywords: Fundus image enhancement · Semi-supervised learning · Contrastive constraint · Importance estimation

1 Introduction

Fundus images are widely used for eye disease screening [5,8]. However, the fundus image quality is inhomogeneous, and low-quality ones may severely affect clinical judgments and decisions [3,16,18,19]. Therefore, it is of great significance to enhance fundus images. Several factors may induce low-quality fundus images, including blurriness, missing focus, uneven illumination, low contrast, and noise [15,19]. The enhancement task is challenging due to the following reasons: (1) The quality of a fundus image is related to not only its intensity profile but also high-level semantic information such as various anatomical landmarks and disease-related lesions [13]. (2) The mapping from low quality to high

Electronic supplementary material The online version of this chapter (https://doi.org/10.1007/978-3-030-87237-3_9) contains supplementary material, which is available to authorized users.

© Springer Nature Switzerland AG 2021
M. de Bruijne et al. (Eds.): MICCAI 2021, LNCS 12908, pp. 87–96, 2021.
https://doi.org/10.1007/978-3-030-87237-3_9

quality is not one-to-one and cannot be easily modeled. (3) Authentic low-quality and high-quality images are typically unpaired.

There are mainly two categories of fundus image enhancement methods, namely non-parametric methods and parametric ones. For example, Cheng et al. proposed a structure-preserving filter for fundus image declouding [2]. This kind of non-parametric method needs a well-designed prior function, and cannot be easily generalized to all cases. Recently, with the development of deep learning [1,6,10,21,24], many data-driven methods have been proposed for fundus image enhancement, mainly focusing on synthesizing low-quality images [15,17,19] or employing an unpaired training framework such as Cycle-GAN [22–24] and CutGAN [14]. Shen et al. designed a correction network utilizing an artificial degradation pipeline [19], but the degradation strategy is relatively simple and may not accommodate well real-life clinical situations. Zhao et al. utilized a CycleGAN variant with unpaired data [23]. However, the cycle-consistency assumption is violated in the high-quality to low-quality fundus image mapping, and structural details cannot be well preserved when using unpaired supervision [11,14]. Most importantly, all these methods consider the enhancing process as an image-level operation and ignore that the importance of each pixel may be different during the enhancing process. For example, enhancing artifacts or vessels should be more important than those that may cause over-enhancement such as macula and optic disc boundary.

In such context, we propose a novel semi-supervised framework for enhancing fundus images, named I-SECRET. Different from existing enhancement methods, I-SECRET consists of a supervised learning component and an unsupervised learning one, which respectively make use of synthetic and authentic data. We first synthesize low-quality fundus images by artificially degrading high-quality ones for the supervised learning component. We then use an authentic dataset composed of large-scale high-quality and low-quality unpaired fundus images for the unsupervised learning component. The supervised learning part provides a task-specific mapping and tends to preserve fundus images' structural details, and the unsupervised learning part improves our method's generalization ability and benefits an extraction of distinctive high-level features. Moreover, we present an innovative importance estimation framework to provide pixel-wise importance maps and to guide both the supervised and the unsupervised components.

The main contributions of this work are four-fold: (1) To the best of our knowledge, the proposed framework is the first semi-supervised method for fundus image enhancement. (2) A novel importance-guided supervised loss is proposed for pixel-wise image translation and its effectiveness has been identified. (3) A novel importance-guided contrastive constraint is employed and validated for fundus image enhancement. (4) Extensive comparison experiments are conducted, both quantitatively and qualitatively. The source code is available at https://github.com/QtacierP/ISECRET.

2   Methods

Given a training set X:$\{x_i\}_{i=1}^{N_x}$ and Y:$\{y_i\}_{i=1}^{N_y}$, we firstly synthesize a degraded dataset $\hat{Y}$:$\{\hat{y}_i\}_{i=1}^{N_y}$, where X is a low-quality dataset, Y is a high-quality dataset

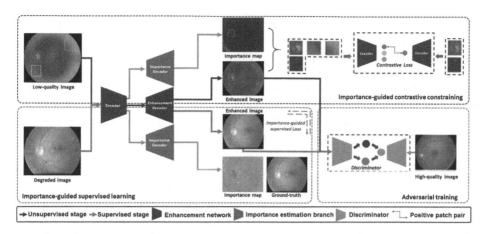

Fig. 1. Flowchart of the proposed I-SECRET. A supervised learning stage builds its basis on degraded image pairs, and an unsupervised stage aims at generalizing the enhancement process. The importance-guided supervised loss estimates each pixel's importance and sets a batch weight in the gradient descent process by summing over the importance of all pixels. Besides, an importance-guided contrastive task is employed for preserving local high-level semantic information consistency based on the local importance. Finally, adversarial training makes the enhanced images more realistic.

and $\hat{Y}$ is an artificially degraded dataset of Y. Our target is to enhance low-quality x and generate enhanced $\hat{x}$. An enhancement network $\mathcal{G}$ is applied for pixel-wise enhancement, and an adversarial discriminator $\mathcal{D}$ is used to distinguish enhanced images from authentic high-quality ones. Additional to adversarial training, a supervised enhancement is conducted based on the artificially degraded image pairs to focus on structural details and pathological features. Figure 1 shows the overall framework of the proposed I-SECRET, consisting of three stages: (1) a supervised learning stage based on an importance-guided supervised loss; (2) an unsupervised learning stage based on an importance-guided contrastive learning constraint; (3) an adversarial training stage.

2.1 Importance-Guided Supervised Learning

In this section, we describe our importance-guided supervised learning. The goal of this stage is to preserve structural details and to avoid information modification which is a common issue in unpaired image translation. Given a real high-quality fundus image y, we firstly synthesize its degraded version $\hat{y}$. In this supervised stage, the enhancement network $\mathcal{G}$ aims at reconstructing the original high-quality image y.

Naive supervised learning considers the learning process as consistent and stable, but the importance of each image pixel apparently varies at different epochs and for different images. For example, the importance of artifacts should be higher than retinal structures like macula. As such, we propose a novel importance-guided supervised loss function (IS-loss), which assigns different weights to different batches based on importance.

The goal of IS-loss is to predict learning weight for each batch based on its importance. To calculate the importance, we add a new decoder branch in the enhancement network to predict pixel-wise importance map. The importance map assigns each pixel a numerical weight. Experimentally, we take an average of the importance of all pixels as the overall weight term, which is then added to the IS-loss function as a regularization term. We thus have

$$\mathcal{L}_{IS}(\theta_{\mathcal{G}}) = \frac{1}{N} \sum_i^N \frac{1}{\exp(\alpha_i)} \mathcal{L}_{\text{MSE}} + \frac{1}{N} \sum_i^N \alpha_i, \tag{1}$$

where N denotes the total number of pixels in the batch, and $\mathcal{L}_{\text{MSE}}$ denotes the batch's mean square error, and α_i denotes the importance of the i-th pixel in the batch. To obtain a positive weight and to guarantee numerical stability, we predict the reciprocal of the exponential term.

The IS-loss delivers a self-adjusted weight at the supervised learning stage. Moreover, it also estimates the importance of each pixel, which can guide the unsupervised learning process. We will present it in the next section.

2.2 Importance-Guided Contrastive Constraint

A contrastive constraint assumes that the local high-level semantic features in a low-quality image and its enhanced image are much closer at the same location compared to those at different locations. Therefore, we construct an internal contrastive task to learn the local consistency, which maps low-quality images and high-quality images into a common latent space.

We utilize the enhancement network $\mathcal{G}$ to embed an original image and the enhanced image into high-level features. $\mathcal{G}$ is U-shaped, which firstly downsamples the input image into low-resolution feature maps. Therefore, the local features of a patch can be represented by a pixel in the high-level feature map, which consists of several feature stacks.

We select several layers $\mathcal{G}_{l\in L}(x)$ from the encoder of the enhancement network $\mathcal{G}$ to extract patches with different sizes, where l indexes the set of selected layers L. Moreover, we apply a stack of multilayer perceptron (MLP) $\{H_{l\in L}\}$ to obtain a stack of features $\{v_{l\in L} = H_{l\in L}[\mathcal{G}_{l\in L}(x)]\}$ and to decouple the semantic features from the specific domain.

We construct a patch pair $v_l = \{H_l(\mathcal{G}_l(x))^{s_1}, H_l(\mathcal{G}_l(x))^{s_2}\}$, where s_1 and s_2 denote the spatial locations of interest. The positive samples v_l^+ are given by pairs with same locations, and the negative samples v_l^- are pairs with mismatched locations. Patches are selected randomly. We formulate the naive patch contrastive loss function based on the InfoNCE loss [12, 14]

$$L_{PC} = -\sum_{l \in L} \log[\frac{\exp(v_l \cdot v_l^+/\tau)}{\exp(v_l \cdot v_l^+/\tau) + \sum \exp(v_l \cdot v_l^-/\tau))}], \tag{2}$$

where τ refers to the temperature coefficient. Furthermore, we apply an identity loss to avoid over-enhancement, which is widely used in unpaired translation frameworks [14,24]. We input a high-quality image y into $\mathcal{G}$ and obtain feature stacks v_l^*. After that, we construct negative samples v_l^{*-} and positive samples v_l^{*+} similarly. The identity loss is calculated as

$$L_{IDT} = -\sum_{l \in L} \log[\frac{\exp(v_l^* \cdot v_l^{*+}/\tau)}{\exp(v_l^* \cdot v_l^{*+}/\tau) + \sum \exp(v_l^* \cdot v_l^{*-}/\tau))}]. \tag{3}$$

Please note the uncertainty in a low-quality fundus image varies from pixel to pixel. It may be impossible to enhance certain pixels, which may influence the unpaired learning. Therefore, the importance of different spatial locations is different. In our previous section, we utilize IS-loss to estimate each pixel's importance. We then utilize the estimated importance to guide our contrastive constraint. Specifically, we construct an importance-guided constraint on the contrastive task by multiplying the importance with the contrastive loss function

$$L_{ICC} = -\sum_{l \in L} \frac{1}{\exp(\alpha_l^+)} \log[\frac{\exp(v_l \cdot v_l^+/\tau)}{\exp(v_l \cdot v_l^+/\tau) + \sum \exp(v_l \cdot v_l^-/\tau))}], \tag{4}$$

where α_l^+ denotes the importance of the positive patch pair. Because the high-level feature map is down-sampled for several times, we apply average pooling to the original importance map to obtain the importance of the entire patch. This importance-guided constraint speeds up convergence and avoids certain information modification.

2.3 Objective Function

The entire enhancement framework aims at three tasks: supervised reconstruction, unsupervised constraint, and adversarial training. We apply Least-squares GAN (LS-GAN) [9] to make the enhanced images more realistic

$$L_{DIS}(\theta_{\mathcal{D}}) = \min_{\mathcal{D}} \frac{1}{2} E_{y \sim Y}[D(y) - 1]^2 + \frac{1}{2} E_{x \sim X}[D(G(x))]^2;$$
$$L_{ADV}(\theta_{\mathcal{G}}) = \min_{\mathcal{G}} \frac{1}{2} E_{x \sim X}[D(G(x)) - 1]^2. \tag{5}$$

The overall loss function is formulated as

$$L = \lambda_{IS} L_{IS} + \lambda_{ADV} L_{ADV} + \lambda_{ICC} L_{ICC} + \lambda_{IDT} L_{IDT}, \tag{6}$$

where L_{IS}, L_{ADV}, L_{ICC}, and L_{IDT} respectively represent the importance-guided supervised loss, adversarial loss, importance-guided contrastive loss, identity loss, λ_{IS}, λ_{ADV}, λ_{ICC}, and λ_{IDT} refer to the corresponding trade-off coefficients. We set the trade-off coefficients as $\lambda_{IS} = \lambda_{ADV} = \lambda_{ICC} = \lambda_{IDT} = 1$ for simplicity.

3 Experiments

3.1 Datasets

We use two kinds of datasets. One is based on authentic low-quality images, for which there are no ground-truth high-quality images. Another one is based on synthetic low-quality images, for which we can use full-reference metrics to measure the enhancement performance.

Authentic Dataset. We utilize EyeQ [3] as our first dataset, which consists of 28792 fundus images with three quality grades ("Good", "Usable", "Reject") and has been divided into a training set, a validation set, and a testing set. We choose images labeled as "Good" to be our high-quality dataset and images labeled as "Usable" to be our low-quality dataset.

Synthetic Dataset. We follow the degradation pipeline in [19] to synthesize a degraded low-quality dataset based on our high-quality dataset (see Appendix Table A1 for detailed parameters). Moreover, we utilize the degraded DRIVE dataset [20] as an additional testing set (see Appendix Fig. A1). Note that the degradation degree on DRIVE is much more severe than EyeQ because the original quality of DRIVE is much higher (see Appendix Fig. A1).

3.2 Implementation

The entire framework is implemented by PyTorch on a workstation equipped with eight NVIDIA RTX 2080Ti. The input images are firstly resized to 512 × 512. We set batch size as 8. Due to the small batch size, we apply instance normalization instead of batch normalization. The generator G is designed with two down-samplings and nine residual blocks. We use Adabelief [25] as the optimizer with an initial learning rate of 0.0001 and cosine decay. The network is trained for 200 epochs. We set the indices of layers L to be $\{1, 5, 9, 12, 16, 18, 20\}$.

3.3 Evaluation

We employ two categories of metrics: full-reference evaluation metrics on the synthetic datasets and non-reference evaluation metrics on the authentic dataset. To be specific, we apply peaky signal-to-noise ratio (PSNR) [4] and structural similarity index measure (SSIM) [4] on the synthetic low-quality datasets. To further demonstrate the effectiveness of the proposed enhancement framework, we utilize a DRIVE-trained Iter-Net [7] to segment retinal vessels in the degraded and enhanced DRIVE testing sets, and compare the segmentation results with the manually-annotated ground truth. We use the vessel segmentation dice (VSD) [19] as another quantitative assessment metric, the results of which are tabulated in Table 1. We also present a visual comparison example in Fig. 2. Experimental results suggest that our proposed enhancement method is meaningful for downstream fundus image analysis tasks such as vessel segmentation.

For non-reference metrics, we propose a specific metric, called fundus image quality assessment score (FIQA). We utilize a pre-trained fundus image quality

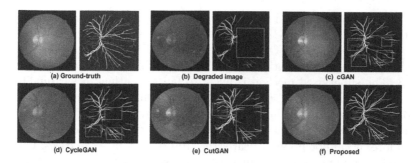

Fig. 2. Visual comparisons on the vessel segmentation task. The red box represents a false positive region and the green box shows a false negative region. (Color figure online)

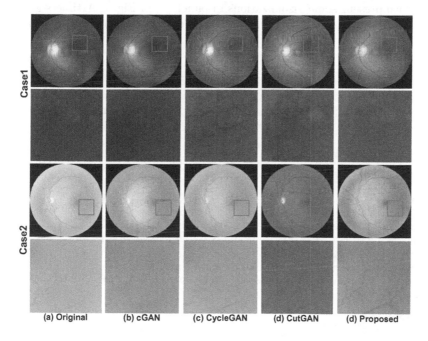

Fig. 3. Visual comparisons on two cases between the proposed method and other representative ones.

assessing network, namely MCF-Net released by [3]. The FIQA score is defined as the ratio of the total number of images predicted as "Good" by MCF-Net to the total number of the entire dataset.

We conduct a set of ablation experiments to evaluate each component's effectiveness, the results of which are also shown in Table 1. Evidently, the proposed IS-loss and the importance-guided contrastive constraint both boost the enhancement performance significantly. The proposed I-SECRET is also compared with other state-of-the-art ones using both non-reference and full-reference metrics in

Table 1. cGAN is a supervised framework, which is trained on our synthetic EyeQ dataset. CycleGAN and CutGAN are both unsupervised methods, trained on our authentic unpaired dataset. Our proposed I-SECRET achieves the best performance in every respect. All other methods tend to fail in certain cases, as shown in Fig. 3. The supervised method is likely to fail on authentic low-quality data because the learning is based on artificially degraded images, which may be unable to accommodate real-life complicated degradation situations. The unsupervised methods often cause information modification and over-enhancement problems. Furthermore, it cannot provide clear structural details in some cases. Our approach can well enhance authentic images with fewer artifacts and more structural details. We also show the learning effectiveness of both IS-loss and contrastive constraining in Fig. 4(b); both components boost the enhancement on the validation set during the entire training phase. To more clearly illustrate the importance estimation, we present some visualizations in panel (a) of Fig. 4. Artifacts generally have high importance whereas retinal structures such as macula and clear optic disc boundary have relatively low importance.

Table 1. Ablation study results and quantitative comparisons of the proposed method with other state-of-the-art ones on both full-reference and non-reference evaluation metrics. − indicates that the metric is not applicable in this case. A higher value in each metric indicates a better enhancement.

	Full-reference					Non-reference
	Degraded EyeQ		Degraded DRIVE			Authentic EyeQ
	PSNR	SSIM	PSNR	SSIM	VSD	FIQA
Original	−	−	−	−	0.8161	0.2038
Degraded	26.28 ± 11.33	0.8896 ± 0.0864	16.00 ± 2.48	0.7934 ± 0.0601	0.5211	−
cGAN [6]	27.24 ± 4.66	0.8925 ± 0.0360	19.94 ± 3.45	0.8569 ± 0.0321	0.6175	0.3039
CycleGAN [24]	24.22 ± 7.91	0.8759 ± 0.0576	18.66 ± 2.29	0.8183 ± 0.0354	0.6407	0.8901
CutGAN [14]	25.70 ± 5.22	0.8881 ± 0.0564	18.50 ± 2.00	0.8610 ± 0.0222	0.6681	0.9188
I-SECRET w.o. IS, ICC	29.58 ± 4.51	0.9058 ± 0.0300	21.25 ± 3.09	0.8481 ± 0.0291	0.6257	0.4058
I-SECRET w.o. ICC	31.32 ± 4.52	0.9187 ± 0.0284	22.38 ± 2.33	0.8887 ± 0.0158	0.6265	0.5078
I-SECRET	**32.18 ± 5.19**	**0.9314 ± 0.0259**	**23.34 ± 2.83**	**0.8980 ± 0.0125**	**0.6865**	**0.9373**

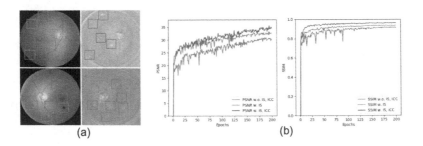

(a)   (b)

Fig. 4. (a) Visualizations of representative importance maps. The green and red boxes respectively represent regions with high and low importance. (b) Metrics (PSNR, SSIM) on the validation set, at different epochs of the training phase. IS denotes the importance-guided supervised loss function, and ICC represents the importance-guided contrastive constraint.

4   Conclusion

In this paper, we propose a novel importance-guided semi-supervised contrastive learning method for fundus image enhancement, named I-SECRET. The estimated importance guides both supervised and unsupervised stages. The supervised learning component aims at preserving structural details and preventing information modification, and the importance-guided unsupervised contrastive learning component makes the enhancing process generalize well to various real-life degradation situations. Based on extensive quantitative and qualitative experiments, the proposed method is identified to perform significantly better than other state-of-the-art enhancement methods.

References

1. Bhattacharjee, D., Kim, S., Vizier, G., Salzmann, M.: DUNIT: detection-based unsupervised image-to-image translation. In: Proceedings of the IEEE Conference on Computer Vision and Pattern Recognition, CVPR, pp. 4787–4796 (2020)
2. Cheng, J., et al.: Structure-preserving guided retinal image filtering and its application for optic disk analysis. IEEE Trans. Med. Imaging TMI **37**(11), 2536–2546 (2020)
3. Fu, H., et al.: Evaluation of retinal image quality assessment networks in different color-spaces. In: Shen, D., et al. (eds.) MICCAI 2019. LNCS, vol. 11764, pp. 48–56. Springer, Cham (2019). https://doi.org/10.1007/978-3-030-32239-7_6
4. Hore, A., Ziou, D.: Image quality metrics: PSNR vs. SSIM. In: Proceedings of 2010 20th International Conference on Pattern Recognition, pp. 2366–2369 (2010)
5. Huang, Y., Lin, L., Li, M., Wu, J., et al.: Automated hemorrhage detection from coarsely annotated fundus images in diabetic retinopathy. In: Proceedings of the IEEE 17th International Symposium on Biomedical Imaging, ISBI, pp. 1369–1372 (2020)
6. Isola, P., Zhu, J.Y., Zhou, T., Efros, A.A.: Image-to-image translation with conditional adversarial networks. In: Proceedings of the IEEE Conference on Computer Vision and Pattern Recognition, CVPR, pp. 1125–1134 (2017)
7. Li, L., Verma, M., Nakashima, Y., Nagahara, H., Kawasaki, R.: IterNet: retinal image segmentation utilizing structural redundancy in vessel networks. In: Proceedings of the IEEE/CVF Winter Conference on Applications of Computer Vision, WACV, pp. 3656–3665 (2020)
8. Lin, L., Li, M., Huang, Y., Cheng, P., Xia, H., et al.: The SUSTech-SYSU dataset for automated exudate detection and diabetic retinopathy grading. Sci. Data **7**(1), 1–1 (2020)
9. Mao, X., Li, Q., Xie, H., Lau, R.Y., Wang, Z., Paul Smolley, S.: Least squares generative adversarial networks. In: Proceedings of the IEEE Conference on Computer Vision and Pattern Recognition, CVPR, pp. 2794–2802 (2017)
10. Mathew, S., Nadeem, S., Kumari, S., Kaufman, A.: Augmenting colonoscopy using extended and directional CycleGAN for lossy image translation. In: Proceedings of the IEEE Conference on Computer Vision and Pattern Recognition, CVPR, pp. 4696–4705 (2020)
11. Nizan, O., Tal, A.: Breaking the cycle-colleagues are all you need. In: Proceedings of the IEEE Conference on Computer Vision and Pattern Recognition, CVPR, pp. 7860–7869 (2020)

12. Oord, A.V.D., Li, Y., Vinyals, O.: Representation learning with contrastive predictive coding. arXiv preprint arXiv:1807.03748
13. Orlando, J.I., Prokofyeva, E., Del Fresno, M., Blaschko, M.B.: An ensemble deep learning based approach for red lesion detection in fundus images. Comput. Meth. Prog. Biomed. **153**(Jan), 115–127 (2018)
14. Park, T., Efros, A.A., Zhang, R., Zhu, J.-Y.: Contrastive learning for unpaired image-to-image translation. In: Vedaldi, A., Bischof, H., Brox, T., Frahm, J.-M. (eds.) ECCV 2020. LNCS, vol. 12354, pp. 319–345. Springer, Cham (2020). https://doi.org/10.1007/978-3-030-58545-7_19
15. Pérez, A.D., Perdomo, O., Rios, H., Rodríguez, F., González, F.A.: A conditional generative adversarial network-based method for eye fundus image quality enhancement. In: Fu, H., Garvin, M.K., MacGillivray, T., Xu, Y., Zheng, Y. (eds.) OMIA 2020. LNCS, vol. 12069, pp. 185–194. Springer, Cham (2020). https://doi.org/10.1007/978-3-030-63419-3_19
16. Raj, A., Tiwari, A.K., Martini, M.G.: Fundus image quality assessment: survey, challenges, and future scope. IET Image Process. **13**(8), 1211–1224 (2019)
17. Sengupta, S., Wong, A., Singh, A., Zelek, J., Lakshminarayanan, V.: DeSupGAN: multi-scale feature averaging generative adversarial network for simultaneous deblurring and super-resolution of retinal fundus images. In: Fu, H., Garvin, M.K., MacGillivray, T., Xu, Y., Zheng, Y. (eds.) OMIA 2020. LNCS, vol. 12069, pp. 32–41. Springer, Cham (2020). https://doi.org/10.1007/978-3-030-63419-3_4
18. Sevik, U., Kose, C., Berber, T., Erdol, H.: Identification of suitable fundus images using automated quality assessment methods. J. Biomed. Opt. **19**(4), 046006 (2014)
19. Shen, Z., Fu, H., Shen, J.: Modeling and enhancing low-quality retinal fundus images. IEEE Trans. Med. Imaging TMI **40**(3), 996–1006 (2020)
20. Staal, J., Abramoff, M.D., Niemeijer, M., Viergever, M.A., van Ginneken, B.: Ridge-based vessel segmentation in color images of the retina. IEEE Trans. Med. Imaging TMI **23**(4), 501–509 (2004). https://doi.org/10.1109/TMI.2004.825627
21. Wang, Y., Khan, S., Gonzalez-Garcia, A., Weijer, J.V.D., Khan, F.S.: Semi-supervised learning for few-shot image-to-image translation. In: Proceedings of the IEEE Conference on Computer Vision and Pattern Recognition, CVPR, pp. 4453–4462 (2020)
22. You, Q., Wan, C., Sun, J., Shen, J., Ye, H., Yu, Q.: Fundus image enhancement method based on CycleGAN. In: Proceedings of 41st Annual International Conference of the IEEE Engineering in Medicine and Biology Society, EMBC, pp. 4500–4503 (2019)
23. Zhao, H., Yang, B., Cao, L., Li, H.: Data-driven enhancement of blurry retinal images via generative adversarial networks. In: Shen, D., et al. (eds.) MICCAI 2019. LNCS, vol. 11764, pp. 75–83. Springer, Cham (2019). https://doi.org/10.1007/978-3-030-32239-7_9
24. Zhu, J.Y., Park, T., Isola, P., Efros, A.A.: Unpaired image-to-image translation using cycle-consistent adversarial networks. In: Proceedings of the IEEE International Conference on Computer Vision, ICCV, pp. 2223–2232 (2017)
25. Zhuang, J., et al.: AdaBelief optimizer: adapting stepsizes by the belief in observed gradients. arXiv preprint arXiv:2010.07468 (2020)

Few-Shot Transfer Learning for Hereditary Retinal Diseases Recognition

Siwei Mai[1], Qian Li[2], Qi Zhao[2], and Mingchen Gao[1(✉)]

[1] Department of Computer Science and Engineering, University at Buffalo,
Buffalo, USA
{siweimai,mgao8}@buffalo.edu
[2] Department of Ophthalmology, Beijing Tongren Eye Center,
Beijing Tongren Hospital, Beijing Key Laboratory of Ophthalmology
and Visual Sciences, Capital Medical University, Beijing, China

Abstract. This project aims to recognize a group of rare retinal diseases, the hereditary macular dystrophies, based on Optical Coherence Tomography (OCT) images, whose primary manifestation is the interruption, disruption, and loss of the layers of the retina. The challenge of using machine learning models to recognize those diseases arises from the limited number of collected images due to their rareness. We formulate the problems caused by lacking labeled data as a Student-Teacher learning task with a discriminative feature space and knowledge distillation (KD). OCT images have large variations due to different types of macular structural changes, capturing devices, and angles. To alleviate such issues, a pipeline of preprocessing is first utilized for image alignment. Tissue images at different angles can be roughly calibrated to a horizontal state for better feature representation. Extensive experiments on our dataset demonstrate the effectiveness of the proposed approach.

Keywords: Hereditary Retinal Diseases Recognition ·
Student-Teacher learning · Knowledge distillation · Transfer learning

1 Introduction

Visual impairment and blindness caused by inherited retinal diseases (IRDs) are increasing due to the global prolonged life expectancy. There was no treatment for IRDs until recently, a number of therapeutic approaches such as gene replacement and induced pluripotent stem cell transplantation have been proposed, developed, and shown promising potential in some of the ongoing therapeutic clinical trials. Spectral-domain Optical coherence tomography (SD-OCT) has been playing a crucial role in the evaluation of the retina of IRDs in diagnosis, progression surveillance as well as strategy exploration and response assessment of the treatment. However, the recognition, interpretation, and comparison of the minimal changes on OCT as shown in IRDs sometimes could be difficult and time-consuming for retinal physicians. Recently automated image analysis

© Springer Nature Switzerland AG 2021
M. de Bruijne et al. (Eds.): MICCAI 2021, LNCS 12908, pp. 97–107, 2021.
https://doi.org/10.1007/978-3-030-87237-3_10

has been successfully applied in the detection of changes on fundus and OCT images of multiple retinal diseases such as diabetic retinopathy and age-related macular degeneration, which are of higher prevalence among the population to enable the acquisition of large volumes of training data for traditional machine learning approaches including deep learning.

On the contrary, for rare diseases like IRDs, acquiring a large volume of high-quality data representative of the patient cohorts is challenging. These datasets also require accompanying annotations generated by experts which are time-consuming to produce. This hinders the applying state-of-the-art image classification, which usually requires a relatively large number of images with annotations for training. The goal of this project is to design a computer-aided diagnosis algorithm when only a very limited number of rare disease samples can be collected.

The methods of diagnosing ocular diseases like age-related macular degeneration (AMD), diabetic macular edema (DME), etc., through the spectral domain OCT images can be roughly categorized into the traditional machine learning methods and deep learning-based methods. There are lots of works on OCT image analysis based on the traditional machine learning methods like Principal Components Analysis (PCA) [1,15], Support Vector Machine (SVM) [12,17], or Random Forest [7], segmenting each layer of the OCT images [18] or learns global representation directly [19,21].

Lots of previous work also focus on the deep-learning-based methods including supervised and unsupervised ways. Existing mature and pre-trained frameworks such as Inception-v3 [8,22], VGG16 [16,22], PCANet [4], GoogLeNet [9,10], ResNet [9,13], DenseNet [9] have been deployed to classify OCT images. Others unify multiple networks together to make classification more robust for diagnosing, for example four-parallel-ResNet system [13] and multi-stage network [14]. Supervised learning has the advantage of learning hierarchical features compared to traditional feature engineering. However, for supervised learning of OCT medical images, satisfactory results are still dependent on large amounts of data.

In addition to the supervised learning methods above, we also try to address the few-shot learning problem based on the contrastive learning. We empirically show that the Siamese network architecture represented by Simple Siamese [2] is able to learn meaningful representations and bypass the limitation of sample size. Also, the embedding features in feature space obtained by the contrastive learning [5] leads to more knowledge learned by the student network in the subsequent S-T architecture.

The goal of this research is to classify a group of macular-involved IRDs from different stages by a limited number of OCT images. Given the limited training data, we plan to assist the classification with an auxiliary dataset in a related task where labeled data are abundant. We propose a Student-Teacher Learning framework to leverage the knowledge from the auxiliary dataset. In the teacher part, the teacher model is firstly trained on a large-scale labeled auxiliary OCT dataset [11] which contains 3 common retinal degenerative diseases with 84484 images. Soft Nearest Neighbor Loss (SNNL) [5] is utilized to maximize the representation entanglement of different classes to help generalization. Transfer

Learning methods is then applied to adapt the teacher model to the target label space. While for the student model, the collected OCT samples are used to serve as the hard labels. The student model can learn from both the teacher model and the hard label information by Knowledge Distillation [6]. We have collected 1128 diseased OCT images (185 of them are normal) from 60 patients (15 of them are normal) with IRDs. The experiments on the collected dataset demonstrated that, even under the circumstance of limited training samples, the student model can catch a better performance than the teacher model and some common few-shot learning methods [24].

2   Methods

The overview of the proposed method is shown in Fig. 1. The proposed pipeline consists of three parts: image preprocessing, training for the teacher model and then the student model. The OCT images are first normalized to reduce the effect of noise on the model during training. The teacher model is designed to adapt to the target OCT dataset based on a projector trained with the auxiliary OCT dataset by Soft Nearest Neighbor Loss (SNNL). The student model learns the knowledge from "soft" labels from the teacher model and the "hard" labels from target dataset. In general, the structure of the student model is smaller than that of the teacher model to prevent overfitting and to increase the training speed. The source code is available in https://github.com/hatute/FSTL4HRDR.

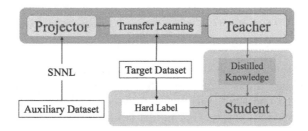

Fig. 1. The overview of the proposed method

The problem of identifying congenital diseases is modeled as a problem of few-shot learning. Unlike the unilateral optimization of model training methods, our approach combines contrastive learning, transfer learning and knowledge distillation to enhance the fast learning ability of the model from various aspects. Second, the teacher-student learning model allows the student to learn more "knowledge" and achieve better performance than the teacher, compared to fine-tuning the original model directly.

2.1   Image Preprocessing

As shown in Fig. 3, the original OCT images show different angles, noise distribution, and size diversity due to the acquisition machine and the patient. This will distract the neural network from the focal area and increase the training time due to the useless data input during training. We adjust all images to the horizontal position without destroying the original pathological information following a adapted OCT image preprocessing strategy from [19]. The main idea of process is to generate a mask to attain retina layered structure.

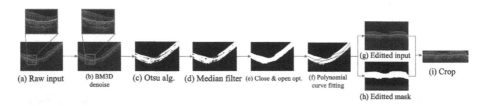

Fig. 2. Pipeline for the image alignment. The process begins with noise reduction as shown in (b) to reduce the irregularly distributed noise with Block-matching and 3D filtering (BM3D) [3] for better capturing the retina structure. (c) The Otsu algorithm allocates the location and morphology of the black background. (d) The median filter further reduces the noise area within the tissue. (e) The morphological operations opening and closing clean noises inside and outside the tissue area. (f) After the contours are obtained, we use a polynomial curve fitting to represent the curvature of the tissue area for adjusting and cropping both the mask and the original image as shown in (i).

2.2   Feature Space Learning

Teacher model is the backbone structure for absorbing and learning the information from an auxiliary dataset, more specifically, the textures, patterns, and pixel distributions in the end-level convolutional layers. Soft Nearest Neighbor Loss (SNNL) [5] is applied for the teacher model training in the feature space before the classifier. SNNL is designed to enhance the separation of class manifolds in representation space. There are bound to be objective differences between the target and auxiliary datasets, and the great separation between the categories in the feature space will facilitate the subsequent transfer learning [5,20] with the target dataset.

Equation 1 shows the total loss function, which consists of the cross-entropy loss on logits and the soft nearest neighbor loss for the representation learning controlled by the hyper-parameter α. i for selected samples in the batch. j for another sample in the same category as i. k for another sample in the same batch as i. In Eq. 2, b is the batch size, T is the temperature. When the temperature is large, the distances between widely separated points can influence the soft nearest neighbor loss more. Moreover, the numerator of the log function implies the distance between the target, and similar samples in each category, while the denominator is the distances between the target and other samples in the batch.

Usually, the use of cosine distances in training results in a smoother training process.

$$\mathcal{L} = \sum_j y_j \log f^k(x_j) + \alpha \cdot \sum_{i \in k-1} l'_{sn}(f^i(x), y) \tag{1}$$

$$l'_{sn} = \arg\min_{T \in \mathbb{R}} -\frac{1}{b} \sum_{i \in 1...b} \log \left(\frac{\sum_{\substack{j \in 1...b \\ j \neq i \\ y_i = y_j}} e^{-\frac{\|x_i - x_j\|^2}{T}}}{\sum_{\substack{k \in 1...b \\ k \neq i}} e^{-\frac{\|x_i - x_k\|^2}{T}}} \right) \tag{2}$$

2.3 Knowledge Distillation and Student-Teacher Learning

In order to overcome the obstacles caused by the lack of training data, we use the combination of Knowledge Distillation and Student-Teacher Learning for knowledge transfer [6,23]. The S-T architecture is designed to give the small-scale (student) model the ability to adapt to small samples and to absorb knowledge from large-scale auxiliary dataset learned by the teacher model. This is mainly designed to eliminate the overfitting problem, when large models cannot learn parameters effectively with a small amount of data.

$$\mathcal{L}(x; W) = \alpha \cdot H(y, \sigma(z_s; T = 1)) + \beta \cdot H(\sigma(z_t; T = \tau), \sigma(z_s; T = \tau)), \tag{3}$$

where α and β control the balance of information coming from the two sources, which generally add up to 1. H is the loss function, σ is the softmax function parameterized by the temperature T, z_s is the logits from student network and z_t is the logits from teacher network. τ denotes the temperature of adapted softmax function, each probability p_i of class i in the batch is calculated from the logits z_i as:

$$p_i = \frac{\exp(\frac{z_i}{T})}{\sum_j \exp\left(\frac{z_j}{T}\right)}, \tag{4}$$

when T increases, the probability distribution of the output becomes "softer", which means the differences among the probability of each class decreased and more information will provide. By the S-T architecture, the smaller size student model with the blank background is able to accept the knowledge from the fine-tuned teacher as well as information from labels.

3 Experiments

3.1 Datasets

Auxiliary Dataset. We use a publicly available dataset of OCT images as shown in Fig. 3 from Cell dataset [11] and BOE dataset [17] for training. The Cell

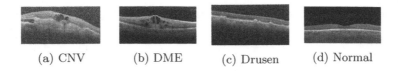

(a) CNV   (b) DME   (c) Drusen   (d) Normal

Fig. 3. Four types of samples in the auxiliary dataset.

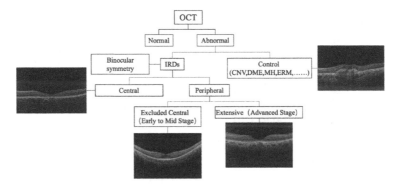

Fig. 4. Relationship of categories in the target dataset

dataset contains four categories including Normal, Choroidal Neo Vascularisation (CNV), Diabetic Macular (DME) and Drusen. They have a total of 109,309 samples, of which 1,000 are used for testing and the rest are used for training. There are two kinds of sizes in those images, $1536 \times 496 \times 1$ and $1024 \times 496 \times 1$. For the experiments, they are all preprocessed and resized to $224 \times 224 \times 1$. The BOE dataset have smaller size than the Cell one. It works for target testing, which acquired from 45 patients. 15 normal patients, 15 patients with dry AMD, and 15 patients with DME.

Target Dataset and Data Acquisition. In the target dataset as shown in Fig. 4, we have 1128 samples from 60 patients' 94 eyes, of which 236 are central IRDs, 204 are excluded central IRDs, 209 are extensive IRDs, 185 are normal and 294 are control samples (CNV, DME, MH, ERM...). The size of the images is $1180 \times 786 \times 1$. Extracted macular OCTs containing at least one OCT scan providing a cross section of the fovea were included in this study. The B scan OCT images with evidence of retinal disease as determined by two retinal specialists were defined as controls. For the experiments, they are all preprocessed and resized to $224 \times 224 \times 1$ because of the limitation of hardware. The ratio of training, testing and validation is 0.70/0.15/0.15. The data were collected from Beijing Tongren Eye Center with a clinical diagnosis of IRDs involving the macular area were included in the current study. SD-OCT data were acquired using a Cirrus HD-OCT 5000 system (Carl Zeiss Meditec Inc., Dublin, CA, USA). This study was performed in line with the principles of the Declaration of Helsinki. Approval was granted by the Ethics Committee of Beijing Tongren Eye Center. (No.TRECKY2017-10, Mar.3,2017).

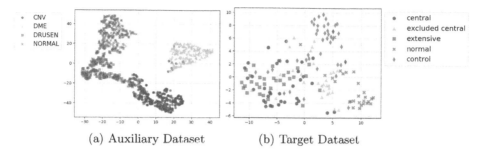

(a) Auxiliary Dataset   (b) Target Dataset

Fig. 5. Feature space representation of teacher (processed by T-SNE). After transfer learning, the teacher model still has excellent clustering and fitting ability in the high-dimensional feature space in the target feature space. The red crosses (normal) appearing in both figures and the purple diamonds (containing CNV, DME, etc.) in the right figure still have good clustering performance. (Color figure online)

3.2   Experimental Settings

Baseline and Data Applicability. It has been shown that the core problems of Few-Shot Learning (FSL) in supervised machine learning are Empirical Risk Minimization and Unreliable Empirical Risk Minimizer [24]. To alleviate these, we usually start with three aspects: data, models, and algorithms. For data, we purposefully design the preprocessing pipeline. We conducted baseline experiments on the state-of-the-art Simple Siamese (SimSiam) network [2]. As shown in Table 1: our preprocessing pipeline mitigates the impact on the model itself due to noise diversity. Also, normalizing this allows the model to exclude redundant concerns.

Feature Space Representation. The SNNL loss function enables the model to get a better projection of the input image during training in the designed feature space, which means that inter-class samples can be clustered while intra-class samples can be separated by the distance function. From Fig. 5, we can see that when the Teacher model (ResNet-50) is trained by the auxiliary dataset, it has the ability to project the test samples from the auxiliary dataset. Meanwhile, to the target dataset, the Teacher also can cluster the normal class and control class which becomes the control class in the target dataset before fine-tuning and transfer learning.

Table 1. Baseline accuracy(%)

Methods	Target dataset	
	Raw	Preprocessed
SimSiam	58.26 ± 1.59	60.5 ± 1.40

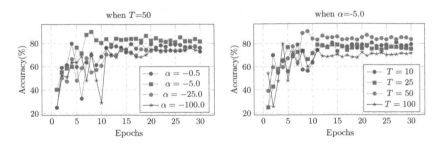

Fig. 6. Teacher model (ResNet-50) Test Experiments

3.3 Student-Teacher Learning

Teacher Model. We choose the ResNet-50 as Teacher Model to handle the auxiliary dataset. The performance is mainly controlled by the hyper-parameter α and Temperature T in Eqs. 1 and 2. In our experiment, we fix the dimension of Feature Space as 128 and pretrain the model with 30 epochs. We decrease the learning rate at epoch 10 and 25 with a factor 0.1. There are two sets of control trials in Fig. 6 optimizing two hyper-parameters α and T. We fix one of them respectively at a time, and optimize the other to get the best accuracy. The best performance is achieved with $T = 50$, and $\alpha = -5.0$.

After training the projector network with the auxiliary dataset by SNNL loss, we perform three different forms of fine-tuning to the target dataset. In the "Features Extraction" way, we freeze the parameters before the last fully-connected layer and replace with a new classifier. In the "High-level" way, we freeze the parameters before the 5th group of convolution layers (the 129_{th} layer in the ResNet-50), left the last group of convolution to learn the high-level features from the new target dataset. In the way of "All Parameters", the model can adjust all the parameters included in ResNet-50. From the data in Table 2, we pick the one with best performance to play the teacher role in the S-T architecture.

Student Model. After accomplished the transfer learning and fine-tuning of Teacher model, We use the ResNet-18 as the Student Model to adapt the smaller size of target data. The ResNet-18 is totally untrained by any data before the S-T learning. From Table 2, we can see that the student model in our trained S-T architecture gets better results than the teacher. This is attributed to the student incorporates knowledge from the teacher's pre-training and information from the hard-label classification. By adjusting the valves of knowledge from both sides, we are able to determine the proportion of prior knowledge that the student model receives from the teacher model versus the feedback from the labels, by adapting this to different data sets. Too much prior knowledge may be counterproductive if the difference between the datasets is greater.

Table 2. Test accuracy (%) comparison of common FSL methods. All the methods based on the pre-trained network with Cell dataset.*Features Extraction* means freezing the pre-trained ResNet-50 and replacing the last layer with a 3-layer classifier. *All Parameters* means the whole ResNet-50 involved in the target-oriented training. *High-level* means only the tail fully connected layers in ResNet-50 involved in the training with the target dataset.

Dataset	Methods				
	Features Extraction	All Parameters	High-level	SimSiam [2]	S-T Learning (ours)
Target(5 Classes)	53.91 ± 1.79	57.17 ± 2.11	59.68 ± 2.59	61.42 ± 2.18	**74.45 ± 1.59**
			Teacher[a]		
BOE(3 Classes)[b]	72.11 ± 0.62	97.83 ± 1.55	92.87 ± 1.96	76.82 ± 1.93	**99.69 ± 0.10**
		Teacher[a]			

[a] chosen as the teacher model in the S-T learning architecture.
[b] BOE dataset has more duplicate labels with the Cell dataset compared to the target dataset. Therefore, it outperforms the target dataset under the same training and network conditions.

4   Conclusion

In this study, we demonstrate a Student-Teacher Learning based classification model on a small dataset to distinguish several retinal diseases. This framework learns the knowledge from both ground truth labels and pretrained Teacher model to make it possible to handle limited data. Data preprocessing also plays a critical role that cannot be ignored before training.

Acknowledgments. This research is partially funded by NSF-IIS-1910492.

References

1. Anantrasirichai, N., Achim, A., Morgan, J.E., Erchova, I., Nicholson, L.: SVM-based texture classification in Optical Coherence Tomography. In: 2013 IEEE 10th International Symposium on Biomedical Imaging, San Francisco, CA, USA, pp. 1332–1335. IEEE (2013)
2. Chen, X., He, K.: Exploring simple Siamese representation learning. In: Proceedings of the IEEE/CVF Conference on Computer Vision and Pattern Recognition, pp. 15750–15758 (2021)
3. Dabov, K., Foi, A., Katkovnik, V., Egiazarian, K.: Image denoising by sparse 3-D transform-domain collaborative filtering. IEEE Trans. Image Proces. **16**(8), 2080–2095 (2007)
4. Fang, L., Wang, C., Li, S., Yan, J., Chen, X., Rabbani, H.: Automatic classification of retinal three-dimensional optical coherence tomography images using principal component analysis network with composite kernels. J. Biomed. Opt. **22**(11), 116011 (2017)

5. Frosst, N., Papernot, N., Hinton, G.: Analyzing and improving representations with the soft nearest neighbor loss. In: International Conference on Machine Learning, pp. 2012–2020. PMLR (2019)
6. Hinton, G., Vinyals, O., Dean, J.: Distilling the knowledge in a neural network. stat 1050, 9 (2015)
7. Hussain, M.A., et al.: Classification of healthy and diseased retina using SD-OCT imaging and random forest algorithm. PloS One **13**(6), e0198281 (2018)
8. Ji, Q., He, W., Huang, J., Sun, Y.: Efficient deep learning-based automated pathology identification in retinal optical coherence tomography images. Algorithms **11**(6), 88 (2018)
9. Ji, Q., Huang, J., He, W., Sun, Y.: Optimized deep convolutional neural networks for identification of macular diseases from optical coherence tomography images. Algorithms **12**(3), 51 (2019)
10. Karri, S.P.K., Chakraborty, D., Chatterjee, J.: Transfer learning based classification of optical coherence tomography images with diabetic macular edema and dry age-related macular degeneration. Biomed. Opt. Express **8**(2), 579–592 (2017)
11. Kermany, D., Zhang, K., Goldbaum, M., et al.: Labeled optical coherence tomography (OCT) and chest X-Ray images for classification (2018)
12. Liu, Y.Y., Chen, M., Ishikawa, H., Wollstein, G., Schuman, J.S., Rehg, J.M.: Automated macular pathology diagnosis in retinal OCT images using multi-scale spatial pyramid and local binary patterns in texture and shape encoding. Med. Image Anal. **15**(5), 748–759 (2011)
13. Lu, W., Tong, Y., Yu, Y., Xing, Y., Chen, C., Shen, Y.: Deep learning-based automated classification of multi-categorical abnormalities from optical coherence tomography images. Transl. Vis. Sci. Technol. **7**(6), 41 (2018)
14. Motozawa, N., et al.: Optical coherence tomography-based deep-learning models for classifying normal and age-related macular degeneration and exudative and non-exudative age-related macular degeneration changes. Ophthalmol. Ther. **8**(4), 527–539 (2019)
15. Sankar, S., et al.: Classification of SD-OCT volumes for DME detection: an anomaly detection approach. In: Medical Imaging 2016: Computer-Aided Diagnosis, vol. 9785, pp. 97852O. International Society for Optics and Photonics (2016)
16. Shih, F.Y., Patel, H.: Deep learning classification on optical coherence tomography retina images. Int. J. Pattern Recogn. Artif. Intell. **34**(08), 2052002 (2020)
17. Srinivasan, P.P., et al.: Fully automated detection of diabetic macular edema and dry age-related macular degeneration from optical coherence tomography images. Biomed. Opt. Express **5**(10), 3568–3577 (2014)
18. Sugmk, J., Kiattisin, S., Leelasantitham, A.: Automated classification between age-related macular degeneration and Diabetic macular edema in OCT image using image segmentation. In: The 7th 2014 Biomedical Engineering International Conference, pp. 1–4. IEEE (2014)
19. Sun, Y., Li, S., Sun, Z.: Fully automated macular pathology detection in retina optical coherence tomography images using sparse coding and dictionary learning. J. Biomed. Opt. **22**(1), 016012 (2017)
20. Tian, Y., Krishnan, D., Isola, P.: Contrastive representation distillation. In: International Conference on Learning Representations (2019)
21. Venhuizen, F.G., et al.: Automated age-related macular degeneration classification in OCT using unsupervised feature learning. In: Hadjiiski, L.M., Tourassi, G.D. (eds.) SPIE Medical Imaging, Orlando, Florida, USA, pp. 94141I (2015)
22. Wang, J., et al.: Deep learning for quality assessment of retinal OCT images. Biomed. Opt. Express **10**(12), 6057–6072 (2019)

23. Wang, L., Yoon, K.-J.: Knowledge distillation and student-teacher learning for visual intelligence: a review and new outlooks. IEEE Trans. Pattern Anal. Mach. Intell., 1 (2021). https://doi.org/10.1109/TPAMI.2021.3055564
24. Wang, Y., Yao, Q., Kwok, J.T., Ni, L.M.: Generalizing from a few examples: a survey on few-shot learning. ACM Comput. Surv. (CSUR) **53**(3), 1–34 (2020)

Simultaneous Alignment and Surface Regression Using Hybrid 2D-3D Networks for 3D Coherent Layer Segmentation of Retina OCT Images

Hong Liu[1,2], Dong Wei[2], Donghuan Lu[2], Yuexiang Li[2], Kai Ma[2], Liansheng Wang[1(✉)], and Yefeng Zheng[2]

[1] Xiamen University, Xiamen, China
liuhong@stu.xmu.edu.cn, lswang@xmu.edu.cn
[2] Tencent Jarvis Lab, Shenzhen, China
{donwei,caleblu,vicyxli,kylekma,yefengzheng}@tencent.com

Abstract. Automated surface segmentation of retinal layer is important and challenging in analyzing optical coherence tomography (OCT). Recently, many deep learning based methods have been developed for this task and yield remarkable performance. However, due to large spatial gap and potential mismatch between the B-scans of OCT data, all of them are based on 2D segmentation of individual B-scans, which may loss the continuity information across the B-scans. In addition, 3D surface of the retina layers can provide more diagnostic information, which is crucial in quantitative image analysis. In this study, a novel framework based on hybrid 2D-3D convolutional neural networks (CNNs) is proposed to obtain continuous 3D retinal layer surfaces from OCT. The 2D features of individual B-scans are extracted by an encoder consisting of 2D convolutions. These 2D features are then used to produce the alignment displacement field and layer segmentation by two 3D decoders, which are coupled via a spatial transformer module. The entire framework is trained end-to-end. To the best of our knowledge, this is the first study that attempts 3D retinal layer segmentation in volumetric OCT images based on CNNs. Experiments on a publicly available dataset show that our framework achieves superior results to state-of-the-art 2D methods in terms of both layer segmentation accuracy and cross-B-scan 3D continuity, thus offering more clinical values than previous works.

Keywords: Optical coherence tomography · 3D coherent layer segmentation · B-scan alignment · 2D-3D hybrid network

---

H. Liu, D. Wei and D. Lu—First three authors contributed equally.

Electronic supplementary material The online version of this chapter (https://doi.org/10.1007/978-3-030-87237-3_11) contains supplementary material, which is available to authorized users.

© Springer Nature Switzerland AG 2021
M. de Bruijne et al. (Eds.): MICCAI 2021, LNCS 12908, pp. 108–118, 2021.
https://doi.org/10.1007/978-3-030-87237-3_11

1   Introduction

Optical coherence tomography (OCT)—a non-invasive imaging technique based on the principle of low-coherence interferometry—can acquire 3D cross-section images of human tissue at micron resolutions [13]. Due to its micron-level axial resolution, non-invasiveness, and fast speed, OCT is commonly used in eye clinics for diagnosis and management of retinal diseases [1]. Notably, OCT provides a unique capability to directly visualize the stratified structure of the retina of cell layers, whose statuses are biomarkers of presence/severity/prognosis for a variety of retinal and neurodegenerative diseases, including age-related macular degeneration [15], diabetic retinopathy [4], glaucoma [14], Alzheimer'4s disease [17], and multiple sclerosis [24]. Usually, layer segmentation is the first step in quantitative analysis of retinal OCT images, yet can be considerably labor-intensive, time-consuming, and subjective if done manually. Therefore, computerized tools for automated, prompt, objective, and accurate retinal layer segmentation in OCT images is desired by both clinicians and researchers.

Automated layer segmentation in retinal OCT images has been well explored. Earlier explorations included graph based [2,10,18,25], contour modeling [5, 20,29], and machine learning [2,18] methods. Although greatly advanced the field, most of these classical methods relied on empirical rules and/or hand-crafted features which may be difficult to generalize. Motivated by the success of deep convolutional neural networks (CNNs) in various medical image analysis tasks [16], researchers also implemented CNNs for retinal layer segmentation in OCT images and achieved superior performance to classical methods [11]. However, most previous methods (both classical and CNNs) segmented each OCT slice (called a B-scan) separately given the relatively big inter-B-scan distance, despite the fact that a modern OCT sequence actually consists of many B-scans covering a volumetric area of the eye [8]. Correspondingly, these methods failed to utilize the anatomical prior that the retinal layers are generally smooth surfaces (instead of independent curves in each B-scan) and may be subject to discontinuity in the segmented layers between adjacent B-scans, potentially affecting volumetric analysis following layer segmentation. Although some works [2,5,6,10,18,20] attempted 3D OCT segmentation, all of them belong to the classical methods that yielded inferior performance to the CNN-based ones, and overlooked the misalignment problem among the B-scans of an OCT volume. Besides the misalignment problem, to develop a CNN-based method for 3D OCT segmentation there is another obstacle: anisotropy in resolution [26]. For example, the physical resolutions of the dataset employed in this work are 3.24 μm (within A-scan, which is a column in a B-scan image), 6.7 μm (cross A-scan), and 67 μm (cross B-scan).

In this work, we propose a novel CNN-based 2D-3D hybrid framework for simultaneous B-scan alignment and 3D surface regression for coherent retinal layer segmentation across B-scans in OCT images. This framework consists of a shared 2D encoder followed by two 3D decoders (the alignment branch and segmentation branch), and a spatial transformer module (STM) inserted to the shortcuts [22] between the encoder and the segmentation branch. Given a B-scan volume as input, we employ per B-scan 2D operations for the encoder for two reasons. First, as suggested by previous studies [27,30], intra-slice feature extraction followed by inter-slice (2.5D or 3D) aggregation is an effective strategy against anisotropic resolution, thus we propose a similar 2D-3D hybrid structure for the anisotropic OCT data. Second, the B-scans in the input volume are subject to misalignment, thus 3D operations across B-scans prior to proper realignment may be invalid. Following the encoder, the alignment branch employs 3D operations to aggregate features across B-scans to align them properly. Then, the resulting displacement field is employed to align the 2D features at different scales and compose well-aligned 3D features by the STM. These 3D features are passed to the segmentation branch for 3D surface regression. Noteworthily, the alignment only insures validity of subsequent 3D operations, but not the cross-B-scan coherence of the regressed layer surfaces. Hence, we further employ a gradient-based, 3D regulative loss [28] on the regressed surfaces to encourage smooth surfaces, which is an intrinsic property of many biological layers. While it is straightforward to implement this loss within our surface regression framework and comes for free (no manual annotation is needed), it proves effective in our experiments. Lastly, the entire framework is trained end-to-end.

In summary, our contributions are as following. First, we propose a new framework for simultaneous B-scan alignment and 3D retinal layer segmentation for OCT images. This framework features a hybrid 2D-3D structure comprising a shared 2D encoder, a 3D alignment branch, a 3D surface regression branch, and an STM to allow for simultaneous alignment and 3D segmentation of the anisotropic OCT data. Second, we further propose two conceptually straightforward and easy-to-implement regulating losses to encourage the regressed layer surfaces to be coherent—not only within but also across B-scans, and also help align the B-scans. Third, we conduct thorough experiments to validate our design and demonstrate its superiority over existing methods.

2 Method

Problem Formulation. Let $\Omega \subset \mathbb{R}^3$, then a 3D OCT volume can be written as a real-valued function $V(x, y, z) : \Omega \to \mathbb{R}$, where the x and y axis are the row and column directions of a B-scan image, and z axis is orthogonal to the B-scan image. Alternatively, V can be considered as an ordered collection of all its B-scans: $V(b) = \{I_b\}$, where $I_b : \Phi \to \mathbb{R}$ is the bth B-scan image, $\Phi \subset \mathbb{R}^2$, $b \in [1, N_B]$, and N_B is the number of B-scans. Then, a retinal layer surface can be expressed by $S = \{r_{b,a}\}$, where $a \in [1, N_A]$, N_A is the number of A-scans, and $r_{b,a}$ is the row index indicating the surface location in the ath A-scan of the bth B-scan. That is, the surface intersects with each A-scan exactly once, which is a common assumption about macular OCT images (*e.g.*, in [11]). The goal of this work is to locate a set of retinal layer surfaces of interest $\{S\}$ in V, preferably being smooth, for accurate segmentation of the layers.

Method Overview. The overview of our framework is shown in Fig. 1. The framework comprises three major components: a contracting path G_f (the shared encoder) consisting of 2D CNN layers and two expansive paths consisting of 3D CNN layers G_a (the alignment branch) and G_s (the segmentation branch), and a functional module: the spatial transformer module (STM). During feature extraction phase, 2D features of separate B-scans in an OCT volume are extracted by G_f. These features are firstly used to generate B-scans alignment displacement by G_a, which is used in turn to align the 2D features via the STM. Then, the well-aligned features are fed to G_s to yield final segmentation. Each of G_a and G_s forms a hybrid 2D-3D residual U-Net [22] with G_f. The entire framework is trained end-to-end. As G_f is implemented as a simple adaption to the encoder in [31] (3D to 2D), below we focus on describing our novel G_a, G_s, and STM.

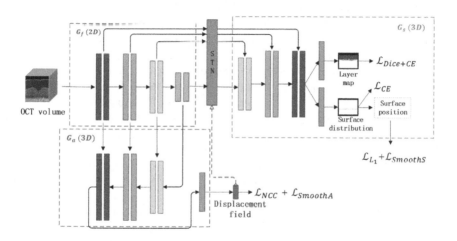

Fig. 1. Overview of the proposed framework.

B-Scan Alignment Branch. Due to the image acquisition process wherein each B-scan is acquired separately without a guaranteed global alignment and the inevitable eye movement, consecutive B-scans in an OCT volume may be subject to misalignment [7]. The mismatch mainly happens along the y axis, and may cause problems for volumetric analysis of the OCT data if unaddressed. Although it is feasible to add an alignment step while preprocessing, a comprehensive framework that couples the B-scan alignment and layer segmentation would mutually benefit each other (supported by our experimental results), besides being more integrated. To this end, we introduce a B-scan alignment branch G_a consisting of an expansive path into our framework, which takes 2D features extracted from a set of B-scans by G_f and stacks them along the cross-B-scan direction to form 3D input. The alignment branch outputs a displacement vector

$\triangle \boldsymbol{d}$, with each element d_b indicating the displacement of the bth B-scan in the y direction. We use the local normalized cross-correlation (NCC) [3] of adjacent B-Scans as the optimization objective (denoted by $\mathcal{L}_{\text{NCC}}$) of G_a.

As smoothness is one of the intrinsic properties of the retinal layers, if the B-scans are aligned properly, ground truth surface positions of the same layer should be close at nearby locations of adjacent B-scans. To model this prior, we propose a supervised loss function to help with the alignment:

$$\mathcal{L}_{\text{SmoothA}} = \sum_{b=1}^{N_B-1} \sum_{a=1}^{N_A} \left((r_{b,a}^g - d_b) - (r_{b+1,a}^g - d_{b+1}) \right)^2, \tag{1}$$

where r^g is the ground truth. The final optimization objective of the alignment branch is $\mathcal{L}_{\text{Align}} = \mathcal{L}_{\text{NCC}} + \mathcal{L}_{\text{SmoothA}}$.

Layer Segmentation Branch. Our layer segmentation branch substantially extends the fully convolutional boundary regression (FCBR) framework by He et al. [11]. Above all, we replace the purely 2D FCBR framework by a hybrid 2D-3D framework, to perform 3D surface regression in an OCT volume instead of 2D boundary regression in separate B-scans. On top of that, we propose a global smoothness guarantee loss to encourage coherent surfaces both within and across B-scans, whereas FCBR only enforces within B-scan smoothness. Third, our segmentation branch is coupled with the B-scan alignment branch, which boost the performance of each other.

The segmentation branch has two output heads sharing the same decoder: the primary head which outputs the surface position distribution for each A-scan, and the secondary head which outputs pixel-wise semantic labels. The secondary head is used only to provide an additional task for training the network, especially considering its pixel-wise dense supervision. Eventually the output of the secondary head is ignored during testing. We follow He et al. to use a combined Dice and cross entropy loss [23] $\mathcal{L}_{\text{Dice+CE}}$ for training the secondary head, and refer interested readers to [11] for more details.

Surface Distribution Head. This primary head generates an independent surface position distribution $q_{b,a}(r|V;\theta)$ for each A-scan, where θ is the network parameters, and a higher value indicates a higher possibility that the rth row is on the surface. Like in [11], a cross entropy loss is used to train the primary head:

$$\mathcal{L}_{\text{CE}} = -\sum_{b=1}^{N_B} \sum_{a=1}^{N_A} \sum_{r=1}^{R} \mathbb{1}(r_{b,a}^g = r) \log q_{b,a}(r_{b,a}^g|V,\theta), \tag{2}$$

where R is the number of rows in an A scan, $\mathbb{1}(x)$ is the indicator function where $\mathbb{1}(x) = 1$ if x is evaluated to be true and zero otherwise. Further, a smooth L1 loss is adopted to directly guide the predicted surface location $\hat{r}$ to be the ground truth: $\mathcal{L}_{L1} = \sum_{b=1}^{N_B} \sum_{a=1}^{N_A} 0.5 t_{b,a}^2 \mathbb{1}(|t_{b,a}| < 1) + (|t_{b,a}| - 0.5)\mathbb{1}(|t_{b,a}| \geq 1)$, where $t_{b,a} = \hat{r}_{b,a} - r_{b,a}^g$, and $\hat{r}_{b,a}$ is obtained via the soft-argmax: $\hat{r}_{b,a} = \sum_{r=1}^{R} r q_{b,a}(r|V,\theta)$.

Global Coherence Loss. Previous studies have shown the effectiveness of modeling prior knowledge that reflects anatomical properties such as the structural smoothness [28] in medical image segmentation. Following this line, we also employ a global smoothness loss to encourage the detected retinal surface $\hat{S}(b,a) = \{\hat{r}_{b,a}\}$ to be coherent both within and across the aligned B-scans based on its gradients:

$$\mathcal{L}_{\text{SmoothS}} = \sum_{b=1}^{N_B} \sum_{a=1}^{N_A} \left\| \nabla \hat{S}(b,a) \right\|^2. \tag{3}$$

Finally, the overall optimization objective of the segmentation branch is $\mathcal{L}_{\text{Seg}} = \mathcal{L}_{\text{Dice+CE}} + \mathcal{L}_{\text{CE}} + \mathcal{L}_{\text{L1}} + \lambda \mathcal{L}_{\text{SmoothS}}$, where λ is a hyperparameter controlling the influence of the global coherence loss.

Spatial Transformer Module. The B-Scans displacement field $\triangle d$ output by the alignment branch G_a is used to align features extracted by G_f, so that the 3D operations of the segmentation branch G_s are valid. To do so, we propose to add a spatial transformer module (STM) [19] to the shortcuts between G_f and G_s. It is worth noting that the STM adaptively resizes $\triangle d$ to suit the size of the features at different scales, and that it allows back prorogation during optimization [19]. In this way, we couple the B-scan alignment and retinal layer segmentation in our framework for an integrative end-to-end training, which not only simplifies the entire pipeline but also boosts the segmentation performance as validated by our experiments.

3   Experiments

Dataset and Preprocessing. The public SD-OCT dataset [9] includes both normal (265) and age-related macular degeneration (AMD) (115) cases. The images were acquired using the Bioptigen Tabletop SD-OCT system (Research Triangle Park, NC). The physical resolutions are 3.24 µm (within A-scan), 6.7 µm (cross A-scan), and 0.067 mm (cross B-scan). Since the manual annotations are only available for a region centered at the fovea, subvolumes of size $400 \times 40 \times 512$ (N_A, N_B, and R) voxels are extracted around the fovea. We train the model on 263 subjects and test on the other 72 subjects (some cases are eliminated from analysis as the competing alignment algorithm [21] fails to handle them), which are randomly divided with the proportion of AMD cases unchanged. The inner aspect of the inner limiting membrane (ILM), the inner aspect of the retinal pigment epithelium drusen complex (IRPE), and the outer aspect of Bruch's membrane (OBM) were manually traced. For the multi-surface segmentation, there are two considerations. First, we employ the topology guarantee module [11] to make sure the correct order of the surfaces. Second, the natural smoothness of these surfaces are different. Therefore, we set different λ (weight of $\mathcal{L}_{\text{SmoothS}}$) values for different surfaces, according to the extents of smoothness and preliminary experimental results. As to preprocessing, an intensity gradient method [18] is employed to flatten the retinal B-Scan image to the estimated Bruch's membrane (BM), which can reduce memory usage.

When standalone B-scan alignment is needed, the NoRMCore algorithm [21] is employed.

For B-scan alignment, we adopt the mean absolute distance (MAD) of the same surface on two adjacent B-scans, and the average NCC between aligned B-scans for quantitative evaluation. For retinal surface segmentation, the MAD between predicted and ground truth surface positions is used. To compare the cross-B-scan continuity of the surfaces segmented by different methods, inspired by [12], we calculate the surface distance between adjacent B-Scans as the statistics of flatness and plot the histogram for inspection.

Implementation. The PyTorch framework (1.4.0) is used for experiments. Implementation of our proposed network follows the architecture proposed in Model Genesis [31], except that the 3D layers of the feature extractor G_f is changed to 2D. To reduce the number of network parameters, we halve the number of channels in each CNN block. All networks are trained form scratch. Due to the memory limit, OCT volumes are cropped into patches of $320 \times 400 \times 40$ voxels for training. We utilize the Adam optimizer and train for 120 epochs. The learning rate is initialized to 0.001 and halved when the loss has not improved for ten consecutive epochs. We train the network on three 2080 Ti GPUs with a mini-batch size of nine patches. Based on preliminary experiments and natural smoothness of the three target surfaces, λ is set to 0, 0.3, and 0.5 for ILM, IRPE, and OBM, respectively. The source code is available at: https://github.com/ccarliu/Retinal-OCT-LayerSeg.git.

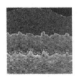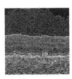

Fig. 2. B-scan alignment results visualized via cross sections. Each B-Scan is repeated eight times for better visualization. Left to right: no alignment (flattened to the BM)/NoRMCore [21]/ours. Yellow: ILM, blue: IRPE, and green: OBM.

Table 1. B-scan alignment results. MAD: mean absolute distance (in pixels). NCC: normalized cross-correlation.

Methods	ILM (MAD)	IRPE (MAD)	OBM (MAD)	Average (MAD)	NCC
No alignment	3.91	4.17	3.93	4.00	0.0781
NoRMCore [21]	1.74	2.19	1.87	1.93	0.0818
Ours	**1.55**	**2.11**	**1.78**	**1.81**	**0.0894**

B-Scan Alignment Results. Figure 2 shows the cross-B-scan sections of an OCT volume before and after alignment. As we can see, obvious mismatches between B-scans can be observed before alignment, and both alignment algorithms make the B-scans more aligned. While it is hard to tell from the visualizations, quantitative results in Table 1 suggest that our framework aligns the B-scans better than the NoRMCore [21], with generally lower MADs and higher NCCs.

Surface Segmentation Results. The results are presented in Table 2. First, we compare our proposed method to FCBR [11] (empirically tuned for optimal performance), which is a state-of-the-art method based on 2D surface regression. As we can see, our method achieves lower average MADs with lower standard deviations (example segmentations in Figs. 3 and S1). In addition, we visualize surface positions of BM as depth fields in Fig S2. For a fair comparison, we visualize the FCBR results aligned by NoRMCore [21]. It can be observed that our method (Fig. S2(d)) produces a smoother depth field than FCBR does (Fig. S2(c)).

Next, we conduct ablation experiments to verify the effectiveness of each module in the proposed framework. Specifically, we evaluate several variants of our model: no_smooth (without the global coherence loss $\mathcal{L}_{\text{SmoothS}}$), no_align (without the alignment branch or pre-alignment), pre_align (without the align-

Table 2. Mean absolute distance (μm) as surface errors ± standard deviation.

Methods	FCBR [11]	Proposed	no_align	pre_align	no_smooth	3D-3D
ILM (AMD)	1.73 ± 2.50	1.76 ± 2.39	2.25 ± 3.77	1.80 ± 2.36	**1.68 ± 1.84**	1.87 ± 2.19
ILM (Normal)	**1.24 ± 0.51**	1.26 ± 0.47	1.40 ± 0.42	1.30 ± 0.49	1.27 ± 0.47	1.31 ± 0.46
IRPE (AMD)	3.09 ± 2.09	**3.04 ± 1.79**	3.14 ± 1.72	3.09 ± 1.79	3.10 ± 1.97	3.12 ± 1.74
IRPE (Normal)	2.06 ± 1.51	2.10 ± 1.36	2.18 ± 1.37	**2.05 ± 1.40**	2.13 ± 1.45	2.13 ± 1.45
OBM (AMD)	4.94±5.35	**4.43 ± 2.68**	4.96 ± 3.26	4.75 ± 3.61	4.84 ± 3.43	4.78 ± 2.99
OBM (Normal)	**2.28 ± 0.36**	2.40 ± 0.39	2.49 ± 0.40	2.34 ± 0.37	2.45 ± 0.41	2.43 ± 0.40
Overall	2.78 ± 3.31	**2.71 ± 2.25**	3.00 ± 2.82	2.77 ± 2.59	2.81 ± 2.48	2.85 ± 2.34

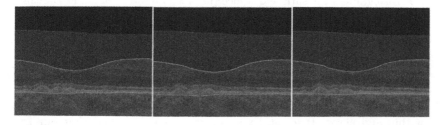

Fig. 3. Visualization of the manual segmentation (left), segmentation by FCBR [11] (middle), and segmentation by our framework (right) of an AMD case. Visualization of a normal control is shown in Fig. S1. Yellow: ILM, blue: IRPE, and green: OBM. (Color figure online)

ment branch but pre-aligned by NoRMCore [21]), 3D-3D (replacing the encoder G_f by 3D CNNs). The results are presented in Table 2, from which several conclusions can be drawn. First, the variant without any alignment yields the worst results, suggesting that the mismatch between B-scans does have a negative impact on 3D analysis of OCT data such as our 3D surface segmentation. Second, our full model with the alignment branch improves over pre_align. We speculate this is because the alignment branch can produce better alignment results, and more importantly, it produces a slightly different alignment each time, serving as a kind of data and feature augmentation of enhanced diversity for the segmentation decoder G_s. Third, removing $\mathcal{L}_{\text{SmoothS}}$ apparently decreases the performance, demonstrating its effectiveness in exploiting the anatomical prior of smoothness. Lastly, our hybrid 2D-3D framework outperforms its counterpart 3D-3D network, indicating that the 2D CNNs can better deal with the mismatched B-scans prior to proper realignment.

B-Scans Connectivity Analysis. As shown in Fig. 4, surfaces segmented by our method has better cross-B-scan connectivity than those by FCBR [11] even with pre-alignment, as indicated by the more conspicuous spikes clustered around 0. This suggests that merely conducting 3D alignment does not guarantee 3D continuity, if the aligned B-scans are handled separately. It is worth noting that our method achieves even better cross-B-scan connectivity than the manual annotations after alignment, likely due to the same reason (*i.e.*, human annotators work with one B-scan at a time).

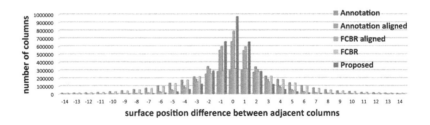

Fig. 4. Histogram of the surface distance (in pixels) between adjacent B-Scans.

4   Conclusion

This work presented a novel hybrid 2D-3D framework for simultaneous B-scan alignment and retinal surface regression of volumetric OCT data. The key idea behind our framework was the global coherence of the retinal layer surfaces both within and across B-scans. Experimental results showed that our framework was superior to the existing state-of-the-art method [11] for retinal layer segmentation, and verified the effectiveness of the newly proposed modules of our framework. In the future, we plan to evaluate our framework on additional datasets with more severe diseases and more annotated layers.

Acknowledgments. This work was supported by the Fundamental Research Funds for the Central Universities (Grant No. 20720190012), Key-Area Research and Development Program of Guangdong Province, China (No. 2018B010111001), and Scientific and Technical Innovation 2030 - "New Generation Artificial Intelligence" Project (No. 2020AAA0104100).

References

1. Abràmoff, M.D., Garvin, M.K., Sonka, M.: Retinal imaging and image analysis. IEEE Rev. Biomed. Eng. **3**, 169–208 (2010)
2. Antony, B.J., Abràmoff, M.D., Harper, M.M., et al.: A combined machine-learning and graph-based framework for the segmentation of retinal surfaces in SD-OCT volumes. Biomed. Opt. Express **4**(12), 2712–2728 (2013)
3. Balakrishnan, G., Zhao, A., Sabuncu, M.R., Guttag, J., Dalca, A.V.: VoxelMorph: a learning framework for deformable medical image registration. IEEE Trans. Med. Imag. **38**(8), 1788–1800 (2019)
4. Bavinger, J.C., Dunbar, G.F., Stem, M.S., et al.: The effects of diabetic retinopathy and pan-retinal photocoagulation on photoreceptor cell function as assessed by dark adaptometry. Invest. Ophthalmol. Vis. Sci. **57**(1), 208–217 (2016)
5. Carass, A., Lang, A., Hauser, M., Calabresi, P.A., Ying, H.S., Prince, J.L.: Multiple-object geometric deformable model for segmentation of macular OCT. Biomed. Opt. Express **5**(4), 1062–1074 (2014)
6. Chen, Z.l., Wei, H., Shen, H.l., et al.: Intraretinal layer segmentation and parameter measurement in optic nerve head region through energy function of spatial-gradient continuity constraint. J. Cent. South Univ. **25**(8), 1938–1947 (2018)
7. Cheng, J., Lee, J.A., Xu, G., Quan, Y., Ong, E.P.: Kee Wong. Motion correction in optical coherence tomography for multi-modality retinal image registration, D.W. (2016)
8. Drexler, W., Fujimoto, J.G.: State-of-the-art retinal optical coherence tomography. Prog. Retin. Eye Res. **27**(1), 45–88 (2008)
9. Farsiu, S., Chiu, S.J., O'Connell, R.V., et al.: Quantitative classification of eyes with and without intermediate age-related macular degeneration using optical coherence tomography. Ophthalmology **121**(1), 162–172 (2014)
10. Garvin, M.K., Abramoff, M.D., Wu, X., Russell, S.R., Burns, T.L., Sonka, M.: Automated 3-D intraretinal layer segmentation of macular spectral-domain optical coherence tomography images. IEEE Trans. Med. Imag. **28**(9), 1436–1447 (2009)
11. He, Y., et al.: Fully convolutional boundary regression for retina OCT segmentation. In: Shen, D., et al. (eds.) MICCAI 2019. LNCS, vol. 11764, pp. 120–128. Springer, Cham (2019). https://doi.org/10.1007/978-3-030-32239-7_14
12. He, Y., Carass, A., Liu, Y., et al.: Structured layer surface segmentation for retina OCT using fully convolutional regression networks. Med. Image Anal. **68**, 101856 (2021)
13. Huang, D., Swanson, E.A., Lin, C.P., et al.: Optical coherence tomography. Science **254**(5035), 1178–1181 (1991)
14. Kansal, V., Armstrong, J.J., Pintwala, R., Hutnik, C.: Optical coherence tomography for glaucoma diagnosis: an evidence based meta-analysis. PloS one **13**(1), e0190621 (2018)
15. Keane, P.A., Liakopoulos, S., Jivrajka, R.V., et al.: Evaluation of optical coherence tomography retinal thickness parameters for use in clinical trials for neovascular age-related macular degeneration. Invest. Ophthalmol. Vis. Sci. **50**(7), 3378–3385 (2009)

16. Ker, J., Wang, L., Rao, J., Lim, T.: Deep learning applications in medical image analysis. IEEE Access **6**, 9375–9389 (2017)
17. Knoll, B., Simonett, J., Volpe, N.J., et al.: Retinal nerve fiber layer thickness in amnestic mild cognitive impairment: case-control study and meta-analysis. Alzheimer's Dementia Diagnosis Assessment Disease Monitoring **4**, 85–93 (2016)
18. Lang, A., Carass, A., Hauser, M., et al.: Retinal layer segmentation of macular OCT images using boundary classification. Biomed. Opt. Express **4**(7), 1133–1152 (2013)
19. Li, H., Fan, Y.: Non-rigid image registration using fully convolutional networks with deep self-supervision. arXiv preprint arXiv:1709.00799 (2017)
20. Novosel, J., Vermeer, K.A., De Jong, J.H., Wang, Z., Van Vliet, L.J.: Joint segmentation of retinal layers and focal lesions in 3-D OCT data of topologically disrupted retinas. IEEE Trans. Med. Imag. **36**(6), 1276–1286 (2017)
21. Pnevmatikakis, E.A., Giovannucci, A.: NoRMCorre: An online algorithm for piecewise rigid motion correction of calcium imaging data. J. Neurosci. Methods **291**, 83–94 (2017)
22. Ronneberger, O., Fischer, P., Brox, T.: U-Net: convolutional networks for biomedical image segmentation. In: Navab, N., Hornegger, J., Wells, W.M., Frangi, A.F. (eds.) MICCAI 2015. LNCS, vol. 9351, pp. 234–241. Springer, Cham (2015). https://doi.org/10.1007/978-3-319-24574-4_28
23. Roy, A.G., et al.: ReLayNet: retinal layer and fluid segmentation of macular optical coherence tomography using fully convolutional networks. Biomed. Opt. Express **8**(8), 3627–3642 (2017)
24. Saidha, S., Syc, S.B., Ibrahim, M.A., et al.: Primary retinal pathology in multiple sclerosis as detected by optical coherence tomography. Brain **134**(2), 518–533 (2011)
25. Shah, A., Abámoff, M.D., Wu, X.: Optimal surface segmentation with convex priors in irregularly sampled space. Med. Image Anal. **54**, 63–75 (2019)
26. Shah, A., Zhou, L., Abrámoff, M.D., Wu, X.: Multiple surface segmentation using convolution neural nets: application to retinal layer segmentation in OCT images. Biomed. Opt. Express **9**(9), 4509–4526 (2018)
27. Wang, S., Cao, S., Chai, Z., et al.: Conquering data variations in resolution: a slice-aware multi-branch decoder network. IEEE Trans. Med. Imag. **39**(12), 4174–4185 (2020)
28. Wei, D., Weinstein, S., Hsieh, M.K., Pantalone, L., Kontos, D.: Three-dimensional whole breast segmentation in sagittal and axial breast MRI with dense depth field modeling and localized self-adaptation for chest-wall line detection. IEEE Trans. Biomed. Eng. **66**(6), 1567–1579 (2018)
29. Yazdanpanah, A., Hamarneh, G., Smith, B., Sarunic, M.: Intra-retinal layer segmentation in optical coherence tomography using an active contour approach. In: Yang, G.-Z., Hawkes, D., Rueckert, D., Noble, A., Taylor, C. (eds.) MICCAI 2009. LNCS, vol. 5762, pp. 649–656. Springer, Heidelberg (2009). https://doi.org/10.1007/978-3-642-04271-3_79
30. Zhang, J., Xie, Y., Zhang, P., Chen, H., Xia, Y., Shen, C.: Light-weight hybrid convolutional network for liver tumor segmentation. In: IJCAI, pp. 4271–4277 (2019)
31. Zhou, Z., et al.: Models genesis: generic autodidactic models for 3D medical image analysis. In: Shen, D., et al. (eds.) MICCAI 2019. LNCS, vol. 11767, pp. 384–393. Springer, Cham (2019). https://doi.org/10.1007/978-3-030-32251-9_42

Computational (Integrative) Pathology

GQ-GCN: Group Quadratic Graph Convolutional Network for Classification of Histopathological Images

Zhiyang Gao, Jun Shi[⊠], and Jun Wang

Shanghai Institute for Advanced Communication and Data Science, School of Communication and Information Engineering, Shanghai University, Shanghai, China
junshi@shu.edu.cn

Abstract. Convolutional neural network (CNN) has achieved superior performance on the computer-aided diagnosis for histopathological images. Although the spatial arrangement of cells of various types in histopathological images is an important characteristic for the diagnosis of cancers, CNN cannot explicitly capture this spatial structure information. This challenge can be overcome by constructing the graph data on histopathological images and learning the graph representation with valuable spatial correlations in the graph convolutional network (GCN). However, the current GCN models for histopathological images usually require a complicated preprocessing process or prior experience of node selection for graph construction. Moreover, there is a lack of learning architecture that can perform feature selection to refine features in the GCN. In this work, we propose a group quadratic graph convolutional network (GQ-GCN), which adopts CNN to extract features from histopathological images for further adaptively graph construction. In particular, the group graph convolutional network (G-GCN) is developed to implement both feature selection and compression of graph representation. In addition, the quadratic operation is specifically embedded into the graph convolution to enhance the representation ability of a single neuron for complex data. The experimental results on two public breast histopathological image datasets indicate the effectiveness of the proposed GQ-GCN.

Keywords: Histopathological images · Computer-aided diagnosis · Group graph convolutional network · Quadratic operation

1 Introduction

The diagnosis from histopathological images remains the "gold standard" for almost all types of cancers in clinical practice, including breast cancer [1]. Computer-aided diagnosis (CAD) for diseases has attracted considerable attention in recent years with the rapid development of artificial intelligence technology [2, 3]. It can relieve the workload of pathologists, providing more objective and reliable diagnosis results [4, 5].

Convolutional neural network (CNN) and its variants have been widely used in various tasks of histopathological images [6, 7]. It can effectively learn local feature

© Springer Nature Switzerland AG 2021
M. de Bruijne et al. (Eds.): MICCAI 2021, LNCS 12908, pp. 121–131, 2021.
https://doi.org/10.1007/978-3-030-87237-3_12

representation since the convolution kernel has the characteristics of local perception and weight sharing [8]. However, convolution layers in CNN are of little use in capturing global contextual information, so as to inevitably ignore the correlation information among different spatial regions [9].

It is known that graph convolutional network (GCN) can obtain the spatial structure feature of the data converted into graph representation [10]. It therefore can be expected that the graph representation of histopathological images reflects the interactions among regions in spatial locations. GCN has been successfully applied in the classification task of histopathological images in several pioneering works. For example, Zhou *et al.* proposed a GCN based on the cell-graph that used the cell nucleus of the histopathological image as nodes to construct the graph [11]; Li *et al.* proposed a GCN for analyzing whole slide images (WSIs) by constructing the graph based on sampling representative patches as node [12]; Adnan *et al.* proposed a GCN that used sub-block features as node embedding and combined multiple instance learning (MIL) to classify lung cancer subtypes [13]. These methods have shown the effectiveness of histopathological image classification by embedding features including global spatial relations in GCN.

However, the existing GCN models for histopathological image classification generally require complicated processing steps to construct the graph, and always suffer from the following problems: 1) The graph construction methods based on either cell nucleus or patches as nodes usually require complex preprocessing procedures and prior experience; 2) In the graph convolution process, graph representation is learned through a simple aggregation of neighborhood node information [14]. There is a lack of explicit learning architecture to selectively compress the node features with redundant information in the process of feature propagation; 3) Histopathological images with a topological spatial structure are highly complex, and therefore, the current GCN models should be further improved to learn effective features from histopathological images.

To tackle the aforementioned issues, a novel group quadratic GCN (GQ-GCN) is proposed for the histopathological image-based CAD. Our GQ-GCN model applies the feature maps generated by CNN for graph construction to avoid the complicated processing steps. In the graph convolutional process, node features of graph representation are grouped to compress and refine the features in group GCN (G-GCN). In addition, the quadratic graph convolution operation is developed to strengthen representation ability for complex histopathological images.

The main contributions of this work are three-fold as follows:

1) A simple yet effective graph construction method is proposed for the classification of histopathological images, in which the nodes are automatically generated from the feature maps of CNN. This constructed graph is then dynamically adjusted to learn superior graph representation under the framework of integrating CNN and GCN.
2) The G-GCN model is developed to group the node features in the graph convolution process. It implicitly learns interactions between different groups of node features to selectively stimulate effective features and suppress redundant features, which can generate discriminative graph representation for classification.

3) The GQ-GCN model is further proposed by introducing a quadratic operation into the graph convolution of G-GCN. It can further enhance the feature representation ability of graph convolution operation for complex histopathological images.

2 Method

Figure 1 shows the flowchart of the proposed GQ-GCN model for histopathological image classification. It consists of two main modules including a CNN and an improved GCN module. The CNN aims to learn and generate feature maps from the input histopathological images for further adaptive graph construction, and the improved GCN module then learns the graph representation to generate features for subsequent classification. The detailed processes are as follows:

1) The histopathological image is fed to CNN to generate high-order semantic feature maps, in which each pixel corresponds to a patch in the histopathological image.
2) Each pixel of the feature map is considered as a node in the graph. The feature vector is regarded as the node embedding of the corresponding patch. The adjacency matrix then can be calculated using k-nearest neighbors (k-NN) method to construct the required graph representation.
3) The generated graph representation is fed to an improved GCN module, which performs the process of node feature grouping and quadratic graph convolution operation to learn the graph representation with spatial structure information.
4) The outputs of the improved GCN module are fed to the pooling layer, fully connected layers, and softmax function to produce the final predictive result. Under the guidance of the cross-entropy loss function, the end-to-end global training and feedback tuning of the entire network is realized.

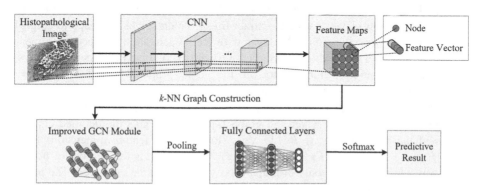

Fig. 1. Flowchart of the proposed GQ-GCN model.

2.1 Adaptive Graph Construction

The adaptive graph construction aims to transform the original histopathological images into a graph. As shown in Fig. 1, the CNN backbone is performed to obtain a set of small multi-channel feature maps from the histopathological image. Each pixel in feature maps is then regarded as a node and represents a corresponding region in the original histopathological image. Therefore, the constructed graph includes spatial correlation information. The feature values of the node are the multi-channel value of the corresponding pixel position, whereas edges are generated in terms of the k-NN. We hypothesize that the pixels in feature maps with smaller Euclidean distances are more likely to interact, the maximum degree of each node is set to k corresponding to its k-NN [11]. The form of graph edges can be expressed as:

$$e_{ij} = \begin{cases} 1 \ if \ v_j \in k - NN(v_i) \ and \ D(v_i, v_j) < d, \\ 0 \qquad\qquad otherwise \end{cases} \tag{1}$$

where v_i, v_j represent the i- th and j- th graph nodes, respectively. $D(\cdot, \cdot)$ denotes Euclidean distance between two nodes feature vectors.

The adaptive graph construction is embedded into the end-to-end network, which can adaptive to adjust the connection between graph nodes according to the update of nodes from CNN during network training. Therefore, the constructed graph can be adaptively learned based on different datasets, so as obtain the optimal graph representation that matches the subsequent classification task well.

2.2 Group Graph Convolutional Network (G-GCN)

G-GCN structure is used to reduce the redundant information extracted by CNN to produce node features and to further select superior fusion feature representation.

As shown in Fig. 2. G-GCN is a symmetrical structure. It has units similar to the gate, which controls the information propagation between adjacent layers. A graph convolution (GraphConv) layer is used to extract linear features, which is used to control the gate, a batch normalization (BN) layer with ReLU activation produces nonlinear features. A multiplier and addition operator is utilized to combine the selected features.

Formally, the node feature vector of the input graph is denoted as $F = \{f_1, f_2, \cdots, f_{T/2}, \cdots, f_{T-1}, f_T\}$, where f_t represents the t-th eigenvalue, $t = 1, \cdots, T$. The input $G_{input} \in R^{N \times F}$ of G-GCN is grouped into two sub-graphs G_1, G_2 along the node feature dimension, where the graph $G_1 \in R^{N \times F_1}$ gets the detailed characteristics of the node and $G_2 \in R^{N \times F_2}$ vary slower in the feature dimensions [15]. $F_1 = \{f_1, f_2, \cdots, f_{(T/2)-1}\}$, $F_2 = \{f_{T/2}, \cdots, f_{T-1} f_T\}$ and N is the number of nodes. In this way, the inherent diversity of graph representation can be enhanced. The information is exchanged and fused between two sub-groups, so as to make the GCN learn more effective and compact feature representation. G_1 goes through a graph convolution layer which produces the linear graph feature map, the output G_1' of which flows into two paths. One path consists of BN and ReLU activation that generate nonlinear graph feature G_1''. The other path is a gate composed of a graph convolution layer and Tanh activation function, which generates output G_{1g}' for feature fusion. Similarly, the other

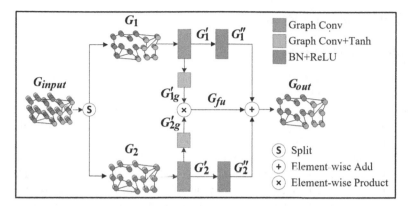

Fig. 2. Illustration of G-GCN structure.

sub-graph G_2 in G-GCN also generates G_2'' and G_{2g}' through the same steps as sub-graph G_1. G_{1g}' and G_{2g}' flow into the multiplier for feature fusion to generate G_{fu}. Finally, G_1'', G_2'' and G_{fu} are combined together with trainable weights and normalized by the *BN* layer to generate the final output G_{out}.

2.3 Quadratic Graph Convolution Operation

The quadratic operation is used to enhance the representation ability of the graph convolutional unit for complex data. We suppose that X is the input of the GCN, and the convolution process of the traditional graph convolution layer can be written as:

$$H(X) = \sigma(\tilde{D}^{-\frac{1}{2}}\tilde{A}\tilde{D}^{-\frac{1}{2}}XW) \tag{2}$$

Where $\tilde{D}$, W are degree matrix and layer-specific trainable weight matrix, respectively. $\sigma(\cdot)$ denotes an activation function, $\tilde{A} = A + I_N$ is the adjacency matrix of the undirected graph with added self-connection, where I_N is the identity matrix [10].

A quadratic neuron summarizes input data as an inner product [16]. We add the quadratic operation into the graph convolutional unit in G-GCN. The quadratic graph convolution can be formulated as follows:

$$H'(X) = \sigma((MXW_r + b_r)(MXW_g + b_g) + MX^2W_b + c) \tag{3}$$

where $M = \tilde{D}^{-\frac{1}{2}}\tilde{A}\tilde{D}^{-\frac{1}{2}}$, b_r, b_g, c are biases and W_r, W_g, W_b are layer-specific trainable weight matrices and X^2 denotes point-wise operation.

3   Experiments and Results

3.1   Datasets and Preprocessing

The proposed GQ-GCN model was evaluated on two datasets, namely BioImaging 2015 challenge (BI) dataset [17] and Databiox dataset [18].

The BI dataset consists of 249 histopathological images for training and 20 histopathological images for testing. There are 4 types of breast histopathological images including normal tissues, benign lesions, in situ carcinomas, and invasive carcinomas. These images are stained by hematoxylin and eosin (H&E) and have high resolution (2048 × 1536 pixels), the magnification factors of the images are 200×. Databiox dataset consists of 922 images obtained by using different magnifications (4×, 10×, 20×, 40×) on breast tumor tissues of 124 patients with invasive ductal carcinoma. We select 40× magnification data and crop the image into 2048 × 1536 pixels to remove the surrounding non-tissue area from datasets for training and testing in the experiment. The images of each class for both datasets are shown in Fig. 3.

We perform the following simple preprocessing: data augmentation by affine transformation including rotation (90°, 180°, 270°), flip horizontally to reduce over-fitting and normalization of the acquired histopathological image datasets.

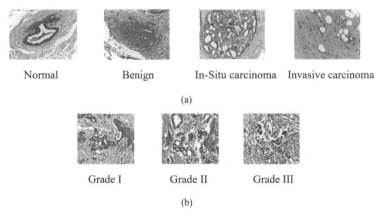

| Normal | Benign | In-Situ carcinoma | Invasive carcinoma |

(a)

Grade I   Grade II   Grade III

(b)

Fig. 3. (a) The images of four types of breast cancer on BI dataset. (b) Grading invasive ductal carcinomas in 40× on Databiox dataset.

3.2   Implementation Details

A set of experiments are presented to evaluate the GQ-GCN model as follows:

1) ResNet18 [19]: A classical CNN that uses residual connections.
2) GCN: GCN uses traditional three graph convolution layers [10] to learn the graph representation, which is generated using adaptive graph construction.

3) G-GCN: An improved GCN model that the graph convolution process utilizes the structure described in Sect. 2.2. The graph representation is generated using an adaptive graph construction method.

4) Q-GCN: An improved GCN model, which uses graph representation based on CNN-based adaptive graph construction and quadratic graph convolution operation layer instead of the traditional graph convolution layer.

In order to further verify the effectiveness of our proposed G-GCN structure using dual-branch (DB) features and fusion (FS) features for weighted addition as the final output features. The ablation experiments of the G-GCN and GQ-GCN are designed as follows:

1) DB: Only the output of the two branches $G_1^{''}$ and $G_2^{''}$ are weighted and added as the final output of the G-GCN structure.

2) FS: Only the fusion features G_{fu} is used as the final output of the G-GCN structure

The 5 fold cross-validation strategy is used to evaluate the proposed model. The widely used accuracy, precision, recall, F-score are selected as evaluation indices. The final results are presented with the format of the mean $\pm$ SD (standard deviation).

In all experiments, the CNN part is created by using the 4 residual blocks of ResNet18 (pre-trained on ImageNet [20]). The 'k' value in k-NN is selected as 8. Graph convolution layer is attached to the CNN, and the feature dimension of output nodes is 128 in the improved GCN module, then the output graph representation is used to predict the final result through the average squeeze pooling and two fully connected layers. Stochastic gradient descent is used optimizer with the batch size of 4, the learning rate is set as 0.001. The weight decay is set as 5e-4. Specifically, the quadratic graph convolution operations use the similar initialization method of the quadratic operation parameter used in [16].

3.3 Results

Table 1 shows the classification results of different models on the BI dataset. It can be found that our proposed GQ-GCN outperforms all the compared models with the best accuracy of $94.38 \pm 0.86\%$, precision of $94.61 \pm 0.80\%$, recall of $94.38 \pm 0.86\%$, F-score of $94.35 \pm 0.86\%$. The model including graph convolution operation has improved in each index as compared with the ResNet18, which shows the effectiveness of the adaptive graph construction module to generate a graph. Using the topological structure of the graph to take into account the spatial structure relationship in the histopathological images is more conducive for classification. Compared with the traditional GCN model, it can be observed that GQ-GCN improves 3.52%, 2.84%, 3.52%, 3.66% on the accuracy, precision, recall, and F-score, respectively.

Table 1. Classification results of different models on BI dataset (Unit: %)

	Accuracy	Precision	Recall	F-score
ResNet18	89.54 ± 1.55	90.61 ± 1.63	89.28 ± 0.95	89.06 ± 1.07
GCN	90.86 ± 1.57	91.77 ± 1.76	90.86 ± 1.57	90.69 ± 1.30
G-GCN	93.34 ± 1.47	93.64 ± 1.47	93.34 ± 1.47	93.31 ± 1.53
Q-GCN	91.93 ± 1.00	92.69 ± 0.89	92.11 ± 0.91	91.98 ± 1.02
GQ-GCN	**94.38 ± 0.86**	**94.61 ± 0.80**	**94.38 ± 0.86**	**94.35 ± 0.86**

Table 2 shows the compared results on the Databiox datasets. The proposed GQ-GCN model achieves the best performance of 83.49 ± 2.53%, 83.50 ± 2.61%, 83.38 ± 3.00%, 83.23 ± 2.82% on the accuracy, precision, recall, and F-score, respectively. Moreover, GQ-GCN improves 4.83%, 3.86%, 5.09%, and 5.02% on classification accuracy, precision, recall, and F-score, respectively as compared with the traditional GCN model.

Figure 4 shows the five indices including the sensitivity and specificity of the proposed models, where Q-GCN and G-GCN gained the overall advantage over GCN on the two datasets. It is obvious that the area of the GQ-GCN model is much larger than traditional GCN and has achieved the best pentagon. The results intuitively show the effectiveness of the model from various indicators.

Table 2. Classification results of different models on Databiox dataset (Unit: %)

	Accuracy	Precision	Recall	F-score
ResNet18	77.73 ± 2.57	78.66 ± 2.24	77.54 ± 2.43	77.67 ± 2.54
GCN	78.66 ± 2.44	79.64 ± 2.91	78.29 ± 2.30	78.21 ± 2.22
G-GCN	81.72 ± 2.23	82.42 ± 2.81	81.72 ± 2.23	81.66 ± 2.17
Q-GCN	79.52 ± 1.93	80.79 ± 2.27	79.49 ± 1.94	79.59 ± 1.91
GQ-GCN	**83.49 ± 2.53**	**83.50 ± 2.61**	**83.38 ± 3.00**	**83.23 ± 2.82**

The classification results using different output features of G-GCN structure in ablation experiments are shown in Table 3 and Table 4. In the G-GCN and GQ-GCN, it can be noticed that the best performance is achieved by using the DB feature and FS feature for weighted addition as the output of the G-GCN structure. The ablation experimental results illustrate the reliability of the G-GCN structure.

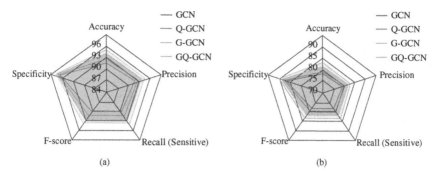

Fig. 4. Radar chart of various indicators comparing GCN improvement module to GCN on (a) BI dataset and (b) Databiox dataset.

Table 3. The ablation experiment results of DB feature output and FS feature output for G-GCN and GQ-GCN on the BI dataset (Unit: %)

	Accuracy	Precision	Recall	F-score
FS (G-GCN)	92.26 ± 2.10	92.86 ± 2.24	92.26 ± 2.10	92.27 ± 2.16
DB (G-GCN)	92.27 ± 1.04	92.55 ± 1.11	92.27 ± 1.12	92.24 ± 1.13
G-GCN	**93.34 ± 1.47**	**93.64 ± 1.47**	**93.34 ± 1.47**	**93.31 ± 1.53**
FS (GQ-GCN)	93.33 ± 2.60	94.07 ± 2.27	93.33 ± 2.60	93.30 ± 2.72
DB (GQ-GCN)	93.65 ± 2.11	93.89 ± 2.32	93.65 ± 2.12	93.61 ± 2.13
GQ-GCN	**94.38 ± 0.86**	**94.61 ± 0.80**	**94.38 ± 0.86**	**94.35 ± 0.86**

Table 4. The ablation experiment results of DB feature output and FS feature output for G-GCN and GQ-GCN on the Databiox dataset (Unit: %)

	Accuracy	Precision	Recall	F-score
FS (G-GCN)	81.06 ± 1.39	82.01 ± 1.64	81.06 ± 1.39	80.99 ± 1.51
DB (G-GCN)	81.28 ± 1.68	81.91 ± 1.57	81.28 ± 1.68	81.18 ± 1.64
G-GCN	**81.72 ± 2.23**	**82.42 ± 2.81**	**81.72 ± 2.23**	**81.66 ± 2.17**
FS (GQ-GCN)	82.38 ± 1.97	82.75 ± 2.50	82.38 ± 1.96	82.44 ± 1.97
DB (GQ-GCN)	82.60 ± 2.22	83.14 ± 2.39	82.60 ± 2.22	82.57 ± 2.13
GQ-GCN	**83.49 ± 2.53**	**83.50 ± 2.61**	**83.38 ± 3.00**	**83.23 ± 2.82**

4 Conclusion

In summary, a novel GQ-GCN model is proposed and achieves excellent performance in histopathological image classification. The GQ-GCN can use the features obtained by CNN to construct graph without any prior knowledge in training. The G-GCN module obtains fused features with stronger expressive ability by grouping the node features of the graph. The Q-GCN can effectively enhance the feature extraction and representation capabilities of the graph convolution neural units. Finally, the effectiveness of the GQ-GCN model combining Q-GCN and G-GCN is verified by experiments on two public datasets.

The current GQ-GCN is developed for the classification of histopathological image patches. In future work, we consider further attempts to combine our GQ-GCN with MIL to apply to the WSI-based CAD.

Acknowledgement. This work is supported by the National Natural Science Foundation of China (81830058, 81627804).

References

1. Gurcan, M.N., Boucheron, L.E., Can, A., et al.: Histopathological image analysis: a review. IEEE Rev. Biomed. Eng. **2**, 147–171 (2009)
2. Shi, J., Zheng, X., Wu, J., et al.: Quaternion Grassmann average network for learning representation of histopathological image. Pattern Recogn. **89**, 67–76 (2019)
3. Shi, J., Wu, J., Li, Y., et al.: Histopathological image classification with color pattern random binary hashing based PCANet and matrix-form classifier. IEEE J. Biomed. Health Inform. **21**(5), 1327–1337 (2017)
4. Veta, M., Pluim, J.P., Van Diest, P.J., et al.: Breast cancer histopathology image analysis: a review. IEEE Trans. Biomed. Eng. **61**(5), 1400–1411 (2014)
5. Komura, D., Ishikawa, S.: Machine learning methods for histopathological image analysis. Comput. Struct. Biotechnol. J. **16**, 34–42 (2018)
6. Wang, C., Shi, J., Zhang, Q., et al.: Histopathological image classification with bilinear convolutional neural networks. In: EMBS, pp. 4050–4053 (2017)
7. Alzubaidi, L., Al-Shamma, O., Fadhel, M.A., et al.: Optimizing the performance of breast cancer classification by employing the same domain transfer learning from hybrid deep convolutional neural network model. Electronics **9**(3), 445 (2020)
8. LeCun, Y., Bengio, Y., Hinton, G.: Deep learning. Nature **521**(7553), 436–444 (2015)
9. Choi, J., Seo, H., Im, S., et al.: Attention routing between capsules. In: ICCV, pp. 1981–1989 (2019)
10. Kipf, T.N., Welling, M.: Semi-supervised classification with graph convolutional networks. In: ICLR, pp. 1–14 (2017)
11. Zhou, Y., Graham, S., Shaban, M., et al.: CGC-Net: cell graph convolutional network for grading of colorectal cancer histology images. In: ICCV, pp. 388–398 (2019)
12. Li, R., Yao, J., Zhu, X., Li, Y., Huang, J.: Graph CNN for survival analysis on whole slide pathological images. In: Frangi, A.F., Schnabel, J.A., Davatzikos, C., Alberola-López, C., Fichtinger, G. (eds.) MICCAI 2018. LNCS, vol. 11071, pp. 174–182. Springer, Cham (2018). https://doi.org/10.1007/978-3-030-00934-2_20

13. Adnan, M., Kalra, S., Tizhoosh, H.R.: Representation learning of histopathology images using graph neural networks. In: CVPR, pp. 988–989 (2020)
14. Xu, K., Hu, W., Leskovec, J., et al.: How powerful are graph neural networks. In: ICLR, pp. 1–17 (2019)
15. Chen, Y., Fan, H., Xu, B., et al.: Drop an octave: reducing spatial redundancy in convolutional neural networks with octave convolution. In: ICCV, pp. 3435–3444 (2019)
16. Fan, F., Shan, H., Kalra, M.K., et al.: Quadratic autoencoder (Q-AE) for low-dose CT denoising. IEEE Trans. Med. Imaging **39**(6), 2035–2050 (2019)
17. Araújo, T., Aresta, G., Castro, E., et al.: Classification of breast cancer histology images using convolutional neural networks. PLoS ONE **12**(6), e0177544 (2017)
18. Bolhasani, H., Amjadi, E., Tabatabaeian, M., et al.: A histopathological image dataset for grading breast invasive ductal carcinomas. Inform. Med. Unlocked **19**, 100341 (2020)
19. He, K., Zhang, X., Ren, S., et al.: Deep residual learning for image recognition. In: CVPR, pp.770–778 (2016)
20. Jia, D., Wei, D., Socher, R., et al.: ImageNet: a large-scale hierarchical image database. In: CVPR, pp. 248–255 (2009)

Nuclei Grading of Clear Cell Renal Cell Carcinoma in Histopathological Image by Composite High-Resolution Network

Zeyu Gao[1,2], Jiangbo Shi[1,2], Xianli Zhang[1,2], Yang Li[1,2], Haichuan Zhang[1,2], Jialun Wu[1,2], Chunbao Wang[3], Deyu Meng[2,4], and Chen Li[1,2(✉)]

[1] School of Computer Science and Technology, Xi'an Jiaotong University, Xi'an, Shaanxi 710049, China
gzy4119105156@stu.xjtu.edu.cn

[2] National Engineering Lab for Big Data Analytics, Xi'an Jiaotong University, Xi'an, Shaanxi 710049, China
cli@xjtu.edu.cn

[3] Department of Pathology, the First Affiliated Hospital of Xi'an Jiaotong University, Xi'an 710061, China

[4] School of Mathematics and Statistics, Xi'an Jiaotong University, Xi'an, Shaanxi 710049, China

Abstract. The grade of clear cell renal cell carcinoma (ccRCC) is a critical prognostic factor, making ccRCC nuclei grading a crucial task in RCC pathology analysis. Computer-aided nuclei grading aims to improve pathologists' work efficiency while reducing their misdiagnosis rate by automatically identifying the grades of tumor nuclei within histopathological images. Such a task requires precisely segment and accurately classify the nuclei. However, most of the existing nuclei segmentation and classification methods can not handle the inter-class similarity property of nuclei grading, thus can not be directly applied to the ccRCC grading task. In this paper, we propose a Composite High-Resolution Network for ccRCC nuclei grading. Specifically, we propose a segmentation network called W-Net that can separate the clustered nuclei. Then, we recast the fine-grained nuclei classification into two cross-category classification tasks that are leaned by two newly designed high-resolution feature extractors (HRFEs). The two HRFEs share the same backbone encoder with W-Net by a composite connection so that meaningful features for the segmentation task can be inherited to the classification task. Last, a head-fusion block is applied to generate the predicted label of each nucleus. Furthermore, we introduce a dataset for ccRCC nuclei grading, containing 1000 image patches with 70945 annotated nuclei. We demonstrate that our proposed method achieves state-of-the-art performance compared to existing methods on this large ccRCC grading dataset.

Keywords: Nuclei grading · Nuclei segmentation · Histopathology

Electronic supplementary material The online version of this chapter (https://doi.org/10.1007/978-3-030-87237-3_13) contains supplementary material, which is available to authorized users.

M. de Bruijne et al. (Eds.): MICCAI 2021, LNCS 12908, pp. 132–142, 2021.
https://doi.org/10.1007/978-3-030-87237-3_13

1   Introduction

Clear cell renal cell carcinoma (ccRCC) is the most common subtype of renal cell carcinoma (RCC), making up about 80% of all cases. Grading of ccRCC has been recognized as a critical prognostic factor, where the overall five-year cancer-specific survival rate varies from 20% to 90% with different grades [1]. Recently, a novel grading guideline only bases upon nucleoli prominence for grades 1–3 is recommended and validated for both ccRCC and papillary (p) RCC by the international society of urologic pathologists (ISUP) and the world health organization (WHO), namely ISUP/WHO grading [2]. Practically, it is unfeasible for pathologists to recognize every single nucleus considering the large size of a tumor slide. Instead, pathologists usually select a few regions for diagnosis, which is rough and may missing some critical diagnostic information. Moreover, pathologists cannot avoid subjectivity and randomness, which may result in inconsistent diagnoses. To tackle these limitations, this paper focuses on developing an accurate computer-aided diagnosis (CAD) system for automatically identify the grade of each nucleus in ccRCC.

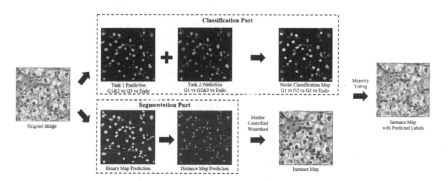

Fig. 1. Overview of the proposed nuclei grading method. G1, G2, and G3 denote tumor nuclei with grades 1 to 3 (green, yellow and red), Endo is the endothelial nuclei (blue). (Color figure online)

Deep learning based methods have been proven to be powerful for medical image analysis [3–5]. Accurate nuclei grading of ccRCC relies on the precise segmentation and the fine-grained classification of each nucleus. For precise segmentation, one popular paradigm is to model the segmentation task as a distance regression task via various methods [6–8], which has shown superior performance in nuclei segmentation. However, directly learn the distance map from the original image is very challenging, which requires a model to focus on both the foreground-background dissimilarity and the spatial information (shape and distance) of each foreground object. As for the nuclei classification, most advanced frameworks generally add a nuclei classification branch to a segmentation network [8,9]. Unlike the coarse-grained classification (e.g., tumor vs.

other types), the fine-grained ccRCC nuclei classification is more challenging because of the inter-class similarity property. Moreover, few existing datasets contain fine-grained labels for the nuclei grading task.

To tackle all the aforementioned limitations, we propose a novel method named Composite High-Resolution Network (CHR-Net) for the ccRCC nuclei grading task, as well as introduce a new dataset containing segmentation annotations and fine-grained labels of ccRCC nuclei. The proposed CHR-Net consists of a backbone encoder to extract features from the input image, a distance regression-based instance segmentation branch to segment each nucleus precisely, and a fine-grained classification branch to predict the grade of each nucleus. The overall framework of CHR-Net is shown in Fig. 1.

Specifically, to make the learning process of distance regression-based instance segmentation task easy and stable, we propose a two-stage network that composes of two U-Net-like networks, namely W-Net. The first network is used to predict the binary maps (i.e., background vs. foreground) that contain the shape information of nuclei. The second is a lightweight U-net, which takes the binary maps as inputs and predicts the distance maps.

In the classification branch, considering the inter-class similarity property of ccRCC nuclei grading, we divide the fine-grained classification task into two sub-tasks based on the ISUP/WHO grading guideline first and then generate the final predictions by a simple fusion block. Another key point for the fine-grained classification is how to maintain fine-grained features in the representation. To this end, we propose a high-resolution feature extractor (HRFE) based on HRNet [10] to maintain high-resolution representations throughout the whole classification branch and a composite connection [11] to inherit meaningful features from the backbone encoder to W-Net.

As a part of this work, we introduce a new dataset for ccRCC nuclei grading, which contains 70945 exhaustively annotated nuclei within four nuclei types (grades 1–3, endothelial). Extensive experiments conducted on this dataset demonstrate the state-of-the-art performance of CHR-Net.

2   Method

In this section we expatiate the proposed CHR-Net, and the architecture details are shown in Fig. 2. The backbone encoder of W-Net is a ResNet-34 [12] with global context attention [13]. The res-block used in HRFE is the same as the backbone encoder, which contains two 3×3 convolution layers and one shortcut layer. The simple-block has two 3×3 convolution layers, and the decoder-block contains one upsample, one shortcut, and two 3×3 convolution layers.

2.1   Instance Segmentation with W-Net

For instance segmentation, the distance regression schema has been proven to be effective. DIST [6] predicts the distance between nuclei pixels and their nearest

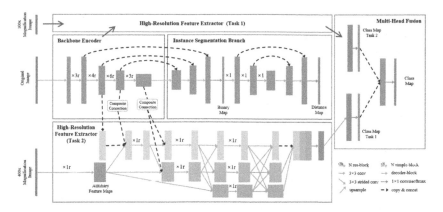

Fig. 2. Architecture details of CHR-Net. The HRFE of Task 1 is hidden for brief display and has the same structure with Task 2.

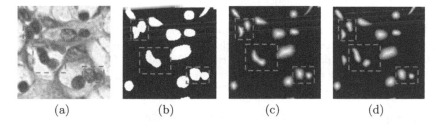

(a)   (b)   (c)   (d)

Fig. 3. Examples of touching nuclei. (a) Original image sub-patch. (b) Ground-truth binary map. (c) Ground-truth distance map. (d) Predicted distance map. Red rectangles indicate touching nuclei. The green rectangle represent a mislabeled nucleus which should be marked as two nuclei. (Color figure online)

background pixels. Center Vector Encoding [7] and HoVer-Net [8] further consider the horizontal and vertical distances. These works directly learn the mapping between the original image and the distance map through an end-to-end neural network, which is hard to capture all valuable features simultaneously.

Instead, we utilize a two-stage learning framework W-Net to accomplish this complex task by dividing it into two sub-tasks. This insight is similar to curriculum learning [14] which has been proven to be effective in histopathology image [15]. In the first stage, a U-Net with ResNet-34 backbone encoder is utilized to mine the dissimilarity between the nuclei and the background while generating the binary maps. In the second stage, we apply a lightweight U-net (LU-Net) to extract the shape and distance-related features from the generated binary maps, meanwhile, convert the binary maps into the distance maps.

As shown in Fig. 3(b), the shape of nuclei are mostly round or oval, but the touching nuclei have an extremely different pattern. We can see from Fig. 3(d) that by leveraging the strict mapping between the nuclei binary map and their distance map, the LU-Net bias the W-Net to separate the touching nuclei, even for the mislabeled one. Since the value of the distance map is continuous, L1 loss L_{dist} is adopted for the regression task in the second stage. And for the binary classification in the first stage, the binary cross-entropy loss L_{bc} is used.

To construct the distance map of each image, we adopt the same approach as DIST [6]. For the pixels of a nucleus, the corresponding values are defined by the distance between each pixel and the closest background pixel. Then we normalize the values of each nucleus to [0, 1].

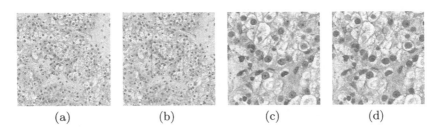

(a)   (b)   (c)   (d)

Fig. 4. Examples of the nuclei grade annotation. (a) Original image at 100x magnification. (b) with annotated masks. (c) Original image at 400x magnification. (d) with annotated masks. The purple, yellow and red masks indicate G1, G2 and G3 tumor nuclei, respectively. The endothelial nuclei are marked by blue. (Color figure online)

2.2   Composite High-Resolution Feature Extractor

For nuclei classification, a popular paradigm in prior works is performing classification after segmentation or detection [16]. Recently, some researches raise that accomplish both tasks (i.e. segmentation and classification) in a unified framework can improve the performance of both tasks. Besides, some public dataset are collected for nuclei classification, such as CoNSeP [8], PanNuke [17] and MoNuSAC [18]. Despite some works that pay attention to nuclei classification, most of them are coarse-grained and rarely focus on the fine-grained nuclei classification that requires grading the tumor nuclei by their appearance.

Furthermore, a major property of nuclei grading is the inter-class similarity that also brings a challenge in nuclei classification, and it appears when observing the tumor nuclei at different magnifications. Specifically, the ISUP grading system for ccRCC is based on the visibility of the nucleoli (as shown in Fig. 4). According to the grading principle, a tumor nuclei belongs to grade 1 if its nucleoli are invisible or small at 400x magnification, it belongs to grade 2 if it has conspicuous nucleoli at 400x magnification but inconspicuous at 100x, and belongs to grade 3 if its nucleoli are visible at 100x magnification. However, the grade 2 tumor nuclei are almost the same as grade 1 at 100x magnification, the same as grade 3 at 400x magnification, which may lead to inaccurate classification. Therefore, ignoring this property may increase the uncertainty of the model, thereby reducing the model performance.

To address this issue, we design two cross-category classification tasks with different auxiliary inputs, and then aggregate the probability maps of these two tasks by an 1×1 convolution layer to generate the final classification output.

The first task merges grade 1 and grade 2 into one category, and the second one merges grade 2 and grade 3. Meanwhile, the feature maps of 100x and 400x magnification images are taken as two auxiliary inputs, respectively. The original images are cropped from the 400x magnification WSIs, then we resize these images to 1/16 of the original size to obtain the 100x magnification images.

Another important point for fine-grained nuclei classification is to extract the semantically strong and spatially precise high-resolution representations. The U-net-like networks, which encode the input image with the high-to-low resolution convolutions and then recover the high-resolution representation from the low-resolution feature maps, have been successfully applied to nuclei segmentation. However, due to the loss of spatial details, the low-resolution feature maps are insufficient for the nuclei classification, especially for small nuclei, even though applying the skip-connection in the networks. Thereby, we propose the HRFE, which consists of a parallel high-to-low resolution convolutions network with three multi-resolution streams for extracting high-resolution features. The structure of HRFE is illustrated in Fig. 2. Different from HRNet [10] that has only one input, the original inputs of two HRFEs are 1) feature maps from the backbone encoder, and 2) the auxiliary feature maps from multi-scale images for different tasks. Furthermore, we adopt an accelerated version of the composite connection [11] that consists of an upsample and a 1×1 convolution layer with batch normalization to combine two HRFEs with the backbone encoder for the feature sharing of the multi-tasks.

The loss function of the classification part is composed of three terms, the categorical cross-entropy losses of the first task L_{mc1}, the second task L_{mc2} and the final classification output L_{mcf}. Finally, the overall loss function of CHR-Net is defined as:

$$L = \underbrace{\lambda_{bc}L_{bc} + \lambda_{dist}L_{dist}}_{segmentation\,part} + \underbrace{\lambda_{mc1}L_{mc1} + \lambda_{mc2}L_{mc2} + \lambda_{mcf}L_{mcf}}_{classification\,part}, \qquad (1)$$

where $\lambda_{bc}, ..., \lambda_{mcf}$ are the weight-balance parameter of each each loss. Empirically, we set $\lambda_{dist} = 2$ and the others to 1.

2.3   Post Processing

With the prediction of the binary and distance map, we perform a marker-controlled watershed to generate the instance segmentation map of each test image. Particularly, the same strategy of [6] is used to find all local maximums of the distance map, and then we take these local maximums as the marker to determine how to split the binary map.

To precisely identify the type of each nucleus, it is necessary to aggregate pixel-level type predictions to generate the type prediction of each nucleus instance. With the processed instance segmentation map, we use majority voting to obtain the most frequently appeared class of each nucleus instance in the nuclei classification map.

3   Experiments and Results

3.1   Dataset

A dataset for nuclei grading of ccRCC is proposed. To balance the data distribution of this dataset, we also include a part of papillary (p) RCC image patches, which follow the same nuclei grading guideline and have more high-grade nuclei. The entire dataset consists of 1000 H&E stained image patches with a resolution of 512×512. Two experienced pathologists are invited to select regions of interest (tumor regions) from 150 ccRCC, 50 pRCC WSIs derived from the KIRC, KIRP project of The Cancer Genome Atlas (TCGA) and scanned at 40x objective magnification. Within the tumor region of ccRCC and pRCC, there are mainly two types of nuclei, endothelial nuclei and tumor nuclei in grades 1 to 3. For each image patch, every nucleus is annotated by three well-trained annotators with OpenHI platform [19]. After annotation, majority voting is adapted to assign the type of each nucleus, and then these results are reviewed by pathologists. This dataset contains 70945 annotated nuclei that consist of 16652 endothelial nuclei and 54293 tumor nuclei (45108, 6406, 2779 for grades 1 to 3, respectively), totally in four classes.

3.2   Evaluation Metrics

The evaluation of the nuclei grading method needs to be executed in instance segmentation and classification, respectively. For instance segmentation, three metrics are applied: the dice coefficient that is a pixel-level metric, the Aggregated Jaccard Index (AJI) that is an object-level metric, and the panoptic quality (PQ) metric that is proposed in [20]. The PQ consists of two parts, detection quality, and segmentation quality. It has been proven to be an accurate and interpretable metric for nuclei segmentation [8,17].

For classification, following the same idea of MoNuSAC [18], the PQ of each class (i.e., PQ_1, PQ_2, PQ_3 and PQ_e) and the average PQ (aPQ) are adopted. The aPQ is the average of each PQ per class.

3.3   Results

We randomly divide the ccRCC grading dataset into training (70%), validation (10%), and testing (20%) set, for training and evaluation. We implement our method with the open-source library TensorFlow on a work-station with two NVIDIA 2080Ti GPUs. For training, data augmentations including flip, rotation, blur are applied to all the models. The dataset and the source code are available at: https://dataset.chenli.group/home/ccrcc-grading and https://github.com/ZeyuGaoAi/Composite_High_Resolution_Network.

Comparisons with State-of-the-Art Methods. We compare the proposed CHR-Net with U-Net, Mask-RCNN [21], Micro-Net [22] and HoVer-Net. For

Table 1. Nuclei classification comparison between our method and the state-of-the-art models on ccRCC Grading dataset.

Methods	Dice	AJI	PQ	aPQ	PQ_1	PQ_2	PQ_3	PQ_e
U-Net	0.8615	0.7344	0.6827	0.4776	0.6001	0.3659	0.5588	0.3857
Mask-RCNN	0.8657	0.7394	0.7126	0.4749	0.6297	0.3338	0.5423	0.3939
Micro-Net	0.8712	0.7375	0.7029	0.5107	0.6432	0.3780	0.6052	0.4163
HoVer-Net	0.8760	0.7440	0.7359	0.5068	0.6319	0.3761	0.5821	0.4370
CHR-Net	**0.8790**	**0.7519**	**0.7497**	**0.5458**	**0.6819**	**0.4027**	**0.6271**	**0.4713**

Table 2. Ablation study of different branches on ccRCC Grading dataset.

Branches	Dice	AJI	PQ	aPQ	PQ_1	PQ_2	PQ_3	PQ_e
SHR	0.8692	0.7233	0.6980	0.5064	0.6376	0.3827	0.5711	0.4342
MHR	0.8604	0.7244	0.7010	0.5156	0.6324	**0.4029**	0.5980	0.4291
MHR+UDist	0.8758	0.7280	0.7227	0.5235	0.6601	0.3950	0.5930	0.4460
MHR+WDist	**0.8790**	**0.7519**	**0.7497**	**0.5458**	**0.6819**	0.4027	**0.6271**	**0.4713**

U-Net and Micro-Net that are originally proposed for segmentation, we use an output dimension of 5 rather than 2. To balance the size of model parameters, the ResNet-34 backbone is used for CHR-Net, and the backbone encoders of U-Net, Mask-RCNN, and HoVer-Net are ResNet-50. We initialize the backbone encoders with pre-trained weights on the ImageNet and freeze their parameters for training 50 epochs, then fine-tune all the models for another 50 epochs. The adam optimizer with a 10^{-4} learning rate (10^{-5} after 25 epochs) is used for the training and fine-tuning.

The comparison results of each method are shown in Table 1. It can be seen that CHR-Net achieves the best performance on both segmentation and classification metrics. For nuclei segmentation, both U-Net and Micro-Net show the worse performance because they do not adopt any learning schema for the instance segmentation. HoVer-Net has the closest performance to CHR-Net (0.7359 vs. 0.7497 on PQ), but the distance map learned from the original image is sensitive to noise, thus leads to an over-segmentation problem in HoVer-Net. For nuclei classification and grading, CHR-Net significantly outperforms any other methods, *i.e.*, U-Net by 6.82%, Mask-RCNN by 7.09%, Micro-Net by 3.51%, and HoVer-Net by 3.9% on aPQ. Note that, Micro-Net achieves the second-best performance among all the methods. We suppose that the multi-resolution inputs of Micro-Net are beneficial to the ccRCC grading task as same as the auxiliary inputs from our method. The qualitative comparisons are provided in the supplementary file.

Ablation Study. We conduct four ablation experiments by using CHR-Net with different branches. SHR indicates the model that only has one HRFE for the four-class nuclei classification without using the segmentation branch. MHR represents the model that has two HRFEs for tasks 1 and 2. UDist and WDist denote two types of segmentation branches which are 1) the branch that learns the distance maps from original images with U-Net and 2) the branch that predicts the binary maps with W-Net, respectively. From Table. 2, we can observe that MHR achieves higher PQ values than SHR on grades 2 and 3, which demonstrates the usefulness of learning the proposed two cross-category classification tasks. Due to the additional branches of instance segmentation, MHR+UDist and MHR+WDist have better segmentation performance than MHR. Compare with MHR+UDist, MHR+WDist utilizes the two-stage learning strategy to achieve a higher Dice, AJI, and PQ. Meanwhile, affected by the segmentation performance, the PQ values of grades 1, 3, and endothelial from MHR+WDist are also significantly increased, and the average PQ is 3.94% higher than the base model SHR. It is worth mentioning that without using the segmentation branch, the PQ_1 and PQ_e of SHR are much higher than U-Net (3.75% and 4.85%), which illustrates the effectiveness of the proposed HRFE.

4   Conclusion

In this paper, we proposed a novel nuclei segmentation and classification method, especially for nuclei grading. A corresponding dataset of ccRCC nuclei grading was introduced and evaluated. Integrating with cancer region detection [23], the whole automatic nuclei grading system can reduce the burden of pathologists and further provide quantitative data (see in supplementary file) for cancer research. We hope that the downstream tasks of nuclei segmentation and classification can draw more attention and our work can inspire other researchers with similar challenges.

Acknowledgements. This work has been supported by the National Key Research and Development Program of China (2018YFC0910404); This work has been supported by National Natural Science Foundation of China (61772409); The consulting research project of the Chinese Academy of Engineering (The Online and Offline Mixed Educational Service System for "The Belt and Road" Training in MOOC China); Project of China Knowledge Centre for Engineering Science and Technology; The innovation team from the Ministry of Education (IRT_17R86); and the Innovative Research Group of the National Natural Science Foundation of China (61721002). The results shown here are in whole or part based upon data generated by the TCGA Research Network: https://www.cancer.gov/tcga.

References

1. Delahunt, B., Eble, J.N., Egevad, L., Samaratunga, H.: Grading of renal cell carcinoma. Histopathology **74**(1), 4–17 (2019). https://doi.org/10.1111/his.13735
2. Delahunt, B., ET AL.: The international society of urological pathology (ISUP) grading system for renal cell carcinoma and other prognostic parameters. Am. J. Surgical Pathol. **37**(10), 1490–1504 (2013)

3. Zhao, R., et al.: Rethinking dice loss for medical image segmentation. In: 2020 IEEE International Conference on Data Mining (ICDM), pp. 851–860 (2020). https://doi.org/10.1109/ICDM50108.2020.00094
4. Xie, C., et al.: Recist-net: Lesion detection via grouping keypoints on recist-based annotation. In: 2021 IEEE 18th International Symposium on Biomedical Imaging (ISBI), pp. 921–924 (2021). https://doi.org/10.1109/ISBI48211.2021.9433794
5. Zhang, X., et al.: Classifying breast cancer histopathological images using a robust artificial neural network architecture. In: Rojas, I., Valenzuela, O., Rojas, F., Ortuño, F. (eds.) IWBBIO 2019. LNCS, vol. 11465, pp. 204–215. Springer, Cham (2019). https://doi.org/10.1007/978-3-030-17938-0_19
6. Naylor, P., Laé, M., Reyal, F., Walter, T.: Segmentation of nuclei in histopathology images by deep regression of the distance map. IEEE Trans. Med. Imaging **38**(2), 448–459 (2019). https://doi.org/10.1109/TMI.2018.2865709
7. Li, J., Hu, Z., Yang, S.: Accurate nuclear segmentation with center vector encoding. In: Chung, A.C.S., Gee, J.C., Yushkevich, P.A., Bao, S. (eds.) IPMI 2019. LNCS, vol. 11492, pp. 394–404. Springer, Cham (2019). https://doi.org/10.1007/978-3-030-20351-1_30
8. Graham, S., et al.: Hover-net: simultaneous segmentation and classification of nuclei in multi-tissue histology images. Med. Image Anal. **58**, 101563 (2019). https://doi.org/10.1016/j.media.2019.101563
9. Qu, H., et al.: Joint segmentation and fine-grained classification of nuclei in histopathology images. In: 2019 IEEE 16th International Symposium on Biomedical Imaging (ISBI 2019), pp. 900–904 (2019). https://doi.org/10.1109/ISBI.2019.8759457
10. Wang, J., et al.: Deep high-resolution representation learning for visual recognition. IEEE Trans. Pattern Anal. Mach. Intell. 1 (2020). https://doi.org/10.1109/TPAMI.2020.2983686
11. Liu, Y., et al.: Cbnet: a novel composite backbone network architecture for object detection. In: Proceedings of the AAAI Conference on Artificial Intelligence, vol. 34, pp. 11653–1166, April 2020. https://doi.org/10.1609/aaai.v34i07.6834
12. He, K., Zhang, X., Ren, S., Sun, J.: Deep residual learning for image recognition. In: The IEEE Conference on Computer Vision and Pattern Recognition (CVPR), June 2016
13. Cao, Y., Xu, J., Lin, S., Wei, F., Hu, H.: Gcnet: non-local networks meet squeeze-excitation networks and beyond. In: Proceedings of the IEEE/CVF International Conference on Computer Vision (ICCV) Workshops, October 2019
14. Bengio, Y., Louradour, J., Collobert, R., Weston, J.: Curriculum learning. In: ICML 2009, p. 41–48. Association for Computing Machinery, New York (2009). https://doi.org/10.1145/1553374.1553380
15. Kang, Q., Lao, Q., Fevens, T.: Nuclei segmentation in histopathological images using two-stage learning. In: Shen, D., et al. (eds.) Medical Image Computing and Computer Assisted Intervention - MICCAI 2019, pp. 703–711. Springer, Cham (2019). https://doi.org/10.1007/978-3-030-32239-7_78
16. Automatic cell nuclei segmentation and classification of breast cancer histopathology images. Signal Process. **122**, 1–13 (2016). https://doi.org/10.1016/j.sigpro.2015.11.011
17. Gamper, J., et al.: Pannuke dataset extension, insights and baselines. arXiv preprint arXiv:2003.10778 (2020)
18. Verma, R., Kumar, N., Patil, A., Kurian, N., Rane, S., Sethi, A.: Multi-organ nuclei segmentation and classification challenge 2020 (2020). https://doi.org/10.13140/RG.2.2.12290.02244/1

19. Puttapirat, P., et al.: Openhi - an open source framework for annotating histopathological image. In: 2018 IEEE International Conference on Bioinformatics and Biomedicine (BIBM), pp. 1076–1082 (2018). https://doi.org/10.1109/BIBM.2018.8621393
20. Kirillov, A., He, K., Girshick, R., Rother, C., Dollár, P.: Panoptic segmentation. In: 2019 IEEE/CVF Conference on Computer Vision and Pattern Recognition (CVPR), pp. 9396–9405 (2019). https://doi.org/10.1109/CVPR.2019.00963
21. He, K., Gkioxari, G., Dollar, P., Girshick, R.: Mask R-CNN. In: Proceedings of the IEEE International Conference on Computer Vision (ICCV), October 2017
22. Raza, S.E.A., et al.: Micro-net: a unified model for segmentation of various objects in microscopy images. Med. Image Anal. **52**, 160–173 (2019). https://doi.org/10.1016/j.media.2018.12.003
23. Gao, Z., Puttapirat, P., Shi, J., Li, C.: Renal cell carcinoma detection and subtyping with minimal point-based annotation in whole-slide images. In: International Conference on Medical Image Computing and Computer-Assisted Intervention, pp. 439–448. Springer (2020). https://doi.org/10.1007/978-3-030-59722-1_42

Prototypical Models for Classifying High-Risk Atypical Breast Lesions

Akash Parvatikar[1], Om Choudhary[1], Arvind Ramanathan[2], Rebekah Jenkins[1], Olga Navolotskaia[3], Gloria Carter[3], Akif Burak Tosun[4], Jeffrey L. Fine[3], and S. Chakra Chennubhotla[1,4(✉)]

[1] Department of Computational and Systems Biology, University of Pittsburgh, Pittsburgh, USA
{akp47,opc3,rcj17,chakracs}@pitt.edu
[2] Data Science and Learning, Argonne National Laboratory, Lemont, IL, USA
ramanathana@anl.gov
[3] Department of Pathology, UPMC Magee-Womens Hospital, Pittsburgh, USA
{navolotskaiao,finejl}@upmc.edu, cartgj@mail.magee.edu
[4] SpIntellx Inc., Pittsburgh, USA
{burak,chakra}@spintellx.com

Abstract. High-risk atypical breast lesions are a notoriously difficult dilemma for pathologists who diagnose breast biopsies in breast cancer screening programs. We reframe the computational diagnosis of atypical breast lesions as a problem of prototype recognition on the basis that pathologists mentally relate current histological patterns to previously encountered patterns during their routine diagnostic work. In an unsupervised manner, we investigate the relative importance of ductal (global) and intraductal patterns (local) in a set of pre-selected prototypical ducts in classifying atypical breast lesions. We conducted experiments to test this strategy on subgroups of breast lesions that are a major source of inter-observer variability; these are benign, columnar cell changes, epithelial atypia, and atypical ductal hyperplasia in order of increasing cancer risk. Our model is capable of providing clinically relevant explanations to its recommendations, thus it is intrinsically explainable, which is a major contribution of this work. Our experiments also show state-of-the-art performance in recall compared to the latest deep-learning based graph neural networks (GNNs).

Keywords: Atypical breast lesions · Prototype-based recognition · Diagnostic explanations · Digital and computational pathology

1 Introduction

Breast cancer screening and early detection can help reduce the incidence and mortality rates [19]. Although effective, screening relies on accurate pathological diagnoses of breast biopsies for more than one million women per year in the

Electronic supplementary material The online version of this chapter (https://doi.org/10.1007/978-3-030-87237-3_14) contains supplementary material, which is available to authorized users.

© Springer Nature Switzerland AG 2021
M. de Bruijne et al. (Eds.): MICCAI 2021, LNCS 12908, pp. 143–152, 2021.
https://doi.org/10.1007/978-3-030-87237-3_14

US [4,18]. Most benign and malignant biopsy diagnoses are straightforward, but a subset are a significant source of disagreement between pathologists and are particularly troublesome for clinicians. Pathologists are expected to triage their patients' biopsies rapidly and accurately, and they have routines for difficult or ambiguous cases (e.g., second-opinion consults, additional stains). Still, disagreement remains an issue; while the literature suggests that diagnosis should be straightforward if diagnostic rules are followed [17], concordance remains elusive in real world diagnosis, reported in one study as low as 48% [4].

Our Approach: In this study, we focus on modeling and differentiating difficult breast lesion subtypes: atypical ductal hyperplasia (ADH), flat epithelial atypia (FEA), columnar cell changes (CCC), and Normal (including usual ductal hyperplasia (UDH) and very simple non-columnar ducts). Our approach originates from the method that pathologists practice, which is to carefully assess alterations in breast ducts before making diagnostic decisions [8,10,19]. Pathologists continually observe tissue patterns and make decisions supported by the morphology. In doing so, they look at an entire duct (*global*) and patterns within portions of the duct (*local*) striving to generate mental associations with prototypical ducts and/or their parts they previously encountered in training or clinical practice. We propose an end-to-end computational pathology model that can imitate this diagnostic process and provide explanations for inferred labels.

We hypothesize that ductal regions-of-interest (ROIs) having similar global and local features will have similar diagnostic labels and some features are more important than others when making diagnostic decisions. Our approach is related to other prototypes-driven image recognition systems that favor visual interpretability [3,6,16].

Contributions: To the best of our knowledge, our work is the first one to: (1) use a diverse set of concordant *prototype* images (diagnostic class agreed by all 3 pathologists) for learning, (2) characterize clinically relevant global and local properties in breast histopathology images, and (3) provide explanations by measuring the relative importance of prototype features, global and local, for the differential diagnosis of breast lesions. We also show that our approach facilitates diagnostic explanations with accuracies comparable to the state-of-the-art methods.

2   Related Work

Although there have been numerous efforts in using prototypes for scene recognition [3,6,16], to date, this idea has not been explored to classify breast lesions. One of the first studies to detect high-risk breast lesions was proposed in [20] which was based on encoding cytological and architectural properties of cells within the ducts. The work in [12] used structural alterations of the ducts as features to classify breast lesions into benign, atypia, ductal carcinoma in-situ (DCIS), and invasive. A different approach was proposed in [13], where the authors used analytical models to find clusters within ROIs with strong histologically relevant structures. However, their approach lacked a good learning strategy to infer the diagnostic label from these clusters. Further, two recent studies approached this problem using attention-based networks to generate global representation of breast biopsy images [11] and biological entity-based graph neural networks (GNNs) [14] (also tested as a baseline method in Table 2). Both methods were tested on an unbalanced dataset like ours and both reported low performance measures in detecting high-risk lesions.

3   Methodology

3.1   Machine Learning Framework

In this paper, we propose an end-to-end computational pathology system that models the entire duct (global) and the patterns occurring within selective portions of the duct (local) with the goal of generating associations with similar ducts and/or parts (prototypical). *We hypothesize that images with one or more ducts having similar global and local features will have similar diagnostic labels and some features are more important than others when making diagnostic decisions.* We will first introduce a composite mapping function to learn the relative importance of global and local features in a prototype set $\mathcal{P}$ for differential diagnoses:

$$h(x; \mathcal{P}) = \sum_{k=1}^{p} \beta_k \left[\exp^{-\lambda_k^G c_k(x)} \times \prod_{j=1}^{m_k} \exp^{-\lambda_{kj}^L f_{kj}(x)} \right]. \tag{1}$$

Here $h(x; \mathcal{P})$ captures the association of a previously unseen image x with a set of prototype images in $\mathcal{P}$. The index k varies over the images in the prototype set $\mathcal{P}$ (size $= p$), while j indexes over a local feature set (size $= m_k$) in a given prototype image indexed by k. β_k determines if the resemblance of a previously unseen image x to the prototype k has a positive (β_+) or negative influence (β_-). λ_k^G and λ_{kj}^L indicate the relative importance of global (ductal) and local (intra-ductal) features in the prototype k respectively. The relative importance can be imagined as a distance measure, so we enforce non-negativity constraints on λ_k^G and λ_{kj}^L values. The functions $c_k(x)$ and $f_{kj}(x)$ compute the global and local differences respectively between x and the prototype set $\mathcal{P}$ (more details below). Finally, in formulating $h(x; \mathcal{P})$ we assume that the prototype images are independent and that the global and local information in each prototype can be functionally disentangled into a product form.

Since our goal is to learn the relative importance of global and local features in a prototype set, we solve the following optimization problem:

$$\underset{\beta, \lambda}{\arg\min} \, \mathcal{L}(\beta, \lambda) = \arg\min \sum_{i=1}^{n} \mathrm{CrsEnt}(\sigma(h(x_i)), y_i) + C_\beta ||\beta||^2 + C_\lambda |\lambda| \tag{2}$$

using gradient descent. We use cross-entropy loss function (CrsEnt) to penalize misclassifications on the training set $\mathcal{X} = \{x_i\}$ and to obtain $\beta_{\text{optimal}} = \{\beta_k\}$ and $\lambda_{\text{optimal}} = \{\lambda_k^G, \lambda_{kj}^L\}$. We use a $tanh(\sigma)$ activation function on $h(x)$ from Eq. 1. To avoid overfitting, we invoke ℓ_2^2 and ℓ_1 regularization with coefficients C_β and C_λ respectively. Following the intuition that a pathologist might pay no attention to some features, e.g., small-round nuclei do not feature typically in the diagnosis of ADH, we choose ℓ_1 regularization for λ to sparsify the weights.

3.2 Encoding Global and Local Descriptions of a Duct

The functions $c_k(x)$ and $f_{kj}(x)$ in Eq. 1 compute the global and local differences between input image x and prototype set $\mathcal{P}$, as outlined in the steps below.

Step 1: For a proof-of-concept, we adopt the approach from [13] to build analytical models of 16 diagnostically relevant histological patterns following the guidelines presented in the WHO classification of tumors of the breast [8].

Analytical model of a cribriform pattern: Fig. 1 illustrates how to model a histological pattern, *cribriform*, that is critical to diagnosing ADH. By considering a spatial neighborhood of 100 µm around each cell (Fig. 1A) in ground-truth annotations of cribriform patterns in ROIs, the model incorporates three different components (Fig. 1B): (1) polarization of epithelial cells around lumen inside the ROI; (2) distance of any given nucleus in the ROI to two nearest lumen; and (3) circularity of lumen structure adjacent to a nucleus inside the ROI. For the ROI in Fig. 1A, the analytical models driving these three components are: (1) mixture of Gaussians (MoG) ($\mu_1 = 0.87, \mu_2 = 0.94, \mu_3 = 0.72$, $\sigma_1 = 0.002, \sigma_2 = 0.002, \sigma_3 = 0.003$, $\pi_1 = 0.44, \pi_2 = 0.35, \pi_3 = 0.21$) for modeling the distribution of clustering coefficients [21]; (2) Gamma distribution ($\alpha = 3.11$, $\beta = 34.37$) for modeling distance values to lumen and (3) a uniform distribution ($a = 0.2$, $b = 0.92$) to model the circularity values of nuclei inside the ROI. We further combine these three components with a mixture model, performing grid-search to optimize the mixing coefficients (Fig. 1B), to form the histological pattern of cribriform (P_{gt}^{crib}).

We pursue a similar approach to modeling other histological patterns using ground-truth ROI annotations: 1. *small*, 2. *large*, 3. *round*, 4. *crowded*, and 5. *spaced*, each modeled as a Gamma distribution; 6. *elliptical*, 7. *large-round*, 8. *small-elliptical*, 9. *spaced-large*, 10. *crowded-small*, 11. *spaced-small*, 12. *crowded-elliptical*, and 13. *spaced-round* each modeled as two-component MoG; and more complex patterns 14. *large-round-spaced*, 15. *picket-fence*, and 16. *cribriform* using a combination of Gamma, MoG, and Uniform distributions. Details on parameter estimation are discussed in [13].

Generating Likelihood Scores: Next, to compare ground-truth model of any histological pattern P_{gt} with a new model generated from the reference nucleus of an input image (P_{new}), we use two distance measures, 2-sample Kolmogorov-Smirnov

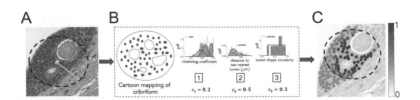

Fig. 1. Modeling cribriform pattern in a sample ROI (A) using parametric models for three component patterns in (B) and generating cell-level likelihood scores (C). Ductal region and intra-ductal lumen are outlined in red in (A). (Color figure online)

test and Kullback-Leibler divergence to compare Gamma and MoG distributions respectively. To map smaller distances that indicate stronger presence of the feature, we compute likelihood scores by applying an inverted S-function on the distances. In Fig. 1C the final likelihood score from evaluating the cribriform pattern is a weighted sum of the likelihood scores of the component patterns. A similar operation is carried out for generating cell-level likelihood scores for the remaining 15 features. The principal advantage of these analytical models is in their ability to handle heterogeneity that emerges from running imprecise low-level image processing routines, such as methods for segmenting nuclei or identifying boundaries of ductal ROIs. The heatmap visualization in Fig. 1C is a mechanism for explaining the model to pathologists, informing where these patterns are and how strongly they influence the overall diagnosis of a ROI.

Step 2: To encode the global description of a duct, we will represent it by a matrix of size $n \times l$ populated with likelihood scores, where n and l refer to the total number of cells and the number of histomorphological patterns respectively ($l = 16$). Additionally, we include the size of the largest duct if the ROI has a cluster of ducts. However, considering only the global information may lead to diagnostic inconsistencies. For example, a duct resembling FEA is better diagnosed as ADH if it contains a local cribriform pattern or as a CCC duct if it contains some hyperplasia (further meriting a comparison of local hyperplastic area with models of FEA/ADH).

Step 3: To encode the local description of a duct, we adopt a strategy followed by most expert pathologists. To this extent, for every histomorphological pattern, we identify islands within the duct where that particular feature is dominant and consider the largest island for further analysis. We detect feature islands by performing non-maxima suppression on cell-level likelihood scores using a threshold (=0.8) based on cross-validation.

Step 4: Finally, we have the machinery to compute the functions $c_k(x)$ and $f_{kj}(x)$ from Eq. 1. We define $c_k(x) = \|d(p_k, x)\|$, where a small value of $c_k(x)$ implies high similarity of image x to prototype p_k. We combine two measures to generate d: Kolmogorov-Smirnov test comparing 16-dim probability distributions of cell-level likelihood scores individually between x and p_k and an inverted S-function on the ratio of the duct sizes between x and p_k. This leads to a 17-dim vector d, which is further compressed by its ℓ_2 norm to obtain a single scalar value $c_k(x)$ for every pair of x and p_k. We further simplify the computation of $f_{kj}(x)$ by applying an inverted S-function on the ratio of the largest feature island sizes from the same histological feature between x and p_k, suitably modified to account for islands that are missing in either x or p_k.

4   Results and Discussion

4.1   Dataset

We collected a cohort of 93 WSIs which were labeled by an expert pathologist on the team to contain at least one ADH ROI. The breast biopsy slides were scanned

Table 1. Statistics of the atypical breast lesion ROI dataset

Prototype Set	PS-1	PS-2	PS-3		Class	NORMAL	CCC	FEA	ADH	Total
No. of ROIs	20	20	30		Train	420	99	116	119	754
No. of feature islands	84	86	145		Test	371	105	33	32	541

at 0.5 μm/pixel resolution at 20× magnification using the Aperio ScanScope XT (Leica Biosystems) microscope from which 1295 ductal ROI images of size $\approx 1K \times 1K$ pixels were extracted using a duct segmentation algorithm described in [13]. Briefly, the algorithm first breaks down the image into non-overlapping superpixels and then evaluates each superpixel's stain level together with its neighboring superpixels and assigns probabilities of them belonging to a duct. These guesses are then used to perform Chan-Vese region-based active contour segmentation algorithm [2] that separates the foreground (i.e., ducts) from the background.

We collected ground truth annotations of extracted ROIs from 3 breast pathology sub-specialists (P1, P2, and P3), who labeled the ROIs with one of the four diagnostic categories: Normal, CCC, FEA, and ADH. The diagnostic concordance for the four categories among P1, P2, and P3 were moderate with a Fleiss' kappa score of ≈ 0.55 [20]. The entire dataset was split into two sets.

i. Prototype set: We formed three prototype sets (PS-1, PS-2, and PS-3) containing ROIs with consensus diagnostic labels from the 3 pathologists having a balanced distribution over the four diagnostic categories. The final set of prototype ROIs were verified by P1 to confirm adequate variability is obtained. The number of aforementioned *islands* are also listed in Table 1.

ii. Train and test set: The training set consists of 754 ROIs labeled by P1 and the test set contains 541 ROIs consensus labeled by P1-P3. The training and test set were separated at WSI level to avoid over-fitting, since ROIs belonging to the same WSI can be correlated histologically. Due to limited number of ROIs belonging to the non-Normal category as seen in Table 1, the ROIs which do not participate in the prototype set were also included in the dataset.

4.2   Model Training and Evaluation

Our ML model (Eq. 1) is trained to minimize the objective function (Eq. 2) using gradient descent (learning rate $= 1 \times 10^{-4}$ and convergence tolerance $= 1 \times 10^{-3}$). Regularization coefficients C_β and C_λ were initialized to 2. To speed up convergence, we shuffle the training data after each iteration so that successive training examples rarely belong to the same class. Prior to training, the model parameters β and λ were initialized with weights randomly drawn from *LeCun normal* [9]. After each iteration, the parametric values of the objective function ($\mathcal{L}$), error-rate (ϵ), β, and λ are stored. After model convergence, we use β_{optimal} and λ_{optimal} parameters in the mapping function (1) to obtain h_{test}. We generate prediction probabilities p by first applying a $tanh$ (σ) activation to h_{test} and then projecting it to the positive octant. If $p \geq 0.5$, the diagnostic label is 1 and 0 otherwise.

4.3 Baseline Models (B1-B3)

Following the method laid out in [14], we define two baseline models, B1 and B2, by re-implementing their cell-graph GNNs. We chose GNNs, a recently emerged state-of-the-art technique for encoding spatial organizations, over pixel-based convolutional neural networks (CNNs) as our experiments with CNNs showed poor performances in capturing the spatial context [13]. B1 is obtained by generating a cell-graph topology and cells within each graph are embedded with cytological features as in [14]. To assess the effect of histological patterns in cell embeddings, we generate B2 by replacing the duct-level cytological features with likelihood scores generated by our method. Finally, B3 is obtained by implementing a Logistic Regression classifier using the duct-level likelihood scores, following a similar strategy as in [13].

Table 2. Diagnostic results from the binary classification task expressed in %

	Model	Baseline			PS-1			PS-2			PS-3		
		B1	B2	B3	G1	L1	GL1	G2	L2	GL2	G3	L3	GL3
HR	R	56±6	68±6	62±3	66±4	71±1	73±4	68±4	72±2	68±3	66±7	74±2	69±3
	wF	77±2	82±3	76±1	65±2	61±1	65±1	67±4	61±1	63±2	63±1	64±1	64±1
ADH	R	38±8	45±7	56±3	70±7	61±8	78±8	59±13	80±4	71±4	72±6	70±11	68±5
	wF	78±4	86±2	79±1	70±3	64±2	67±5	64±3	62±1	60±6	64±2	67±1	64±1
FEA	R	48±12	40±6	35±4	54±6	64±5	68±7	58±6	60±3	63±5	63±6	67±2	62±5
	wF	81±5	82±3	78±1	71±2	65±2	69±3	66±4	66±3	69±3	66±2	69±2	66±3

4.4 Classification Results

For the sake of differential diagnosis of atypical breast lesions, we implemented several models using global (G), local (L), and both global and local information (GL) from three prototype sets (PS1-PS3) and compared it with the baseline models (B1-B3) (see Table 2). During the training step of each model, we created a balanced training set by randomly subsampling ROIs from each category so that we have equal number of ROIs for each classification category. To check for statistical significance, for each classification task, we run our ML algorithm on 10 training sets wherein the images are randomly selected and we report the classification scores as the mean and standard deviation over 10 runs (Table 2). The top panel of Table 2 (HR row) compares the classification performance of low-risk (Normal+CCC, −ve class) vs high-risk (FEA+ADH, +ve class) cases. For each diagnostic category (+ve class), we further implemented a different binary classifier for each modeling strategy proposed. The bottom panel of Table 2 (ADH and FEA row) shows the comparative performances of ADH- and FEA-vs-rest diagnostic classification. We highlight results from high-risk category because ADH lesion presents both - a risk of currently existing cancer (about 4%) and there is a high absolute future risk of about 1% per year, up to 30% lifetime risk [5]. FEA lesion combines the nuclear atypia seen in ADH, but lacks hyperplasia and has simpler architecture [7]. Some patients with FEA will be offered surgery and they would also be treated as high-risk in the future.

Performance Metrics: For each classification scenario, we use *recall* (R) as the performance metric to focus on the correct detection of positive class, since there is a significant class imbalance (see Table 1) and the consequence of misdiagnosis (false negative) implies increased chance of developing cancer with lack of providing early treatment. We include *weighted F-measure* (wF) as an additional metric which gives importance to the correct detection of both positive and negative classes [15]. The class specific weights in wF are proportional to the number of positive and negative examples present in the test set.

Classification Performance: We highlight the best *recall* performances in Table 2, that are achieved using state-of-the-art baseline models against our method in black and gray boxes, respectively. Our method shows significant improvement ($p < 0.01$) in detecting diagnostically critical high-risk ADH and FEA ROIs compared to the baseline methods (the best average recall achieved is 80% for ADH classifier and 68% for FEA). We also observe that baseline models are performing better on detecting Normal ROIs (see Supp. Table 1 for comparative results of CCC-, and Normal-vs-rest classification). This behaviour explains higher weighted F-measure of baseline models in low- vs. high-risk classification, since in the testing set low-risk ROIs are 7-fold more than high-risk ROIs (i.e., baseline models are biased to detect low-risk lesions even when the training set was balanced). It is critical to note that real-life clinical observance of high-risk lesions is also around 15% [8], which is naturally reflected in our testing set, and it is crucial to catch these less-seen high-risk lesions for pre-cancer interventions while being able to provide diagnostic explanations to given recommendations.

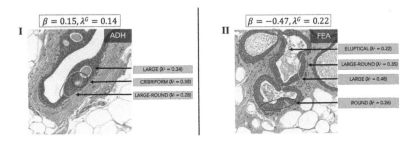

Fig. 2. Highlighting the relative importance of the global and local features from different prototypes (I and II) in ADH-vs-rest classifier.

4.5   Discussion

The explainability of our model is depicted in Fig. 2, which shows that our model leverages both global (λ_G) and local (λ_L) information of the ductal ROIs of two prototypical images, I and II, in detecting ADH from one of the experiments using GL3 classifier built using prototype set PS3. The values of model parameters: absolute change in the objective function ($\Delta\mathcal{L}$), training error-rate (ϵ),

β, and λ after each iteration are shown in Supp. Figure 1 and more examples of explainability are shown in Supp. Figure 2. Figure 2-I positively guides in detecting ADH category ($\beta = 0.15$) whereas Fig. 2-II is counterintuitive in detecting ADH lesions ($\beta = -0.47$). Although two of the histological feature islands, large and large-round present within these ROIs overlap, we assert that the absence of complex architectural pattern such as cribriform within Fig. 2-II might have led to a negative influence of this prototype's influence to detect ADH. Although it is possible that an FEA type lesion could be upgraded to ADH pathologically without cribriform architecture, this would require thickening of the duct lining to more than 5 cell layers which is uncommon in clinical practice.

Computational Cost: The entire pipeline is implemented in native Python 3.8. Total time required to obtain a diagnostic label with computation of all features for a previously unseen ROI is less than $30s$ on a 64-bit single $3.4\,GHz$ Intel Xeon processor.

Limitations: (1) Features like *bulbous micropapillae* and *rigid cellular bars* which are diagnostically relevant to high-risk lesions are missing; (2) Selection of prototypes was made on the basis of expert visual inspection. There is a need for more sophisticated statistical approaches [1] for prototype selection and (3) for a more detailed ablation study to test the robustness and reliability of our ML framework; (4) To offset the issue of unbalanced datasets, we are collecting expert annotations on additional high-risk lesion images.

Future Work: Our intent is to create an approach that generalizes, not only to other, more straightforward breast diagnoses but also to tissue histologies from other organs. Explainable machine learning approaches like ours will support pathologists during their transition to digital and computational pathology.

Acknowledgments. The grant NIH-NCI U01CA204826 to SCC supported this work. The work of AP and OC was partially supported by the sub-contracts 9F-60178 and 9F-60287 from Argonne National Laboratory (ANL) to the University of Pittsburgh from the parent grant DE-AC02-06CH1135 titled, Co-Design of Advanced Artificial Intelligence Systems for Predicting Behavior of Complex Systems Using Multimodal Datasets, from the Department of Energy to ANL.

References

1. Bien, J., Tibshirani, R.: Prototype selection for interpretable classification. Ann. Appl. Statist. **5**, 2403–2424 (2011)
2. Chan, T.F., et al.: Active contours without edges. IEEE Trans. Image Process. **10**(2), 266–277 (2001)
3. Chen, C., Li, O., Tao, D., Barnett, A., Rudin, C., Su, J.K.: This looks like that: deep learning for interpretable image recognition. In: Advances in Neural Information Processing Systems, pp. 8930–8941 (2019)
4. Elmore, J.G., et al.: Diagnostic concordance among pathologists interpreting breast biopsy specimens. JAMA **313**(11), 1122–1132 (2015)

5. Hartmann, L.C., Degnim, A.C., Santen, R.J., Dupont, W.D., Ghosh, K.: Atypical hyperplasia of the breast–risk assessment and management options. New England J. Med. **372**(1), 78–89 (2015)
6. Hase, P., Chen, C., Li, O., Rudin, C.: Interpretable image recognition with hierarchical prototypes. In: Proceedings of the AAAI Conference on Human Computation and Crowdsourcing, vol. 7, pp. 32–40 (2019)
7. Hugar, S.B., Bhargava, R., Dabbs, D.J., Davis, K.M., Zuley, M., Clark, B.Z.: Isolated flat epithelial atypia on core biopsy specimens is associated with a low risk of upgrade at excision. Am. J. Clin. Pathol. **151**(5), 511–515 (2019)
8. Lakhani, S.R.: WHO Classification of Tumours of the Breast. International Agency for Research on Cancer (2012)
9. LeCun, Y.A., Bottou, L., Orr, G.B., Müller, K.-R.: Efficient BackProp. In: Montavon, G., Orr, G.B., Müller, K.-R. (eds.) Neural Networks: Tricks of the Trade. LNCS, vol. 7700, pp. 9–48. Springer, Heidelberg (2012). https://doi.org/10.1007/978-3-642-35289-8_3
10. Li, B., et al.: Classifying breast histopathology images with a ductal instance-oriented pipeline
11. Mehta, S., Lu, X., Weaver, D., Elmore, J.G., Hajishirzi, H., Shapiro, L.: Hatnet: an end-to-end holistic attention network for diagnosis of breast biopsy images. arXiv preprint arXiv:2007.13007 (2020)
12. Mercan, E., Mehta, S., Bartlett, J., Shapiro, L.G., Weaver, D.L., Elmore, J.G.: Assessment of machine learning of breast pathology structures for automated differentiation of breast cancer and high-risk proliferative lesions. JAMA Netw. Open **2**(8), e198777–e198777 (2019)
13. Parvatikar, A., et al.: Modeling histological patterns for differential diagnosis of atypical breast lesions. In: Martel, A.L., et al. (eds.) MICCAI 2020. LNCS, vol. 12265, pp. 550–560. Springer, Cham (2020). https://doi.org/10.1007/978-3-030-59722-1_53
14. Pati, P., et al.: HACT-Net: a hierarchical cell-to-tissue graph neural network for histopathological image classification. In: Sudre, C.H., et al. (eds.) UNSURE/GRAIL -2020. LNCS, vol. 12443, pp. 208–219. Springer, Cham (2020). https://doi.org/10.1007/978-3-030-60365-6_20
15. Pedregosa, F., et al.: Scikit-learn: machine learning in Python. J. Mach. Learn. Res. **12**, 2825–2830 (2011)
16. Quattoni, A., Torralba, A.: Recognizing indoor scenes. In: 2009 IEEE Conference on Computer Vision and Pattern Recognition, pp. 413–420. IEEE (2009)
17. Schnitt, S.J., Connolly, J.L.: Processing and evaluation of breast excision specimens: a clinically oriented approach. Am. J. Clin. Pathol. **98**(1), 125–137 (1992)
18. Silverstein, M.: Where's the outrage? J. Am. College Surgeons **208**(1), 78–79 (2009)
19. American Cancer Society: Breast cancer facts & figures 2019–2020. Am. Cancer Soc. 1–44 (2019)
20. Tosun, A.B., et al.: Histological detection of high-risk benign breast lesions from whole slide images. In: Descoteaux, M., et al. (eds.) MICCAI 2017. LNCS, vol. 10434, pp. 144–152. Springer, Cham (2017). https://doi.org/10.1007/978-3-319-66185-8_17
21. Zhou, N., Fedorov, A., Fennessy, F., Kikinis, R., Gao, Y.: Large scale digital prostate pathology image analysis combining feature extraction and deep neural network. arXiv preprint arXiv:1705.02678 (2017)

Hierarchical Attention Guided Framework for Multi-resolution Collaborative Whole Slide Image Segmentation

Jiangpeng Yan[1,2], Hanbo Chen[2], Kang Wang[3], Yan Ji[2], Yuyao Zhu[3], Jingjing Li[4], Dong Xie[4], Zhe Xu[1], Junzhou Huang[2], Shuqun Cheng[3(✉)], Xiu Li[1(✉)], and Jianhua Yao[2(✉)]

[1] Tsinghua University, Beijing, China
li.xiu@sz.tsinghua.edu.cn
[2] Tencent AI Lab, Shenzhen, China
jianhuayao@tencent.com
[3] Eastern Hepatobiliary Surgery Hospital, Shanghai, China
chengshuqun@aliyun.com
[4] Shanghai Institute of Nutrition and Health, Shanghai, China

Abstract. Segmentation of whole slide images (WSIs) is an important step for computer-aided cancer diagnosis. However, due to the gigapixel dimension, WSIs are usually cropped into patches for analysis. Processing high-resolution patches independently may leave out the global geographical relationships and suffer slow inference speed while using low-resolution patches can enlarge receptive fields but lose local details. Here, we propose a Hierarchical Attention Guided (HAG) framework to address above problems. Particularly, our framework contains a global branch and several local branches to perform prediction at different scales. Additive hierarchical attention maps are generated by the global branch with sparse constraints to fuse multi-resolution predictions for better segmentation. During the inference, the sparse attention maps are used as the certainty guidance to select important local areas with a quadtree strategy for acceleration. Experimental results on two WSI datasets highlight two merits of our framework: 1) effectively aggregate multi-resolution information to achieve better results, 2) significantly reduce the computational cost to accelerate the prediction without decreasing accuracy.

Keywords: Segmentation · Whole slide image · Deep Learning · Acceleration

1 Introduction

The semantic segmentation of whole slide images (WSIs) plays an essential role in lesion detection and tumor staging. But evaluating gigapixel WSIs manually is labor-intensive and error-prone. It is reported that the number of WSIs for

---

J. Yan, H. Chen and K. Wang—contributed equally

© Springer Nature Switzerland AG 2021
M. de Bruijne et al. (Eds.): MICCAI 2021, LNCS 12908, pp. 153–163, 2021.
https://doi.org/10.1007/978-3-030-87237-3_15

clinical applications increases significantly in recent years while skilled pathologists are in shortage [9]. Inspired by the recent success of Deep Learning [10] in medical image analysis [17,20,21], researchers resort to artificial intelligence techniques to assist pathologists [4,13,22].

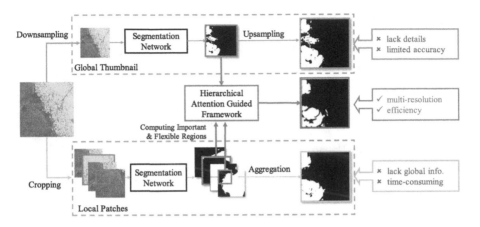

Fig. 1. Current WSI segmentation methods have trade-off between efficiency and accuracy. Our proposed HAG framework unifies multi-resolution analysis and efficiency.

However, it is infeasible to directly feed gigapixel WSIs into popular deep semantic segmentation models such as FCN [12] or U-net [17] due to the current GPU memory limitation. One possible solution is to downsample the original WSI to a lower resolution (Fig. 1 top row), where the discriminative details might be lost leading to degradation of the final performance. Alternatively, WSI can be cropped into patches for analysis and the final segmentation masks are aggregated from patch-level predictions (Fig. 1 bottom row). However, this approach suffers two major limitations: 1) processing these patches independently without considering the geographical relationships between each other may leave out some useful context information; 2) cropping gigapixel WSI may result in hundreds of patches which is time-consuming to analyze. Some recent studies [8,13,16,18,19] attempt to solve the first problem by fusing features from different resolutions. However, those methods require additional computations. The trade-off between the efficiency and performance must be made. An efficient ML framework is presented in [11], where the stain normalization and I/O process were accelerated while the patch-based inference pipeline was not optimized. In a work by Dong et al. [6], the speed problem was solved by training a reinforcement-learning based agent to select fixed-size local regions for zooming in. However, the agent training is a challenging task and only two resolutions are considered.

To solve the problem, here we propose a Hierarchical Attention Guided (HAG) framework (Fig. 2). It is inspired by the top-to-bottom attentive mechanism from pathologists' diagnosis process. When pathologists evaluate a WSI,

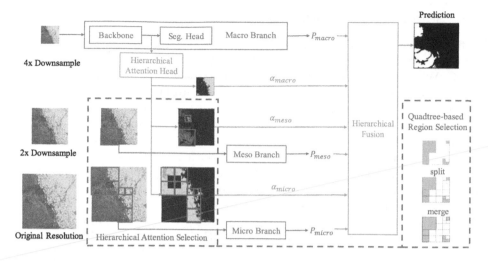

Fig. 2. Illustration of the HAG framework. Key components of three phases are high-lighted in different colors: phase 1) segmentation branch pre-training (green), phase 2) hierarchical attention based fusion (orange), and phase 3) quadtree-based hierarchical region selection during inference (red). A quadtree based important regions selection method is presented for acceleration. (Color figure online)

they first check images in low magnitude and only zoom in the uncertain regions for details. Accordingly, our framework contains a global segmentation branch and several local branches that perform patch-based segmentation at different resolutions. During the training phase, the global branch also generates sparse spatial attention maps to fuse patch-based predictions from local branches. With such hierarchical fusion, multi-scale predictions collaborate with each other to improve results. During the inference process, these sparse attention maps are then used as the certainty guidance to select necessary local patches with a quadtree based region selection strategy. Our method unifies multi-resolution analysis and inference speed-up by fusing three-scale segmentation with attention maps and use the same maps for region selection. Our experiments show that the proposed framework can: 1) effectively aggregate multi-resolution information to achieve better results, 2) significantly reduce the computational cost to accelerate the prediction without decreasing accuracy.

2   Methods

The HAG framework includes following three phases: 1) segmentation branch pre-training, 2) hierarchical attention based fusion, and 3) quadtree-based hierarchical region selection during inference, shown in Fig. 2. We will introduce our framework following this order.

2.1   Segmentation Branch Pre-training

Different from general images, discriminative details in WSI vary with the resolutions. Thus, in practice, models are usually trained at a fixed magnitude [3,15]. Without loss of generality, we pre-train the segmentation network in three different resolutions, namely the macro/meso/micro branch. For simplicity, we set the resolution scale between two adjacent branches to 2x, shown in Fig. 2. The cropping operation is considered due to the constraint of GPU memory. To avoid prediction artifacts at boundary, images are cropped into patches of size $m * m$ with extra p pixel overlap between adjacent edges such that the input image size will be $(m + 2p) * (m + 2p)$. Linknet [2], the efficient variant of U-net[17], is adopted as the backbone for all segmentation branches. The common cross-entropy loss is used to supervise the training, defined as: $L_{ce}(Y, P) = -\sum_i [y^i log(p^i) + (1 - y^i)log(1 - p^i)]$, where i is the pixel location, Y is the binary ground-truth mask and P the predicted results.

2.2   Hierarchical Attention Based Fusion

Given segmentation at each branch as P_{macro}, P_{meso} and P_{micro}, we fuse them to generate the final segmentation result P. An intuitive solution is to re-sample them to the same size and then average them by: $P = (P_{macro}^{\uparrow 4} + P_{meso}^{\uparrow 2} + P_{micro})/3$, where P_{meso} and P_{micro} are aggregated from corresponding local patches, $\uparrow k$ represents bilinear interpolation operation which up-samples the image by k times. However, this requires complete computation of P_{meso} and P_{micro}, which is time-consuming. Our experience with WSI data suggests that different types of tissue regions have certain resolution preference. Thus, we propose to conduct more flexible fusion based on spatial attention maps:

$$P = \alpha_{macro} \cdot P_{macro}^{\uparrow 4} + \alpha_{meso} \cdot P_{meso}^{\uparrow 2} + \alpha_{micro} \cdot P_{micro}, \tag{1}$$

where α_i is the corresponding spatial attention map for scale i and $\sum \alpha_i = 1$. In additional to achieve the optimal segmentation prediction, α can also play as the importance map. With it, redundant computations can be skipped for inference speedup, which will be elaborated in the next session. To achieve this goal, two criteria need be met for α: (1) α_{meso} and α_{micro} are sparse - this is critical in reducing the call frequency of the corresponding branch; (2) the computational cost of α is low.

To meet criteria (2), we compute α at the macro scale. This is also motivated by pathologists' top-to-bottom attentive mechanism - by looking at a sample in low resolution first, the pathologist can decide whether to zoom-in for close inspection. Because the decision of zoom-in is highly correlated with tissue segmentation task, the same set of image features could be shared between the two tasks. As shown in Fig. 2, in our implementation, the hierarchical attention generation head is connected to the macro branch such that the attention module shares the feature extraction backbone of the segmentation network. In this way, the computational cost of generating α could be negligible. Note the feature maps produced by the macro branch as F, α is obtained by:$\alpha = softmax(\mathcal{A}(F))$, where $\mathcal{A}$ is a fully convolution module to generate the 3-channel output. Since all three attention maps computed in this way are of the same resolution as macro scale image, α_{meso} and α_{micro} needs to be up-sampled accordingly to have the uniform size. We update Eq. 1 as:

$$P = (\alpha_{macro} \cdot P_{macro})^{\uparrow 4} + (\alpha_{meso})^{\uparrow 4} \cdot (P_{meso})^{\uparrow 2} + (\alpha_{micro})^{\uparrow 4} \cdot P_{micro}. \qquad (2)$$

Notably, $\mathcal{A}$ needs to be trained independently rather than end-to-end together with three branches because it takes 1, 4, and 16 inference times for the macro, meso, and micro branch to produce the prediction.

Cross-entropy loss L_{ce} is also adopted when training attention head. To meet criteria (1), we borrow the idea of LASSO and apply additional L1 regularization on α_{meso} and α_{micro}. The final objective loss function is defined as:

$$\mathcal{L} = L_{ce}(Y, P) + \lambda_{meso}||\alpha_{meso}||_1 + \lambda_{micro}||\alpha_{micro}||_1, \qquad (3)$$

where λ is the regularization coefficient.

2.3   Quadtree-Based Hierarchical Region Selection During Inference

After the above training, we obtain hierarchical attention maps which can favor better prediction regions at the certain scale. Therefore, we can selectively process higher resolution patches with the guidance of the sparse α_{meso} and α_{micro} instead of processing all the patches. Since the computation time of α is negligible and the network architecture of different branches are identical, the computational time t is linearly correlated with the total number of pixels of input images: $t = O(\sum(|I|))$. To effectively select patches, a quadtree-based method has been adopted.

Quadtree structure method [7] was proposed originally for creating vector data spatial indexing. As shown in the right bottom of Fig. 2, it can be adopted to split the sparse foreground object in an image into sub-regions with different sizes. Guided by α_{meso} and α_{micro}, the quadtree can hierarchically select important sub-regions that need to be further computed. To construct a quadtree, we define two hyper-parameters to determine when the split should be stopped and one rule to prune the tree from over-splitting. First, the split will be stopped when the node size is smaller than a certain size. Given that the cropped images are overlapped by p pixels, we empirically set $2p$ as the minimum size of the nodes. Second, a threshold T of the average attention value inside the minimum region units $2p * 2p$ will decide whether the child patch needs to be activated for analysis. When each child contains either activated or inactivated minimum region units, we know that the split can be stopped. After splitting, we need to prune the leaves where the computational time of processing them is more than processing their parent node. To understand this rule, we need to compute and compare the number of input pixels before and after splitting a region. Intuitively, the input pixels of a patch should be equal to or more than its child.

Table 1. Distribution of two datasets in the experiment.

	Cases	Images	Cancerous	Noncancerous
Camelyon16	270	2099	993	1016
HCC	90	1244	980	264

However, since we expand the cropping with size $\widetilde{m} * \widetilde{m}$ by p pixels, its computation time will be:$t_p = O((\widetilde{m} + 2p)^2)$. While computation time of its child is:$t_c = O(\sum_{i \in S}(\widetilde{m}_i + 2p)^2)$, where S is the set of sub-regions selected for computation, and $\widetilde{m}_i = \widetilde{m}/2^l$, where l is decided by which level the sub-region is from. When p is comparable to $\widetilde{m}$ and S is densely selected, we will have $t_p < t_c$ and pruning its children could further save the computational cost.

Since it takes 4 and 16 inference times to process corresponding patches for generating P_{meso} and P_{micro}, we build the quadtree for α_{meso} and α_{micro} with the initial depth of 2 and 3 separately. The regions selected for meso branch analysis will be skipped in the micro branch. Firstly, one quadtree is built in α_{meso} to choose the local area set S_{meso}. Then, the selected regions are mapped to α_{micro} and deactivate corresponding attention values. After that, the other quadtree is adopted to select the local area set S_{micro}. Finally, the prediction results can be approximately obtained by:

$$P = (\alpha_{macro} \cdot P_{macro})^{\uparrow 4} + (I^i - \alpha^i_{macro})^{\uparrow 4} \cdot (P^i_{meso})^{\uparrow 2} + (I^j - \alpha^j_{macro})^{\uparrow 4} \cdot P^j_{micro}, \quad (4)$$

where $i \in S_{meso}$ and $j \in (S_{micro} - S_{meso})$, I^i and I^j are 0–1 matrices in which 1-value only exists in selected regions.

3   Experimental Analysis

3.1   Dataset and Pre-processing

Two datasets are adopted including the public Camelyon16 dataset [1] and an in-house Hepatocellular Carcinoma (HCC) dataset collected from our collaborating hospital. **The Camelyon16 dataset:** contains 270 hematoxylin-eosin (H&E) stained WSIs focusing on sentinel lymph nodes [1]. **The HCC dataset:** contains 90 H&E stained WSIs. Sample collection, fixation, processing and pathological diagnosis of HCC followed the Practice Guidelines for the Pathological Diagnosis of Primary Liver Cancer[5]. The study was approved by the Institutional Ethics Committee of the hospital. Both datasets contain lesion-level annotations.

Similar to [6,18], we generated the 2048 × 2048 patches from the Camelyon16/HCC dataset with the specimen-level pixel size of 1335 nm/1840 nm to get a proper view of biological tissues. The following strategy was adopted: A sliding window of size 2048 × 2048 with stride of 1792 (256 pixels overlap) was used to crop the WSIs. We filtered background crops by setting pixels with chroma ($max[RGB] - min[RGB] > 64$) as foreground and only kept the crops containing > 5% foreground pixels. The distribution of the generated images are listed in Table 1. We followed the hold-out strategy to divide two datasets by cases into the training, validation, and test sets with the proportion of 6:2:2. Notably, as the non-cancerous region in the Camelyon16 dataset is much larger than the cancerous region, we use a randomly sample sub-set of non-cancerous patches. Cancerous tissues in the HCC dataset spread more sparsely than those in the Camelyon16, so it is more difficult to generate noncancerous images. We over-sampled the noncancerous images for 4 times when training. The following three resolutions were then considered: the macro resolution where one image was downsampled to 512×512 pixels directly, the meso resolution where one image was downsampled 2 times then cropped into 4 tiles with an overlap region of 64 pixels, the micro resolution where one image was divided into 16 tiles with the same overlapping. In other words, we set $m = 512$, $p = 64$.

3.2 Implementation Details

Environment. We implemented all methods with an NVIDIA P40 GPU and Pytorch [14].

Network Architecture. We chose ResNet18 [10] as the backbone of Linknet [2]. We set the attention head having the same architecture as the segmentation head but with different channels for their target outputs.

Hyper-parameter Settings. Three branches were first pre-trained with the corresponding resolution with 250 epochs with data augmentation strategies including rotation, color jittering, etc. The Adam optimizer was adopted with a learning rate of 0.001. After pre-training, models with the best performance on the validation set were remained and the attention head was trained with Eq. 3 for another 100 epochs. For λ_{meso} and λ_{micro} in Eq. 3, we performed grid-searching and chose $[\lambda_{meso}, \lambda_{micro}] = [0, 1e{-}4]/[0, 1e{-}2]$ for Camelyon16/HCC. We also grid searched for the threshold to construct quardtrees on α_{meso} and α_{micro} and we had $[T_{meso}, T_{micro}] = [0.5, 0.6]/[0.3, 0.8]$ for Camelyon16/HCC.

Test Metrics. For segmentation performance, two common metrics are adopted including Accuracy and Dice between the predicted and ground-truth cancerous pixels of the whole test set. For computational cost comparisonal, we report average floating operations (FLOPs) in all the convolutional layers of different methods. Lower values of FLOPs represent faster speed.

3.3 Experimental Results

Quantitative results are presented in Table 2. It can be concluded that our proposed HAG framework benefits from fusing all the single scale baselines with non-selective fusion via Eq. 2. With the help of selection inference, the average FLOPs are significantly reduced with marginal performance trade-in via Eq. 4. Intriguingly, the Camelyon16 and HCC dataset show different scale preferences. For the Camelyon16 dataset, a finer resolution can help the deep model predict better results. For the HCC dataset, more false positive predictions are observed when inference at the micro branch - a higher pixel-level accuracy but a lower

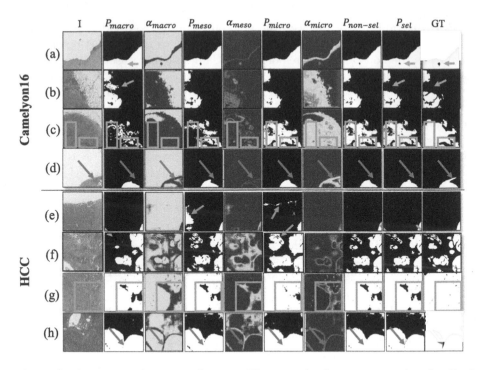

Fig. 3. Qualitative results on two datasets. The attention heatmaps are also visualized where yellow regions indicate high values. From the right to left, we present images, prediction results along with attention maps of the macro/meso/micro branch, non-selective fusion results via Eq. 2, selective fusion results via Eq. 4 and GTs. Orange boxes show where errors exist in manual annotations but corrected in our segmentation. Green and blue arrows address where visual quality improves by fusing the prediction from three resolutions and red arrows point to uncertain areas discovered. (Color figure online)

dice score. Both situations can be handled by fusing predictions in different scale and the best performance is achieved by complete non-selective fusion. However, this is the most computational expensive approach as well. Our proposed selective fusion framework significantly reduces the computational cost and keeps similar performance in comparison with non-selective framework. Notably, more inference speed-up has been achieved for HCC dataset since it favors macro-scale.

Qualitative results are shown in Fig. 3. Generated attention maps reasonably ignore background areas where there does not exist biological tissues. For the Camelyon16 dataset, the attention maps tend to favor predictions at the micro branch with higher activated attention values, while the meso branch is preferred for the HCC dataset. This is consistent with the quantitative results because more false positive predictions occur in the HCC dataset with a finer resolution. This is due to cancerous cells in the HCC dataset have obvious different appearances from normal ones and thus are more easily identified in a

Table 2. Quantitative performance on two dataset. The macro branch can be regarded as a downsampling-based baseline and the meso/micro branch can be regarded as patch-based baselines with different resolutions.

	Camelyon16				HCC			
	Accuracy	Dice	FLOPs	Ratio	Accuracy	Dice	FLOPs	Ratio
Macro Branch (4x Downsample)	81.6%	84.1%	36.8G	0.06x	86.5%	89.3%	36.8G	0.06x
Meso Branch (2x Downsample, 2 × 2 Crop)	86.9%	87.9%	147.2G	0.25x	88.5%	89.3%	147.2G	0.25x
Micro Branch (4 × 4 Crop)	89.1%	90.5%	588.9G	1x	89.6%	87.7%	588.9G	1x
Non-selective Fusion	89.0%	90.6%	784.8G	1.33x	89.3%	90.6%	784.8G	1.33x
Selective Fusion	88.9%	90.4%	204.3G	0.35x	88.8%	90.3%	87.7G	0.15x

coarser scale. However, this does not mean analyzing in the coarse scale only is sufficient. As highlighted by the green arrows in Fig. 3, macro-branch performs poorly on small structures which can be corrected by our methods. As highlighted by blue arrows in Fig. 3, the HAG framework can make the right selection to avoid errors in meso and micro branches as well. Intriguingly, as addressed by the red arrows in Fig. 3, even when all the branches can not produce satisfying predictions for fusion, the learned attention maps can highlight uncertain areas where errors occur. Notably, annotation error exists in both datasets because labeling gigapixel WSIs is very challenging. As highlighted by orange boxes in Fig. 3, the case (d) and (e) from two datasets both show that predicted segmentation results can identify normal tissues and cancerous tissues better than manual labels.

4   Conclusion

In this work, we propose a HAG framework where we integrate hierarchical attention mechanism into WSI segmentation pipeline. Motivated by pathologists' top-to-bottom attentive mechanism, we add an additive module to generate hierarchical and sparse attention maps with the potential for different clinical applications. Experimental results show that the generated attention can act as: 1) a weighted fusion map to effectively aggregate multi-resolution information for a better result. 2) a selection guide map to reduce the inference areas and accelerate the prediction process without decreasing performance. The major limitation is that the scales are empirically selected, we will incorporate more flexible scale-searching to further improve the performance in the future.

Acknowledgement. This research was partly supported by the National Natural Science Foundation of China (Grant No. 41876098), the National Key R&D Program of China (Grant No. 2020AAA0108303), and Shenzhen Science and Technology Project (Grant No. JCYJ20200109143041798).

References

1. Bejnordi, B.E., et al.: Diagnostic assessment of deep learning algorithms for detection of lymph node metastases in women with breast cancer. JAMA **318**(22), 2199–2210 (2017)
2. Chaurasia, A., Culurciello, E.: Linknet: exploiting encoder representations for efficient semantic segmentation. In: Proceedings of the IEEE Visual Communications and Image Processing, pp. 1–4 (2017)
3. Tosun, A.B., et al.: Histological detection of high-risk benign breast lesions from whole slide images. In: Descoteaux, M., et al. (eds.) MICCAI 2017. LNCS, vol. 10434, pp. 144–152. Springer, Cham (2017). https://doi.org/10.1007/978-3-319-66185-8_17
4. Chen, H., Qi, X., Yu, L., Dou, Q., Qin, J., Heng, P.A.: Dcan: deep contour-aware networks for object instance segmentation from histology images. Med. Image Anal. **36**, 135–146 (2017)
5. Cong, W.M., et al.: Practice guidelines for the pathological diagnosis of primary liver cancer: 2015 update. World J. Gastroenterol. **22**(42), 9279 (2016)
6. Dong, N., et al.: Reinforced auto-zoom net: towards accurate and fast breast cancer segmentation in whole-slide images. In: Stoyanov, D., et al. (eds.) DLMIA/MLCDS -2018. LNCS, vol. 11045, pp. 317–325. Springer, Cham (2018). https://doi.org/10.1007/978-3-030-00889-5_36
7. Finkel, R.A., Bentley, J.L.: Quad trees a data structure for retrieval on composite keys. Acta Informatica **4**(1), 1–9 (1974)
8. Gu, F., Burlutskiy, N., Andersson, M., Wilén, L.K.: Multi-resolution networks for semantic segmentation in whole slide images. In: Stoyanov, D., et al. (eds.) OMIA/COMPAY -2018. LNCS, vol. 11039, pp. 11–18. Springer, Cham (2018). https://doi.org/10.1007/978-3-030-00949-6_2
9. Harrold, I.M., Bean, S.M., Williams, N.C.: Emerging from the basement: the visible pathologist. Arch. Pathol. Laboratory Med. **143**(8), 917–918 (2019)
10. He, K., Zhang, X., Ren, S., Sun, J.: Deep residual learning for image recognition. In: Proceedings of the IEEE Conference on Computer Vision and Pattern Recognition, pp. 770–778 (2016)
11. Ioannou, N., et al.: Accelerated ML-assisted tumor detection in high-resolution histopathology images. In: Shen, D., et al. (eds.) MICCAI 2019. LNCS, vol. 11764, pp. 406–414. Springer, Cham (2019). https://doi.org/10.1007/978-3-030-32239-7_45
12. Long, J., Shelhamer, E., Darrell, T.: Fully convolutional networks for semantic segmentation. In: Proceedings of the IEEE Conference on Computer Vision and Pattern Recognition, pp. 3431–3440 (2015)
13. Mehta, S., Mercan, E., Bartlett, J., Weaver, D., Elmore, J.G., Shapiro, L.: Y-Net: joint segmentation and classification for diagnosis of breast biopsy images. In: Frangi, A.F., Schnabel, J.A., Davatzikos, C., Alberola-López, C., Fichtinger, G. (eds.) MICCAI 2018. LNCS, vol. 11071, pp. 893–901. Springer, Cham (2018). https://doi.org/10.1007/978-3-030-00934-2_99
14. Paszke, A., et al.: Pytorch: An imperative style, high-performance deep learning library. In: Advances in Neural Information Processing Systems, pp. 8026–8037 (2019)

15. Qu, H., Yan, Z., Riedlinger, G.M., De, S., Metaxas, D.N.: Improving nuclei/gland instance segmentation in histopathology images by full resolution neural network and spatial constrained loss. In: Shen, D., et al. (eds.) MICCAI 2019. LNCS, vol. 11764, pp. 378–386. Springer, Cham (2019). https://doi.org/10.1007/978-3-030-32239-7_42

16. van Rijthoven, M., Balkenhol, M., Siliņa, K., van der Laak, J., Ciompi, F.: Hooknet: multi-resolution convolutional neural networks for semantic segmentation in histopathology whole-slide images. Med. Image Anal. **68**, 101890 (2021)

17. Ronneberger, O., Fischer, P., Brox, T.: U-Net: convolutional networks for biomedical image segmentation. In: Navab, N., Hornegger, J., Wells, W.M., Frangi, A.F. (eds.) MICCAI 2015. LNCS, vol. 9351, pp. 234–241. Springer, Cham (2015). https://doi.org/10.1007/978-3-319-24574-4_28

18. Schmitz, R., et al.: Multi-scale fully convolutional neural networks for histopathology image segmentation: from nuclear aberrations to the global tissue architecture. Med. Image Anal. **70**, 101996 (2021)

19. Tokunaga, H., Teramoto, Y., Yoshizawa, A., Bise, R.: Adaptive weighting multifield of view CNN for semantic segmentation in pathology. In: Proceedings of the IEEE Conference on Computer Vision and Pattern Recognition, pp. 12597–12606 (2019)

20. Wang, Y., et al.: Double-uncertainty weighted method for semi-supervised learning. In: Martel, A.L., et al. (eds.) MICCAI 2020. LNCS, vol. 12261, pp. 542–551. Springer, Cham (2020). https://doi.org/10.1007/978-3-030-59710-8_53

21. Yan, J., Chen, S., Zhang, Y., Li, X.: Neural architecture search for compressed sensing magnetic resonance image reconstruction. Comput. Med. Imaging Graph. **85**, 101784 (2020)

22. Yao, J., Zhu, X., Jonnagaddala, J., Hawkins, N., Huang, J.: Whole slide images based cancer survival prediction using attention guided deep multiple instance learning networks. Med. Image Anal. **65**, 101789 (2020)

Hierarchical Phenotyping and Graph Modeling of Spatial Architecture in Lymphoid Neoplasms

Pingjun Chen[1] , Muhammad Aminu[1], Siba El Hussein[2], Joseph D. Khoury[3], and Jia Wu[1(✉)]

[1] Department of Imaging Physics, Division of Diagnostic Imaging,
The University of Texas MD Anderson Cancer Center, Houston, TX, USA
jwu11@mdanderson.org
[2] Department of Pathology, University of Rochester Medical Center,
Rochester, NY, USA
[3] Department of Hematopathology, Division of Pathology and Lab Medicine,
The University of Texas MD Anderson Cancer Center, Houston, TX, USA

Abstract. The cells and their spatial patterns in the tumor microenvironment (TME) play a key role in tumor evolution, and yet the latter remains an understudied topic in computational pathology. This study, to the best of our knowledge, is among the first to hybridize local and global graph methods to profile orchestration and interaction of cellular components. To address the challenge in hematolymphoid cancers, where the cell classes in TME may be unclear, we first implemented cell-level unsupervised learning and identified two new cell subtypes. Local cell graphs or supercells were built for each image by considering the individual cell's geospatial location and classes. Then, we applied supercell level clustering and identified two new cell communities. In the end, we built global graphs to abstract spatial interaction patterns and extract features for disease diagnosis. We evaluate the proposed algorithm on H&E slides of 60 hematolymphoid neoplasms and further compared it with three cell level graph-based algorithms, including the global cell graph, cluster cell graph, and FLocK. The proposed algorithm achieved a mean diagnosis accuracy of 0.703 with the repeated 5-fold cross-validation scheme. In conclusion, our algorithm shows superior performance over the existing methods and can be potentially applied to other cancer types.

Keywords: Spatial pattern analysis · Cell phenotyping · Supercell · Graph modeling · Hematolymphoid cancer

1 Introduction

The tumor is a complex ecosystem that emerges and evolves under selective pressure from its microenvironment, involving trophic, metabolic, immunolog-

---

P. Chen, M. Aminu and S. El Hussein—Equal Contribution.
J. Khoury and J. Wu—Co-supervision.

© Springer Nature Switzerland AG 2021
M. de Bruijne et al. (Eds.): MICCAI 2021, LNCS 12908, pp. 164–174, 2021.
https://doi.org/10.1007/978-3-030-87237-3_16

ical, and therapeutic factors. The relative influence of these factors orchestrates the abundance, localization, and functional orientation of cellular components within the tumor microenvironment (TME) with resultant phenotypic and geospatial variations, a phenomenon known as intratumoral heterogeneity (ITH) [8,26]. As such, ITH provides a substrate from which neoplastic cells emerge, escape immunologic surveillance, undergo genetic evolution, and develop pathways that lead to therapy resistance. In routine practice, such attributes are evaluated microscopically primarily using tumor tissue sections stained with the hematoxylin and eosin stain (H&E). With the advent of digital pathology, machine learning-empowered computational pipelines have been proposed to profile TME using H&E tissue sections to enhance cancer diagnosis and prognostication [12,16,27].

Most studies published to date have focused on phenotyping the textural patterns of tissue slides in a top-down manner, through either conventional hand-crafted features (Gabor, Fourier, LBP, GLCM, etc.) or deep convolutional neural networks (CNN) to extract versatile features specifically tailored for particular clinical scenarios [3–5,11,19,28,30]. Though these studies have achieved promising performance, they missed connection to individual cellular components in TME, thereby limiting their ability to capture neoplastic cell characteristics in their microenvironment milieu and capitalizing on critical diagnostic aspects and prognostic predictions. To bridge this gap, few bottom-up studies focused on profiling cellular architectures from digital pathology slides have emerged using graph theory approach and graph convolution network (GCN) approach [13,18,20,22,24,29]. The graph theory approach first constructs either local or global graph structures and then extracts hand-crafted features to test their clinical relevance. By contrast, the GCN approach aims to automatically learn representations from the global graph formed at the cellular level and abstract the features via multiple layers of graph convolution and pooling operations, similar to the CNN approach. However, a common limitation to these algorithms is their lack of ability to differentiate known cellular populations. Pilot studies have been proposed to address this limitation in the colorectal cancer [14,23], a solid tumor with a well-studied TME that contains vascular structures, immune cells, fibroblasts, and extracellular matrix [15,17]. There are no studies exploring this approach in hematolymphoid neoplasms.

Diffuse large B-cell lymphoma (DLBC) is an aggressive lymphoid malignancy that may arise through a series of clonal evolution steps, occasionally from a low-grade lymphoid neoplasm called chronic lymphocytic leukemia/small lymphocytic lymphoma (CLL/SLL) [2,6]. The latter is among the most prevalent lymphoid neoplasms and is associated with a favorable survival rate (5-year survival rate around 83%). In a subset of patients, CLL/SLL can pursue a more aggressive clinical course referred to as "accelerated CLL/SLL" (aCLL). Patients with CLL/SLL and/or aCLL can also develop a full-blown DLBCL, called Richter transformation DLBCL (RT-DLBL), a complication that is associated with a high mortality rate with a median overall survival of 9 months [1,6]. Unlike solid tumors with a well-defined TME, there is no standard way to categorize cells into biological subtypes in hematolymphoid tumors. To diagnose these patients, pathologists make diagnoses based on their empirical knowledge of tumor cell morphology, normal histology, and deviations from normal tissue architectures. By default, such an approach is subjective and prone to inter- and intra-reader variations.

To improve the diagnostic accuracy of tissue examination of lymphoid neoplasms, we propose an innovative computational framework that integrates unsupervised clustering and graph modeling algorithms as a knowledge discovery approach to hierarchically decode cellular and clonal level phenotypes in TME. In particular, we dissect the process into four key steps (Fig. 1). First, we segment each cell and based on their features to identify intrinsic subtypes. Second, we focus on spatial interaction among neighboring cells by building local graphs factoring in their subtypes, so that closely-interacting cells are merged to form supercells. Third, we pool the supercells together to discover the cellular community at a population level. Lastly, we build global graphs incorporating community information to extract features for diagnostic purposes.

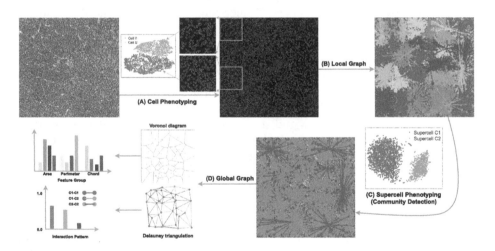

Fig. 1. Illustration of the proposed hierarchical cell phenotyping and graph modeling algorithm to profile the cellular architecture for analyzing lymphoid pathology images. (A) Cell phenotyping via spectral clustering algorithm. (B) Cell local graph construction to obtain supercells via a Ranking Operation-based Clustering (ROC) algorithm. (C) Supercell phenotyping (community detection) via spectral clustering algorithm. (D) The construction of global graphs based on supercells for extracting features.

To sum up, the main contributions of our work are as follows: (1) We use clustering as a knowledge discovery approach to explore intrinsic cellular and clonal phenotypes of TME to advance our understanding of hematolymphoid cancers. (2) We develop a novel hierarchical graph construction algorithm to comprehensively characterize interaction patterns at both the local cellular level and global community level for cellular architectures. (3) The proposed algorithm attains superior diagnostic performance compared with three state-of-the-art graph theory-based methods to enhance blood cancer diagnosis. To the best of our knowledge, this is the first study using such a design in the digital hematopathology field. We believe that our design has opened a new direction to quantify intratumoral heterogeneity, an aspect that has particular clinical implications in terms of risk stratification and prediction.

2   Method

2.1   Cell Phenotyping via Unsupervised Learning

Given a digital H&E slide, segmentation of nuclei is a prerequisite step for cellular-based analysis. We adopt a multiple-pass adaptive voting (MPAV) algorithm to segment the nuclei in digitized tissue images [21] To discover cell subtypes, we first characterize the morphology, intensity, and regional patterns of individual nuclei with a set of features (n = 24, "Cell features" in Table 1). To eliminate redundant features, we apply the Laplacian score method to select the top informative ones for the downstream analysis [10]. By treating each cell as an instance and randomly sampling cells across three disease subtypes, we embed pooled cells in a two-dimensional t-SNE feature space and then apply the spectral clustering to discover inter- and intra-disease cell subtypes. After repeating the sampling process multiple times, we observe that two intrinsic cell phenotypes are consistently identified. We train a classifier via an ensemble of learners aggregated with the bagging method [7] based on sampled cells for clustering, so that the cell subtypes can be propagated to unsampled ones.

Table 1. Summary of manual-crafted cell and graph features.

Category	No.	Feature names
Cell features	24	**Area, EquivDiameter, {Major;Minor} AxisLength, Perimeter, Mean {Inside;Outside} BoundaryIntensity, IntegratedIntensity, NormalizedBoundarySaliency,** Normalized {Inside;**Outside**} BoundaryIntensity, Eccentricity, Orientation, Intensity {Mean;Range;Deviation}, Solidity, Circularity, EllipticalDeviation, BoundarySaliency, {Inside;Outside} BoundaryIntensity {Range;Deviation}
Voronoi features	12	{Area;Perimeter;Chord} {Mean;Deviation;Disorder}, {Area;Perimeter;Chord} Ratio of Minimum to Maximum

2.2 Supercell via Local Graph

In the local cell graph construction, the cell centroids together with the obtained cell subtypes information are used to identify cell clusters $\{C\}$, where the Ranking Operation-based Clustering (ROC) algorithm applied (detailed in Fig. 2) [9]. The ROC algorithm is insensitive to the scale of features and type of distance metric used which makes it well-fitted for cell cluster identification. Given a set of n cells, their feature vectors represented as $X = \{x_i\}_{i=1}^{n}$ where $x_i \in \mathbb{R}^3$, the ROC algorithm first computes the pairwise distances $\{d^k\}_{k=1}^{3}$ from X. It then computes ranking matrices $\{r^k\}_{k=1}^{3}$ containing the ranking indices of the elements of $\{d^k\}_{k=1}^{3}$. The cumulative sparse ranking of each cell feature $\{s^k\}_{k=1}^{3}$ is then computed and all the local maxima $\{m\}$ of the cumulative sparse ranking are identified and used to group the cells into clusters $\{C\}$.

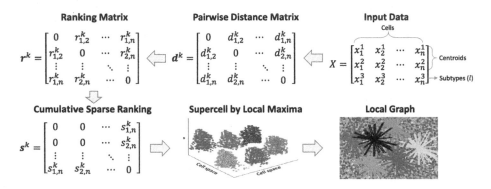

Fig. 2. The procedures of local graph construction via the ROC algorithm.

2.3 Cell Community Identification by Clustering of Supercells

We take the convex hull-covered polygon as each supercell's boundary. Unlike the individual cell, neighboring supercells often have overlapped regions, where the different cell classes interaction and confrontation occur (Fig. 3(A)). To discover the supercell groups (we term as cell community), we perform unsupervised phenotyping at supercell level. We characterize an individual supercell by looking into: 1) the encompassed cell features (i.e., compute mean feature values of individual cells) as well as 2) the cellular spatial orchestration and interaction (i.e., build a Voronoi diagram within supercell and extract related features). With these features (n=22, bolded cell features, and all Voronoi features in Table 1), we implement clustering to identify supercell subtypes (identical to cellular level clustering in Sect. 2.1). As previously stated, t-SNE is first adopted to reduce the feature space and embed supercells. Then we use spectral clustering to define similar intra- and interpatient supercells (i.e., cell community). For the evaluated lymphocytic images, two types of cell communities are identified.

Supercell phenotyping outcomes can be visualized from the two demo examples displayed in Fig. 3(B).

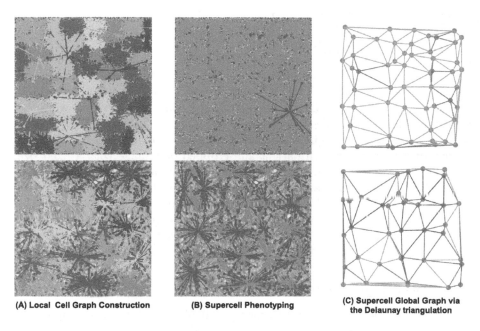

(A) Local Cell Graph Construction   (B) Supercell Phenotyping   (C) Supercell Global Graph via the Delaunay triangulation

Fig. 3. Exemplar intermediate results of the proposed algorithm. Column (A) shows the constructed local graphs (Supercells). Column (B) shows the supercell phenotyping results. Column (C) shows the built global graphs via the Delaunay triangulation, in which different edge colors represent different supercell interaction patterns.

2.4 Global Supercell Graph Construction and Feature Extraction

We build global graphs to characterize interactions among labeled supercells inside each image. Two global graphs, including the Delaunay triangulation and the Voronoi diagram, are constructed based on the supercell and cell community to complement each other. In the Delaunay scheme, the area is tessellated into triangular cells, which nodes are centroids of supercells. While in the Voronoi scheme, the area is split into sets of convex and adjacent polygonal cells, in which anchors are supercell centroids. Figure 3(C) shows two demos of the built global graph via the Delaunay triangulation. We extract features from the Delaunay graph through characterizing node-to-node interaction (i.e., edge) patterns. Assume there is k different type of nodes (inherit from supercell labels), the overall number of edge types is $k(k+1)/2$. We accumulate each edge type's counts and propose the percentages of different edge types as the global graph features. As for the global Voronoi graph, 12 features, as indicated in Table 1, are extracted. We combine the features from both the Delaunay graph and the

Voronoi diagram and test their performance in the diagnosis of different hematological malignancy subtypes (CLL vs aCLL vs RT-DLBL).

3 Experiments and Results

3.1 Dataset Description

Digitized clinical tumor tissue slides collected at The University of Texas MD Anderson Cancer Center (UTMDACC) were used a study dataset. The study was approved by the UTMDACC Review Board and conducted following the Declaration of Helsinki. The glass slides were scanned using an Aperio AT2 scanner at 20x optical magnification, with each pixel equaling 0.5 μm. We chose the best quality slide for each patient and cropped one image with a fixed size of $1,000 \times 1,000$ pixels from level 0 of each pyramidal formatted slide. The image was cropped by a board-certified pathologist with subspecialty expertise who annotated the region of interest (ROI)'s central part. Each patient only has one sample image in this design to facilitate the k-fold cross-validation analysis. After excluding slides with server artifacts, we were left with 20 images of each diagnosis to maintain the balance among CLL, aCLL, and RT-DLBL.

3.2 Implementation Details

The implementation includes four aspects: cell phenotyping, local graph construction, supercell phenotyping, and image classification. Since each image with the size $1,000 \times 1,000$ pixels contains thousands of cells, we randomly select 3,000 cells from each disease and pool 9,000 cells from all patients together to conduct the cell clustering. To propagate cell clustering labels to unsampled ones, we train the cell classifier with an ensemble of learners aggregated with the bagging method. In the local graph construction, there are two parameters to set for the ROC algorithm. We set the sparse ranking matrices' sparsity as 0.9 and the number of neighbors for local maxima identification as 10. The total number of supercells generated at the population level is 2,794, and we use all of them for supercell phenotyping, which employs the same clustering and classification manners as in cell phenotyping. As for the image classification, we conduct repeated 5-fold cross-validation with the Support Vector Machine (SVM). We mainly employ two metrics to evaluate the performance, including accuracy and area under the curve (AUC) for each diagnosis with the one-vs-rest strategy. We report the mean values of these metrics with 100 times randomization. The code is released at https://github.com/WuLabMDA/HierarchicalGraphModeling.

3.3 Results and Discussions

We compare the proposed method with three cell-level graph-based algorithms, including the Global Cell Graph (GCG) [24], Local Cell Graph (LCG) [18], and FLocK [20]. The GCG is built using the Voronoi diagram; The LCG is constructed using the mean shift algorithm [25] utilizing the cell centroids; The

FLocK is built with mean shift utilizing centroids as well as area and intensity of the cell. To have a fair comparison, we try our best to adjust the hyper-parameters used in these three compared methods to report their best results. The comparison results are shown in Table 2. Our proposed algorithm shows superior performance on these evaluated metrics among all the compared methods. The proposed method obtains the mean accuracy of 0.703 under 5-fold cross-validation with a 100 times randomization scheme for the three category disease diagnoses. Using only the local or the global graph fails to separate CLL from the other clinically relevant subtypes. By contrast, combining the local and global graph can improve the performance by a significant margin with a 0.4 increase in accuracy on the CLL. Further investigations find that the newly identified two cell communities have significantly different distributions between CLL and aCLL+RT (p-value=3.54e-08).

The two local graph methods (LCG and FLock) show better performance than the GCG. These results show that the local graph can better mine the cellular patterns than the global graph. Similar to the local graph methods, our method also firstly builds the local graph. Unlike them, LCG only utilizes the cell's centroid information, and FLocK uses the centroids with some cell features. While the proposed method considers the cell type when building the local graph. Moreover, we construct another layer of cell community detection for the global graph on top of the created local graph to further abstract the cellular features. We assume that this two-layer graph algorithm is better at extracting the multi-scale (both local and global) cellular interactions and intratumoral heterogeneity, thus surpass the compared methods. To the best of our knowledge, this study is among the first to hybridize local and global graph methods to study cellular patterns. Hereby, we hypothesize that the proposed hybrid design can overcome the limitation inherent in the adoption of the global or local graph approaches solely to more meaningfully profile tumor composition and intratumoral heterogeneity. Indeed, the global approach misses the cellular level details while the local graph ignores the high-level interaction patterns between communities.

Table 2. Performance of the three compared graph theory based methods and the proposed method

Method	Accuracy	AUC (CLL)	AUC (aCLL)	AUC (RT-DLBL)
GCG [24]	0.436 ± 0.037	0.421 ± 0.054	0.730 ± 0.027	0.770 ± 0.023
LCG [18]	0.471 ± 0.042	0.555 ± 0.049	0.669 ± 0.050	0.763 ± 0.032
FLocK [20]	0.601 ± 0.045	0.545 ± 0.054	**0.816 ± 0.025**	0.847 ± 0.022
Proposed	**0.703 ± 0.030**	**0.915 ± 0.009**	0.724 ± 0.033	**0.866 ± 0.028**

We take advantage of the clustering algorithm to attain the type of both cell and supercell (cell community) in hematolymphoid cancers, given that their cellular components in TME are unclear and that is distinct from solid tumors with well-studied TME. We attach great importance to cell type information and hypothesize that cells belonging to different types and communities play distinct functions. The unsupervised manner would also save tremendous workload for obtaining medical experts cell labeling and shed light on uncovering new insight into cell subtypes and communities.

We propose a novel supercell concept in this study. The supercell is anticipated to be an excellent bridge to connect the neighboring cell interaction (local graph) and cell community interaction (global graph). Here, we just scratch the surface of supercells properties, through merely exploiting supercells central coordinates to build global graphs. Indeed, each supercell contains rich information of the local TME, and their overlapped region may manifest interplay mechanisms of differing tumor subclones or habitats. We anticipate that future studies will help derive more biological insight based on the supercell context. Our approach in this analysis uses manually designed features from the supercell-based global graph for diagnosis due to limited image samples. However, future approaches should permit taking each supercell as the node to use the graph convolution network (GCN) to further improve diagnostic accuracy when sufficient images are available.

4   Conclusion

We present a hierarchical cell phenotyping and graph modeling algorithm to profile the spatial patterns of neoplastic lymphoid cells distributed within the tumor microenvironment. Using this global graph's manual-crafted features, we achieve promising results based on clinical tumor images from various types of hematolymphoid tumors of different grades. We anticipate that the proposed cell phenotyping and supercell design can adapt to a broader category of cancers.

References

1. Agbay, R.L.M.C., Jain, N., Loghavi, S., Medeiros, L.J., Khoury, J.D.: Histologic transformation of chronic lymphocytic leukemia/small lymphocytic lymphoma. Am. J. Hematol. **91**(10), 1036–1043 (2016)
2. Agbay, R.L.M.C., Loghavi, S., Medeiros, L.J., Khoury, J.D.: High-grade transformation of low-grade b-cell lymphoma. Am. J. Surgi. Pathol. **40**(1), e1–e16 (2016)
3. Campanella, G., et al.: Clinical-grade computational pathology using weakly supervised deep learning on whole slide images. Nat. Med. **25**(8), 1301–1309 (2019)
4. Chen, P., Liang, Y., Shi, X., Yang, L., Gader, P.: Automatic whole slide pathology image diagnosis framework via unit stochastic selection and attention fusion. Neurocomputing **453**, 312–325 (2021)
5. Chen, P., Shi, X., Liang, Y., Li, Y., Yang, L., Gader, P.D.: Interactive thyroid whole slide image diagnostic system using deep representation. Comput. Methods Program. Biomed. **195**, 105630 (2020)
6. El Hussein, S., et al.: Artificial intelligence strategy integrating morphologic and architectural biomarkers provides robust diagnostic accuracy for disease progression in chronic lymphocytic leukemia. J. Pathol. (2021)

7. Friedman, J., Hastie, T., Tibshirani, R.: The Elements of Statistical Learning. Series in Statistics New York, vol. 1. Springer, New York (2001)
8. Gerlinger, M., et al.: Intratumor heterogeneity and branched evolution revealed by multiregion sequencing. N. Engl. J. Med. **366**, 883–892 (2012)
9. Gu, X., Angelov, P., Zhao, Z.: A distance-type-insensitive clustering approach. Appl. Soft Comput. **77**, 622–634 (2019)
10. He, X., Cai, D., Niyogi, P.: Laplacian score for feature selection. In: Advances in Neural Information Processing Systems, vol. 18, pp. 507–514 (2005)
11. Hou, L., Samaras, D., Kurc, T.M., Gao, Y., Davis, J.E., Saltz, J.H.: Patch-based convolutional neural network for whole slide tissue image classification. In: Proceedings of the IEEE Conference on Computer Vision and Pattern Recognition, pp. 2424–2433 (2016)
12. Janowczyk, A., Madabhushi, A.: Deep learning for digital pathology image analysis: a comprehensive tutorial with selected use cases. J. Pathol. Inform. **7** (2016)
13. Jaume, G., et al.: Towards explainable graph representations in digital pathology. arXiv preprint arXiv:2007.00311 (2020)
14. Javed, S., et al.: Cellular community detection for tissue phenotyping in colorectal cancer histology images. Med. Image Anal. **63**, 101696 (2020)
15. Joyce, J.A., Fearon, D.T.: T cell exclusion, immune privilege, and the tumor microenvironment. Science **348**(6230), 74–80 (2015)
16. Komura, D., Ishikawa, S.: Machine learning methods for histopathological image analysis. Comput. Struct. Biotechnol. J. **16**, 34–42 (2018)
17. Korneev, K.V., Atretkhany, K.S.N., Drutskaya, M.S., Grivennikov, S.I., Kuprash, D.V., Nedospasov, S.A.: Tlr-signaling and proinflammatory cytokines as drivers of tumorigenesis. Cytokine **89**, 127–135 (2017)
18. Lewis, J.S., Jr., Ali, S., Luo, J., Thorstad, W.L., Madabhushi, A.: A quantitative histomorphometric classifier (quhbic) identifies aggressive versus indolent p16-positive oropharyngeal squamous cell carcinoma. Am. J. Surgi. Pathol. **38**(1), 128 (2014)
19. Li, Y., Chen, P., Li, Z., Su, H., Yang, L., Zhong, D.: Rule-based automatic diagnosis of thyroid nodules from intraoperative frozen sections using deep learning. Artif. Intell. Med. **108**, 101918 (2020)
20. Lu, C., et al.: Feature-driven local cell graph (flock): new computational pathology-based descriptors for prognosis of lung cancer and hpv status of oropharyngeal cancers. Med. Image Anal. **68**, 101903 (2021)
21. Lu, C., Xu, H., Xu, J., Gilmore, H., Mandal, M., Madabhushi, A.: Multi-pass adaptive voting for nuclei detection in histopathological images. Sci. Rep. **6**(1), 1–18 (2016)
22. Pati, P., et al.: HACT-Net: a hierarchical cell-to-tissue graph neural network for histopathological image classification. In: Sudre, C.H., et al. (eds.) UNSURE/GRAIL -2020. LNCS, vol. 12443, pp. 208–219. Springer, Cham (2020). https://doi.org/10.1007/978-3-030-60365-6_20
23. Schürch, C.M., et al.: Coordinated cellular neighborhoods orchestrate antitumoral immunity at the colorectal cancer invasive front. Cell **182**(5), 1341–1359 (2020)
24. Shin, D., et al.: Quantitative analysis of high-resolution microendoscopic images for diagnosis of esophageal squamous cell carcinoma. Clin. Gastroenterol. Hepatol. **13**(2), 272–279 (2015)
25. Tuzel, O., Porikli, F., Meer, P.: Kernel methods for weakly supervised mean shift clustering. In: 2009 IEEE 12th International Conference on Computer Vision, pp. 48–55. IEEE (2009)

26. Vitale, I., Shema, E., Loi, S., Galluzzi, L.: Intratumoral heterogeneity in cancer progression and response to immunotherapy. Nat. Med. 1–13 (2021)
27. Wu, J., Mayer, A.T., Li, R.: Integrated imaging and molecular analysis to decipher tumor microenvironment in the era of immunotherapy. In: Seminars in Cancer Biology. Elsevier (2020)
28. Zhang, Z., Chen, P., Shi, X., Yang, L.: Text-guided neural network training for image recognition in natural scenes and medicine. IEEE Trans. Pattern Anal. Mach. Intell. **43**(5), 1733–1745 (2021)
29. Zhou, Y., Graham, S., Alemi Koohbanani, N., Shaban, M., Heng, P.A., Rajpoot, N.: Cgc-net: cell graph convolutional network for grading of colorectal cancer histology images. In: Proceedings of the IEEE/CVF International Conference on Computer Vision Workshops (2019)
30. Zhu, X., Yao, J., Zhu, F., Huang, J.: Wsisa: making survival prediction from whole slide histopathological images. In: Proceedings of the IEEE Conference on Computer Vision and Pattern Recognition, pp. 7234–7242 (2017)

A Computational Geometry Approach for Modeling Neuronal Fiber Pathways

S. Shailja$^{(\boxtimes)}$, Angela Zhang , and B. S. Manjunath

University of California, Santa Barbara, CA 93117, USA
{shailja,angela00,manj}@ucsb.edu

Abstract. We propose a novel and efficient algorithm to model high-level topological structures of neuronal fibers. Tractography constructs complex neuronal fibers in three dimensions that exhibit the geometry of white matter pathways in the brain. However, most tractography analysis methods are time consuming and intractable. We develop a computational geometry-based tractography representation that aims to simplify the connectivity of white matter fibers. Given the trajectories of neuronal fiber pathways, we model the evolution of trajectories that encodes geometrically significant events and calculate their point correspondence in the 3D brain space. Trajectory inter-distance is used as a parameter to control the granularity of the model that allows local or global representation of the tractogram. Using diffusion MRI data from Alzheimer's patient study, we extract tractography features from our model for distinguishing the Alzheimer's subject from the normal control. Software implementation of our algorithm is available on GitHub (https://github.com/UCSB-VRL/ReebGraph).

Keywords: Computational geometry · Computational pathology · Reeb graph · Trajectories · Brain fibers · Connectome

1 Introduction

Diffusion MRI (dMRI) tractography [2] constructs morphological 3D neuronal fibers represented by 3D images called tractograms. In recent years, analysis of fibers in dMRI tractography data has received wide interest due to its potential applications in computational pathology, surgery, and studies of diseases, such as brain tumors [3,10], Alzheimer's [4], and schizophrenia [13]. Tractography datasets are huge and complex consisting of millions of fibers arising and terminating at different functional regions of the brain. Computational analysis of these fibers is challenging owing to their complex topological structures in three dimensions. Tractography produces white matter pathways that can be deduced as spatial trajectories represented by a sequence of 3D coordinates. To model the geometry of these trajectories, we utilize the concept of Reeb graphs [17] that

Supported by NSF award: SSI # 1664172 and NIH award # 5R01NS103774-02.

M. de Bruijne et al. (Eds.): MICCAI 2021, LNCS 12908, pp. 175–185, 2021.
https://doi.org/10.1007/978-3-030-87237-3_17

have been successfully used in a wide variety of applications in computational geometry and graphics, such as shape matching, topological data analysis, simplification, and segmentation. We assume that the groups of trajectories that are spatially close to each other share similar properties. Therefore, we compute a model to encode the arising & ending and the merging & splitting behavior for groups of trajectories (as shown in Fig. 1) along with their point correspondence. With these computations in place, we develop a finite state machine that can be used to query the state of any trajectory or its shared groups. The resulting model has tunable granularity that can be used to derive models with the desired level of geometrical details or abstract properties.

2 Related Work

Brain tractography datasets are constructed from the dMRI of an individual's brain [23,24]. One way to analyze the fiber tracts is to generate a connectivity matrix that provides a compact description of pairwise connectivity of regions of interest (ROI) derived from anatomical or computational brain atlases. For example, the connectivity matrices can be used to compute multiple graph theory-based metrics to distinguish between the brains of healthy children and those with recent traumatic brain injury [21]. However, such methods overlook the geometrical characteristics within a region of interest. A number of inter-fiber distance-based approaches have been used to analyze the fibers [1,5,8,11,12,26] for clustering and segmentation but have some limitations. For example, one needs prior information about the number of clusters to be segmented in [8]. More sophisticated methods produce high-dimensional representations that are not efficient [20,25]. Due to the complex nature of tractography algorithms, another way to compare bundles is by using tract profiling techniques that quantifies diffusion measures along each fiber tract [22]. Notably, researchers in [7] introduced a representation that is sparse and can be integrated with learning methods for further study. However, their approach leads to possible loss of critical points of fibers (due to polynomial fitting) and ignores multi-fiber tractography. Our design addresses this by sequentially processing the group behavior emerging due to events of individual trajectories. Our method builds on previous work on time-dependent trajectory analysis using a Reeb graph. A deterministic algorithm for Reeb graph computation in $O(n \log n)$ time is shown in [14]. Reeb graph can be used to model the trajectory grouping structure defined by time as a parameter [6]. For tractography analysis, the concept of "bundling" and "unbundling" structure of trajectory data to compute a sparse graph is proposed in [18]. They show graph representation of brain tractography but do not present the algorithm or proofs for the computation, focusing instead on the novel problem definition.

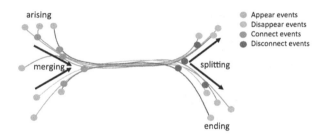

Fig. 1. A basic example of a set of trajectories displaying the arising, merging, splitting, and ending behaviour. These qualitative behaviors of group of trajectories emerge due to the events (appear, connect, disconnect, and disappear) of individual trajectory. Events of trajectories are used to define behavior of the group of trajectories.

3   Preliminaries

In the three dimensional Euclidean space $\mathbb{R}^3$, we define the following terms that would help in setting up the problem in this section.

Trajectory: A trajectory T is as an ordered sequence of points in $\mathbb{R}^3$. We denote a trajectory T as a sequence of points $\{p_1, p_2, ..., p_m\}$, where m is the number of points in T and $p_i \in \mathbb{R}^3$.

ε-(dis)connected Points: For any pair of points p_1 and p_2 in $\mathbb{R}^3$, we define $d(p_1, p_2)$ as the Euclidean distance between the two points:

$$d(p_1, p_2) = \|p_1 - p_2\|_2 \, ,$$

where $\|\cdot\|_2$ represents the Euclidean norm. Two points p_1, p_2 are ϵ-connected if $d(p_1, p_2) \leq \epsilon$. Similarly, two points p_1, p_2 are ϵ-disconnected if $d(p_1, p_2) > \epsilon$.

Appear Event: For each trajectory T, the initial point of its ordered sequence is labeled for the occurrence of the *appear event*. For example, for trajectory $T_1 = \{p_1, p_2, ..., p_m\}$, we observe the appear event at the point p_1.

Disappear Event: For each trajectory T, the final point of its ordered sequence is labeled for the occurrence of the *disappear event*. For example, for trajectory $T_1 = \{p_1, p_2, ..., p_m\}$, we observe the disappear event at p_m.

Connect Events: To define *connect events* for a pair of trajectories, consider two trajectories

$$T = \{p_1, p_2, ..., p_m\}, \quad T^{'} = \{p_1^{'}, p_2^{'}, ..., p_m^{'}\},$$

then a connect event for the pair $(T, T^{'})$ is defined by $(p_i, p_j^{'})$ such that $p_i \in T, p_j^{'} \in T^{'}$ and,

$$d(p_i, p_j^{'}) \leq \epsilon, \quad d(p_{i-1}, p_{j-1}^{'}) > \epsilon, \quad \text{for } i > 1 \text{ and } j > 1.$$

If there is no such pair of points, it implies that T and $T^{'}$ are disjoint. Moreover, if T and $T^{'}$ are ϵ-connected at $(p_i, p_j^{'})$ and if $T^{'}$ and T^* are also ϵ-connected

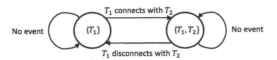

Fig. 2. An example of state diagram for trajectory T_1. T_1 is either directly (dis)connected with T_2 or ϵ-step (dis)connected.

at (p'_j, p^*_l) where $p^*_l \in T^*$, then we say that T and T^* are ϵ-*step connected* at (p_i, p^*_l).

Disconnect Events: Given a pair of trajectories (T, T') with a connect event at (p_i, p'_j), we define a *disconnect event* by (p_{i+k}, p'_{j+k}) such that,

$$d(p_{i+k}, p'_{j+k}) > \epsilon, \quad d(p_{i+k-1}, p'_{j+k-1}) \leq \epsilon.$$

Max-width ϵ-Connected Trajectories: For an input $\mathcal{I}$, there are many possible ϵ-step connected trajectories. The maximal group of trajectories at a given step k are called *max-width ϵ-step connected* and there is no other possible set of sub-trajectories that can intersect with the maximal group at k.

Note that the trajectories estimated from dMRI tractography do not have a specific beginning or ending, as dMRI is not sensitive to the direction of connections. So, reversing the order of the points of a streamlines will produce similar results. Two events appear and disappear are used for convenience in describing the algorithm and its implementation.

3.1   Problem Formulation

We set up the following central problem for this paper:

Input: A set of trajectories $\mathcal{I} = \{T_1, T_2, ..., T_n\}$, such that $T_i \in \mathbb{R}^3$ for all $i \in \{1, 2, ..., n\}$ where n is the number of trajectories.

Output: A finite state machine (FSM) S that models the evolution of trajectories and their critical points of interaction with all other trajectories.

$$S = (A, O, V, \mathcal{R}),$$
$$\mathcal{R} : (S \times A) \longrightarrow (S \times O),$$

where A is the set of events associated with each trajectory $T_i \in \mathcal{I}$, O is the set of outputs encoding the location information of the critical events, V is the set of states that corresponds to a group of trajectories. $\mathcal{R}$ is the state-transition and output function. When the machine is in a current state $v \in V$ and receives an input $a \in A$ it moves to the next state specified by R and produces an output location $o \in O$ as shown in Fig. 2.

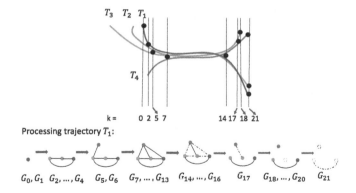

Fig. 3. The figure shows an input $\mathcal{I} = \{T_1, T_2, T_3, T_4\}$ exhibiting arising, merging, splitting, and ending behaviour. After processing the sequence of points in T_1, at $k = 0, 2, 5, 7, 14, 17, 18, 21$ steps, we modify the G_k respectively. Connect, disconnect, appear, and disappear events associated with T_1 are marked by black circles. Delete node and edge queries are represented by dashed circle and dashed line in G_k.

4 Reeb Graph

The central part of solving the problem as stated above is to compute $\mathcal{R}$—the state transition and output function. Towards that end, we compute an undirected graph $\mathcal{R}$ called the Reeb graph. In this section, we define the Reeb graph and then proceed to develop an algorithm that can compute this graph for a set of trajectories. Formally, a Reeb graph $\mathcal{R}$ is defined on a manifold $\mathcal{M} \in \mathbb{R}^3$ using the evolution of level sets L [9]. To adapt this definition of $\mathcal{R}$ for the case of neuronal fiber trajectory evolution problem, we define a manifold $\mathcal{M}$ in $\mathbb{R}^3$ as the union of all points in the tractogram. The set of points of trajectories at step k is the level set of k. The connected components in the level set of k correspond to the max-width ϵ-connected trajectories at step k. Unlike previous studies [6], here, any number of trajectories can become ϵ-(dis)connected at the same location. Reeb graph $\mathcal{R}$ describes the evolution of the connected components over sequential steps. At every step k, the changes in connected components (states of FSM) are represented by vertices in $\mathcal{R}$.

4.1 Computing the Reeb Graph

In Sect. 3, for a given trajectory, we defined appear and disappear events. For a pair of trajectories, we defined connect and disconnect events. These events $(a \in A)$ describe the branching structure of the trajectories. To compute the Reeb graph, we process these events sequentially. We maintain a graph $G = (V', E')$ where the vertices represent the set of trajectories. G is a graph that changes with steps representing the connect and disconnect relations between different trajectories. At each step k, we insert new nodes at appear events and delete nodes at disappear events. At connect events, we insert edges in G and at

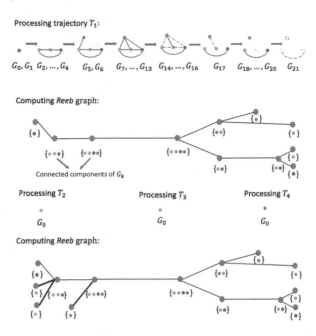

Fig. 4. Continuing the same example from Fig. 3, we show representation of $\mathcal{R}$ from G_k. Edges of $\mathcal{R}$ encodes the maximal group of trajectories and vertices of $\mathcal{R}$ records the significant points of the trajectories.

disconnect events, we delete edges. At each step k, an edge (T_1, T_2) in G shows that T_1 and T_2 are directly connected. Therefore the max-width ϵ-connected trajectories correspond to the connected components in G at step k.

Initialization: We spend $O(N^2)$ time to store the appear, disappear, connect, and disconnect events for all pair of the trajectories. We store a mapping M from the current components in G to the corresponding vertices in $\mathcal{R}$. We start from one of the trajectories and add other trajectories of interest on the way of following its points sequentially. We maintain a data structure to flag the points for which the events are already processed and store their mappings to the vertices of the Reeb graph in D. Note that although the computational time is $O(N^2)$, this step is massively parallelizable.

Split and Merge: To handle a disconnect event of trajectories T_1 and T_2 at step k, we delete the edge (T_1, T_2) from G_k. Similarly, for a connect event of trajectories T_1 and T_2 at step k, we add the edge (T_1, T_2) to G_k. We do this for all the connect and disconnect events as shown in Fig. 3 for trajectory T_1. For the disconnect event, we query G_{k-1} to get the connected component C consisting of trajectories T_1 and T_2 and locate the corresponding u in $\mathcal{R}$. We query G_k to get the connected components C_1 and C_2 consisting of trajectories T_1 and T_2, respectively. $C_1 = C_2$ implies that the trajectories T_1 and T_2 are still ϵ-step connected. If $C_1 \neq C_2$, we add a new split vertex v to $\mathcal{R}$ and a new edge (u, v) and update M accordingly.

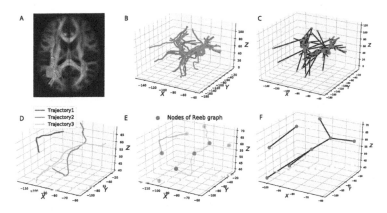

Fig. 5. (A) shows the fiber tracts created by DSI Studio (http://dsi-studio.labsolver. org/Manual/Fiber-Tracking) for an example ROI. (B) shows the example white matter fiber tracts in 3D. (C) exhibits the corresponding $\mathcal{R}$ for the example fibers. (D) shows three fibers from R to form a qualitative impression of our proposed algorithm. (E) indicates the nodes of $\mathcal{R}$ overlapped on the trajectories. (F) represents the proposed grouping structure with the vertices and edges.

Computing $\mathcal{R}$ from G: We query G_k and G_{k-1} to get the connected components at step k and $k-1$ respectively. For each connected component C_c in G_k, if C_c is present in the connected components of G_{k-1}, then we do not modify $\mathcal{R}$. This implies that no such event occurred in the trajectories of C_c which could result in any critical points. Otherwise, using M, we locate the corresponding nodes in $\mathcal{R}$ for the connected components in G_{k-1}, we call it previous connected components. The corresponding nodes in $\mathcal{R}$ for the connected components in G_k are called present connected components. For each component in present connected components, we add a node v in $\mathcal{R}$ if not already present in the previous connected component and assign the location ($o \in O$) as the coordinates of one of the points in the connected components. If that is the case, we also add an edge (u, v), where u is the node corresponding to previous connected component C_1 and v is the node corresponding to present connected component C_2, if $|C_1 \cap C_2| > 0$. Finally, we update M accordingly.

At next step $k+1$, if we encounter the point of a trajectory T for which the events have already been processed, we query D to locate the vertex u and v in $\mathcal{R}$ for p_k and p_{k+1} respectively. We add an edge (u, v) to $\mathcal{R}$ as shown in Fig. 4 and delete the node corresponding to trajectory T in G and update M.

Theorem 1. *For a given set of trajectories, $\mathcal{I} = \{T_1, T_2, ..., T_n\}$ with a total of N points, the Reeb graph $\mathcal{R}$ of $\mathcal{I}$ can be computed in $O(N \log N)$ time.*

Proof. It is possible to compute the connected components of a graph $G(V', E')$ with $|V'|$ vertices and $|E'|$ edges using Breadth First Search (BFS) or Depth First Search (DFS) in $O(N^2)$ time. But, since we know all of the points of the

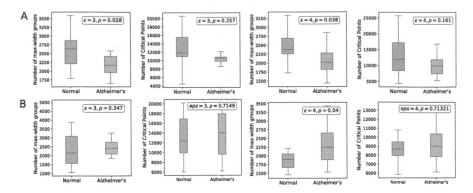

Fig. 6. Statistical analysis results for different values of ϵ showing the comparison between normal and Alzheimer's subjects across properties of $\mathcal{R}$ for ROI A) Posterior Cingulate Gyrus and B) Middle Occipital Gyrus

given input $\mathcal{I}$ at which any event occurs, we can use a dynamic graph connectivity approach [14] to improve the computation time. This method allows connectivity operations, inserts, and deletes, in $O(logN)$ time. In the worst case, we modify and query the graph G to get the connected components for all the points in $\mathcal{I}$. Hence, the total time required for the construction of $\mathcal{R}$ is $O(NlogN)$.

5   Examples and Applications

To the best of our knowledge, there are no existing modeling methods in the literature for brain fibers that can be used to compare our method directly. To provide the proof of concept and demonstrate utility, we evaluate our proposed algorithm on real data and validate manually as illustrated in Fig. 5. To design a case study demonstrating the utility of $\mathcal{R}$, we randomly select 22 subjects (11 Normal and 11 Alzheimer's patient) from the publicly available Alzheimer's Disease Neuroimaging Initiative (ADNI) [15] dataset (http://adni.loni.usc.edu/). We evaluate the qualitative representation of critical points using our model on fibers for random ROIs. All the analytically significant points are captured by $\mathcal{R}$ through nodes and edges, which are highly consistent across subjects. The proposed model can be employed in the existing deep learning and machine learning algorithms to provide new insights into the structure and the function of the brain. Similar to recent research works where graph theory-based features are utilized for classification tasks, we compute the total number of max-width ϵ-connected groups that is $|E|$ and the aggregate of significant points on fibers that is $|V|$. We also calculate network properties such as clustering, centrality, modularity, and efficiency of $\mathcal{R}$. We choose two ROIs: Posterior Cingulate Gyrus and Middle Occipital Gyrus from the left hemisphere based on the Automated Anatomical Labelling (AAL) atlas [16,19] and compute tractography consisting of 1000 fibers in each ROI for each subject. We used Q-Space Diffeomorphic

Reconstruction as implemented in DSI Studio [23] to compute the fibers. In Fig. 6, we show the distribution of a set of properties that can be used to facilitate comparisons between Alzheimer's and normal subjects. By comparing the p-value for the ROIs shown in Fig. 6, we can conclude that Posterior Cingulate Gyrus (lesser p-value) is a more significant ROI than Middle Occipital Gyrus. This is in accordance with the study [16] that highlights the relevant ROIs for Alzheimer's disease. The average run time of our implementation for examples consisting of 132,000 points on average was 42 s on Intel Core CPU 4 GHz processor with 32 GB RAM.

6   Conclusion

Our paper proposes the study of the spatial evolution of neuronal trajectories including the algorithmic analysis. We also demonstrate how our proposed reduced graph encodes the critical points of the pathways. Point correspondence of the critical coordinates in the 3D brain space calculated in our algorithm is an essential requirement of the tract-orientated quantitative analysis which is overlooked in the previous works. This aids in localizing and underpinning the points of interest in white matter tracts. Through our preliminary experiments, we show a set of properties of the Reeb graph that can be used to distinguish between the Alzheimer's patients and control subjects. In future, we plan to utilize graph-theoretic concepts to analyze the Reeb graph models of white matter fibers. We intend to further evaluate the reproducibility of our approach on additional datasets. Integrating graph-theoretic features of the Reeb graph with data-driven learning approaches can greatly improve our understanding of various human disease pathways.

References

1. Andersson, M., Gudmundsson, J., Laube, P., Wolle, T.: Reporting leaders and followers among trajectories of moving point objects. GeoInformatica 12(4), 497–528 (2008)
2. Basser, P.J., Pajevic, S., Pierpaoli, C., Duda, J., Aldroubi, A.: In vivo fiber tractography using DT-MRI data. Magn. Reson. Med. 44(4), 625–632 (2000)
3. Berman, J.I., Berger, M.S., Mukherjee, P., Henry, R.G.: Diffusion-tensor imaging–guided tracking of fibers of the pyramidal tract combined with intraoperative cortical stimulation mapping in patients with gliomas. J. Neurosurg. 101(1), 66–72 (2004)
4. Bozzali, M., et al.: White matter damage in Alzheimer's disease assessed in vivo using diffusion tensor magnetic resonance imaging. J. Neurol. Neurosurg. Psychiatry 72(6), 742–746 (2002)
5. Brun, A., Knutsson, H., Park, H.-J., Shenton, M.E., Westin, C.-F.: Clustering fiber traces using normalized cuts. In: Barillot, C., Haynor, D.R., Hellier, P. (eds.) MICCAI 2004. LNCS, vol. 3216, pp. 368–375. Springer, Heidelberg (2004). https://doi.org/10.1007/978-3-540-30135-6_45

6. Buchin, K., Buchin, M., van Kreveld, M., Speckmann, B., Staals, F.: Trajectory grouping structure. In: Dehne, F., Solis-Oba, R., Sack, J.-R. (eds.) WADS 2013. LNCS, vol. 8037, pp. 219–230. Springer, Heidelberg (2013). https://doi.org/10.1007/978-3-642-40104-6_19

7. Cabeen, R.P., Toga, A.W., Laidlaw, D.H.: Tractography processing with the sparse closest point transform. Neuroinformatics, 1–12 (2020)

8. Dodero, L., Vascon, S., Murino, V., Bifone, A., Gozzi, A., Sona, D.: Automated multi-subject fiber clustering of mouse brain using dominant sets. Front. Neuroinform. **8**, 87 (2015)

9. Doraiswamy, H., Natarajan, V.: Efficient algorithms for computing Reeb graphs. Comput. Geom. **42**(6–7), 606–616 (2009)

10. Kao, P.Y., Shailja, S., Jiang, J., Zhang, A., Khan, A., Chen, J.W., Manjunath, B.: Corrigendum: improving patch-based convolutional neural networks for MRI brain tumor segmentation by leveraging location information. Front. Neurosci. **14** (2020)

11. Moberts, B., Vilanova, A., Van Wijk, J.J.: Evaluation of fiber clustering methods for diffusion tensor imaging. In: VIS 05. IEEE Visualization, pp. 65–72. IEEE (2005)

12. O'Donnell, L.J., Schultz, T.: Statistical and machine learning methods for neuroimaging: examples, challenges, and extensions to diffusion imaging data. In: Hotz, I., Schultz, T. (eds.) Visualization and Processing of Higher Order Descriptors for Multi-Valued Data. MV, pp. 299–319. Springer, Cham (2015). https://doi.org/10.1007/978-3-319-15090-1_15

13. Park, H.J., et al.: White matter hemisphere asymmetries in healthy subjects and in schizophrenia: a diffusion tensor MRI study. Neuroimage **23**(1), 213–223 (2004)

14. Parsa, S.: A deterministic $o(m\log(m))$ time algorithm for the Reeb graph. Discrete Comput. Geom. **49**(4), 864–878 (2013)

15. Petersen, R.C., et al.: Alzheimer's disease neuroimaging initiative (ADNI): clinical characterization. Neurology **74**(3), 201–209 (2009). https://doi.org/10.1212/wnl.0b013e3181cb3e25

16. Rondina, J.M., et al.: Selecting the most relevant brain regions to discriminate Alzheimer's disease patients from healthy controls using multiple kernel learning: a comparison across functional and structural imaging modalities and atlases. NeuroImage Clin. **17**, 628–641 (2018). https://doi.org/10.1016/j.nicl.2017.10.026

17. Shinagawa, Y., Kunii, T.L., Kergosien, Y.L.: Surface coding based on Morse theory. IEEE Comput. Graph. Appl. **11**(5), 66–78 (1991)

18. Sun, J., Cieslak, M., Grafton, S., Suri, S.: A reeb graph approach to tractography. In: Proceedings of the 23rd SIGSPATIAL International Conference on Advances in Geographic Information Systems, pp. 1–4 (2015)

19. Tzourio-Mazoyer, N., et al.: Automated anatomical labeling of activations in SPM using a macroscopic anatomical parcellation of the MNI MRI single-subject brain. NeuroImage **15**(1), 273–289 (2002). https://doi.org/10.1006/nimg.2001.0978

20. Wang, Q., Yap, P.-T., Wu, G., Shen, D.: Fiber modeling and clustering based on neuroanatomical features. In: Fichtinger, G., Martel, A., Peters, T. (eds.) MICCAI 2011. LNCS, vol. 6892, pp. 17–24. Springer, Heidelberg (2011). https://doi.org/10.1007/978-3-642-23629-7_3

21. Watson, C.G., DeMaster, D., Ewing-Cobbs, L.: Graph theory analysis of DTI tractography in children with traumatic injury. NeuroImage Clin. **21**, 101673 (2019). https://doi.org/10.1016/j.nicl.2019.101673

22. Yeatman, J.D., Dougherty, R.F., Myall, N.J., Wandell, B.A., Feldman, H.M.: Tract profiles of white matter properties: automating fiber-tract quantification. PLoS ONE **7**(11), e49790 (2012)
23. Yeh, F.C., Tseng, W.Y.I.: NTU-90: a high angular resolution brain atlas constructed by Q-space diffeomorphic reconstruction. NeuroImage **58**(1), 91–99 (2011). https://doi.org/10.1016/j.neuroimage.2011.06.021
24. Yeh, F.C., Verstynen, T.D., Wang, Y., Fernández-Miranda, J.C., Tseng, W.Y.I.: Deterministic diffusion fiber tracking improved by quantitative anisotropy. PLoS ONE **8**(11), e80713 (2013). https://doi.org/10.1371/journal.pone.0080713
25. Yendiki, A., Panneck, P., Srinivasan, P., Stevens, A., Zöllei, L., Augustinack, J., Wang, R., Salat, D., Ehrlich, S., Behrens, T., et al.: Automated probabilistic reconstruction of white-matter pathways in health and disease using an atlas of the underlying anatomy. Front. Neuroinform. **5**, 23 (2011)
26. Zhang, S., Correia, S., Laidlaw, D.H.: Identifying white-matter fiber bundles in DTI data using an automated proximity-based fiber-clustering method. IEEE Trans. Vis. Comput. Graph. **14**(5), 1044–1053 (2008)

TransPath: Transformer-Based Self-supervised Learning for Histopathological Image Classification

Xiyue Wang[1], Sen Yang[2], Jun Zhang[2], Minghui Wang[1], Jing Zhang[3(✉)], Junzhou Huang[2], Wei Yang[2], and Xiao Han[2]

[1] College of Computer Science, Sichuan University, Chengdu, China
haroldhan@tencent.com
[2] Tencent AI Lab, Shenzhen, China
[3] College of Biomedical Engineering, Sichuan University, Chengdu, China
jing_zhang@scu.edu.cn

Abstract. A large-scale labeled dataset is a key factor for the success of supervised deep learning in histopathological image analysis. However, exhaustive annotation requires a careful visual inspection by pathologists, which is extremely time-consuming and labor-intensive. Self-supervised learning (SSL) can alleviate this issue by pre-training models under the supervision of data itself, which generalizes well to various downstream tasks with limited annotations. In this work, we propose a hybrid model (*TransPath*) which is pre-trained in an SSL manner on massively unlabeled histopathological images to discover the inherent image property and capture domain-specific feature embedding. The *TransPath* can serve as a collaborative local-global feature extractor, which is designed by combining a convolutional neural network (CNN) and a modified transformer architecture. We propose a token-aggregating and excitation (TAE) module which is placed behind the self-attention of the transformer encoder for capturing more global information. We evaluate the performance of pre-trained *TransPath* by fine-tuning it on three downstream histopathological image classification tasks. Our experimental results indicate that *TransPath* outperforms state-of-the-art vision transformer networks, and the visual representations generated by SSL on domain-relevant histopathological images are more transferable than the supervised baseline on ImageNet. Our code and pre-trained models will be available at https://github.com/Xiyue-Wang/TransPath.

Keywords: Self-supervised learning · Transformer · Histopathological image

1 Introduction

Benefiting from a massive amount of labeled data, deep learning has obtained success in medical image analysis. However, such careful annotations are very scarce in histopathological whole-slide images (WSIs). Gigapixel size of the image

© Springer Nature Switzerland AG 2021
M. de Bruijne et al. (Eds.): MICCAI 2021, LNCS 12908, pp. 186–195, 2021.
https://doi.org/10.1007/978-3-030-87237-3_18

creates a large search space for labeling, and the wide variations, even between the same class, further increase the annotation challenge. Extracting effective features from unlabeled histopathological images can promote the development of digital pathology and aid pathologists for faster and more precise diagnoses.

To address these issues, transfer learning from large labeled ImageNet [14] are proven to be an effective training strategy [12]. However, a large domain shift exists between natural images and histopathological images. The desired approach to tackle this domain shift is pre-training or training from scratch on the domain-relevant data, which is limited by the annotation-lacking problem. To address this, self-supervised pre-training is a possible alternative, which learns the image representation using the supervision signal produced from the data itself. Self-supervised learning (SSL) has achieved superior performance in the field of natural images for image classification, semantic segmentation, and object detection tasks [2,6].

For the histopathological image analysis, there have been several works that apply SSL techniques (e.g. CPC, SimCLR, and MoCo) to improve the classification performance [3,8,9,11,15]. However, there are still two aspects that could be improved. First, these works lack a large domain-specific histopathological image dataset for self-supervised pre-training, and their pre-trained image patches were cropped from a small number of WSIs (up to 400 WSIs). The small dataset results in a lack of sample diversity and prevents robust and generic representation learning. Second, only CNN structures are applied. CNN has a good capacity to learn low-level texture content features (local features) which is a crucial determinant in the classification task. The learning of global context features is often limited by the receptive field. The cropped histopathological image patches are usually enough to capture both the cell-level structure (e.g., cellular microenvironment) and tissue-level context (e.g., tumor microenvironment). Thus, both the local and global features are required for digital pathology. To learn global features, the transformer-based architecture may be a viable alternative, which originates from the natural language processing (NLP) field and has shown great potential in the computer vision field [4].

In this work, we collected the current largest histopathological image dataset for self-supervised pre-training, which comprises approximately 2.7 million images with the size of 2048×2048 cropped from a total of 32,529 WSIs from the cancer genome atlas (TCGA[1]) and pathology AI platform (PAIP[2]) datasets. The utilized datasets guarantee sample diversity and cover multi-sites (over 25 anatomic sites) and multi-cancer subtypes (over 32 classes). We propose a hybrid CNN-transformer framework to enhance the local structure and global context features extraction, where the transformer is modified by adding a customized TAE module into the self-attention block of the transformer. CNN extracts local features by convolutional computation. Transformer captures global dependencies through the information interaction among the tiled patches (tokens) from

---

[1] https://www.cancer.gov/about-nci/organization/ccg/research/structural-genomics/tcga/.

[2] http://www.wisepaip.org/paip/.

the generated features by CNN. The customized TAE is designed to further enhance global weight attention by taking all tokens into account. The combination of CNN and transformer networks can provide a robust and generalized feature extractor to capture both local fine structure and global context for the histopathological image analysis.

Our main contributions can be summarized as follows:

(1) To the best of our knowledge, this is the first self-supervised pre-training work carried out on the current largest public histopathological image dataset, which guarantees the sample diversity and helps the network capture sufficient domain-specific features.
(2) A novel hybrid architecture, which combines CNN and transformer to simultaneously capture the local structure and global context, is proposed to perform the histopathological image classification.
(3) We modified the self-attention layer of the vanilla transformer encoder by inserting our customized TAE module to strengthen the global feature learning ability further.
(4) Benefiting from the above design, our model outperforms state-of-the-art vision transformer networks on three public histopathological datasets. The proposed model can serve as a feature extractor for the downstream pathology image analysis. Our code and pre-trained model have been released online to facilitate reproductive research.

2   Methods

The overview of the proposed framework is provided in Fig. 1. There are two key points in our algorithm, namely construction of backbone and self-supervised pre-training, which will be introduced in the following.

2.1   Proposed Hybrid Network Backbone (*TransPath*)

The proposed hybrid network backbone *TransPath* aims to utilize both the local feature mining ability of CNN and the global interaction ability of the transformer. As shown in Fig. 1, the input image x is augmented as x_1 and x_2, which are then input to our designed backbone. In the backbone, CNN is first used to extract features ($\frac{H}{32} \times \frac{W}{32} \times 1024$). The produced features are the grid outputs $\frac{H}{32} \times \frac{W}{32} \times D$, where each grid element has a feature representation of length D. We denote each grid element as a token (i.e. token or word as in NLP), and the two-dimensional elements are flattened to a sequence of tokens $N \times D$, where $N = \frac{H}{32} \times \frac{W}{32}$. Besides the image features, we also provide the corresponding learnable position embeddings (*pos*). Then, similar to the ViT, an extra learnable classifier embedding (*cls*) as a single token is added to the transformer input to form a new input X with $N + 1$ patches. The final state of *cls* is acted as the final features generated by the transformer.

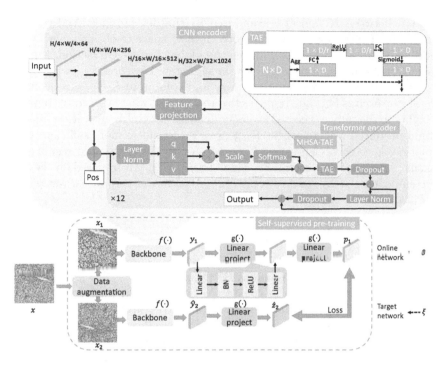

Fig. 1. Overview of the proposed CNN-transformer-based self-supervised pre-training procedure. BYOL architecture is used for self-supervised learning due to its negative sample independence [5]. The CNN block utilized in this work is ResNet50, which can be replaced by any CNN architecture. The transformer encoder is modified by inserting our customized TAE module for more sufficient global feature learning. BN: batch normalization.

Different from previous studies, the multi-head self-attention (MHSA) is modified in this work by adding our customized token-aggregating and excitation (TAE) module to produce a new MHSA block called MHSA-TAE, which is computed as follows.

$$\text{Linear projection} : \boldsymbol{Q} \leftarrow W_q X, \boldsymbol{K} \leftarrow W_k X, \boldsymbol{V} \leftarrow W_v X$$

$$\text{Self-attention} : F_{MHSA} = \text{Softmax}\left(\boldsymbol{Q}\boldsymbol{K}^\top / \sqrt{d}\right) \boldsymbol{V}$$

$$\text{Attention aggregation} : F_{agg} = \frac{1}{N+1} \sum_{i=1}^{N+1} F_{MHSA}(i,j) \tag{1}$$

$$\text{Output} : F_{MHSA-TAE} = \sigma(W' \times \sigma(W \times F_{agg})) \times F_{MHSA}$$

where the input X is linearly projected into 3 subspaces with weights W_k, W_q, and W_v to get $\boldsymbol{K}$, $\boldsymbol{Q}$, and $\boldsymbol{V}$, which consider all tokens, thereby helping generate global attention vectors. In the self-attention computation process, the interaction between K and Q is computed by the dot product. And then, the weight is scaled with factor b and projected into V space to obtain a new feature embedding F_{MHSA}. To further enhance the global feature extraction, the TAE module averages the input tokens to obtain aggregated features F_{agg} with the size of $1 \times D$, where the i and j denote the row and column in F_{MHSA}, respectively. The final step excites F_{agg} and re-projects it to F_{MHSA}, where W and W' represent the weights in the fully connected layers, σ denotes the ReLU activation function. The final produced feature weight $F_{MHSA-TAE}$ considers more sufficient global information since each element in $F_{MHSA-TAE}$ is the aggregated result across all tokens. After that, the attention weight $F_{MHSA-TAE}$ is imposed on the input feature embedding X by residual connection to form the output features y of our *TransPath*.

2.2   Self-supervised Pre-training

Self-supervised pre-training aims to learn a visual representation of raw data without manual supervision. We adopt BYOL architecture [5], which avoids the definition of negative samples in contrastive learning. As illustrated in Fig. 1, there are two parallel paths that share a similar structure but different network weights. The backbone adopts our proposed *TransPath*. We train the online network with parameter θ and to-be-updated parameter ξ of target network by $\xi \leftarrow \tau\xi + (1 - \tau)\theta$.

Given a random histopathological image x, its two augmentations (x_1 and x_2) are then alternately fed to the two parallel paths. When x_1 and x_2 respectively pass through our *TransPath* (formulated as $f(\cdot)$) in the online and target networks, which generates visual representations $y_1 = f^\theta(x_1)$, $\hat{y}_2 = f^\xi(x_2)$. Then, linear projection head $g(\cdot)$ is adopted to transform the representations to other latent spaces, e.g. $p_1 = g^\theta(g^\theta(y_1))$ in online network, $\hat{z}_2 = g^\xi(\hat{y}_2)$ in target network. Symmetrically, the swapped prediction separately feeds x_1 and x_2 to the target and online networks, obtaining $y_2 = f^\theta(x_2)$, $\hat{y}_1 = f^\xi(x_1)$, $p_2 = g^\theta(g^\theta(y_2))$, $\hat{z}_1 = g^\xi(\hat{y}_1)$. The objective function is optimized by minimizing the distance error of ℓ_2-norm between online and target networks:

$$L(p, z) = -\frac{p}{\|p\|_2} \cdot \frac{z}{\|z\|_2} \tag{2}$$

where $\|\cdot\|_2$ denotes the ℓ_2-norm. The symmetric objective function L_{loss} is calculated as:

$$L_{loss} = \frac{1}{2}L(p_1, \hat{z}_2) + \frac{1}{2}L(p_2, \hat{z}_1) \tag{3}$$

After self-supervised pre-training, the pre-trained backbone can then be fine-tuned to various downstream tasks.

3   Datasets

The datasets used for pre-training and fine-tuning are collected from different projects. The pre-trained histopathological image dataset is collected from two

WSI-level datasets: TCGA and PAIP. We crop these WSIs as approximately 2.7 million unlabeled images (2048 × 2048 pixels). After the self-supervised pre-training process, we fine-tune our CNN-transformer network to prove its classification ability on three public histopathological image datasets: NCT-CRC-HE, PatchCamelyon, and MHIST. The following will introduce them in detail.

TCGA. TCGA includes 30,072 WSIs covering over 25 anatomic sites and over 32 cancer subtypes. We crop these WSIs into images with the size of 2048 × 2048 pixels. After excluding images without tissues, we randomly select M images from each WSI. When the number of images in a WSI is less than M, all images available will be used. It is worth noting that because our image size is large enough, $M = 100$ can almost cover the entire WSI area. Finally, we generate a TCGA pre-training dataset with 2,476,964 unlabeled histopathological images.

PAIP. PAIP releases 2457 WSIs, including 6 cancer types (liver, renal, colorectal, prostatic, pancreatic, and cholangio cancers). Following the same image extraction strategy as the TCGA dataset, we produce a PAIP pre-training dataset with 223,557 unlabeled histopathological images.

NCT-CRC-HE. NCT-CRC-HE is provided by National Center for Tumor Diseases (NCT) to identify 8 colorectal cancer tissues and 1 normal tissue. A total of 100,000 images with 224 × 224 pixels are extracted from 86 WSIs [7], which is used as the training set in the fine-tuning process. The test set contains 7180 images extracted from 50 patients with colorectal adenocarcinoma.

PatchCamelyon. PatchCamelyon (PCam) contains 327,680 images (96 × 96) [1] for breast cancer detection, which are extracted from Camelyon16 challenge dataset with 400 WSIs. The data splitting in our fine-tuning experiment follows the PCam, resulting in 245,760, 40,960, and 40,960 images for training, validation, and test, respectively.

MHIST. MHIST is designed to classify colorectal polyps as benign and pre-cancerous [18], which consists of 3,152 images with the size of 224 × 224 pixels. Following the official data splitting, 2,175 images (1,545 benign and 630 precancerous) are used for training and 977 images (617 benign and 360 precancerous) are used for evaluation.

4   Experimental Results and Discussions

4.1   Experimental Setup

In the pre-training process, we use BYOL architecture to train our *TransPath*. The input images are downsampled as 512 × 512 pixels and batch size is set as 256. The data augmentation strategies keep the same as SimCLR [2]. The network is optimized by an SGD optimizer [10] with an initial learning rate of 0.03 and its weight decay of 0.0001. Our pre-trained model is implemented in PyTorch [13] framework and with 32 Nvidia V100 GPUs, which takes 100 epochs and around 200 h to converge. In the fine-tuning process, the input image size keeps consistent with the corresponding datasets. SGD is used as the default optimizer with a batch size of 64 and an initial learning rate of 0.0003.

4.2 Ablation Study

We conduct a set of ablation studies to investigate the effects of three key components (CNN encoder, transformer encoder, and TAE module) within our proposed *TransPath*. The results are listed in Table 1. In this experiment, CNN is initialized by ImageNet pre-training. It is seen that CNN can obtain a satisfactory classification result, especially in the NCT-CRC-HE dataset. To alleviate the weak global feature extraction problem of CNN, we then integrate CNN and transformer (ViT), which generates consistent performance gains across three datasets in terms of three metrics (AUC +2%, ACC +3%, and F1-score +3%). To further enhance the global context features in the transformer, we insert a customized TAE module into the MHSA block, which further improves the classification performance by 3% in terms of the F1-score on MHIST. The above-reported results demonstrate that the combination of CNN with local feature capture ability and transformer with global dependence learning ability can produce robust visual representation for the histopathological image analysis.

Table 1. Ablation study

Networks	Datasets and metrics							
	MHIST			**NCT-CRC-HE**		**PatchCamelyon**		
	F1-score	ACC	AUC	F1-score	ACC	F1-score	ACC	AUC
CNN	0.7957	0.8095	0.9188	0.9099	0.9081	0.8227	0.844	0.9311
CNN+Trans	0.8277	0.8302	0.9378	0.9313	0.9319	0.8587	0.8605	0.9536
CNN+Trans+TAE (ours)	0.8586	0.8651	0.9476	0.9486	0.9483	0.8661	0.8766	0.9631
CNN+Trans+TAE +SSL (our full method)	0.8993	0.8968	0.9727	0.9582	0.9585	0.8983	0.8991	0.9779

4.3 Comparisons with Vision Transformer Networks

This subsection compares our *TransPath* with current state-of-the-art vision transformer networks, including pure transformer-based architectures (ViT [4] and T2T-ViT-24 [20]) and hybrid CNN-transformer paradigms (VT-ResNet [19] and BoTNet-50 [16]). In this experiment, our model is initialized by ImageNet pre-training and other models keep consistent as their publications. As shown in Fig. 2, the hybrid paradigms consistently achieve better performance compared with the pure-transformer across three datasets. Our method follows the design of CNN-transformer and achieves the best performance in these histopathological image classification tasks.

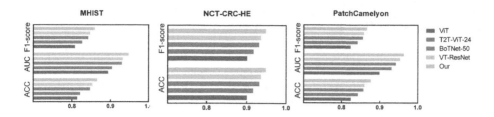

Fig. 2. Comparisons with current state-of-the-art vision transformer networks evaluated on three public datasets.

4.4   Comparisons with Various Pre-training Strategies

This subsection fine-tunes our *TransPath* under different pre-training strategies, including random parameter initialization, ImageNet pre-training, and self-supervised pre-training. As shown in Table 2, when the network is trained from scratch (random parameter initialization), the lowest performance can be seen in all three databases. The pre-trained *TransPath* on domain-relevant data in a self-supervised manner outperforms ImageNet pre-training by 4% of F1-score and 3% of ACC and AUC on MHIST, which demonstrates the potential of SSL on the histopathological image analysis.

Table 2. Comparisons with various pre-training strategies

Networks	Datasets and metrics							
	MHIST			NCT-CRC-HE		PatchCamelyon		
	F1-score	ACC	AUC	F1-score	ACC	F1-score	ACC	AUC
Random	0.8183	0.8206	0.8789	0.9332	0.9322	0.856	0.8567	0.9354
ImageNet	0.8586	0.8651	0.9476	0.9486	0.9483	0.8662	0.8766	0.9631
SSL (ours)	0.8993	0.8968	0.9727	0.9582	0.9585	0.8983	0.8991	0.9779

5   Conclusion

We proposed a customized CNN-transformer architecture for histopathological image classification. Our approach makes use of both local and global receptive fields to extract discriminating and rich features. The proposed TAE module is inserted in the transformer structure to better capture global information. The self-supervised pre-trained model on large domain-specific histopathological images can benefit various downstream classification tasks through transfer learning. Experimental results on three public datasets for three different classification tasks demonstrated the effectiveness of our proposed method and the pre-trained model. Future work will investigate the effects of various SSL methods, other data augmentation methods tailored for histopathological images [17], and whether it is beneficial to separate the frozen slides from the formalin-fixed paraffin-embedded (FFPE) slides in the TCGA dataset.

Acknowledgements. This research was funded by the National Natural Science Foundation of China (No. 61571314), Science & technology department of Sichuan Province, (No. 2020YFG0081), and the Innovative Youth Projects of Ocean Remote Sensing Engineering Technology Research Center of State Oceanic Administration of China (No. 2015001).

References

1. Bejnordi, B.E., et al.: Diagnostic assessment of deep learning algorithms for detection of lymph node metastases in women with breast cancer. JAMA **318**(22), 2199–2210 (2017)
2. Chen, T., Kornblith, S., Norouzi, M., Hinton, G.: A simple framework for contrastive learning of visual representations. In: International Conference on Machine Learning, pp. 1597–1607. PMLR (2020)
3. Dehaene, O., Camara, A., Moindrot, O., de Lavergne, A., Courtiol, P.: Self-supervision closes the gap between weak and strong supervision in histology. arXiv preprint arXiv:2012.03583 (2020)
4. Dosovitskiy, A., et al.: An image is worth 16x16 words: transformers for image recognition at scale. arXiv preprint arXiv:2010.11929 (2020)
5. Grill, J.B., et al.: Bootstrap your own latent: a new approach to self-supervised learning. arXiv preprint arXiv:2006.07733 (2020)
6. He, K., Fan, H., Wu, Y., Xie, S., Girshick, R.: Momentum contrast for unsupervised visual representation learning. In: IEEE Conference on Computer Vision and Pattern Recognition, pp. 9729–9738 (2020)
7. Kather, J.N., et al.: Predicting survival from colorectal cancer histology slides using deep learning: a retrospective multicenter study. PLoS Med. **16**(1), 1–22 (2019)
8. Koohbanani, N.A., Unnikrishnan, B., Khurram, S.A., Krishnaswamy, P., Rajpoot, N.: Self-path: self-supervision for classification of pathology images with limited annotations. arXiv preprint arXiv:2008.05571 (2020)
9. Li, B., Li, Y., Eliceiri, K.W.: Dual-stream multiple instance learning network for whole slide image classification with self-supervised contrastive learning. arXiv preprint arXiv:2011.08939 (2020)
10. Loshchilov, I., Hutter, F.: SGDR: stochastic gradient descent with warm restarts. arXiv preprint arXiv:1608.03983 (2016)
11. Lu, M.Y., Chen, R.J., Wang, J., Dillon, D., Mahmood, F.: Semi-supervised histology classification using deep multiple instance learning and contrastive predictive coding. arXiv preprint arXiv:1910.10825 (2019)
12. Mormont, R., Geurts, P., Marée, R.: Multi-task pre-training of deep neural networks for digital pathology. IEEE J. Biomed. Health Inform. **25**(2), 412–421 (2020)
13. Paszke, A., et al.: Pytorch: an imperative style, high-performance deep learning library. Adv. Neural Inf. Process. Syst. **32**, 8026–8037 (2019)
14. Russakovsky, O., et al.: ImageNet large scale visual recognition challenge. Int. J. Comput. Vis. **115**(3), 211–252 (2015)
15. Srinidhi, C.L., Kim, S.W., Chen, F.D., Martel, A.L.: Self-supervised driven consistency training for annotation efficient histopathology image analysis. arXiv preprint arXiv:2102.03897 (2021)

16. Srinivas, A., Lin, T.Y., Parmar, N., Shlens, J., Abbeel, P., Vaswani, A.: Bottleneck transformers for visual recognition. arXiv preprint arXiv:2101.11605 (2021)
17. Tellez, D., et al.: Quantifying the effects of data augmentation and stain color normalization in convolutional neural networks for computational pathology. Med. Image Anal. **58**, 1–9 (2019)
18. Wei, J., et al.: A petri dish for histopathology image analysis. arXiv preprint arXiv:2101.12355 (2021)
19. Wu, B., et al.: Visual transformers: token-based image representation and processing for computer vision. arXiv preprint arXiv:2006.03677 (2020)
20. Yuan, L., et al.: Tokens-to-Token ViT: training vision transformers from scratch on ImageNet. arXiv preprint arXiv:2101.11986 (2021)

From Pixel to Whole Slide: Automatic Detection of Microvascular Invasion in Hepatocellular Carcinoma on Histopathological Image via Cascaded Networks

Hanbo Chen[1]([✉]), Kang Wang[2], Yuyao Zhu[2], Jiangpeng Yan[3,4], Yan Ji[3], Jingjing Li[5], Dong Xie[5], Junzhou Huang[3], Shuqun Cheng[2], and Jianhua Yao[3]

[1] Tencent AI Lab, Bellevue, US
hanbochen@tencent.com
[2] Eastern Hepatobiliary Surgery Hospital, Shanghai, China
[3] Tencent AI Lab, Shenzhen, China
[4] Tsinghua University, Beijing, China
[5] Shanghai Institute of Nutrition and Health, Chinese Academy of Sciences, Shanghai, China

Abstract. Microvascular invasion (MVI) is a histological feature of hepatocellular carcinoma (HCC). It is the strongest feature related to HCC recurrence and survival after liver resection. However, its diagnosis is time consuming which requires pathologist to examine histopathological images at high resolution. A computer aided MVI detection system that improves the diagnosis efficiency and consistency is in demand. There are two challenges in MVI detection (1) MVI is formed by the same type of tumor cells as common cancer tissue (CCT) and (2) both MVI and CCT's size varies significantly – from a few cells to thousands of cells. Inspired by pathologists' routine reading procedure, we propose a 3-stage solution composed by cascaded networks to tackle this problem. In this framework, images are first analyzed by pixel-level cancer tissue segmentation, followed by region-level instance feature extraction, and then by slide-level comparison to detect MVI. To reduce inter-stage error accumulation, the system is designed in the way that later stage can learn and correct errors in the previous stages. To effectively conduct slide-level analysis, a novel convolutional graph neural network with short cut (sc-GCN) is proposed to solve the over-smoothing problem in classic GCN methods. Testing results on 90 WSI samples show that the proposed system achieves state-of-the-art performance on MVI detection.

Keywords: Microvascular invasion in hepatocellular carcinoma · Whole slide image · Deep learning · Segmentation network · Graph neural network

---

H. Chen, K. Wang, Y. Zhu—co-first author; S. Cheng, J. Yao—co-corresponding author

---

Electronic supplementary material The online version of this chapter (https://doi.org/10.1007/978-3-030-87237-3_19) contains supplementary material, which is available to authorized users.

© Springer Nature Switzerland AG 2021
M. de Bruijne et al. (Eds.): MICCAI 2021, LNCS 12908, pp. 196–205, 2021.
https://doi.org/10.1007/978-3-030-87237-3_19

1   Introduction

Hepatocellular carcinoma (HCC) causes over 600,000 death annually and has been classified as the sixth most common malignancy worldwide [1]. Microvascular invasion (MVI) is a histological feature of HCC. It is tumor cells forming a plug or polyp inside microvascular (Fig. 1(a–e)). Recent clinical evidence suggests MVI to be the strongest feature related to tumor recurrence and survival after liver resection [2]. Accurate diagnosis of MVI is crucial for prognostic evaluation and treatment planning for HCC patients. However, it is quite challenging and time consuming to locate MVI, as its size is relatively smaller than normal cancer tissue. Even seasoned pathologists need to screen the sample at high resolution to avoid missing diagnosis.

Recent advance in computational pathology could potentially ease such burden. Accompanied by the growing amount of whole-slide imaging (WSI) collection, the emerging deep learning based algorithms are widely applied in digital pathology image analysis applications [3, 4], including normal/abnormal tissue segmentation [5–10] and classification [11], cancer staging [12], and survival analysis [13–16]. The major challenges in conducting WSI analysis include (1) training and inference on gigapixel WSI image; (2) sparsely distributed lesion tissues and imbalanced training samples; (3) lack of accurately annotated data. Previous works have resolved those challenges by cropping WSI into patches and optimizing patch-based training process.

In a recent patch-based analysis of HCC samples, a pretrained convolutional neural network (CNN) successfully extracts features to predict after resection survival [16]. However, a system that can detect MVI is still absent. In our view, compared with other WSI applications, there are two major obstacles in designing MVI detection system: (1) MVI is formed by the same kind of tumor cells as the common cancer tissue (CCT) (Fig. 1(e)); (2) Both MVI and CCT's size varies significantly – from a few tumor cells to thousands of tumor cells (Fig. 1). Thus, the classic patch-based analysis method is not applicable for MVI detection, as some patches may only catch parts of the MVI and contain other tissues. Local information inside a patch is not sufficient to detect MVI and distinguish it from CCT.

When pathologists diagnose MVI, they will browse the whole slide first to locate cancer regions and then examine each instance and its surroundings. Inspired by this process, in the paper we propose a cascade of deep learning networks (Fig. 2). We first identify tumor cells with a pixel-wise segmentation network. Then we group segmentations into tumor regions and extract region-wise features with CNN and hand-crafted descriptors. Finally, a convolutional graph neural network (GCN) is adopted to fine-tune the classification in slide-level by comparing each proposed region with its neighbors. The major draw-back of the multi-stage system is error accumulation. To solve this problem, we design the system in the way that later stage can learn and correct errors in the previous stages. We also propose a novel GCN model with short cut (sc-GCN) to solve the over-smoothing problem of classic GCN methods. Our results show that the proposed system works reasonably well in automatic MVI detection.

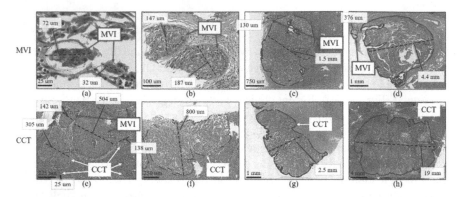

Fig. 1. Examples of MVIs and CCTs with size varies from small (left) to big (right). MVIs and CCTs are pointed by green/white arrows accordingly. Diameters are measured by black dash lines. Images are in different scales with scale bar on the bottom left. (Color figure online)

2   Methods

To conduct analysis on gigapixel WSIs, our proposed framework is composed by three stages (Fig. 2): 1) cancer tissue segmentation; 2) region feature extraction; and 3) graph convolutional neural network classifier. Each stage is trained and inferenced separately. In this section, we will first introduce our experimental data and then cover details of each stage accordingly.

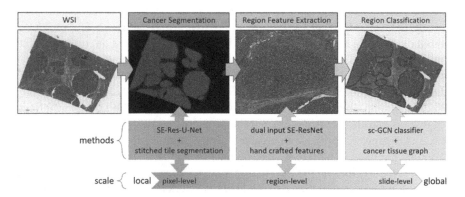

Fig. 2. Illustration of our proposed cascaded networks.

2.1   Experimental Data

190 hematoxylin-eosin H&E stain of hepatocellular carcinoma tissue from 190 patients has been collected in this study. Sample collection, fixation, processing and patholog-ical diagnosis of HCC follow the practice guidelines for the pathological diagnosis of primary liver cancer: 2015 update [17]. The study is approved by the Institutional Ethics

Table 1. Number of samples and their area mean/standard deviation (mm^2) in each group.

	Training			Validation			Testing		
	CCT	MVI	UCT	CCT	MVI	UCT	CCT	MVI	UCT
Count	233	607	93	21	47	17	354	488	59
Area Mean	23	0.39	2.8	34	0.32	1.6	16	0.28	1.9
Area std.	39	1.2	4.1	46	0.73	3.3	32	0.82	3.3

Committee of the hospital. Experienced pathologists manually annotate all the cancer tissues with ASAP (https://computationalpathologygroup.github.io/ASAP/) and label them as: MVI, CCT (common cancer tissue), or UCT (uncertain type that cannot be diagnosed by pathologists). Since experts only annotate the boundary of tissue, white backgrounds inside tissue are not excluded in the annotation. Mask of white regions on WSI are automatically generated by thresholding chroma to mask out blank area inside annotations. We randomly split the data into training (90 WSIs), validation (10 WSIs), and testing (90 WSIs). Details of data stats are in Table 1.

2.2 Cancer Tissue Segmentation

Since conducting neural network analysis on the gigapixel WSI exceeds the memory limitation of common computing infrastructures, WSIs either need to be down-sampled or cropped into small tiles before analysis. Because MVI could be a cluster of a few cancer cells (Fig. 1a), image needs to be inspected in high resolution to preserve cellular-level structures. We choose to crop WSI into 512 × 512 tiles at 20x magnitude when conducting segmentation. During inference time, a sliding window of dimension 512 × 512 and step 256 will be applied to generate samples. In this way, 50% overlap is observed between adjacent tiles. Overlapped predictions will be weighted by their distance to the tile edge to smooth the border discontinuity of segmentation network. Since MVI and CCT are composed by the same type of tumor cells, they cannot be differentiated by inspecting at cellular level (Fig. 1e). In this stage, we combine MVI, CCT, and UCT and train a network to segment cancer tissues. To force clear separation between adjacent tissues, we follow previous work [6, 7, 10] and add a third class of 5 μm-thick tissue border into our segmentation target. Instead of binary segmentation, we conduct 3-class segmentation: foreground, background, and edge.

A customized network based on U-Net architecture is utilized. U-Net is a U-shape fully convolutional neural network designed for segmentation task [5, 9, 18]. It features a set of skip connections concatenating low-order features with high-order features which helps preserve sharp and accurate edges of target. Later works show that the performance of U-Net can be further improved by replacing encoder with more powerful backbones [5]. In this work, we choose squeeze-and-excitation ResNet (SE-ResNet) [19] as the encoder and the final architecture is named as SE-Res-U-Net. The reason we favor SE-ResNet is because it allows self-adjustment of the feature map based on its global averaging. For a H&E stained slide, its color, contrast, and brightness could be affected by the processing protocol. Such variance is consistent across the whole image and thus can be potentially corrected by the squeeze-and-excitation module in SE-ResNet.

2.3 Region Feature Extraction

After stitching tiles of tumor cell segmentation, a complete binary mask of cancer tissues is obtained for each WSI image. We follow the previous works [7] and adopt connected component algorithm to extract cancer tissue instance. Our goal is to classify each instance into MVI or CCT.

As we need to train a classifier to classify these tumor tissue instances, a label needs to be assigned to each instance. This has been achieved by comparing the overlap between instances and expert annotations. Since our annotation is relatively coarse, some annotated regions could be split into smaller regions after segmentation. When 90% of an instance belongs to a certain type of tissue, i.e. CCT, MVI, or normal tissue (NMT), the corresponding label will be assigned. Those segmentations that do not meet any above criteria are labeled as uncertain (UCT) which will be ignored during training. The reason we consider NMT as a classification target is because false positive segmentations in stage 1 are inevitable. Detecting them in later stages allows our system to learn and correct them.

Based on the definition of MVI, we can decide if a tumor region is MVI by checking whether there are endothelial cells surrounding it. However, in practice, it is challenging to identify and annotate endothelial cells on H&E stained slides. Experienced pathologists make diagnosis by comparing a potential MVI with its neighbors in terms of its shape and surrounding tissues. To imitate this procedure, we extract morphology features of each region including area, perimeter, radius ($\sqrt{area/\pi}$), perimeter over radius, eccentricity, and solidity (ratio of pixels in the region to pixels of the convex hull image). Because the shape of tissue fragments next to the cutting border may be truncated, we also measure each instance's distance to the tissue border as a feature.

In addition to hand crafted features, a convolutional neural network (SE-ResNet) is trained to extract high-order tissue shape features and global texture information of each instance. To achieve this, both the segmentation mask of each instance and the corresponding raw image are feed into the network. We name the network dual input SE-ResNet. Specifically, a squared shape bounding box that is 10% larger than the instance is used to crop the image and its mask. Since the sizes of tissue instances vary, they are all resized into 256×256. Then the mask is concatenated with the image as the 4th color channel as the network input. Each input sample will be classified as MVI, CCT, or NMT. The predicted probability will be concatenated with 6 hand crafted features (i.e. instance feature dimension is 7) to generate the final prediction of MVI. Notably, all features are normalized to the range of (0, 1) before analysis.

2.4 Graph Convolutional Neural Network Classifier

When searching for MVI, pathologists will compare a suspicious tissue with its surrounding neighbors to make the final decision. However, most existing computational pathology algorithms largely ignore such information and make decision for each region independently. Recent studies suggest that such gap can be bridged with the help of graph neural network [12–14]. Intuitively, by taking each cancer tissue instance as a vertex, a graph can be generated by connecting instance with edge-to-edge distance shorter than threshold (<1mm). Notably, different from [12–14], which take image patches as graph vertices, we take previously detected tissue instances as vertices.

We then adopt GCN with similar structures as the one proposed in [14] to train the vertex classifier. GCN is an efficient and practical graph neural network composed by a cascade of graph convolution layers [20]. Within each layer, the features of a vertex are accumulated with its neighbors to approximate 1-order Chebyshev polynomial in the spatial domain:

$$H^{(l+1)} = \sigma(D^{-\frac{1}{2}}AD^{-\frac{1}{2}}H^{(l)}W^l) \tag{1}$$

where H is the hidden variable of vertices, A is the adjacency matrix with self-loop, $D = \sum_j A_{ij}$ is the degree diagonal matrix, W is the model weights, and $\sigma(.)$ is the activation function. However, different with [14] which classify the whole WSI image (the graph), our goal is to classify the tissue instance (the vertex). This can be achieved by removing the last pooling layer and modify the lose function. In addition, we introduce a short-cut inside the network to concatenate the GCN output with the initial graph input as the input to a multi-layer perceptron (MLP) to generate the final results (Fig. 3). As GCN only considers 1-order connections, it relies on cascaded layers to increase its receptive field. However, this could smooth-out the vertex feature and cause over-smoothing problem. By introducing this short-cut, we want to compare each tissue instance with its neighbors and easy over-smoothing problem. We name this GCN with short-cut as sc-GCN.

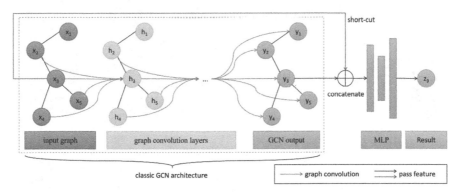

Fig. 3. Illustration of the proposed sc-GCN architecture. It has 2 differences with classic GCN: 1) a short-cut is introduced by concatenating raw node features with hidden variables after convolution; 2) an additional MLP fuses the concatenated features to classify each vertex.

2.5 Training Configurations

When training SE-Res-U-Net and SE-ResNet, random data augmentation including shift, zoom, brightness, contrast, HSV shift, smoothing and flip have been utilized. To balance the samples, when training SE-Res-U-Net, the ratio of foreground, background, and boundary samples is approximately 1:1:1 in each mini batch. In practice, we maintain separate pools for each type of sample and randomly pick samples from each pool in turn when constructing a mini batch. When training SE-ResNet, MVI, CCT, and NMT are also sampled by ratio 1:1:1 with the same approach. When training sc-GCN, to reduce the impact of over-whelming noisy small segmentation fragments, vertices are weighted by their radius when computing loss. To avoid overfit, model with the lowest validation loss will be saved for further analysis. More details of network and training parameters can be found in the supplemental materials.

3   Results

In this section, the analyses on 90 testing data are reported. Figure 4 shows two examples of the prediction results. By visual inspection, the proposed segmentation framework works reasonably well in detecting tumor cells and isolating adjacent tumor tissues. As highlighted by the green arrows, automatic segmentation results can separate tissues in close vicinity which may sometimes be marked as one region in coarse annotation. However, as highlighted by white arrows, when two tissues are too close, the tissue border segmentation does not work very well in separating some touching regions. By visual inspection (Fig. 4b), we find the prediction of the border class looks reasonable but weak (azure arrows), except when the border is between tissue and white background

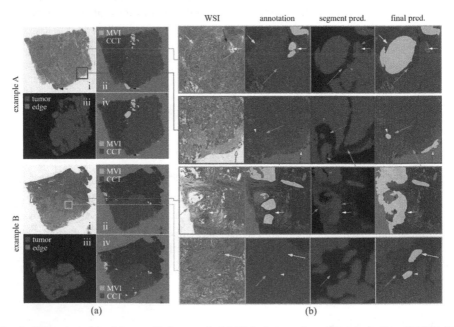

Fig. 4. Two examples of the prediction result. (a) Global view of examples including (i) WSI, (ii) manual annotation overlaid, (iii) segmentation result, and (iv) final prediction result. (b) Zoom-in view responding to the boxes in (i). Arrow highlights are discussed in the paper. (Color figure online)

(pink arrows). This observation suggests that the weak border prediction is caused by the annotation quality – the borders between different type of tissues drawn by hand is often not precise. Notably, coarse annotation (red arrows) also causes segmentation artifact at tissue borders (orange arrows).

Table 2. Quantitative analysis in each stage. For stage 1, we evaluate cancer tissue detection. For stage 2 and 3, we evaluate MVI detection. For area weighted metrices, samples are weighted by its instance region area such that larger instance has higher weight.

Stage	Task	Method	None weighted			Area weighted		
			Recall	Prec	F1	Recall	Prec	F1
1	Cancer	Se-Res-U-Net	0.961	0.072	0.133	1.000	0.992	0.996
2	MVI	SE-ResNet	0.660	0.518	0.580	0.778	0.290	0.422
2	MVI	Hand features MLP	0.391	0.293	0.335	0.835	0.359	0.502
3	MVI	All features MLP	0.516	0.656	0.578	0.637	0.755	0.691
3	MVI	**sc-GCN**	0.512	0.767	**0.614**	0.616	0.825	**0.705**

Cancer segmentation achieves 0.92 IOU (intersect over union). False positive (FP) and false negative predictions (FN) are also evaluated. Since the segmentation could split a coarse annotation into finer sub-regions, when a manual annotation is covered by any predicted region, it is counted as true positive (TP), otherwise as FN. If a predicted region is not covered by any annotation, it is counted as FP. Recall, precision, and F1 are then computed accordingly. As shown in Table 2, 96% of tumor regions have been detected in stage 1. However, a large number of FPs have been detected at the same time resulting in a low precision. If we weight the samples by their area, recall will be very close to 1 and the precision can be as high as 0.992. This is because most of the large tumor areas have been detected and most of the false positive detections are small fragment segmentations. Intuitively, we can filter small fragments by their size. However, this will exclude small MVIs and CCTs (Fig. 1) as well. In stage 2 and 3, most false positive detections can be filtered out by learning algorithms.

In Table 2, we show the MVI detection performance in the stage 2 by SE-ResNet and the final prediction by sc-GCN. To compare hand crafted features with learnt features, and to show that neighborhood features fused by graph neural network can effectively improve region classification performance, a multi-layer perceptron with the same size of fully connected layers as sc-GCN is adopted to analyze the hand crafted features or the whole set of region features to classify MVI, CCT, and NMT. It is evident that the FP can be significantly eliminated in the later stages. sc-GCN achieves the best balance between FP and FN and improves F1 score from its previous stages. Yellow arrows in Fig. 4 highlight some examples of FP detection of MVI. After reviewed by pathologists, 2 of 5 are reasonable detections with MVI features (yellow arrows with white edge). FN detections of MVI are also observed (black arrows). One of them is caused by the wrong segmentation connecting MVI with adjacent CCT. Another one highlighted by black arrows with white edge is close to the tissue border and has incomplete boundary, which makes it hard to diagnose.

Table 3. Ablation study of sc-GCN on classifying manual annotated instance into MVI VS. CCT. Size: use region size as score to classify CCT. GCN + MLP: sc-GCN without short-cut connection.

Method	Size	MLP	GCN	GCN + MLP	sc-GCN
AUC	0.654	0.858	0.807	0.811	**0.887**
F1	–	0.805	0.761	0.831	**0.878**

To our best knowledge, it is the first time sc-GCN has been proposed for pathology analysis. To show the effectiveness of this approach, an ablation study has been conducted and the classic GCN is compared. To isolate the impact of other networks, this analysis is based on the manual annotation and hand-crafted features only. In addition to GCN, we also compare with MLP, and GCN + MLP. The same set of parameters are selected, and details can be found in Supplemental Materials. As shown in Table 3, GCN has a performance drop in comparison with MLP due to over-smoothing. By introducing a short cut, our proposed sc-GCN achieves the best performance.

4 Conclusion

In this paper, a 3-stage system with cascaded networks is proposed to detect MVI on WSI of HCC tissues. Analysis is conducted from pixel-level, to region-level, and then to slide-level. For slide-level analysis, a novel sc-GCN model is introduced to solve the over-smoothing problem in classic GCN methods. Later stage can significantly correct false positive predictions in the early stage. However, a certain level of errors can still be observed. Some are caused by coarse annotations. In the future, we will improve the system to make the training process more robust to annotation noise [21]. Multi-scale features will also be considered to generate more accurate predictions [9].

References

1. Torre, L.A., Bray, F., Siegel, R.L., Ferlay, J., Lortet-Tieulent, J., Jemal, A.: Global cancer statistics, 2012. CA. Cancer J. Clin. **65**, 87–108 (2015)
2. Rodríguez-Perálvarez, M., Luong, T.V., Andreana, L., Meyer, T., Dhillon, A.P., Burroughs, A.K.: A systematic review of microvascular invasion in hepatocellular carcinoma: diagnostic and prognostic variability. Ann. Surg. Oncol. **20**, 325–339 (2013)
3. Deng, S., et al.: Deep learning in digital pathology image analysis: a survey. Front. Med. **14**(4), 470–487 (2020). https://doi.org/10.1007/s11684-020-0782-9
4. Srinidhi, C.L., Ciga, O., Martel, A.L.: Deep neural network models for computational histopathology: a survey. Med. Image Anal. **67**, 101813 (2021)
5. Mehta, S., Mercan, E., Bartlett, J., Weaver, D., Elmore, J.G., Shapiro, L.: Y-Net: joint segmentation and classification for diagnosis of breast biopsy images. In: Frangi, A.F., Schnabel, J.A., Davatzikos, C., Alberola-López, C., Fichtinger, G. (eds.) MICCAI 2018. LNCS, vol. 11071, pp. 893–901. Springer, Cham (2018). https://doi.org/10.1007/978-3-030-00934-2_99

6. Zhou, Y., Onder, O.F., Dou, Q., Tsougenis, E., Chen, H., Heng, P.-A.: CIA-Net: robust nuclei instance segmentation with contour-aware information aggregation. In: Chung, A.C.S., Gee, J.C., Yushkevich, P.A., Bao, S. (eds.) IPMI 2019. LNCS, vol. 11492, pp. 682–693. Springer, Cham (2019). https://doi.org/10.1007/978-3-030-20351-1_53

7. Chen, H., Qi, X., Yu, L., Dou, Q., Qin, J., Heng, P.-A.: DCAN: deep contour-aware networks for object instance segmentation from histology images. Med. Image Anal. **36**, 135–146 (2017)

8. Mukhopadhyay, S., et al.: Whole slide imaging versus microscopy for primary diagnosis in surgical pathology: a multicenter blinded randomized noninferiority study of 1992 cases (pivotal study). Am. J. Surg. Pathol. **42**, 39–52 (2018)

9. Schmitz, R., Madesta, F., Nielsen, M., Krause, J., Steurer, S., Werner, R., Rösch, T.: Multi-scale fully convolutional neural networks for histopathology image segmentation: from nuclear aberrations to the global tissue architecture. Med. Image Anal. **70**, 101996 (2021)

10. Xu, Y., Li, Y., Liu, M., Wang, Y., Lai, M., Chang, E.-C.: Gland instance segmentation by deep multichannel side supervision. In: Ourselin, S., Joskowicz, L., Sabuncu, M.R., Unal, G., Wells, W. (eds.) MICCAI 2016. LNCS, vol. 9901, pp. 496–504. Springer, Cham (2016). https://doi.org/10.1007/978-3-319-46723-8_57

11. Li, W., Nguyen, V.-D., Liao, H., Wilder, M., Cheng, K., Luo, J.: Patch transformer for multi-tagging whole slide histopathology images. In: Shen, D., Liu, T., Peters, T.M., Staib, L.H., Essert, C., Zhou, S., Yap, P.-T., Khan, A. (eds.) MICCAI 2019. LNCS, vol. 11764, pp. 532–540. Springer, Cham (2019). https://doi.org/10.1007/978-3-030-32239-7_59

12. Raju, A., Yao, J., Haq, M.M., Jonnagaddala, J., Huang, J.: Graph attention multi-instance learning for accurate colorectal cancer staging. In: Martel, A.L., et al. (eds.) MICCAI 2020. LNCS, vol. 12265, pp. 529–539. Springer, Cham (2020). https://doi.org/10.1007/978-3-030-59722-1_51

13. Li, R., Yao, J., Zhu, X., Li, Y., Huang, J.: Graph CNN for survival analysis on whole slide pathological images. In: Frangi, A.F., Schnabel, J.A., Davatzikos, C., Alberola-López, C., Fichtinger, G. (eds.) MICCAI 2018. LNCS, vol. 11071, pp. 174–182. Springer, Cham (2018). https://doi.org/10.1007/978-3-030-00934-2_20

14. Zhu, X., Yao, J., Zhu, F., Huang, J.: WSISA: making survival prediction from whole slide histopathological images. In: The IEEE Conference on Computer Vision and Pattern Recognition (CVPR), pp. 7234–7242 (2017)

15. Yao, J., Zhu, X., Huang, J.: Deep multi-instance learning for survival prediction from whole slide images. In: Shen, D., Liu, T., Peters, T.M., Staib, L.H., Essert, C., Zhou, S., Yap, P.-T., Khan, A. (eds.) MICCAI 2019. LNCS, vol. 11764, pp. 496–504. Springer, Cham (2019). https://doi.org/10.1007/978-3-030-32239-7_55

16. Saillard, C., et al.: Predicting survival after hepatocellular carcinoma resection using deep learning on histological slides. Hepatology **72**, 2000–2013 (2020)

17. Cong, W.M., et al.: Practice guidelines for the pathological diagnosis of primary liver cancer: 2015 update. World J. Gastroenterol. **22**, 9279 (2016)

18. Ronneberger, O., Fischer, P., Brox, T.: U-Net: convolutional networks for biomedical image segmentation. In: Navab, N., Hornegger, J., Wells, W.M., Frangi, A.F. (eds.) MICCAI 2015. LNCS, vol. 9351, pp. 234–241. Springer, Cham (2015). https://doi.org/10.1007/978-3-319-24574-4_28

19. Hu, J., Shen, L., Sun, G.: Squeeze-and-excitation networks. In: The IEEE Conference on Computer Vision and Pattern Recognition (CVPR), pp. 7132–7141 (2018)

20. Kipf, T.N., Welling, M.: Semi-supervised classification with graph convolutional networks. In: 5th International Conference on Learning Representations (ICLR) (2017)

21. Jungo, A., Reyes, M.: Assessing reliability and challenges of uncertainty estimations for medical image segmentation. In: Shen, D., et al. (eds.) MICCAI 2019. LNCS, vol. 11765, pp. 48–56. Springer, Cham (2019). https://doi.org/10.1007/978-3-030-32245-8_6

DT-MIL: Deformable Transformer for Multi-instance Learning on Histopathological Image

Hang Li[1,2], Fan Yang[2], Yu Zhao[2], Xiaohan Xing[2,3], Jun Zhang[2],
Mingxuan Gao[1,2], Junzhou Huang[2], Liansheng Wang[1(✉)], and Jianhua Yao[2(✉)]

[1] School of Informatics, Xiamen University, Xiamen, China
`lswang@xmu.edu.cn`
[2] AI Lab, Tencent, Shenzhen, China
[3] The Department of Electronic Engineering,
The Chinese University of Hong Kong, Shatin, Hong Kong, China

Abstract. Learning informative representations is crucial for classification and prediction tasks on histopathological images. Due to the huge image size, whole-slide histopathological image analysis is normally addressed with multi-instance learning (MIL) scheme. However, the weakly supervised nature of MIL leads to the challenge of learning an effective whole-slide-level representation. To tackle this issue, we present a novel embedded-space MIL model based on deformable transformer (DT) architecture and convolutional layers, which is termed DT-MIL. The DT architecture enables our MIL model to update each instance feature by globally aggregating instance features in a bag simultaneously and encoding the position context information of instances during bag representation learning. Compared with other state-of-the-art MIL models, our model has the following advantages: (1) generating the bag representation in a fully trainable way, (2) representing the bag with a high-level and nonlinear combination of all instances instead of fixed pooling-based methods (e.g. max pooling and average pooling) or simply attention-based linear aggregation, and (3) encoding the position relationship and context information during bag embedding phase. Besides our proposed DT-MIL, we also develop other possible transformer-based MILs for comparison. Extensive experiments show that our DT-MIL outperforms the state-of-the-art methods and other transformer-based MIL architectures in histopathological image classification and prediction tasks. An open-source implementation of our approach can be found at https://github.com/yfzon/DT-MIL.

Keywords: Deformable transformer · Multi-instance learning · Key-value attention · Histopathological image analysis

---

H. Li, F. Yang and Y. Zhao—Contributed equally to this work.

M. de Bruijne et al. (Eds.): MICCAI 2021, LNCS 12908, pp. 206–216, 2021.
https://doi.org/10.1007/978-3-030-87237-3_20

1   Introduction

Histopathological image analysis plays a crucial role in modern medicine, especially cancer treatment, where it has been employed as the gold standard for diagnosis. With the development of the digital slide scanner, these images can be digitized into whole slide images (WSIs), which paves a way for computer-aided analysis [18,19,23,29,31]. Due to the huge size of a WSI, the analysis of histopathological images is usually formulated into multi-instance learning (MIL) task [1,4,26,30] where a WSI is regarded as a bag and tiled into hundreds or thousands of patches that are regarded as instances. As the applications of artificial intelligence (AI) in histopathological image analysis move forward, in addition to tasks matching the standard multiple instance (SMI) assumption [17] (e.g., cancer classification), it has gradually entered the applications such as metastasis prediction and disease prognosis and needs comprehensive consideration of the tumor micro-environment, including fibroblasts, immune cells, and vessels, etc. on the entire WSI [11].

Existing MIL methods consist of three main paradigms: bag-space (BS), instance-space (IS) and embedded-space (ES) MIL [1,27]. BS paradigm [6] treats each bag as a single entity and exploits bag-to-bag distance for classification, which is not common in histopathological image analysis due to the huge image size. In IS methods, the learning process mainly lies at the instance level, and the bag-level prediction is obtained by simply aggregating instance predictions. IS-paradigm methods are normally two-stage approaches and often exhibit inferior performance to the other paradigms [4,14,15]. The ES paradigm, on the other hand, embeds all instances into low-dimensional representations firstly and then integrates them to generate a bag-level representation, which has the potential to comprehensively embed information of the entire WSI for tackling specific analysis tasks. Therefore, designing an effective bag embedding module is a key to enhance the performance of ES MIL methods.

The first attempts for bag embedding are fixed pooling-based methods such as max pooling, average pooling, and log-sum-exp pooling [27] or parameterized pooling-based methods such as dynamic pooling [28], noisy-and pooling [16] and adaptive pooling [32]. These methods are either fixed or partially trainable with limited flexibility. Later, Ilse *et al.* introduced the attention mechanism into the bag embedding of the MIL, which is fully trainable [13]. Shi *et al.* [22] further improved the attention-based MIL by connecting the attention mechanism with the loss function and adding a specific regulation to improve the allocated weights of the attention mechanism. However, these single attention-based methods embed the bag as a weighted sum of instance features, which is just a linear combination rather than a high-level feature embedding. Besides, all the above-mentioned methods fail to encode the position and context information of tiled patches (instances) in the WSI (bag). Campanella *et al.* [3] adopted recurrent neural network (RNN) as the bag embedding module and treated extracted patch features as a one-dimensional sequence during bag representation learning, which partly encodes the position and context information. However, the one-dimensional-sequence formalization cannot fully represent 2D positions of patches inside a WSI, and the RNN model processes instance embeddings sequentially instead of parallelly. Besides, the RNN has limited ability to capture long-range information. As one of the most advanced sequence-to-sequence architectures, Transformer [25], is rapidly replacing RNN in natural language processing tasks [9,25]. The self-attention layers in the transformer allow it to update each element of a sequence by aggregating all elements in the sequence simultaneously, and the positional encoding procedure allows the model to leverage the position information [5,25]. Besides the above-mentioned advantages of transformer, the characteristics of computational efficiency and scalability offer its potential value in computer vision applications [5,10,33].

In this work, we introduce the Transformer into histopathological image analysis for the first time. We propose a novel ES-MIL model using deformable transformer encoder, transformer decoder, and convolutional layers to build a fully trainable bag embedding module for generating high-level representation. Besides our proposed DT-MIL, we also implement other possible transformer-based MIL architectures for comparison. The main contributions of our work are summarized as follows:

- We propose a novel end-to-end embedded-space MIL model integrated with deformable transformer for histopathological image analysis, which incorporates the position relationship and context information of instances into bag embedding.
- We propose a position-encoded feature image to efficiently represent a huge WSI, where each super-pixel in a certain position is the feature vector extracted from the corresponding patch by a convolutional encoder.
- We enable our MIL method to effectively conduct instance selection via associated attention weights and instance-feature calibration simultaneously by introducing the deformable self-attention and multiple head attention mechanisms into bag embedding.
- Extensive experiments on histopathological image analysis tasks demonstrate the superiority of our DT-MIL compared with other transformer based MIL architectures and other state-of-the-art methods.

2   Methods

The framework of the proposed DT-MIL is illustrated in Fig. 1. It consists of three main components including the position preserving dimension reduction (PPDR), transformer-based bag embedding (TBBE), and classification. In the PPDR component, a convolutional-neural-network (CNN) encoder is involved to down-sample a WSI into a small feature image, where each patch in the original WSI is embedded as a super-pixel (extracted instance-level features) located at the corresponding position. Then it comes our designed bag embedding module, which is composed of a 1×1 convolutional layer for automatically instance-level feature selection and a deformable transformer encoder-decoder for generating a high-level bag representation which comprehensively refers to all instance features and leverages the 2D position information. The self-attention mechanism in the transformer allocates variable weights for different instance features

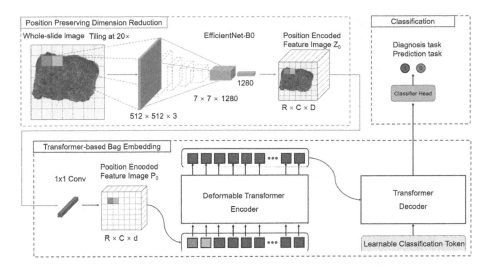

Fig. 1. Overview of the proposed deformable transformer multi-instance learning model (DT-MIL), which is composed by three parts, i.e., the position preserving dimension reduction (PPDR), transformer-based bag embedding (TBBE), and classification. The classification token is similar to the [class] token in BERT [9], which is a learnable embedding to make the model perform classification.

during bag embedding, achieving adaptive instance selection. The deformable attention module in the deformable transformer encoder can further reduce the model complexity and allow our bag embedding module to focus more on the key informative instances. Finally, after obtaining an informative high-level bag representation, a classification head is followed to conduct the final prediction.

WSI Dimension Reduction and Instance-level Feature Selection: To process a gigapixel WSI, the first step in our DT-MIL is to reduce its scale. To this end, we use a pre-trained EfficientNet B0 [24] (on ImageNet) to extract features from patches tiled from the region-of-interest (ROI, if there is) within a WSI. These features are regarded as superpixels and then stitched together to form a position-encoded feature image. To be specific, assuming the tiled patches from a WSI $\mathbf{I}$ are $\{\mathbf{x}_1, \mathbf{x}_2, \cdots, \mathbf{x}_N\}$, where $\mathbf{x}_i \in \mathbb{R}^{W \times H \times 3}$, W and H denote the width and height of the patch, respectively. The corresponding embedded features are denoted as $\{\mathbf{e}_1, \mathbf{e}_2, \cdots, \mathbf{e}_N\}$, where $\mathbf{e}_i \in \mathbb{R}^D$. Suppose the WSI is composed with patches in R rows and C columns, then the down-scaled position-encoded feature image is denoted as $\mathbf{Z}_0 \in \mathbb{R}^{R \times C \times D}$, where D depends on the output size of the feature extraction network. Then, a 1×1 convolution is utilized for instance-level feature selection, which reduces the channel dimension of the position-encoded feature image from D to a smaller dimension d, generating a new position-encoded feature image $\mathbf{P}_0 \in \mathbb{R}^{R \times C \times d}$. Therefore, each WSI is significantly compressed in a factor of $\frac{W \times H \times D \times 3}{d}$ (Typical values we use are $W, H = 512$ (or 256), $D = 1280$ and $d = 512$).

Deformable Transformer Encoder: The deformable transformer encoder in our bag embedding module works for updating each instance representation with globally aggregating instance representations in $\mathbf{P}_0$ simultaneously and referring to the position context information. The encoder is a stack of repeated blocks, where each block is composed with a multi-head deformable self-attention module (MDSA) and a feed-forward network (FFN) together with residual connections and Layer Normalization [2] (LN), i.e.:

$$EB(\mathbf{P}_i) = LN(\mathbf{H} + FFN(\mathbf{H})), \tag{1}$$

$$\mathbf{H} = LN(\mathbf{P}_{i-1} + MDSA(\mathbf{P}_{i-1})), \tag{2}$$

where $\mathbf{P}_i$ is the feature maps after i^{th} encoder block. Different from the conventional self-attention mould in transformer that globally aggregates all instance representations when updating one of them, the deformable self-attention module only globally attends to a small set of key instances. Given an input $\mathbf{P}_i \in \mathbb{R}^{R \times C \times d}$, let q index a query element with content feature $\mathbf{f}_q$ and 2D reference point $\mathbf{r}_q$, the MDSA is defined as:

$$MDSA(\mathbf{f}_q, \mathbf{r}_q, \mathbf{P}_i) = \sum_{m=1}^{M} \mathbf{W}_m[\sum_{k=1}^{K} A_{mqk} \cdot \mathbf{W}'_m \mathbf{P}_i(\mathbf{r}_q + \Delta \mathbf{r}_{mqk})], \tag{3}$$

where m indexes the attention head, k indexes the sampled keys, and K is the total sampled key number ($K \ll RC$). $\mathbf{W}'_m \in \mathbb{R}^{C_v \times d}$ and $\mathbf{W}_m \in \mathbb{R}^{C_v \times d}$ ($C_v = d/M$ by default) are learnable weights. $A_{mqk} \in [0, 1]$ and $\Delta \mathbf{r}_{mqk} \in \mathbb{R}^2$ represent the attention weight and the sampling offset of the kth sampling point in the mth attention head and the attention weight A_{mqk} is normalized by $\sum_k^K A_{mqk} = 1$.

In transformer encoder, the position information is embedded with a positional encoding module. Here, we extend the original module in Transformer [25] for the 2D case. For the coordinates of each dimension, we utilize $\Omega/2$ sine and cosine functions with different frequencies:

$$PE(pos, i) = \begin{cases} sin(pos \cdot \omega_j), & for \quad i = 2j, \\ cos(pos \cdot \omega_j), & for \quad i = 2j + 1; \end{cases} \tag{4}$$

where $\omega_j = 1/10000^{2j/\frac{\Omega}{2}}$, pos denotes the position in the corresponding dimension, i indicates the order of patches in a dimension of 2D position encoding, and j is used to indicate whether it is the odd or even number.

Transformer Decoder: In the decoder part, we follow the standard architecture of the transformer. The decoder is composed of repeated blocks with concatenated multi-head self-attention, multi-head encoder-decoder attention and FFN layers together with residual connections and Layer Normalization. Different from the original transformer that uses six blocks as the decoder, here we utilize two blocks to further reduce the model complexity. To perform classification, we set a learnable embedding as the classification token. The attention

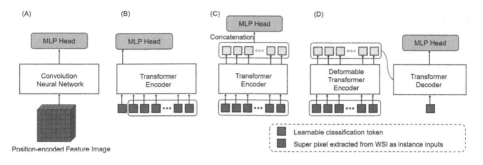

Fig. 2. Diagrams of different bag-embedding modules. (A) CNN-MIL, (B) ViT-MIL, (C) DTEC-MIL, (D) DT-MIL

mechanism in transformer decoder is typical key-value attention [25], which can be defined as follows:

$$Att(Q, K, V) = softmax(\frac{QK^T}{\sqrt{d_k}})V, \tag{5}$$

where Q, K, and V are matrices packing a set of queries, keys, and values. d_k is the dimension of keys and queries and d_v is the dimension of the values. The multi-head attention employs the key-value attention multiple times for allowing the model to jointly attend to information from different representation subspace at different positions, which is defined as:

$$
\begin{aligned}
MHA(Q, K, V) &= Concat(Head_1, \cdots, Head_M)W^O, \\
Head_i &= Att(QW_i^Q, KW_i^K, VW_i^V);
\end{aligned}
\tag{6}
$$

and the above projections are parameter matrices $W_i^Q \in \mathbb{R}^{d_{model} \times d_k}$, $W_i^K \in \mathbb{R}^{d_{model} \times d_k}$, $W_i^V \in \mathbb{R}^{d_{model} \times d_v}$, $W^O \in \mathbb{R}^{Md_v \times d_{model}}$, d_{model} is the feature embedding dimensions of the model. In multi-head self attention $V = K = Q$ and in multi-head encoder-decoder attention, $K = V$ is the output of the encoder and Q is the query matrix from the decoder.

Classification Head: The classification head maps the bag-level embedding to the final prediction, which is implemented by a multilayer perceptron (MLP) with one hidden layer.

Besides our proposed DT-MIL, we also develop three ES-MIL methods with different bag-embedding modules that work on the top of the position-encoded feature image to generate the bag representation. As shown in Fig. 2, the first method utilizes convolutional layers for generating the bag representation (CNN-MIL, Fig. 2 A). The second one, termed ViT-MIL, uses the classification transformer architecture in vision transformer (ViT) [10] (Fig. 2 B). And, the third method, denoted DTEC-MIL, uses a deformable transformer encoder together with a concatenation for bag embedding (Fig. 2 C).

3   Experiment

In this study, we applied the proposed DT-MIL method in two datasets as described below.

BREAST-LNM Dataset: Biopsy slides of breast cancer patients for lymph node metastasis prediction. We collected 3957 H&E stained preoperative core biopsy slides of breast patients. The slides were scanned as WSIs at 20 × magnification (0.5 μm/pixel). The lymph node metastasis condition was concluded by consensus of two expert pathologists based on the tissue slides generated after surgical removal of the cancer tissue. The dataset contained 1840 positive samples and 2117 negative samples.

CPTAC-LUAD Dataset: Tissue slides of lung adenocarcinoma patients for cancer diagnosis. The data of lung adenocarcinoma cases were collected from Clinical Proteomic Tumor Analysis Consortium (NCI/NIH) [7]. The data were publicly available and contained 1065 WSIs, including 684 tumor tissue and 381 normal tissues. The tissue H&E slides were scanned at 20× magnification (0.5 μm/pixel). The diagnosis result of each case was annotated in the clinical report of this cohort.

Implementation Details. We used the same experimental setup for both the BREAST-LNM prediction and CPTAC-LUAD diagnosis tasks. The datasets were randomly split into a training, validation, and test set (60% vs 20% vs 20%). The best model was chosen according to the performance on the validation set. For preprocessing, the original WSI was tiled into non-overlapping patches with the size of 512 × 512 in a grid sampling manner and the OTSU algorithm [20] was utilized to mask out the tissue-free background. The DT-MIL model was implemented in Pytorch [21] and was trained on Tesla P40 GPU server. EfficientNet-B0 [24] pre-trained with ImageNet [8] was employed as the feature extractor and the last few layers of the CNN model were fine-tuned to learn task-relevant features. The transformer part was randomly initiated [12]. For both tasks, the DT-MIL model was trained in an end-to-end manner employing the Adam optimizer with learning rate 2×10^{-4}, weight decay 1×10^{-4}, and a batch size of 2. We implemented the group normalization, which is not sensitive to batch size and is effective for convergence on small batch size.

Evaluation. For both BREAST-LNM prediction and CPTAC-LUAD diagnosis tasks, the performance of the proposed DT-MIL was compared with the state-of-the-art methods including the attention-based MIL [13] and RNN-based MIL [3], and our developed methods including CNN-MIL, transformer-based ViT-MIL, and DTEC-MIL. These models were evaluated by Area Under the Curve of the receiver operating characteristic curve (AUC), F1-score, precision, and recall on the test data set.

4   Results and Discussion

Table 1 shows the model performance on the BREAST-LNM dataset and the CPTAC-LUAD dataset. The results validate the superiority of the proposed DT-MIL method, compared with the state-of-the-art methods (A-MIL and RNN) on both the diagnosis of lung cancer and the metastasis prediction of breast cancer. The comparison between DT-MIL and A-MIL validates the superior of the proposed DT-MIL that can efficiently conduct instance selection, instance-feature calibration, and generate a high-level bag embedding, while the A-MIL is a single attention-based method that embeds the bag as a weighted sum of instance features. The comparison results of DT-MIL and RNN show the superiority of the proposed model that fully considers the 2D positions of patches inside the WSI and captures useful long-range context information, comparing to the one-dimensional-sequence formalization in RNN. Notably, all the methods achieve much better results on the cancer diagnosis task than the metastasis prediction task since the diagnosis task is simpler. In the diagnosis task, the model only needs to differentiate the tumor tissues from normal tissues. However, in the metastasis prediction task, the tumor progression depends more on the changes in the micro-environment instead of local morphological features. Therefore, there are patches weakly correlated with the metastasis results, and mining the informative patches based on weak supervision signals is critical. Our proposed DT-MIL method achieves superior performance on the prediction task, proving the efficientness of the well-designed deformable transformer attention method that distinguishes informative patches from a global view and efficiently embeds them for bag representation.

Table 1. Model performance on the prediction task of the BREAST-LNM dataset and the cancer diagnosis task of the CPTAC-LUAD dataset.

Model	BREAST-LNM				CPTAC-LUAD			
	AUC	F1-score	Precision	Recall	AUC	F1-score	Precision	Recall
A-MIL [13]	54.28	59.30	45.63	**85.39**	98.09	95.85	**99.22**	92.70
RNN [3]	61.85	60.09	51.59	71.94	97.56	95.44	95.83	95.04
CNN-MIL	54.23	53.97	48.20	61.30	97.45	93.91	90.00	98.18
ViT-MIL	64.63	58.36	54.32	63.04	95.67	**96.92**	95.45	98.43
DTEC-MIL	71.87	61.97	60.94	63.04	98.05	95.84	92.70	**99.21**
DT-MIL	**72.88**	**63.93**	**61.10**	67.05	**99.06**	**96.92**	98.44	95.45

Comparing our DT-MIL with CNN-MIL, transformer-based ViT-MIL and DTEC-MIL, we find that the DT-MIL achieves superior performance on both the prediction and diagnosis tasks, showing the DT-MIL architecture has the potential to efficiently capture the instance-level feature and interaction via deformable transformer encoder and generate optimal global bag embedding via transformer decoder. Comparing to DTEC-MIL, our proposed DT-MIL uses a multi-head attention-based transformer decoder to integrate encoded features of instances obtained after the transformer encoder rather than a simple concatenation. And comparing to ViT-MIL, our DT-MIL applies the deformable mechanism, which allows the network to globally focus on the key related instances during feature updating, instead of calculating all the instances. Besides the advantage of reducing the computing complexity, this procedure may also alleviate the influence of involving unrelated instances during feature updating.

5   Conclusions

In this work, we propose a novel MIL model for histopathological image analysis. Our proposed DT-MIL introduces the deformable transformer encoder and decoder architecture for bag representation learning for the first time. Extensive experiments on the lung cancer and breast cancer datasets illustrate that DT-MIL achieves state-of-the-art performance in diagnosis and metastasis prediction tasks, showing the potential of our model to be a general and efficient MIL solution for further applications in histopathological image analysis.

Acknowledgements. This work was partially funded by National Key R&D Program of China (2018YFC2000702).

References

1. Amores, J.: Multiple instance classification: review, taxonomy and comparative study. Artif. Intell. **201**, 81–105 (2013)
2. Ba, J.L., Kiros, J.R., Hinton, G.E.: Layer normalization. arXiv preprint arXiv:1607.06450 (2016)
3. Campanella, G., et al.: Clinical-grade computational pathology using weakly supervised deep learning on whole slide images. Nat. Med. **25**(8), 1301–1309 (2019)
4. Cao, R., et al.: Development and interpretation of a pathomics-based model for the prediction of microsatellite instability in colorectal cancer. Theranostics **10**(24), 11080 (2020)
5. Carion, N., Massa, F., Synnaeve, G., Usunier, N., Kirillov, A., Zagoruyko, S.: End-to-end object detection with transformers. In: Vedaldi, A., Bischof, H., Brox, T., Frahm, J.-M. (eds.) ECCV 2020. LNCS, vol. 12346, pp. 213–229. Springer, Cham (2020). https://doi.org/10.1007/978-3-030-58452-8_13
6. Cheplygina, V., Tax, D.M., Loog, M.: Multiple instance learning with bag dissimilarities. Pattern Recognit. **48**(1), 264–275 (2015)
7. Clark, K., et al.: The cancer imaging archive (TCIA): maintaining and operating a public information repository. J. Digit. Imaging **26**(6), 1045–1057 (2013)
8. Deng, J., Dong, W., Socher, R., Li, L.J., Li, K., Fei-Fei, L.: ImageNet: a large-scale hierarchical image database. In: 2009 IEEE Conference on Computer Vision and Pattern Recognition, pp. 248–255. IEEE (2009)
9. Devlin, J., Chang, M.W., Lee, K., Toutanova, K.: BERT: pre-training of deep bidirectional transformers for language understanding. arXiv preprint arXiv:1810.04805 (2018)

10. Dosovitskiy, A., et al.: An image is worth 16x16 words: transformers for image recognition at scale. arXiv preprint arXiv:2010.11929 (2020)
11. Garrett, W.S.: Cancer and the microbiota. Science **348**(6230), 80–86 (2015)
12. Glorot, X., Bengio, Y.: Understanding the difficulty of training deep feedforward neural networks. In: Proceedings of the Thirteenth International Conference on Artificial Intelligence and Statistics, pp. 249–256. JMLR Workshop and Conference Proceedings (2010)
13. Ilse, M., Tomczak, J., Welling, M.: Attention-based deep multiple instance learning. In: International Conference on Machine Learning, pp. 2127–2136. PMLR (2018)
14. Kandemir, M., Hamprecht, F.A.: Computer-aided diagnosis from weak supervision: a benchmarking study. Comput. Med. Imaging Graph. **42**, 44–50 (2015)
15. Kather, J.N., et al.: Deep learning can predict microsatellite instability directly from histology in gastrointestinal cancer. Nat. Med. **25**(7), 1054–1056 (2019)
16. Kraus, O.Z., Ba, J.L., Frey, B.J.: Classifying and segmenting microscopy images with deep multiple instance learning. Bioinformatics **32**(12), i52–i59 (2016)
17. Lee, H., Battle, A., Raina, R., Ng, A.Y.: Efficient sparse coding algorithms. In: Advances in Neural Information Processing Systems, pp. 801–808 (2007)
18. Li, R., Yao, J., Zhu, X., Li, Y., Huang, J.: Graph CNN for survival analysis on whole slide pathological images. In: Frangi, A.F., Schnabel, J.A., Davatzikos, C., Alberola-López, C., Fichtinger, G. (eds.) MICCAI 2018. LNCS, vol. 11071, pp. 174–182. Springer, Cham (2018). https://doi.org/10.1007/978-3-030-00934-2_20
19. Mehta, S., Mercan, E., Bartlett, J., Weaver, D., Elmore, J.G., Shapiro, L.: Y-Net: Joint segmentation and classification for diagnosis of breast biopsy images. In: Frangi, A.F., Schnabel, J.A., Davatzikos, C., Alberola-López, C., Fichtinger, G. (eds.) MICCAI 2018. LNCS, vol. 11071, pp. 893–901. Springer, Cham (2018). https://doi.org/10.1007/978-3-030-00934-2_99
20. Ostu, N.: A threshold selection method from gray-level histograms. IEEE Trans. Syst. Man Cybern. **9**(1), 62–66 (1979)
21. Paszke, A., et al.: Automatic differentiation in pytorch (2017)
22. Shi, X., Xing, F., Xie, Y., Zhang, Z., Cui, L., Yang, L.: Loss-based attention for deep multiple instance learning. In: AAAI, vol. 34, pp. 5742–5749 (2020)
23. Srinidhi, C.L., Ciga, O., Martel, A.L.: Deep neural network models for computational histopathology: a survey. Med. Image Anal., 101813 (2020)
24. Tan, M., Le, Q.: EfficientNet: rethinking model scaling for convolutional neural networks. In: International Conference on Machine Learning, pp. 6105–6114. PMLR (2019)
25. Vaswani, A., et al.: Attention is all you need. In: Guyon, I., et al. (eds.) NIPS, vol. 30. Curran Associates, Inc. (2017)
26. Wang, T., et al.: Microsatellite instability prediction of uterine corpus endometrial carcinoma based on h&e histology whole-slide imaging. In: 2020 IEEE 17th International Symposium on Biomedical Imaging (ISBI), pp. 1289–1292. IEEE (2020)
27. Wang, X., Yan, Y., Tang, P., Bai, X., Liu, W.: Revisiting multiple instance neural networks. Pattern Recognit. **74**, 15–24 (2018)
28. Yan, Y., Wang, X., Guo, X., Fang, J., Liu, W., Huang, J.: Deep multi-instance learning with dynamic pooling. In: Asian Conference on Machine Learning, pp. 662–677 (2018)
29. Yao, J., Zhu, X., Huang, J.: Deep multi-instance learning for survival prediction from whole slide images. In: Shen, D., Liu, T., Peters, T.M., Staib, L.H., Essert, C., Zhou, S., Yap, P.-T., Khan, A. (eds.) MICCAI 2019. LNCS, vol. 11764, pp. 496–504. Springer, Cham (2019). https://doi.org/10.1007/978-3-030-32239-7_55

30. Zhao, Y., et al.: Predicting lymph node metastasis using histopathological images based on multiple instance learning with deep graph convolution. In: CVPR, pp. 4837–4846 (2020)
31. Zhou, Y., Onder, O.F., Dou, Q., Tsougenis, E., Chen, H., Heng, P.-A.: CIA-Net: robust nuclei instance segmentation with contour-aware information aggregation. In: Chung, A.C.S., Gee, J.C., Yushkevich, P.A., Bao, S. (eds.) IPMI 2019. LNCS, vol. 11492, pp. 682–693. Springer, Cham (2019). https://doi.org/10.1007/978-3-030-20351-1_53
32. Zhou, Y., Sun, X., Liu, D., Zha, Z., Zeng, W.: Adaptive pooling in multi-instance learning for web video annotation. In: ICCV, pp. 318–327 (2017)
33. Zhu, X., Su, W., Lu, L., Li, B., Wang, X., Dai, J.: Deformable DETR: deformable transformers for end-to-end object detection. In: ICLR (2021)

Early Detection of Liver Fibrosis Using Graph Convolutional Networks

Marta Wojciechowska[1,2(✉)] [iD], Stefano Malacrino[2,3] [iD],
Natalia Garcia Martin[2] [iD], Hamid Fehri[1,2] [iD], and Jens Rittscher[1,2,4] [iD]

[1] Institute of Biomedical Engineering, Department of Engineering Science,
University of Oxford, Oxford, UK
`marta.wojciechowska@lincoln.ox.ac.uk`
[2] Big Data Institute, University of Oxford, Li Ka Shing Centre for Health
Information and Discovery, Oxford, UK
[3] Nuffield Department of Surgical Sciences, University of Oxford, Oxford, UK
[4] NIHR Oxford Biomedical Research Centre, Oxford, UK

Abstract. Detection of early onset of fibrosis is critical to detecting long term damage to identify potential loss of organ function. While formal grading systems for fibrosis have been established, we argue that a quantitative analysis of fibrosis patterns will improve diagnostic quality and help to standardise clinical reporting. Here we are using deep learning to identify elementary fibrosis patterns. Subsequently, a graphical model is utilised to model the spatial organisation of the fibrosis patterns. Our experimental results demonstrated that this approach correlates well with established clinical grading. The presented method holds the potential to be applied to histology in other organs (e.g. kidney).

Keywords: Digital pathology · Fibrosis · Graph neural networks

1 Introduction

In the context of chronic diseases, fibrosis refers to the deposition of collagen in tissue. Fibrosis can lead to organ dysfunction and even to organ failure. Typically, histochemical stains are being used to visualise collagen which would otherwise be hard to quantify. Assessing the level of fibrosis plays an important role in the diagnosis of liver disease in general and Non-alcoholic Steatohepatitis (NASH) in particular. NASH is a progressive liver disease characterised by inflammation and fibrosis, and has strong links to diabetes, obesity, and cardiovascular diseases. By 2030, the number of NASH patients is expected to increase by 60% and the number of liver deaths related to NASH by 178% [4]. NASH is a histological definition that groups together defects in diverse biochemical processes causing hepatic fat accumulation, inflammation, necrosis and fibrosis.

While the measurement of the Collagen Proportionate Area (CPA) [6] provides a very basic assessment of the collagen content per unit area, it has already been shown that the assessment of morphometrical features allows for a more

M. de Bruijne et al. (Eds.): MICCAI 2021, LNCS 12908, pp. 217–226, 2021.
https://doi.org/10.1007/978-3-030-87237-3_21

accurate histological staging of fibrosis [2]. Here, we propose to utilise deep learning to identify collagen deposition patterns that will form the basis of a more objective and standardised assessment of the fibrosis progression in liver biopsies as defined by the METAVIR standard (see Fig. 1). Rather than simply training a deep neural network and utilising the learnt model for a global prediction [18], our proposed method identifies the macro-patterns and characterises the different fibrosis stages through modelling the level of bridging.

2   Previous Work

Whole Slide Images (WSIs) are typically split into smaller patches and the tile-level representations are later aggregated to predict the label of the entire slide. Such an approach has been used in diseases where information present at the cell-level is important to form a diagnosis - e.g. in cancer.

The assessment of fibrosis, however, is unique in that the grading system describe changes (bridging) which occur at a macroscopic scale as opposed to cellular scale (see Fig. 1) [5]. In the case of liver disease, a single fibrotic bridge might even span the width of a typical biopsy. For this reason, current approaches use either downsampled WSIs [18] or very large patches of tissue [9] as inputs to a CNN classifier. The limitation of such methods is that they rely on large sections of tissue, the collection of which is not possible in a clinical setting. Other approaches used handcrafted features and leveraged the knowledge of tissue architecture to achieve more interpretable results [17]. The downside of the patch-based methods is that such representations do not take into account the tissue topology at the macroscopic scale.

Graphs provide a unique way of describing spatial relationships between objects [14]. More recently, Graph Convolutional Networks (GCNs) have been applied to histopathology. While CNNs operate on patches directly, GCNs apply the convolutions to predefined graph nodes. Such nodes can represent biological entities as in the case of cell-graphs [20], or larger tissue regions - superpixels [13] or groups of tiles of similar appearance [19]. We propose a novel tissue representation that combines the robustness of deep learning with the prior knowledge of tissue architecture by employing a graph-based model. Such a representation resembles a human reader's understanding of the slide, leading to more interpretable analysis of fibrosis.

3   Data

A set of 271 percutaneous liver biopsies from patients with NAFLD, representing varying stages of fibrosis (Fig. 1) was provided by Perspectum Ltd. The slides have been stained with Picrosirius Red (PSR), which dyes tissue collagen red. Each biopsy has been assigned a fibrosis grade by an expert pathologist in accordance to the METAVIR standard (F0-F4) [5]. The slides have been scanned with an Aperio scanner at 20x magnification. The dataset has been divided into training and testing folds with a 80:20 ratio.

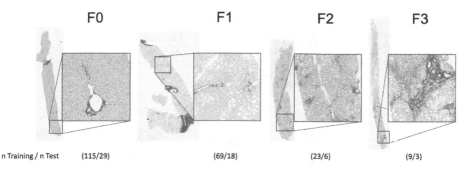

Fig. 1. Liver fibrosis stages (METAVIR standard). Healthy liver (grade F0) shows little collagen (red stain), which is almost only present in portal tract walls. During the initial stages of fibrosis (F1-F2) a network of fine collagen strands appears in the parenchyma. In the higher stages (F3-F4) the pathological fibres form "bridges" connecting portal tracts and central veins, resulting in a cobweb-like macro-pattern. It should be noted that the highest grade (F4 - cirrhosis) is not present in the dataset. (Color figure online)

4   Methodology

The task of fibrosis detection can be modelled as a multi-class classification problem. Each slide is decomposed into a set of tiles and one of C classes is assigned to the whole sample. The classes are derived directly from the pathology staging system. In this work, we propose a novel method of tissue graph construction based on the identification of liver tissue landmarks (portal tracts and central veins) and partitioning of the slide into regions centred around said landmarks. Firstly, all slides are pre-processed by segmenting the tissue collagen at full image resolution. The landmarks are identified by a tile clustering pipeline.

A tissue graph is then constructed using the labelled tile representations as nodes. Regions of dense collagen identified by the clustering pipeline are used as input landmarks for a tessellation algorithm. The resulting graph consists of star-like structures, each one containing a biologically relevant region of the tissue (e.g. a single portal tract or region of fibrosis). As a baseline method we used the approach from Yu et al. [18] with a ResNet18 applied to the whole pre-processed and downsampled slides [8]. In order to satisfy the memory limitations, the WSIs were here downsampled by a factor of 32.

4.1   Tile Subtyping

A CNN trained on dense annotations created using QuPath [1] is used to identify regions that contain collagen. To address the problem of variation in staining slides are binarised using a specifically trained collagen segmentation CNN. Regions of high collagen content are identified using the tile subtyping pipeline

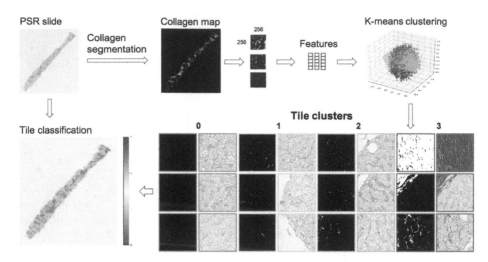

Fig. 2. Tile subtyping pipeline. 4 clusters of collagen tiles have been identified, each representing a different level of collagen content. The classified tiles are coloured according to their predicted cluster. Regions with high collagen content (cluster 3) are later used as Voronoi centres in tissue graph construction. The tile size of 256×256 px was specifically chosen to capture the local pattern of the collagen fibres and at the same time to limit the field of view to only contain one type of collagen pattern at a time.

(Fig. 2). Features from small tiles (256×256 px) are extracted from the full resolution slides using an ImageNet pretrained ResNet18 model, and the resulting feature vectors $\in \mathbb{R}^{512}$ are clustered using a k-means clustering algorithm. About 10% of tiles randomly sampled from the whole dataset are used to learn the fibre representation. Experimenting on different numbers of clusters, we found that setting $k = 4$ results in easily interpretable clusters with tiles containing increasing amount of collagen. In particular, tiles from cluster 3 contained regions of dense collagen: liver vasculature and regions of fibrosis.

4.2   Graph Construction

The graph construction pipeline is presented in Fig. 3. Firstly, regions of high collagen content are identified using the tile labels generated by the tile subtyping pipeline (i.e. tiles with collagen in cluster 3 - see Fig. 2). Next, centroids of each dense collagen region are used as centre points for Voronoi tessellation. The final tissue graph is constructed using features extracted with an ImageNet pretained ResNet18 model from each tile as node features X. The Euclidean distance D from each tile to its corresponding Voronoi centre is encoded as edge weight w. The graph construction was implemented using NetworkX package [7].

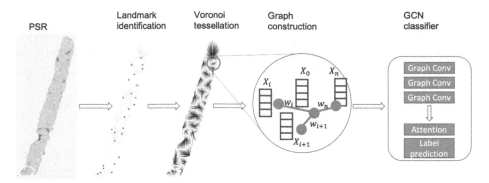

Fig. 3. The slide classification pipeline. First, tissue landmarks are identified and are used as centres for a Voronoi tessellation of image tiles. Next, a tissue graph is constructed using features extracted from individial tiles and the tessellation weights. Finally, the graph representing the whole slide serves as an input to the GCN classifier.

4.3 Graph Convolutional Layers

Given the constructed graph $G(V, E)$ with N nodes, the associated features matrix $X \in \mathbb{R}^{N,512}$ and adjacency matrix $A \in \mathbb{R}^{N,N}$ are used as an input to a 3-layer GNN. At each layer, a graph convolutional operator from GCN [11] is applied, followed by a non-linear activation function. The final nodes features matrix $H \in \mathbb{R}^{N,64}$ contains nodes representations that encode both the local graph structure and the features of the nodes. Here G^* denotes each of the convolutional layers:

$$H' = ReLu(G^*(X, A)) \quad H'' = ReLu(G^*(H', A)) \quad H = tanh(G^*(H'', A)). \quad (1)$$

As alternatives we also tested GAT [16] and GIN [15] and results can be found in Table 1.

4.4 Attention Layer

After the last graph layer, an attention layer is used to aggregate the node vectors into a set of 4 vectors, each vector being a representation of the input slide with respect to one of the output classes. For each class, a set of attention scores is computed for the input vectors: each attention score represents the importance of an input vector for that class. The sum of the input vectors weighted by their corresponding attention scores generates the final vector representation of the slide with respect to the class.

Formally, attention for a class c is computed as a function of the input sequence H and a query vector u_c, jointly learned by the network during training. Similarity between each input element H_i and the query vector u_c is computed through dot product to obtain the corresponding attention weight $\hat{\alpha}_{ci}$. A softmax function is then applied to the vector of weights $\hat{\alpha}_c$ to obtain normalised weights α_c. Finally, the attention weights are used to compute a weighted sum of the input values and obtain the final slide representation v_c.

$$v_c = \sum_i \alpha_{ci} \mathbf{H}_i \qquad \text{with} \qquad \alpha_c = Softmax(\mathbf{H}u_c^\top). \qquad (2)$$

Each slide vector v_c is passed to a fully connected layer for the final classification. The classifier has a separate set of weights to compute the raw score for each class $\hat{y}_c$. The class scores $\hat{y}_c$ are then concatenated and Softmax is used to obtain the likelihood vector $\hat{y}$.

$$\hat{y} = Softmax(\hat{y}_0, ..., \hat{y}_C) \qquad \text{with} \qquad \hat{y}_c = \mathbf{W}_c^\top v_c + b_c. \qquad (3)$$

The cross-entropy loss is computed from the likelihood vector $\hat{y}$ and the ground truth y. Training was performed to minimise the loss function by backpropagation.

5   Results

The proposed models were implemented using PyTorch [12] and PyTorch Geometric [3]. Training was performed using the Adam optimiser [10] with initial learning rate of $1e-02$, $\beta_0 = 0.9$, $\beta_1 = 0.999$, $\epsilon = 1e-08$. For the GCN, we use a weight decay factor of $1e-5$. Models were trained for at least 300 epochs and training was stopped when the change of the loss function was negligible. When training the GCN, we applied dropout with probability 0.2 before the final classifiers. We use a batch size of 64 for the GCN and a batch size of 1 for the baseline ResNet18 due to memory limitations. The results reported in Table 1 are averaged across three runs. All models have been trained on an NVIDIA Quadro RTX 6000 GPU. The source code of our analysis is available at https://github.com/mkatw/gnn-fibrosis.

The results of the quantitative analysis of slide fibre content using the identified tile subtypes are presented in Fig. 4. The weighted fibrosis score is calculated using the formula from Eq. (4):

$$WFS = \frac{1}{C-1} \sum_{c=0}^{C-1} cp_c, \qquad (4)$$

where C is the number of classes and p_c is the fraction of tiles of class c in a given slide. A large variation in the overall fibrosis score can be seen within each of the pathology grades. The variation in the weighted score is expected, as a similar phenomenon is present in CPA measurements across the progressing stages of fibrosis [6]. Measuring the distribution of tile subtypes allows for a more fine-grained quantitative analysis of fibrosis in a slide. Typical examples of graphs

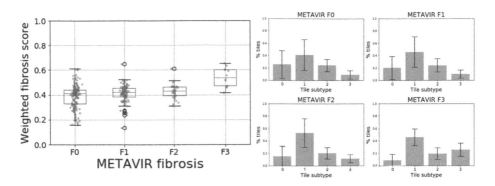

Fig. 4. The weighted fibrosis score across fibrosis stages and the distribution of tile subtypes across each METAVIR stage. The weighted fibrosis score, which is not informed by tissue topology, does not separate between classes F0 and F1 (Wilcoxon signed-rank test coefficients: $W = -1.798$, $p = 0.072$) and classes F1 and F2 ($W = -0.775$, $p = 0.438$). However, class F3 can be differentiated from all the other classes: F0 ($W = -4.436$, $p < 0.001$), F1 ($W = -4.181$, $p < 0.001$), F2 ($W = -3.559$, $p < 0.001$), and class F2 can be differentiated from F0 ($W = -2.062$, $p = 0.039$).

Table 1. F1 scores across fibrosis classes. Results expressed in %.

Model	F0	F1	F2	F3
ResNet18	53.81 ± 6.36	21.40 ± 12.73	16.93 ± 15.00	24.44 ± 21.43
GCN	65.09 ± 5.50	19.75 ± 11.63	**28.15 ± 24.48**	70.71 ± 12.02
ATN-GCN	51.63 ± 2.83	27.27 + 15.62	21.99 ± 6.72	**75.56 ± 7.70**
GAT	**71.32 ± 8.56**	**34.50 ± 21.11**	0.00 ± 0.00	44.44 ± 38.49
ATN-GAT	59.15 ± 9.09	33.23 ± 28.91	22.22 ± 38.49	19.05 ± 16.49
GIN	68.31 ± 0.23	13.33 ± 23.09	0.00 ± 0.00	13.33 ± 23.09
ATN-GIN	68.18 ± 0.00	0.00 ± 0.00	0.00 ± 0.00	0.003 ± 0.00
	F0–F1	–	F2	F3
ResNet18	67.98 ± 2.26		26.07 ± 7.74	0.00 ± 0.00
GCN	**93.01 ± 0.53**		18.79 ± 18.21	0.80 ± 0.00
ATN-GCN	89.26 ± 2.58		**28.28 ± 11.00**	**78.57 ± 6.18**
GAT	92.07 ± 1.40		27.78 ± 25.46	61.11 ± 9.62
ATN-GAT	86.22 ± 6.98		0.00 ± 0.00	0.00 ± 0.00
GIN	90.02 ± 0.00		0.00 ± 0.00	0.00 ± 0.00
ATN-GIN	90.02 ± 0.00		0.00 ± 0.00	0.00 ± 0.00
	F0–F1–F2	–	–	F3
ResNet18	74.19 ± 1.78			6.36 ± 5.53
GCN	99.03 ± 0.00			85.71 ± 0.00
ATN-GCN	**99.36 ± 0.55**			**88.57 ± 10.30**
GAT	96.85 ± 1.08			38.89 ± 34.69
ATN-GAT	96.90 ± 1.04			0.00 ± 0.00
GIN	96.30 ± 0.00			0.00 ± 0.00
ATN-GIN	96.30 ± 0.00			0.00 ± 0.00

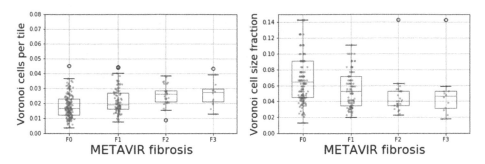

Fig. 5. The number and size of the Voronoi cells across the fibrosis stages. It can be seen that the size of a Voronoi cell relative to the area of the biopsy can change by an order of magnitude, therefore allowing to capture biological objects of varying sizes.

are presented in Fig. 6. Selected properties of the constructed tissue graphs are shown in Fig. 5.

The F1 scores of the trained models are gathered in Table 1. Here, we have tested three distinct classification setups. In the first, all fibrosis stages (F0-F3) were used directly as prediction classes. In the second and third setup, classes (F0-F1) and (F0-F2) were merged, respectively. This was done because stage F0, F1, and F2 cases have a similar macroscopic appearance and are often difficult to distinguish even for a trained pathologist. The experiments demonstrate that our GCN performs better than ResNet18 in each of the classification tasks.

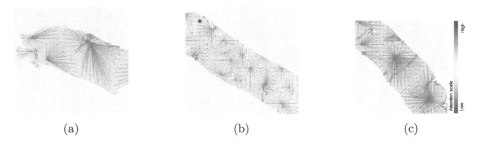

(a)   (b)   (c)

Fig. 6. Examples of tissue graphs superimposed on the original images. Node size and colour reflect attention activation for the predicted slide class. Notice that the edge length in the individual sub-graphs corresponds to the underlying pattern of fibrosis and that the sub-graphs capture biologically meaningful regions, e.g. (6a) Stage F0 with no signs of fibrosis. (6b) Stage F2 with early fibrotic clusters in the parenchyma. (6c) Stage F3 with prominent bridging.

6   Conclusion

We have proposed a new model that facilitates a quantitative analysis of fibrosis in liver biopsies. The developed pipeline allows for an explicit separation of fibres in the slide into localised fibrosis patterns and the individual regions can be inspected by a pathologist. This representation fully aligns with established fibrosis scoring such as METAVIR. Importantly, this approach can be integrated into an interactive scoring system where pathologists can eliminate specific graphs form the analysis. The method could easily be extended to different fibrosis stainings and to other organs.

Acknowledgements. MW is funded by the UK Engineering and Physical Sciences Research Council and Medical Research Council (EP/L016052/1) and in part by Perspectum Ltd. NGM is supported by CRUK Oxford Centre Prize DPhil Studentship (C2195/A27450). HF is funded by NIH 5R01CA193694-02. SM and JR are supported by the PathLAKE Centre of Excellence for digital pathology and artificial intelligence which is funded from the Data to Early Diagnosis and Precision Medicine strand of the HM Government's Industrial Strategy Challenge Fund, managed and delivered by Innovate UK on behalf of UK Research and Innovation (UKRI). Views expressed are those of the authors and not necessarily those of the PathLAKE Consortium members, the NHS, Innovate UK or UKRI. Grant ref: File Ref 104689/application number 18181. JR is in part funded by the National Institute for Health Research Oxford Biomedical Research Centre.

References

1. Bankhead, P., et al.: QuPath: open source software for digital pathology image analysis. Sci. Rep. **7**(1), 16878 (2017)
2. Calvaruso, V., et al.: Computer-assisted image analysis of liver collagen: relationship to Ishak scoring and hepatic venous pressure gradient. Hepatology **49**(4), 1236–1244 (2009)
3. Fey, M., Lenssen, J.E.: Fast graph representation learning with pytorch geometric (2019)
4. Friedman, S.L., Neuschwander-Tetri, B.A., Rinella, M., Sanyal, A.J.: Mechanisms of NAFLD development and therapeutic strategies. Nat. Med. **24**(7), 908–922 (2018)
5. Goodman, Z.D.: Grading and staging systems for inflammation and fibrosis in chronic liver diseases. J. Hepatol. **47**(4), 598–607 (2007)
6. Goodman, Z.D., Becker, R.L., Pockros, P.J., Afdhal, N.H.: Progression of fibrosis in advanced chronic hepatitis C: evaluation by morphometric image analysis. Hepatology **45**(4), 886–894 (2007)
7. Hagberg, A.A., Schult, D.A., Swart, P.J.: Exploring network structure, dynamics, and function using networkX. In: Varoquaux, G., Vaught, T., Millman, J. (eds.) Proceedings of the 7th Python in Science Conference, pp. 11–15. Pasadena, CA USA (2008)
8. He, K., Zhang, X., Ren, S., Sun, J.: Deep residual learning for image recognition. In: Proceedings of the IEEE Computer Society Conference on Computer Vision and Pattern Recognition 2016-December, pp. 770–778 (2016)

9. Heinemann, F., Birk, G., Stierstorfer, B.: Deep learning enables pathologist-like scoring of NASH models. Sci. Rep. **9**(1), 1–10 (2019)
10. Kingma, D.P., Ba, J.: Adam: a method for stochastic optimization. In: 3rd International Conference for Learning Representations, San Diego, 2015 (2017)
11. Kipf, T.N., Welling, M.: Semi-supervised classification with graph convolutional networks. In: International Conference on Learning Representations (ICLR) (2017)
12. Paszke, A., et al.: Pytorch: an imperative style, high-performance deep learning library. In: Advances in Neural Information Processing Systems 32, pp. 8024–8035. Curran Associates, Inc. (2019)
13. Pati, P., et al.: HACT-Net: a hierarchical cell-to-tissue graph neural network for histopathological image classification. In: Sudre, C.H., et al. (eds.) UNSURE/GRAIL -2020. LNCS, vol. 12443, pp. 208–219. Springer, Cham (2020). https://doi.org/10.1007/978-3-030-60365-6_20
14. Sharma, H., Zerbe, N., Lohmann, S., Kayser, K., Hellwich, O., Hufnagl, P.: A review of graph-based methods for image analysis in digital histopathology. Diagnost. Pathol. **1**(1), 1–51 (2015)
15. Veličković, P., Casanova, A., Liò, P., Cucurull, G., Romero, A., Bengio, Y.: Graph attention networks. In: 6th International Conference on Learning Representations, ICLR 2018 - Conference Track Proceedings, pp. 1–12 (2018)
16. Xu, K., Jegelka, S., Hu, W., Leskovec, J.: How powerful are graph neural networks? In: 7th International Conference on Learning Representations, ICLR 2019, pp. 1–17 (2019)
17. Xu, S., et al.: QFibrosis: a fully-quantitative innovative method incorporating histological features to facilitate accurate fibrosis scoring in animal model and chronic hepatitis B patients. J. Hepatol. **61**(2), 260–269 (2014)
18. Yu, Y., et al.: Deep learning enables automated scoring of liver fibrosis stages. Sci. Rep. **8**(1), 1–10 (2018)
19. Zheng, Y., Jiang, B., Shi, J., Zhang, H., Xie, F.: Encoding histopathological WSIS using GNN for scalable diagnostically relevant regions retrieval. In: Shen, D., et al. (eds.) MICCAI 2019. LNCS, vol. 11764, pp. 550–558. Springer, Cham (2019). https://doi.org/10.1007/978-3-030-32239-7_61
20. Zhou, Y., Graham, S., Alemi Koohbanani, N., Shaban, M., Heng, P.A., Rajpoot, N.: CGC-net: cell graph convolutional network for grading of colorectal cancer histology images. In: Proceedings - 2019 International Conference on Computer Vision Workshop, ICCVW 2019, pp. 388–398 (2019)

Hierarchical Graph Pathomic Network for Progression Free Survival Prediction

Zichen Wang[1,2], Jiayun Li[1,2], Zhufeng Pan[1,3], Wenyuan Li[1,4], Anthony Sisk[1,5], Huihui Ye[1,5], William Speier[1,2,6], and Corey W. Arnold[1,2,4,5,6(✉)]

[1] Computational Diagnostics Lab, UCLA, Los Angeles, USA
cwarnold@ucla.edu
[2] The Department of Bioengineering, UCLA, Los Angeles, USA
[3] The Department of Computer Science, UCLA, Los Angeles, USA
[4] The Department of Electrical and Computer Engineering, UCLA, Los Angeles, USA
[5] The Department of Pathology and Laboratory Medicine, UCLA, Los Angeles, USA
[6] The Department of Radiological Sciences, UCLA, Los Angeles, USA

Abstract. High resolution histology images contain information related to disease prognosis. However, survival prediction based on current clinical grading systems, which rely heavily on a pathologist's histological assessment, has significant limitations due to the heterogeneity and complexity of tissue phenotypes. To address these challenges, we propose a deep learning framework that leverages hierarchical graph-based representations to enable more precise prediction of progression-free survival in prostate cancer patients. Unlike conventional approaches that analyze patch-based or cell-based pathomic features alone without considering their spatial connectivity, we explore multi-scale topological structures of whole slide images in an integrative context. Extensive experiments have demonstrated the effectiveness of our model for better progression prediction.

Keywords: Progression free survival · Graph convolutional neural network · Self-supervised learning · Hierarchical graph representations

1 Introduction

Prostate cancer (PCa) is the most common and second deadliest non-skin cancer in American men [1]. Prostate cancer progression following surgery is measured through changes in histological and biochemical measures. The ability to predict progression-free survival (PFS) could assist physicians in selecting treatment options for patients, with patients at a higher risk for progression receiving more aggressive treatment. The Gleason grading system is the current best method for PCa diagnosis and is a critical component in clinical survival assessment and treatment planning [2]. Gleason grades are assigned by pathologists

---

Z. Wang and J. Li—Contributed equally to this work.

Electronic supplementary material The online version of this chapter (https://doi.org/10.1007/978-3-030-87237-3_22) contains supplementary material, which is available to authorized users.

© Springer Nature Switzerland AG 2021
M. de Bruijne et al. (Eds.): MICCAI 2021, LNCS 12908, pp. 227–237, 2021.
https://doi.org/10.1007/978-3-030-87237-3_22

based on visual interpretation of tumor architecture. This process suffers from inter-observer variability and is constrained by its categorization system, which cannot fully capture the disease's continuous feature spectrum. To address this issue, previous machine learning methods on survival prediction focus mainly on extracting features from manually selected regions of interest (ROIs) and use pre-defined aggregation methods to generate slide-level embeddings [3–5]. However, there are two major limitations with current approaches. First, current methods ignore spatial connectivity of patches and thus fail to learn global topological representations of WSIs and may not account for tumor heterogeneity. Second, ROI-based methods often require annotations from human experts, which are expensive and can be infeasible to collect.

Deep learning methods have opened a new paradigm for automated whole slide image (WSI) analysis. However, due to image sizes, data availability, and hardware limitations, patch sampling of WSIs is necessary. To address the above challenges, graph convolutional network (GCN)-based approaches model WSIs as graph structured data, which combine global context and local connectivity with parameter efficiency. Many recent studies can be categorized into patch-based and cell-based approaches. Patch-based methods [6–9] focus on learning global topological representations of WSIs. For example, Li et al. [7] proposed a graph model for survival prediction by rendering the optimal graph representations of WSIs. Graph nodes were selected patches and node features were initialized by a VGG-16 network. Graph edges were constructed by thresholding the Euclidean distances between node features. Cell-based methods [10–12] aim to construct feature maps of patches by exploring the topological structure of cells and the micro-environment. As opposed to patch-based methods, cell-based methods emphasize the biological significance of WSIs. For example, Chen et al. [12] proposed a multimodal fusion model for cancer survival prediction. They applied GCNs as a complementary method to convolutional neural networks (CNNs) for feature extraction. They used segmented nuclei as nodes and initialized the node attributes with handcrafted features. The edges between two nodes were thresholded by a fixed spatial distance while the maximum degree of each node was set to k corresponding to its k-nearest neighbors.

Existing GCN-based methods for WSI analysis are limited in two aspects. First, patch-based methods rely on pretrained deep learning models or handcrafted features, which ignore the informative signals from cell graphs. Second, cell-based methods are inefficient in modeling WSIs with large numbers of cells, and thus typically require laborious patch-level labeling. We propose to unify patch-based and cell-based methods with a hierarchical GCN framework, balancing efficiency and granularity. We hypothesize that analyzing WSIs through multi-scale graph representations, from fine to coarse grained, will outperform current approaches for PFS prediction using WSIs. The main contributions of our paper are summarized as follows:

- To the best of our knowledge, we propose the first hierarchical GCN framework, termed graph pathomic network, for cancer survival prediction using

WSIs, which models nuclei-level and patch-level graph structures in an integrative context.

- We propose an efficient self-supervised learning method to pretrain our graph pathomic network, yielding improved performance over trained-from-scratch counterparts.
- We develop a deep learning system for PCa PFS prediction that does not rely on manually selected ROIs and patch-level labels.

2 Method

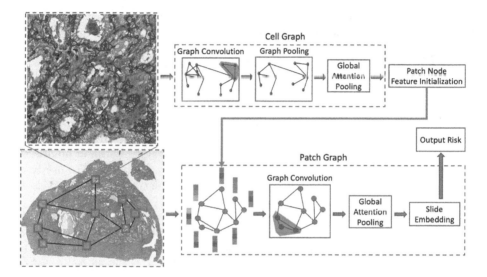

Fig. 1. Model architecture of the hierarchical graph pathomic network. Given a WSI, we sample patches using the tumor detection model to construct a patch graph, each node of which is represented by its corresponding cell graph. Our model learns hierarchical graph representations of WSIs from nuclei-level to patch-level.

2.1 Tumor Region Detection

Unlike previous studies, which rely on manually selected ROIs [3–5], we utilize a patch-level CNN trained on weakly-labeled slides to sample cancerous patches. Specifically, we formulate the problem of training a tumor detection model with slide-level labels as a multiple instance learning (MIL) task [13]. According to the basic assumption of the MIL, top patches within a malignant slide will have probabilities closer to 1, while patches from a benign slide should have probabilities closer to 0 [13]. The patches with the highest predicted probabilities in each slide inherit the slide-level label. The patch-level model is further optimized with these pseudo patch-level labels. The process is iterated until convergence. The model is then finetuned on a small dataset with coarse contour annotations.

2.2 Graph Pathomic Network

Nuclei Segmentation and Cell Feature Extraction. Accurate nuclei instance segmentation is important in defining reliable cell features that would be indicative of cancer progression. We train a Mask R-CNN [14] using the dataset from [15] to segment nuclei. After obtaining nuclei masks, we define an eight-pixel width of the ring-like neighborhood region around each nucleus as its cytoplasm area. We then extract nuclear morphometry features and imaging features (including intensity, gradient and Haralick features) for nuclear and cytoplasm regions respectively, resulting in 108-dimensional feature descriptors for each cell.

Hierarchical Graph Representation of WSIs

- **Cell Graph.** To learn complex relationships between cells for patch representation, we construct cell graphs by defining each cell as a node and an edge as the potential interaction between two cells. The intuition is that cells that are closer to each other are more likely to interact. We use the k-nearest neighbors algorithm to construct adjacency matrices of cell graphs. Specifically, we assign an edge between two nuclei if they are within a fixed spatial distance from each other. In addition, the maximum neighborhood number of each node is set to K corresponding to its k-nearest neighbors. We use K=5 to model topological information of cell graph structures, and 60 pixels at 40x resolution to set the largest distance.
- **Patch Graph.** For each WSI, we define a patch graph to aggregate patch-level features and extract topological properties of the WSI. Given a set of selected patches by the tumor region detection model, we define each patch as a node in a patch graph, and initialize its features with cell graph representations. Similar to cell graph construction, we use the k-nearest neighbors algorithm (K = 3) to construct edge sets based on spatial distance between two patches.

Graph Convolutional Network. We use the GCN with attention, also referred as the graph attention network (GAT) [16] to perform graph convolution operations to extract and propagate features along edges of the graph. Specifically, a graph $\mathcal{G} \in \mathbb{G}$ can be denoted by $\mathcal{G}(\mathcal{V}, \mathcal{E})$ consisting of a vertex set $\mathcal{V} = \{v_i\}_{i=1}^{N_\mathcal{V}}$ and edge set $\mathcal{E} = \{e_j\}_{j=1}^{N_\mathcal{E}}$, $\vec{h}_{v_i} \in \mathbb{R}^N$ is the node feature of vertex v_i. A general GCN layer can be defined as follows:

$$g_\mathcal{E}(v_i) = \text{ReLU}\left(W \cdot \text{Mean}\left(\{h_{v_j} | v_j \in \mathcal{N}_{v_i}^\mathcal{E} \cup \{v_i\})\}\right)\right). \tag{1}$$

where $W \in \mathbb{R}^{M \times N}$ is a learnable matrix transforming N-dimensional features to M-dimensional features, the Mean is an element-wise mean-pooling operation. $\mathcal{N}_{v_i}^\mathcal{E}$ is the neighborhood of the node v_i connected by $\mathcal{E}$ in $\mathcal{G}$. GAT uses an attention mechanism on node features to construct the weighting kernel as $W_{v_i,v_j} = \alpha_{v_i,v_j} W$. The weighting coefficients can be expressed as:

$$\alpha_{v_i,v_j} = \frac{\exp\left(\rho\left(\vec{a}^T\left[W\vec{h}_{v_i}\|W\vec{h}_{v_j}\right]\right)\right)}{\sum_{v_k\in\mathcal{N}_{v_i}^{\mathcal{E}}}\exp\left(\rho\left(\vec{a}^T\left[W\vec{h}_{v_i}\|W\vec{h}_{v_k}\right]\right)\right)} \tag{2}$$

where T represents transposition and $\|$ is the concatenation operation.

Graph Pooling. To coarsen the graph and generate high-level representation, self-attention graph pooling [17] based on both graph features and topology are used to reduce the number of nodes with a fixed pooling ratio k. After each graph pooling layer, the top k% nodes are selected based on their attention scores, and the remaining nodes are removed from the graph.

Model Architecture. Figure 1 shows an overview of our proposed model. In order to model cell-level and patch-level graph structure of WSIs in an integrative context, we build a multi-scale GCN framework using hierarchical graph representations of WSIs. Our model consists of two consecutive steps. In the first step, our model operates directly on cell graphs of all selected patches from the same slide to generate node representations for a patch graph. We use three model layers to update node features and the topological structure of cell graphs. Each layer consists of a GAT and graph pooling operations. The graph embedding $\mathbf{r_i}$ of a cell graph is obtained by applying a global soft attention-based aggregation operation [18] on updated node features $\mathbf{x_n}$, which can be expressed as:

$$\mathbf{r}_i = \sum_{n=1}^{N_i} \text{softmax}\left(h_{\text{gate}}\left(\mathbf{x}_n\right)\right) \odot \mathbf{x}_n \tag{3}$$

where h_{gate} is a neural network that computes attention scores by mapping node feature vectors to scalars. In the second step, we apply two GAT layers to further update the patch graph, which is initialized by features from cell graphs. Finally, we apply the same global soft attention-base aggregation operation to generate slide embeddings for PFS prediction.

2.3   Model Training for Progression Free Survival Prediction

We utilize the negative logarithm of Cox partial likelihood proposed in the Deep-Surv model [19] as the loss function for model optimization. Given the event e_i is observed for patient i at T_i, the Cox loss can be computed by Eq. 4.

$$l(\beta) = -\sum_{i:e_i=1}\left(h_\theta(\mathbf{z}) - log\sum_{j\in R_{(T_i)}}\exp(h_\theta(\mathbf{z}))\right) \tag{4}$$

where $\mathbf{z}$ is the slide embedding of a patient, $j \in R_{(T_i)}$ represents a set of patients with events that have not occurred at T_i. $h(\cdot)_\theta$ is a non-linear function (*e.g.*, a multi-layer perceptron).

2.4 Momentum Contrast for Unsupervised Pre-training of Cell Graph

Training an accurate GCN model often requires a large collection of labeled data and expressive features. However, we have limited patient-level labels in this study. Several recent works have demonstrated that pre-trained GCN models can benefit downstream applications by providing useful features or parameter initialization [20,21]. We generalize the Momentum Contrastive (MoCo) model [22] to graph data for pretraining the cell graph module of our proposed framework.

The main assumption for the MoCo model is that features from augmented versions of the same input should be more similar than features from different inputs. Specifically, input data can be projected into feature vectors k_i by a key encoding function $f_k(\cdot)$, which can be considered as keys in a dataset. Given the encoded representation q_i of a query data generated by the query encoding function $f_q(\cdot)$, there exists one matched key, which has the largest similarity value to q_i. The similarity between a pair of feature vectors can be measured using the cosine distance: $\mathrm{sim}(q_i, k_i) = \frac{q_i k_i}{\|q_i\|\|k_i\|}$. The contrastive loss is defined by Eq. 5.

$$\mathcal{L}_q = -\log \frac{\exp(\mathrm{sim}(q_i k_i)/\gamma)}{\exp(\mathrm{sim}(q_i k_i)/\gamma) + \sum_{j \neq i}^{N} \exp(\mathrm{sim}(q_i k_j)/\gamma)} \tag{5}$$

where γ is the temperature parameter. q_i and k_i are feature vectors from different views of the same data i. Importantly, MoCo improves conventional contrastive learning by building a dynamic dictionary with a queue and a moving-averaged encoder. This enables building a large and consistent dictionary on-the-fly that facilitates contrastive unsupervised learning. Specifically, we define two augmentation methods to generate different views of the same cell graph. (1) Node dropping: we randomly drop cell nodes with a fixed percent number (5%) from the original graph. (2) Graph structure perturbation: we randomly set hyperparameters for cell graph construction from a fixed range of values, which also reduces model sensitivity to parameters. In this study, hyperparameters include maximum neighborhood number (5–7) and the largest distance between connected nodes (55–70 px).

3 Experiment

3.1 Dataset and Preprocessing

Three datasets are used in this experiment. (1) A UCLA prostate biopsy dataset containing 20,229 slides from prostate needle biopsies from 830 patients [13]. (2) A Cedars-Sinai dataset consisting of 30 slides from prostatectomies of 30 patients, which were annotated with coarse contour annotations [23]. (3) The PFS prediction is performed on the publicly available TCGA-PRAD dataset [24] using patches of size 512×512 at 40x magnification(0.25 um per pixel). Datasets (1) and (2) are used to train the tumor detection model. For dataset (3), clinical data and H&E stained diagnostic slides were retrieved using the Genomic Data Commons (GDC) data portal. Additional follow-up data are obtained from the TCGA Pan-Cancer Clinical Data Resource (TCGA-CDR) [24]. The recommended progression-free interval (PFI) is used as the clinical endpoint [24]. 399 cases with available diagnostic slides are included in this study. Five-fold cross validation stratified by events is utilized for model training and validation. Within each fold, we further split the training data into 80% for training and 20% for validation. Model performance is evaluated on testing data for each fold to avoid overfitting.

3.2 Methods Comparison

To evaluate the effectiveness of our hierarchical graph pathomic network, we performed experiments on different typos of features, aggregation methods, and linear Cox models.

Clinical Features. We utilized clinical variables including age, PSA value, Gleason grade group (GG), and pathologic T stage to fit a baseline Cox model.

Linear Cox Model. We compared our model with linear Cox models, including Lasso-Cox (*i.e.,,* with $\mathcal{L}_1$ penalty) and ElasticNet-Cox (*i.e.,* with $\mathcal{L}_2$ penalty). Different types of features as described in the following sections were used as covariates for linear Cox models.

Attention MIL-Based Aggregation. We compared the GCN-based aggregation with the attention MIL method, which demonstrated promising results in GG prediction [13]. Specifically, a trainable attention module was incorporated to summarize patch-level features into slide embeddings.

Texture-Based Features. We extracted 90 first-order statistics and texture-based features with the Pyradiomics package [25]. Texture-based features were utilized as predictors in *ElasticNet-Cox-texture* and *Lasso-Cox-texture* experiments.

Self-supervised CNN Features. We adopted the MoCo model with ResNet50 as the backbone [22] to learn CNN features from patches. The trained query encoder of the MoCo model was used as the feature extractor to generate a 128×1 feature vector for each patch. Self-supervised learning features were utilized as covariates in the *Lasso-Cox-deep* and *ElasticNet-Cox-deep* experiments. *Deep-Att-MIL* denotes the deep survival model that leverages self-supervised CNN features and attention MIL-based aggregation. *Deep-GCN* denotes the variant of our proposed method, which includes only the patch graph module and uses self-supervised CNN features as initial node embeddings.

Handcrafted Cell Graph Features. To validate the effectiveness of the cell graph, we extract pre-defined cell graph features for the ablation study. We compute global features of the nuclei with the given centroids based on the partitioning of the space into Voronoi cells and on the induced graph structure. This type of feature only captures the topological structure of cell graph.

3.3   Model Training and Evaluation

We selected 200 patches from each slide for analysis. We used a learning rate of 0.001 and a batch size of 64 for Deep-Att-MIL model training. The learning rate and batch size for Deep-Att-MIL-clinical were set at 0.001 and 12, respectively. All GCN-based models were trained with a batch size of 16 and a learning rate of 0.0005. Adam optimizer was used in all experiments. PFS analysis models were evaluated with the concordance index (c-index), which was computed with the lifelines package [26]. The c-index measures the effectiveness of predicted risk scores on ranking survival times, with 1 indicating the perfect concordance and 0.5 representing results from random predictions. For cases with multiple slides, average hazards were utilized. All models were implemented with PyTorch, trained and validated with one Tesla V100 GPU.

Table 1. Concordance index of models on predicting progression free survival for prostate cancer patients following radical prostatectomy.

Models	c-index ↑
Clinical features	0.7254 ± 0.042
Lasso-Cox-texture	0.6818 ± 0.067
Lasso-Cox-graph	0.6857 ± 0.092
Lasso-Cox-deep	0.7046 ± 0.111
ElasticNet-Cox-texture	0.6671 ± 0.052
ElasticNet-Cox-graph	0.6892 ± 0.084
ElasticNet-Cox-deep	0.7254 ± 0.101
Deep-Att-MIL	0.7420 ± 0.089
Deep-GCN	0.7441 ± 0.123
Graph pathomic network	0.7539 ± 0.103
Pre-trained graph pathomic network	$\mathbf{0.7636 \pm 0.091}$
Deep-Att-MIL + clinical	0.7586 ± 0.076
Deep-GCN + clinical	0.7743 ± 0.122
Graph pathomic network + clinical	0.7831 ± 0.105
Pre-trained graph pathomic network + clinical	$\mathbf{0.7934 \pm 0.082}$

4   Results

Average c-index and 95% confidence interval for model experiments are shown in the Table 1. The baseline Cox model with clinical features obtained an average c-index of 72.54%. The pre-trained graph pathomic network that combined clinical variables achieved the highest average c-index of 79.34%, which was around 7% higher than the baseline model with only clinical features. The spatial distribution of nuclei is important for prostate progression estimation. As shown in the Table 1, models with handcrafted graph-based features showed better performances than those with texture-based features. Models with deep learning representations demonstrated superior performance compared with handcrafted features. The GCN based aggregation method showed better results in predicting progression compared to Att-MIL aggregation. The graph pathomic network outperformed all baseline models, demonstrating the effectiveness of learning features from hierarchical graphs. Graph MoCo pre-training brought around 1% c-index improvement than trained from-scratch counterparts. We also observed that pre-trained graph pathomic network converged faster during model training.

In summary, we developed a deep learning system with novel hierarchical graph-based representations for PFS prediction of PCa patients. By building hierarchical graph representations, our proposed model shows promising results on predicting PFS. In addition, combining clinical factors and pathomic features is superior to the baseline model with clinical features only, suggesting the potential of leveraging quantitative pathomic features for better progression prediction. However, we only evaluated our model on the TCGA-PRAD dataset. Validation on large prospective datasets is needed to further validate pathomic features. Reinforcement learning may also be investigated in future work to enable adaptive patch selection and end-to-end training.

References

1. Siegel, R.L., Miller, K.D., Jemal, A.: Cancer statistics, 2019. CA Cancer J. Clin. **69**(1), 7–34 (2019)
2. Epstein, J.I., et al.: A contemporary prostate cancer grading system: a validated alternative to the Gleason score. Euro. Urol. **69**(3), 428–435 (2016)
3. Chandramouli, S., et al.: Computer extracted features from initial H&E tissue biopsies predict disease progression for prostate cancer patients on active surveillance. Cancers **12**(9), 2708 (2020)
4. Leo, P., et al.: Computerized histomorphometric features of glandular architecture predict risk of biochemical recurrence following radical prostatectomy: a multisite study (2019)
5. Cheng, L., et al.: Nuclear shape and orientation features from H&E images predict survival in early-stage estrogen receptor-positive breast cancers. Lab. Invest. **98**(11), 1438–1448 (2018)

6. Zhao, Y., et al.: Predicting lymph node metastasis using histopathological images based on multiple instance learning with deep graph convolution. In: Proceedings of the IEEE/CVF Conference on Computer Vision and Pattern Recognition, pp. 4837–4846 (2020)

7. Li, R., Yao, J., Zhu, X., Li, Y., Huang, J.: Graph CNN for survival analysis on whole slide pathological images. In: Frangi, A.F., Schnabel, J.A., Davatzikos, C., Alberola-López, C., Fichtinger, G. (eds.) MICCAI 2018. LNCS, vol. 11071, pp. 174–182. Springer, Cham (2018). https://doi.org/10.1007/978-3-030-00934-2_20

8. Adnan, M., Kalra, S., Tizhoosh, H.R.: Representation learning of histopathology images using graph neural networks. In: Proceedings of the IEEE/CVF Conference on Computer Vision and Pattern Recognition Workshops, pp. 988–989 (2020)

9. Ding, K., Liu, Q., Lee, E., Zhou, M., Lu, A., Zhang, S.: Feature-enhanced graph networks for genetic mutational prediction using histopathological images in colon cancer. In: Martel, A.L., et al. (eds.) MICCAI 2020. LNCS, vol. 12262, pp. 294–304. Springer, Cham (2020). https://doi.org/10.1007/978-3-030-59713-9_29

10. Zhou, Y., Graham, S., Koohbanani, N.A., Shaban, M., Heng, P.-H., Rajpoot, N.: CGC-net: cell graph convolutional network for grading of colorectal cancer histology images. In: Proceedings of the IEEE/CVF International Conference on Computer Vision Workshops (2019)

11. Wang, J., Chen, R.J., Lu, M.Y., Baras, A., Mahmood, F.: Weakly supervised prostate TMA classification via graph convolutional networks. In: 2020 IEEE 17th International Symposium on Biomedical Imaging (ISBI), pp. 239–243. IEEE (2020)

12. Chen, R.J., et al.: Pathomic fusion: an integrated framework for fusing histopathology and genomic features for cancer diagnosis and prognosis. IEEE Trans. Med. Imaging (2020)

13. Li, J., et al.: A multi-resolution model for histopathology image classification and localization with multiple instance learning. In: Computers in Biology and Medicine, p. 104253 (2021)

14. He, K., Gkioxari, G., Dollár, P., Girshick, R.: Mask R-CNN. In: Proceedings of the IEEE International Conference on Computer Vision, pp. 2961–2969 (2017)

15. Kumar, N., et al.: A multi-organ nucleus segmentation challenge. IEEE Trans. Med. Imaging **39**(5), 1380–1391 (2019)

16. Veličković, P., Cucurull, G., Casanova, A., Romero, A., Lio, P., Bengio, Y.: Graph attention networks. arXiv preprint arXiv:1710.10903 (2017)

17. Lee, J., Lee, I., Kang, J.: Self-attention graph pooling. In: International Conference on Machine Learning, pp. 3734–3743. PMLR (2019)

18. Li, Y., Tarlow, D., Brockschmidt, M., Zemel, R.: Gated graph sequence neural networks. arXiv preprint arXiv:1511.05493 (2015)

19. Katzman, J.L., Shaham, U., Cloninger, A., Bates, J., Jiang, T., Kluger, Y.: Deep survival: a deep cox proportional hazards network. Stat **1050**(2) (2016)

20. Hu, W., et al.: Strategies for pre-training graph neural networks. arXiv preprint arXiv:1905.12265 (2019)

21. Qiu, J., et al.: GCC: graph contrastive coding for graph neural network pre-training. In: Proceedings of the 26th ACM SIGKDD International Conference on Knowledge Discovery & Data Mining, pp. 1150–1160 (2020)

22. He, K., Fan, H., Wu, Y., Xie, S., Girshick, R.: Momentum contrast for unsupervised visual representation learning. In: Proceedings of the IEEE/CVF Conference on Computer Vision and Pattern Recognition, pp. 9729–9738 (2020)

23. Ing, N., et al.: Semantic segmentation for prostate cancer grading by convolutional neural networks. In: Medical Imaging 2018: Digital Pathology, vol. 10581, pp. 105811B. International Society for Optics and Photonics (2018)

24. Liu, J., et al.: An integrated TCGA pan-cancer clinical data resource to drive high-quality survival outcome analytics. Cell **173**(2), 400–416 (2018)
25. Van Griethuysen, J.J.M., et al.: Computational radiomics system to decode the radiographic phenotype. Cancer Res. **77**(21), e104–e107 (2017)
26. Davidson-Pilon, C., et al.: Camdavidsonpilon/lifelines: v0. 24.15. Zenodo (2020)

Increasing Consistency of Evoked Response in Thalamic Nuclei During Repetitive Burst Stimulation of Peripheral Nerve in Humans

Jessica S. L. Vidmark[1]([✉]) [iD], Estefania Hernandez-Martin[1] [iD],
and Terence D. Sanger[1,2] [iD]

[1] University of California—Irvine, Irvine, CA 92697, USA
jvidmark@uci.edu
[2] Children's Health Orange County, Orange, CA 92868, USA

Abstract. *Objective.* Peripheral nerve stimulation has been proposed as a noninvasive treatment for patients with movement disorders such as essential tremor, Parkinson's disease, and dystonia. While the outcomes have shown clinical effect, the mechanism behind the effect is not yet clear. The goal of this work was to study the brain's responses to peripheral stimulation bursts and explain the therapeutic results. *Approach.* We performed peripheral stimulation of the median nerve(s) in 12 pediatric patients undergoing deep brain stimulation for dystonia. Stimulation was given in bursts (50–200 Hz stimulation in blocks of 100 ms, separated by 100 ms without stimulation) and intracranial activity was simultaneously recorded from deep brain stimulation leads implanted in thalamic nuclei. After using a novel method to remove stimulus artifacts, sequences of neural responses during and after the bursts were analyzed. *Results.* Peripheral burst stimulation induced increasing consistency of successive evoked responses in thalamic nuclei. *Significance.* We propose that this phenomenon is due to progressive synchronization of small populations of thalamic neurons, so that over time there is phase locking of the response in an increasing number of neurons in the population. Clinical efficacy could thus be due to "synchronization blockade", in which the synchronized response of the population prevents transmission of intrinsic abnormal signals due to tremor or dystonia. Further studies are necessary to confirm this model of clinical effect. Enhanced understanding will increase the potential for use of peripheral stimulation as a noninvasive alternative or adjunct to deep brain stimulation.

Keywords: Peripheral burst stimulation · Evoked response · Neural synchronization

1 Introduction

Peripheral nerve stimulation (PNS) has been proposed as a noninvasive treatment method [1] to modulate neural activity at the subcortical level in subjects with movement disorders such as essential tremor [2, 3], Parkinson's disease [4], and dystonia [5, 6]. Prior

---

Electronic supplementary material The online version of this chapter (https://doi.org/10.1007/978-3-030-87237-3_23) contains supplementary material, which is available to authorized users.

© Springer Nature Switzerland AG 2021
M. de Bruijne et al. (Eds.): MICCAI 2021, LNCS 12908, pp. 238–247, 2021.
https://doi.org/10.1007/978-3-030-87237-3_23

work has shown that there is a robust evoked response to peripheral stimulation in thalamic nuclei, including ventral intermediate (VIM) and ventral posterolateral anterior (VPLa) nuclei [7]–[10], likely mediated through cerebello- and spinothalamic pathways. This response has led to the conjecture that PNS could have a similar effect to thalamic deep brain stimulation (DBS), and might thus ameliorate movement disorders where intracranial thalamic stimulation has been effective.

Neural responses generated by electrical stimulations are commonly mixed with stimulus artifacts [11, 12]. While these artifacts can serve as a marker to aid in the alignment of neural responses to their respective trigger, electrical stimulations often cause problems, not only by saturating the recording contacts, but also because the capacitive components in the contacts give rise to a capacitive discharge phase, prolonging the time required for the recording contact to return to baseline [12]. This complexity of stimulus artifacts may explain why many PNS studies use low-frequency stimulation (<10 Hz), allowing for ample time between stimuli [10, 13–16].

However, while the saturation period typically leads to a complete loss of neural recordings, neural responses generally can be recorded during the capacitive discharge phase. The concern here is instead separating the neural activity from this "decay artifact". Decaying exponential models have been previously implemented to remove decay artifacts [17, 18], and have proven more successful at removing artifacts than other common methods, including independent component analysis (ICA).[1] Expanding on these models, we here present a novel method that incorporates complex exponentials to fit to and accurately remove oscillating decay artifacts. This method allows us to reduce the stimulus artifact influence and avoid the noise mixed with the neural response.

The robustness and reliability of the method were tested on DBS contact recordings from thalamic nuclei during high frequency peripheral stimulation in pediatric patients with movement disorders, including generalized dystonia and hemidystonia. The results promote the method's ability to extract clear neural responses, not only *after* the last pulse in the burst, but also *between* pulses, in studies with high-frequency stimulations. Furthermore, results show a new phenomenon of progressive increase in consistency, consistent with a model of neural population synchronization in response to repetitive stimulation.

2   Materials and Methods

2.1   Patient Selection

Subjects for clinical DBS surgery were chosen based on the inclusion criteria of all of the following: presence of movement disorder, significantly limiting or interfering with normal function or care; potential stimulation targets, identifiable with magnetic resonance imaging; and low success from symptomatic or etiologic medical therapy. Prior to the study, subjects or their legal guardians provided HIPAA authorization for research use of protected health information, as well as written informed consent both for surgical procedures conforming to standard hospital practice, and for research use

---

[1] The stimulus artifact and the evoked potential always correlate, since one causes the other. Hence, ICA is inherently not an applicable approach for stimulus artifact removal.

of electrophysiological data. All research use of data was approved by the institutional review boards of Children's Hospital Los Angeles (CHLA) and Children's Health Orange County (CHOC).

Data from 12 pediatric patients (7 male, 5 female, 6–20 years old, median age: 16) were used in this study (Table S1, Supplementary Material).

2.2 Data Acquisition

During surgery to establish optimal permanent DBS lead placement, up to 10 temporary Adtech MM16C depth leads (Adtech Medical Instrument Corp., Oak Creek, WI, USA) were implanted into potential DBS targets, identified prior to surgery through a collaborative consultation between the departments of Neurology and Neurosurgery at CHLA or CHOC. Typical target areas included the thalamus (VIM, VPLa, and ventral oralis anterior/posterior, Voa/Vop) and basal ganglia, due to prior studies of clinical efficacy in dystonic patients when lesioned or electrically stimulated [19–23]. Each implanted lead consisted of 6 low-impedance "macro-contacts", and 10 high-impedance "micro-contacts". These intracranial leads were linked to the amplifier inputs via Adtech Cabrio™ connectors, through shielded cables.

Concurrently with contralateral median nerve stimulation, data was recorded through the micro-contacts, sampled at ~ 22 kHz and band-pass filtered at 0.3–9 kHz. Recordings were gathered using either a system consisting of a PZ5M 256-channel digitizer, an RZ2 processor, and an RS4 high speed data storage (Tucker-Davis Technologies Inc., Alachua, FL, USA), or a NeuroOmega™ 96-channel system (AlphaOmega Co USA Inc., Alpharetta, GA, USA).

2.3 Peripheral Burst Stimulation

In the 2–5 days following lead implantation, after allowing the patient to fully recover from the effects of the general anesthesia administered for surgery, testing and data collection were performed. Peripheral stimulation was applied to the median nerve at the wrist through 1-cm adhesive disk electrodes, with the cathodic electrode placed proximally. Current-controlled stimulations were provided through a STMISOLA (Biopac Systems Inc., Goleta, CA, USA) isolated stimulator, driven by a pulse train generated by a Power1401 digital to analog converter (Cambridge Electronic Design Inc., Cambridge, UK).

Peripheral burst stimulations consisted of biphasic pulses in frequencies of approximately 50, 100, 150, and 200 Hz, active in 100-ms bursts, separated by 100 ms without stimulation (Fig. S1, Supplementary Material). Thus, the burst frequency was 5 Hz, and the within-burst frequency varied from approximately 50 to 200 Hz. For each stimulation frequency, the amplitude of the stimulus was slowly increased until a palpable twitch was evoked in the subject's thenar muscles, or until just before the subject experienced discomfort (typically 4.8 ± 1.7 mA for left side stimulation and 4.4 ± 1.2 mA for right). Thereafter, four minutes of stimulation were performed for each frequency and in each stimulated wrist, generating approximately 1200 stimulation bursts per condition.

2.4 Data Treatment

All data analysis was performed in MATLAB (The MathWorks, Inc., Natick, MA, USA). The recorded neural activity was defined as the relative response between two nearby contacts, i.e., local bipolar recordings, and was time-averaged and time-locked to the last stimulus in the burst. To ensure accuracy and avoid time delays in synchronization pulses between different equipment, we identified the stimulus time by looking for the occurrence of stimulus artifacts in the recorded data.

The raw data were upsampled, searched for stimulus artifacts, and split into 200-ms segments (100 ms on-stim, 100 ms off). All segments not flagged as outliers were then aligned to each other through cross-correlation of the last artifact in the stimulation burst, with time "0" defined at this last artifact. The resulting ~ 1000 stimulation bursts per frequency and side were finally averaged, greatly increasing the signal-to-noise ratio (SNR) of the final average response.

2.5 Artifact Removal

After data treatment, decay artifacts were removed. Decay artifact shapes are affected by factors including stimulation and recording contacts, and may also vary between subjects. For non-oscillatory "simple" exponential decay artifacts (Fig. 1A), we concur with [18] that the addition of *two* separate exponential decays is necessary to accurately model the capacitive discharge. Hence, the following simple exponential decay artifact model (SEDAM) was used to fit to and remove these types of decay artifacts:

$$\text{SEDAM} := A_1 e^{\lambda_1 t} + A_2 e^{\lambda_2 t} + C \tag{1}$$

where A_1 and A_2 denote the amplitudes and λ_1 and λ_2 the decay constants of the two exponential components, and C denotes the baseline offset.

However, for oscillating decay artifacts (Fig. 1B), the simple exponential does not suffice to model and remove the artifact. Hence, we here present a novel artifact removal method, which uses the complex exponential $\alpha e^{\beta t}$ [24], where α and β are complex numbers, and the magnitude of α is denoted A:

$$\alpha = |\alpha| e^{i\theta} = A e^{i\theta} \tag{2}$$

$$\beta = \lambda + i\omega_0 \tag{3}$$

Expanding the exponential using Euler's formula,

$$e^{i\varphi} = \cos(\varphi) + i \, \sin(\varphi), \tag{4}$$

and using the definitions from Eqs. (2) and (3), the complex exponential can be separated into real and imaginary components:

(A) Simple exponential decay artifact

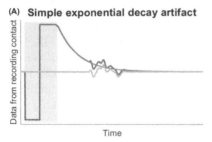

Time

(B) Complex exponential decay artifact

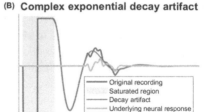

Fig. 1. Examples of simple and complex exponential decay artifacts and how they can corrupt the underlying neural response. Common types of decay artifacts (orange traces) can complicate the detection of the underlying neural response (yellow) from the raw recording (blue). Plot (A) portrays a recording with a simple exponential decay artifact, while (B) shows a complex exponential decay artifact. The grey box highlights the region where the stimulus artifact saturates the recording contact, during which the contact is unable to record neural activity. (Color figure online)

$$\alpha e^{\beta t} = A e^{i\theta} e^{(\lambda+i\omega_0)t} = A e^{\lambda t} e^{i(\omega_0 t+\theta)} = A e^{\lambda t}(\cos(\omega_0 t+\theta) + i\,\sin(\omega_0 t+\theta)) =$$
$$\underbrace{A e^{\lambda t}\cos(\omega_0 t+\theta)}_{\mathrm{Re}(\alpha e^{\beta t})} + i\,\underbrace{A e^{\lambda t}\sin(\omega_0 t+\theta)}_{\mathrm{Im}(\alpha e^{\beta t})} \tag{5}$$

For our purposes, only the real component of the complex exponential, corresponding to a damped oscillator, is relevant for the modeling of the decay artifact. Similar to the simple exponential model, a combination of *two* real complex exponentials was necessary to accurately model all oscillatory decay artifacts in our data, leading to the final definition of the complex exponential decay artifact model (CEDAM):

$$\mathrm{CEDAM} := A_1 e^{\lambda_1 t}\cos(\omega_{01}t+\theta_1) + A_2 e^{\lambda_2 t}\cos(\omega_{02}t+\theta_2) + C \tag{6}$$

where, similar to the simple exponentials, A_1 and A_2 denote the amplitudes of the two complex exponentials, λ_1 and λ_2 the decay constants of the respective exponential components, ω_{01} and ω_{02} the angular frequencies of the respective sinusoidal components, and θ_1 and θ_2 their angular offsets. C denotes the baseline offset.

Note that in order to prevent overfitting to the neural response, rather than fitting to just the decay artifact, the fit should ideally only be based on the segment *before* the first neural response (referred to as an evoked potential, EP). Using this first fit to remove all stimulus artifacts in the burst ensures that the fit is only based on, and hence will only remove, components due to the stimulus artifact.[2]

Hence, the appropriate decay artifact removal model (simple or complex exponential) was fit to the data segment after the first stimulus artifact's saturated region and until the (expected) EP or the next stimulation, whichever came first. This fit was then used

---

[2] This assumes that the decay artifacts of all stimulations in the burst are identical. This is, however, a fair assumption, considering that they are generated by stimulations of the same shape and size, originating from the same contacts, and recorded from the same contacts.

to remove the decay artifacts throughout the whole burst, when suitable.[3] After removal of the decay artifacts, the saturated regions of the stimulus artifacts (from 0.3 ms before to 2.8 ms after the start of the stimulation) were interpolated, and the average segment high-pass filtered with a cutoff of 50 Hz. The saturated regions were thereafter blanked for visualization purposes. R^2 values were calculated between the decay artifact fit and the data segment used for fitting to determine goodness of fit (GoF).

2.6 Evoked Potential Characterization

Due to differences in impedance and target region accuracy[4] between the contacts on each DBS lead, some contact recordings displayed clearer EPs than others. Hence, for each subject, hemisphere, and recording region, if EPs were detected, the contact combination with the clearest response was used in the subsequent analysis.

After visual inspection, an SNR threshold of 0.8 was empirically selected to automate the process of including only clear data samples: only those recordings containing at least one EP above this threshold after detrending were included in the analysis.

2.7 Analysis Methods

The synchronization change throughout each burst was investigated by calculating the cross-correlation between each adjacent EP[5]. The trend of cross-correlation between adjacent EPs throughout each burst frequency was determined and tested for a monotonic trend in a population analysis using the seasonal Kendall test [25].

The analysis above was also repeated after adding white noise to higher-amplitude EPs to make all EP SNRs in each burst equal (or equal to 1, whichever was greatest). This allowed us to test if any of the observed correlation trends were merely attributed to differences in SNR between EPs, and would hence disappear when SNR was equal.

3 Results

The dual exponential fit methods (SEDAM and CEDAM) successfully modeled and removed the decay artifacts of both simple and complex exponential shapes (Fig. 2 and Fig. S2, Supplementary Material), with R^2 measures up to and greater than 0.99, allowing for clear analysis of the underlying within-burst EPs.

---

[3] In the rare cases that the first fit was not a good approximation of the subsequent decay artifacts, individual fits were implemented and removed.

[4] The length of the DBS lead is larger than the target brain region, which may cause some contacts to be outside the target region.

[5] To ensure equivalent comparisons, only data regions containing EPs after stimulations (and of equal overlap, if applicable) were included in the analysis.

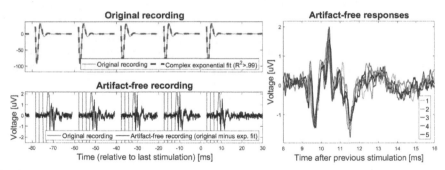

Fig. 2. Removal of complex exponential decay artifacts. The top left plot shows the underdamped oscillatory decay artifact fit (black dashes) under the original data (grey), from a ~ 50-Hz stimulation burst. When the decay artifact is removed, the underlying neural responses can be seen (bottom left, black tracing). The right-most plot shows these EPs overlayed to highlight their strong correlation. *Note: stimulus artifact saturated regions have been blanked.*

For all investigated frequencies and recording regions, significant monotonic increases in cross-correlation throughout the burst were detected, indicating progressively increasing consistency in the shape of the EP (Fig. 3). Even after adding noise to even out the SNRs of the EPs within each burst, significant monotonic increases in consistency were seen for all recorded regions and frequencies, with only one exception[6] (Fig. S3, Supplementary Material).

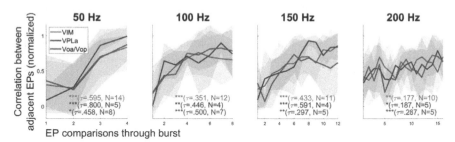

Fig. 3. Correlations between adjacent evoked potentials (EPs) increase with time during the stimulation bursts. Correlation trends from all subjects & hemispheres were normalized before calculating mean (lines) and standard deviation (shadings) for each stimulation frequency group (subplot titles). Statistical monotonic increases in correlation were seen in all recording locations (VIM, green; VPLa, blue; Voa/Vop, red) and over all stimulation frequencies, shown by the positive and significant tau value results from the seasonal Kendall test (listed in subplots). *Symbols: τ, Kendall's tau (measure of monotonic strength); *, $p < 0.05$; **, $p < 0.01$; ***, $p < 0.001$; N, number of samples (subjects and hemispheres) with clear EPs.* (Color figure online)

---

[6] This exception displayed a p-value of .0532, just above the significance threshold (.05).

4   Discussion

Our results show the reliability and accuracy of the presented decay artifact removal method, which allows us to detect EPs during high-frequency stimulation. In addition to the very high GoF measures, the similarities of the EPs to previous studies (e.g. [13–16]) along with the electrical basis of the artifact model, differing from typical EP shapes and models, provide even stronger proof of success. We also highlight the importance of fitting to the decay artifact portion *before* the first EP whenever possible, which ensures that the fit is only based on, and hence will only remove, artifactual recordings (Fig. S2B, Supplementary Material). Many studies display difficulties in removing decay artifacts [7, 13–16, 26], generating unusable data portions that our novel method could greatly reduce.

Using this new method for stimulus artifact removal, we have shown that there is a consistent pattern of evoked responses, with increasing consistency in subsequent responses within a burst. This phenomenon has not previously been reported for centrally recorded EPs, and it suggests that the evoked response to short bursts of stimulation may be substantially different from the steady-state response to prolonged stimulation. While our data do not provide a mechanism for this effect, the results are strongly reminiscent of what would be expected by progressive synchronization of a population of independent neural responses [13]. In other words, subsequent pulses may progressively recruit and align the phases of otherwise independent neural oscillators, and the increasing phase-locking with each stimulus would lead to increased consistency of the total evoked response.

Thus, the increasing correlation of the EPs throughout the burst may be a sign of the peripheral stimulations inducing progressive synchronization in thalamic nuclei. This phenomenon would be expected to cause a "synchronization blockade" in which the induced regular firing of neural populations at high frequency would prevent propagation of the intrinsic pathological signals normally present in that population. Hence, while synchronized neural activity has been detected in movement disorders [27, 28], it is possible that artificial synchronization helps by "fighting fire with fire". For example, in the context of ET, artificially enhanced synchronization could prevent the tremor frequency from propagating and could be responsible for the observed benefit of peripheral stimulation in recent studies [2, 3].

No matter what the mechanism, synchronization of neural firing due to peripheral stimulation could at least partially mimic synchronization of neural firing due to local DBS. This suggests potential efficacy of peripheral stimulation as a noninvasive treatment for movement disorders such as ET, Parkinson's disease, and dystonia, which would function at least in part by activation of the same treatment mechanisms activated by invasive DBS.

5   Conclusion

Our novel decay artifact removal method has allowed us to demonstrate a previously unreported phenomenon: the progressive increase in consistency of thalamic evoked potentials in response to peripheral stimulation. While understanding this phenomenon may be important for elucidating network dynamics within the thalamus, it also provides a potentially noninvasive alternative to DBS for disorders that respond to electrical stimulation in the thalamus.

Acknowledgements. We thank our volunteers and their parents for participating in this study. We also thank Diana Ferman and Jennifer MacLean for their assistance with neurologic examinations, as well as Ruta Deshpande and Enrique Argüelles for helping gather much of the data.

Conflicts of Interest. Dr. Terence Sanger serves as a paid consultant and owns stock in Cala Health Inc., a company that develops and manufactures noninvasive electrical stimulation devices for treatment of movement disorders.

References

1. Klostermann, F., Funk, T., Vesper, J., Curio, G.: Spatiotemporal characteristics of human intrathalamic high-frequency (> 400 Hz) SEP components. NeuroReport **10**(17), 3627–3631 (1999)
2. Pahwa, R., et al.: An acute randomized controlled trial of noninvasive peripheral nerve stimulation in essential tremor. Neuromodulation Technol. Neural Interface **22**(5), 537–545 (2019)
3. Chalah, M.A., Lefaucheur, J.-P., Ayache, S.S.: Non-invasive central and peripheral stimulation: new hope for essential tremor? Front. Neurosci. **9**, 440 (2015)
4. Sandoval, E.: Cala health receives FDA breakthrough device designation for cala trio^{TM} therapy to treat action tremors in parkinson's disease. Business Wire (2020)
5. Bending, J., Cleeves, L.: Effect of electrical nerve stimulation on dystonic tremor. Lancet **336**(8727), 1385–1386 (1990)
6. Tinazzi, M., et al.: Effects of transcutaneous electrical nerve stimulation on motor cortex excitability in writer's cramp: neurophysiological and clinical correlations. Mov. Disord. Off. J. Mov. Disord. Soc. **21**(11), 1908–1913 (2006)
7. Hernandez-Martin, E., Arguelles, E., Deshpande, R., Sanger, T.D.: Evoked potentials during peripheral stimulation confirm electrode location in thalamic subnuclei in children with secondary dystonia. J. Child Neurol. **35**(12), 0883073820931970 (2020)
8. Klostermann, F., Gobbele, R., Buchner, H., Curio, G.: Dissociation of human thalamic and cortical SEP gating as revealed by intrathalamic recordings under muscle relaxation. Brain Res. **958**(1), 146–151 (2002)
9. Shima, F., Morioka, T., Tobimatsu, S., Kavaklis, O., Kato, M., Fukui, M.: Localization of stereotactic targets by microrecording of thalamic somatosensory evoked potentials. Neurosurgery **28**(2), 223–230 (1991)
10. Klostermann, F., Vesper, J., Curio, G.: Identification of target areas for deep brain stimulation in human basal ganglia substructures based on median nerve sensory evoked potential criteria. J. Neurol. Neurosurg. Psychiatry **74**(8), 1031–1035 (2003)
11. McLean, L., Scott, R.N., Parker, P.A.: Stimulus artifact reduction in evoked potential measurements. Arch. Phys. Med. Rehabil. **77**(December), 1286–1292 (1996)
12. Hua, Y., Lovely, D.F., Doraiswami, R.: Factors affecting the stimulus artifact tail in surface-recorded somatosensory-evoked potentials. Med. Biol. Eng. Comput. **44**(3), 226–241 (2006)
13. Hanajima, R., et al.: Very fast oscillations evoked by median nerve stimulation in the human thalamus and subthalamic nucleus. J. Neurophysiol. **92**(6), 3171–3182 (2004)

14. Morioka, T., Shima, F., Kato, M., Fukui, M.: Origin and distribution of thalamic somatosensory evoked potentials in humans. Electroencephalogr. Clin. Neurophysiol. **74**(3), 186–193 (1989)
15. Hanajima, R., Dostrovsky, J.O., Lozano, A.M., Chen, R.: Dissociation of thalamic high frequency oscillations and slow component of sensory evoked potentials following damage to ascending pathways. Clin. Neurophysiol. **117**(4), 906–911 (2006)
16. Kim, N., et al.: Activation of the thalamic parafascicular nucleus by electrical stimulation of the peripheral vestibular nerve in rats. Exp. Brain Res. **235**(5), 1617–1625 (2017)
17. Sinclair, N.C., et al.: Deep brain stimulation for Parkinson's disease modulates high-frequency evoked and spontaneous neural activity. Neurobiol. Dis. **130**, 384–388 (2019)
18. Casula, E.P., et al.: TMS-evoked long-lasting artifacts: a new adaptive algorithm for EEG signal correction. Clin. Neurophysiol. **128**(9), 1563–1574 (2017)
19. Wichmann, T., Dostrovsky, J.O.: Pathological basal ganglia activity in movement disorders. Neuroscience **198**, 232–244 (2011)
20. Sanger, T.D., Tarsy, D., Pascual-Leone, A.: Abnormalities of spatial and temporal sensory discrimination in writer's cramp. Mov. Disord. **16**(1), 94–99 (2001)
21. Sanger, T.D., Kukke, S.N.: Abnormalities of tactile sensory function in children with dystonic and diplegic cerebral palsy. J. Child Neurol. **22**(3), 289–293 (2007)
22. Sanger, T.D., Merzenich, M.M.: Computational model of the role of sensory disorganization in focal task-specific dystonia. J. Neurophysiol. **84**(5), 2458–2464 (2000)
23. Cif, L., Coubes, P.: Historical developments in children's deep brain stimulation. Eur. J. Paediatr. Neurol. **21**(1), 109–117 (2017)
24. Arslan, G.: Exponential and sinusoidal signals (2009). http://www2.hawaii.edu/~gurdal/EE315/class2.pdf
25. Hirsch, R.M., Slack, J.R.: A nonparametric trend test for seasonal data with serial dependence. Water Resour. **20**(6), 727–732 (1984)
26. Sinclair, N.C., et al.: Subthalamic nucleus deep brain stimulation evokes resonant neural activity. Ann. Neurol. **83**(5), 1027–1031 (2018)
27. Chu Chen, C., Kühn, A.A., Trottenberg, T., Kupsch, A., Schneider, G.H., Brown, P.: Neuronal activity in globus pallidus interna can be synchronized to local field potential activity over 3–12 Hz in patients with dystonia. Exp. Neurol. **202**(2), 480–486 (2006)
28. Rubchinsky, L.L., Park, C., Worth, R.M.: Intermittent neural synchronization in Parkinson's disease. Nonlinear Dyn. **68**(3), 329–346 (2012)

Weakly Supervised Pan-Cancer Segmentation Tool

Marvin Lerousseau[1,2(✉)], Marion Classe[2,3], Enzo Battistella[1,2],
Théo Estienne[1,2], Théophraste Henry[2], Amaury Leroy[2,4], Roger Sun[2],
Maria Vakalopoulou[1,2], Jean-Yves Scoazec[3], Eric Deutsch[2],
and Nikos Paragios[4]

[1] Paris-Saclay University, CentraleSupélec, 91190 Gif-sur-Yvette, France
[2] Paris-Saclay University, Gustave Roussy, Inserm, Molecular Radiotherapy
and Novel Therapeutics, 94800 Villejuif, France
[3] Gustave Roussy, Department of Laboratory Medicine and Pathology,
94800 Villejuif, France
[4] TheraPanacea, 75014 Paris, France

Abstract. The vast majority of semantic segmentation approaches rely on pixel-level annotations that are tedious and time consuming to obtain and suffer from significant inter and intra-expert variability. To address these issues, recent approaches have leveraged categorical annotations at the slide-level, that in general suffer from robustness and generalization. In this paper, we propose a novel weakly supervised multi-instance learning approach that deciphers quantitative slide-level annotations which are fast to obtain and regularly present in clinical routine. The extreme potentials of the proposed approach are demonstrated for tumor segmentation of solid cancer subtypes. The proposed approach achieves superior performance in out-of-distribution, out-of-location, and out-of-domain testing sets.

Keywords: Whole slide image tumor segmentation · Weak supervision

1 Introduction

Semantic segmentation relies on supervised learning where images are paired with manually curated maps [7]. This has also been the case for medical imaging [18], and computational pathology [16]. In digital pathology, despite efforts to annotate and provide ground-truth segmentations for some cancer types, the lack of fine-grained annotations hinders the development of automatic segmentation tools for solid cancers. Unfortunately, pathologists-curated datasets are fairly small, given that the biggest open-source dataset with pixelwise annotations contains 400 whole slide images [17]. Consequently, the generalization performance of the learnt models is limited and they fail to grasp the underlying clinical heterogeneity regarding tissue preparation, slide digitization, and

Electronic supplementary material The online version of this chapter (https://doi.org/10.1007/978-3-030-87237-3_24) contains supplementary material, which is available to authorized users.

© Springer Nature Switzerland AG 2021
M. de Bruijne et al. (Eds.): MICCAI 2021, LNCS 12908, pp. 248–256, 2021.
https://doi.org/10.1007/978-3-030-87237-3_24

tissue structures [1]. The lack of pixelwise annotations could be explained by the tedious and cumbersome facet of the task, aggravated by the lack of availability of pathologists [20].

Despite this expertise shortage, we observe an increasing availability of whole slide images [25,28]. In recent years, more and more efforts are devoted towards publicly available data. The Cancer Genome Atlas (TCGA) [26] which counts 30072 whole slide images from 32 cancer subtypes is the most prominent example. Whole slide images lack in general annotations but are routinely associated with weak clinical variables such as labels at the slide-level. Slide labels are abundant weak annotations for WSIs.

There exists a rich literature on segmentation models trained from using categorical labels at the slide-level [1–3,9,11,14,21,24]. Most of them rely on multiple instance learning (MIL) [5,6] where an embedder maps instances in an embedding space, which are further processed by a pooling operator.

In this work, we exploit eyeball estimates of percentages of tumor in whole slide images for training tumor segmentation models. Such quantities are routinely obtained during tumor purity estimation, a process ensuring that a tissue sample has enough neoplastic material for further genetic tests. We harness such labels through a highly modular algorithm derived from MIL to train segmentation models (Sect. 2). Large-scale experiments involving almost all types of solid primary tumors are performed on entirely public data, including the percentages estimates (Sect. 3).

2 Methods

Let us consider a set of training whole slide images (x_k). Specifically, each whole slide image x_k is denoted by its constituents $(x_{k,i})$, such as pixels or tiles. Our goal is to learn a θ-parametrized model f_θ that maps any x_k to its (unknown) tumor segmentation map $\hat{y}_k$, apparent to a coarse map $(\hat{y}_{k,i})_i$. Each training sample x_k has a label $p_k \in [0, 100]\%$ representing the percentage of tumor within x_k. We denote by $\max_{p_k}\{f_\theta(x_k)\}$ the $p_k\%$ maximal values of the predicted coarse map $\{f_\theta(x_{k,i}); x_{k,i} \in x_k\}$ and by $\min_{100-p_k}\{f_\theta(x_k)\}$ the $100 - p_k\%$ minimal values.

We now present WESEG (**W**eakly sup**E**rvised **Seg**mentation), an algorithm whose goal is to train f_θ by ensuring that the percentage of predicted tumor is equal to the percentage annotation. To do so, we adopt a recursive training mechanism for each sample x_k. Specifically, WESEG builds a proxy ground-truth map that contains $p_k\%$ of tumor pixels by assigning a value of 1 to the $p_k\%$ of pixels with maximum predicted probabilities $(f_\theta(x_{k,i}))_i$, otherwise 0.

Equivalently, given an elementwise loss function L such as binary cross-entropy, WESEG aims at minimizing the following empirical risk for a sample x_k with percentage annotation p_k:

$$e = \sum_{i \in \max_{p_k}\{f_\theta(x_k)\}} L\left(f_\theta(x_{k,i}), 1\right) + \sum_{i \in \min_{100-p_k}\{f_\theta(x_k)\}} L\left(f_\theta(x_{k,i}), 0\right)$$

By construction, this methodology ensures that an error signal of 0 for a sample (x_k, p_k) implies that $p_k\%$ of output probabilities are of value 1, and $100 - p_k\%$ of value 0, which is precisely the meaning of the percentage annotation. After training, the learned segmentation model can be inferred on new WSIs without any percentage annotation. Besides, while our notation uses percentage annotations, this approach can be used with count-based weak annotations.

As illustrated by the public annotations used in our experiments, the percentage annotations can be noisy. This is notably a consequence of the difficulty of estimating a surface to the human eye. To take this uncertainty into account, we introduce four parameters r_{low}, r_{high}, a_{low} and a_{high} such that for a sample with percentage annotation p_k:

- probabilities below the $((1 - r_{low}) * p_k - a_{low})$th percentile are assigned 0
- probabilities above the $((1 + r_{high}) * p_k + a_{high})$th percentile are assigned 1
- remaining probabilities are discarded from the error signal computation

With $r_{low} = r_{high} = a_{low} = a_{high} = 0$ this formulation is equivalent to the original version above. Generally speaking, the r (resp. a) parameters control a relative (resp. absolute) margin around the annotation. In practice, these values are selected either empirically or by finding bias in annotations.

Our approach refers to a modular, scalable and network architecture-free framework. Its main strength lies in the ability to progressively construct ground truth from very weakly annotated data, and recursively update the associated network architecture towards better and better performance. The underlying principle employs the concept Highest Confidence First where progressively throughout this recursive process, data samples are labeled with accurate labels and fed back to the network for end-to-end retraining. For demonstration purposes we have adopted a conventional ResNet [8] architecture, that by no means restricts the nature of architectures that can be accommodated such as Unet [23], GAN, etc. from the proposed versatile paradigm.

3   Experiments

Large-scale experiments are conducted for pan-cancer tumor segmentation in WSIs. Several weakly supervised learning frameworks are benchmarked (Sect. 3.1) by optimizing the same architecture with common-hyperparameters (Sect. 3.3) on a shared training set (Sect. 3.2). Results are reported (Sect. 3.4) for multiple testing sets (Sect. 3.2).

3.1   Benchmarked Approaches

- **AttentionMIL** [10] classifies WSIs with an attention module. As suggested by the authors, for a given set of tiles with computed attention weights (a_k), the scores are obtained by min-max scaling the weights. Additionally, if a WSI is predicted as normal, all tile predictions are set to 0. The attention module was a two layer feedforward neural network with 128 hidden neurons.

- **AlphaBetaMIL** [14] learns an instance-level MIL model with two parameters α and β which are fixed and common for all training samples. For WSIs with label 0, their approach assigns all pixels to 0. Otherwise, $\alpha\%$ of pixels with highest probability are assigned 1, while the $\beta\%$ lowest are assigned 0. 10 configurations were uniformly sampled for parameters α and β.
- A **supervised** approach is emulated by considering all slides with annotation of either 0% or 100% and discarding others. With a 0% annotation, the ground-truth map can be inferred as filled with benign tissue. On the contrary, with an annotation of 100%, the ground-truth can be inferred as filled with 1. This approach is therefore apparent to a supervised learning one with pixelwise ground truth segmentation maps.
- The **proposed** approach is trained with all percentages annotations. The values of r_{low}, r_{high}, a_{low} and a_{high} were set to 0.

3.2   Datasets

Training Data. The training set was built using the snap-frozen whole slide images TCGA data referring to the 32 most common solid cancer subtypes with 3 of them being excluded from training and used as testing set, leading to a training set of 18306 WSIs from 10903 patients. The distribution of the number of whole slide images and patients per subtype can be found at the supplementary Table 1. The 10903 patients were further split into 70%, 10%, and 20% cases for training, validation, and test sets respectively.

Two types of annotations were retrieved. Firstly, binary labels indicating whether each WSI is of normal type (0), *i.e.* with no apparent neoplastic tissue, otherwise 1. 2248 out of the 12783 WSIs are found normal. Secondly, we retrieved publicly available annotations of percentages of tumor for all but 235 out of the 18306 WSIs. These annotations were available in the TCGA repository and identified by *"percent_tumor_cells"*.

Testing Performance. In order to derive a meaningful assessment of the generalization capabilities of the benchmarked models, several testing sets were constituted. First, 175 WSIs were sampled from the hold-out testing set of the training cohort, *i.e.* 5 WSIs from each of the 29 training subtypes. 2 pathologists curated ground-truth tumor maps with exhaustive annotations. This set is identified as the out-of-distribution testing set.

Similarly, 24 pixelwise WSI annotations were curated on the 3 cancer subtypes excluded from the training cohort, *i.e.* cervix squamous cell, rectum adenocarcinoma, and glioblastoma multiforme. Both rectum and cervix locations are unseen in the training set. Besides, the training set contains only low grade glioblastoma for the brain location. Consequently, these 3 testing cohorts provide insight about the out-of-location performance.

Finally, out-of-domain performance was assessed on formalin-fixed paraffin-embedded (FFPE) slides from 2 open-source datasets with public pixelwise ground-truth: DigestPath for colon adenocarcinoma [15], and PAIP2019 for liver hepatocellular carcinoma [12]. FFPE tissue displays dissimilarity with frozen tissue, therefore providing insight about out-of-domain generalization.

WSI Pre-processing. All WSI were tiled at a magnification of 10x into 512 pixel-wide tiles with 128 overlapping pixels on each side using [19]. Tiles detected as background were completely discarded from the study (including performance measures), *i.e.* those where at least 90% of pixels have both red, green, and blue channels above 200.

3.3   Optimization Details

All approaches are used to train a ResNet50 [8] architecture pretrained on Imagenet [4]. At each training step, 30 tiles were randomly sampled for each of 8 whole slide images, for a total batch size of 240. Each tile was data-augmented with random vertical and horizontal flips, color jitter with brightness 0.1, contrast 0.1, saturation 0.1, and hue 0.01, standard scaled with mean and variance computed from the training set, and random cropped into 224 pixel-wide tiles. In order to produce segmentation of higher granularity, the penultimate layer of ResNet50 was discarded, *i.e.* global adaptive pooling. For a 224 pixel-width input, the output features maps are thus of size 7×7. A final linear classification layer was applied elementwise, producing outputs of size 7×7 instead of 1. Early stopping was triggered when no validation loss improvement was found for 50 epochs. Error signals were computed with binary cross-entropy and weights were updated with the Adam optimizer [13]. An independent random search was performed for all learning algorithms for learning rate selection within a range of $[1e^{-6}, 1e^{-3}]$ in a log-uniform fashion. Final learning rates were selected with the best achieved validation losses. Each random search was given a budget of 5 days on 2 V100. The total training time of our experiments is 117 V100·days. All experiments was performed with pytorch [22] v1.7.1.

Table 1. Performance of all benchmarked approaches on all datasets in area under the ROC curve. All results are computed on tissue pixels, *i.e.* by completely discarding background pixels. **Bold** results highlight the best method for each testing cohort.

Method	Out-of-distribution	Out-of-location	Out-of-domain	
			DigestPath [15]	PAIP [12]
AlphaBetaMIL [14]				
($\alpha = 50, \beta = 0$)	0.880	0.917	0.728	0.667
($\alpha = 50, \beta = 50$)	0.847	0.876	0.562	0.612
($\alpha = 75, \beta = 0$)	0.881	0.884	0.717	0.654
Average	0.845	0.885	0.685	0.642
AttentionMIL [10]	0.892	0.864	0.540	0.545
Supervised	0.905	0.886	0.534	0.620
Proposed	**0.932**	**0.946**	**0.779**	**0.671**

3.4   Results

Testing results are reported in Table 1. Each model was inferred on all testing samples from both out-of-distribution, out-of-location, and out-of-domain testing sets. Then, each predicted whole slide image map was compared with the

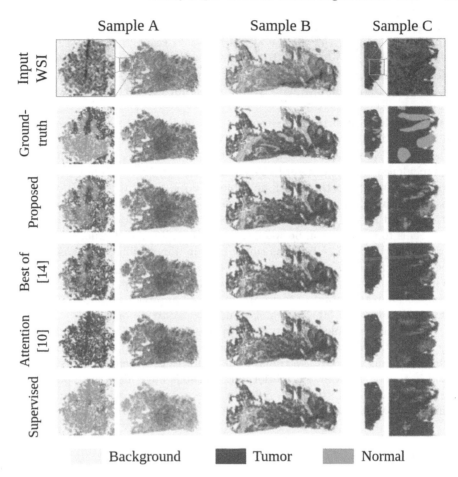

Fig. 1. Example of out-of-distribution segmentation maps for three testing whole slide images (Sample A, Sample B and Sample C). The lines display, in that order, input WSIs, the pathologists curated ground-truth annotations, results from the proposed approach, results from the best performing configuration of [14], results from the attention-based MIL [10], and results from the supervised approach.

pathologists' curated ground-truth annotations, and AUC was computed on non-background pixels. For [14], the 3 best performing configurations are displayed, with the "Average" representing the mean of all configurations; all results are displayed in supplementary Table 2.

The proposed approach achieved the best performance on all testing sets except for PAIP [12] where it ranked second. Indeed, the error was reduced by more than 37% compared to the best performing method that used binary annotations. The proposed approach also appeared to better leverage percentage annotations with an error reduction higher than 28% compared to the supervised approach that uses percentages. Furthermore, the proposed approach obtained better generalization performances than the counterparts. Indeed, the proposed approach is the top performer for all testing sets except for PAIP [12] where it ranked second. Notably, while AttentionMIL and the supervised approach loses performance in the out-of-location testing sets, the proposed approach achieved better than on holdout testing sets from tissue locations that were included in the training set.

We were interested in understanding the quality of the public percentages annotations that were used by the proposed approach. Statistical exploration revealed 44.9% of non-0% annotations were multiple of 20%, whereas the ground-truth incidence should be closer to 5%, indicating that human annotators tending to round estimates to the closer multiple of 20%. Similarly, 89.1% of annotations were found to be multiple of 5% where incidence should be close to 20%. Moreover, pathologist inspection of the percentages annotations indicates that there seems to be confusion between tumor cells and tumor tissue. For instance, stromal tissue is often counted as tumor cells in annotations, whereas it can be considered as tumor tissue as a byproduct of tumor. An histogram of percentages annotations is displayed in supplementary Fig. 1 along with other distribution measures. From this point of view, the proposed approach achieved remarkable performance although labels are noisy and bear systemic bias.

Some testing samples outputs are displayed in Fig. 1. Upon visual pathologists' qualitative inspection of the produced testing maps, most errors seemed to come from discriminating stromal from tumor cells, which are generally interlocked in tissues. Besides, less performing methods have more false positives on inflammatory cells which might reflect a bias in most locations, which is that immune cells are recruited in neoplastic tissues and are absent in normal tissues.

4   Conclusion

In this work, we leveraged weak annotations for training a tumor segmentation model for virtually all solid cancer subtypes. Experiments illustrate that the proposed approach performs better than traditional weakly supervised approaches, highlighting that the percentages annotations translate into performance gain. Besides, the proposed approach seems robust with respect to bias and noise in percentages annotations and leads to tumor segmentation models of higher quality for performance and generalization.

Numerous extensions could be considered to further improve the performance of our versatile framework. First, performance could be enhanced by refining the input percentages annotations of the proposed approach and retraining with the same approach, in a transductive learning [27] fashion. In another perspective, although this work leveraged human annotations of percentages, the proposed approach could be used with input percentages computed by a model trained only with WSI binary annotations. The proposed approach would act as an annotation-free refining strategy for segmentation in WSI. Finally, even though our work involves whole slide images, our generic approach could be used off-the-shelf for other modalities.

References

1. Campanella, G., et al.: Clinical-grade computational pathology using weakly supervised deep learning on whole slide images. Nat. Med. **25**(8), 1301–1309 (2019)
2. Campanella, G., Silva, V.W.K., Fuchs, T.J.: Terabyte-scale deep multiple instance learning for classification and localization in pathology. arXiv preprint arXiv:1805.06983 (2018)
3. Coudray, N., et al.: Classification and mutation prediction from non-small cell lung cancer histopathology images using deep learning. Nat. Med. **24**(10), 1559–1567 (2018)
4. Deng, J., Dong, W., Socher, R., Li, L.J., Li, K., Fei-Fei, L.: Imagenet: a large-scale hierarchical image database. In: 2009 IEEE Conference on Computer Vision and Pattern Recognition, pp. 248–255. IEEE (2009)
5. Dietterich, T.G., Lathrop, R.H., Lozano-Pérez, T.: Solving the multiple instance problem with axis-parallel rectangles. Artif. Intell. **89**(1–2), 31–71 (1997)
6. Foulds, J.R., Frank, E.: A review of multi-instance learning assumptions (2010)
7. Garcia-Garcia, A., Orts-Escolano, S., Oprea, S., Villena-Martinez, V., Garcia-Rodriguez, J.: A review on deep learning techniques applied to semantic segmentation. arXiv preprint arXiv:1704.06857 (2017)
8. He, K., Zhang, X., Ren, S., Sun, J.: Deep residual learning for image recognition. In: Proceedings of the IEEE Conference on Computer Vision and Pattern Recognition, pp. 770–778 (2016)
9. Hou, L., Samaras, D., Kurc, T.M., Gao, Y., Davis, J.E., Saltz, J.H.: Patch-based convolutional neural network for whole slide tissue image classification. In: Proceedings of the IEEE Conference on Computer Vision and Pattern Recognition, pp. 2424–2433 (2016)
10. Ilse, M., Tomczak, J.M., Welling, M.: Attention-based deep multiple instance learning. arXiv preprint arXiv:1802.04712 (2018)
11. Kim, R.H., et al.: A deep learning approach for rapid mutational screening in melanoma. bioRxiv, p. 610311 (2019)
12. Kim, Y.J., et al.: PAIP 2019: liver cancer segmentation challenge. Med. Image Anal. **67**, 101854 (2020)
13. Kingma, D.P., Ba, J.: Adam: a method for stochastic optimization. arXiv preprint arXiv:1412.6980 (2014)
14. Lerousseau, M., et al.: Weakly supervised multiple instance learning histopathological tumor segmentation. In: Martel, A.L., et al. (eds.) MICCAI 2020. LNCS, vol. 12265, pp. 470–479. Springer, Cham (2020). https://doi.org/10.1007/978-3-030-59722-1_45
15. Li, J., et al.: Signet ring cell detection with a semi-supervised learning framework. In: Chung, A.C.S., Gee, J.C., Yushkevich, P.A., Bao, S. (eds.) IPMI 2019. LNCS, vol. 11492, pp. 842–854. Springer, Cham (2019). https://doi.org/10.1007/978-3-030-20351-1_66
16. Li, Z., et al.: Deep learning methods for lung cancer segmentation in whole-slide histopathology images-the acdc@ lunghp challenge 2019. arXiv preprint arXiv:2008.09352 (2020)
17. Litjens, G., et al.: 1399 H&E-stained sentinel lymph node sections of breast cancer patients: the camelyon dataset. GigaScience **7**(6), giy065 (2018)
18. Litjens, G., et al.: A survey on deep learning in medical image analysis. Med. Image Anal. **42**, 60–88 (2017)

19. Martinez, K., Cupitt, J.: Libvips: a fast image processing library with low memory needs (2007)
20. Metter, D.M., Colgan, T.J., Leung, S.T., Timmons, C.F., Park, J.Y.: Trends in the us and Canadian pathologist workforces from 2007 to 2017. JAMA Netw. Open **2**(5), e194337–e194337 (2019)
21. Oquab, M., Bottou, L., Laptev, I., Sivic, J.: Is object localization for free?-weakly-supervised learning with convolutional neural networks. In: Proceedings of the IEEE Conference on Computer Vision and Pattern Recognition, pp. 685–694 (2015)
22. Paszke, A., et al.: Automatic differentiation in pytorch (2017)
23. Ronneberger, O., Fischer, P., Brox, T.: U-Net: convolutional networks for biomedical image segmentation. In: Navab, N., Hornegger, J., Wells, W.M., Frangi, A.F. (eds.) MICCAI 2015. LNCS, vol. 9351, pp. 234–241. Springer, Cham (2015). https://doi.org/10.1007/978-3-319-24574-4_28
24. Schmauch, B., et al.: A deep learning model to predict RNA-seq expression of tumours from whole slide images. Nat. Commun. **11**(1), 1–15 (2020)
25. Stathonikos, N., Veta, M., Huisman, A., van Diest, P.J.: Going fully digital: perspective of a Dutch academic pathology lab. J. Pathol. Inf. **4**, 15 (2013)
26. Tomczak, K., Czerwińska, P., Wiznerowicz, M.: The cancer genome atlas (TCGA): an immeasurable source of knowledge. Contemp. Oncol. **19**(1A), A68 (2015)
27. Vapnik, V.N.: An overview of statistical learning theory. IEEE Trans. Neural Netw. **10**(5), 988–999 (1999)
28. Zarella, M.D., et al.: A practical guide to whole slide imaging: a white paper from the digital pathology association. Arch. Pathol. Lab. Med. **143**(2), 222–234 (2019)

Structure-Preserving Multi-domain Stain Color Augmentation Using Style-Transfer with Disentangled Representations

Sophia J. Wagner[1,2,4], Nadieh Khalili[5], Raghav Sharma[3], Melanie Boxberg[1,4], Carsten Marr[3], Walter de Back[5], and Tingying Peng[1,2,4(✉)]

[1] Technical University Munich, Munich, Germany
Tingying.peng@helmholtz-muenchen.de
[2] Helmholtz AI, Oberschleißheim, Germany
[3] Institute for Computational Biology, HelmholtzZentrum Munich, Germany
[4] Munich School of Data Science (MuDS), Munich, Germany
[5] ContextVision AB, Stockholm, Sweden

Abstract. In digital pathology, different staining procedures and scanners cause substantial color variations in whole-slide images (WSIs), especially across different laboratories. These color shifts result in a poor generalization of deep learning-based methods from the training domain to external pathology data. To increase test performance, stain normalization techniques are used to reduce the variance between training and test domain. Alternatively, color augmentation can be applied during training leading to a more robust model without the extra step of color normalization at test time. We propose a novel color augmentation technique, HistAuGAN, that can simulate a wide variety of realistic histology stain colors, thus making neural networks stain-invariant when applied during training. Based on a generative adversarial network (GAN) for image-to-image translation, our model disentangles the content of the image, i.e., the morphological tissue structure, from the stain color attributes. It can be trained on multiple domains and, therefore, learns to cover different stain colors as well as other domain-specific variations introduced in the slide preparation and imaging process. We demonstrate that HistAuGAN outperforms conventional color augmentation techniques on a classification task on the publicly available dataset Camelyon17 and show that it is able to mitigate present batch effects (Code and model weights are available at https://github.com/sophiajw/HistAuGAN.).

Keywords: Color augmentation · Style-transfer · Disentangled representations

1 Introduction

Modern cancer diagnosis relies on the expert analysis of tumor specimen and biopsies. To highlight its structure and morphological properties, conventionally,

© Springer Nature Switzerland AG 2021
M. de Bruijne et al. (Eds.): MICCAI 2021, LNCS 12908, pp. 257–266, 2021.
https://doi.org/10.1007/978-3-030-87237-3_25

the tissue is stained with hematoxylin and eosin (H&E) [5]. The path from the raw tissue to the final digitized image slide however consists of many different processing steps that can introduce variances, such as tissue fixation duration, the age and the composition of the H&E-staining, or scanner settings. Therefore, histological images show a large variety of colors, not only differing between laboratories, but also within one laboratory [3].

This variability can lead to poor generalization of algorithms that are trained on WSIs from a single source. One strategy to account for this is stain color normalization. Traditionally, this is either done by aligning the color distribution of the test images to a reference tile in the training domain [12] or by decomposing the color space of a reference tile into hematoxylin and eosin components [10,17]. Then, H&E components of the test tiles can be aligned while keeping the structure intact.

Recently, the focus shifted toward the application of style-transfer methods such as cycle-consistent generative adversarial networks, cycleGAN [19], for stain normalization [16]. However, these models aim to match the target distribution possibly leading to undesired changes in the morphological structure [6]. To circumvent this, other approaches propose color space transformations [14], structural similarity loss functions [9], or residual learning [4].

We propose a novel histological color transfer model, HistAuGAN, based on a GAN architecture for image-to-image translation. In contrast to previous approaches, HistAuGAN disentangles the content of a histological image, i.e., the morphological tissue structure, from the stain color attributes, hence preserving the structure while altering the color. Therefore, HistAuGAN can be used as a stain augmentation technique during training of a task-specific convolutional neural network (CNN). We demonstrate that this helps to render the trained network color-invariant and makes it transferable to external datasets without an extra normalization step at test time. Applied as an augmentation technique, HistAuGAN significantly outperforms other color augmentation techniques on a binary tumor-classification task. Furthermore, clustering results suggest that HistAuGAN can capture sources of domain shifts beyond color variations, such as noise and artefacts introduced in the staining or digitization process, e.g., image compression or blurring.

To the best of our knowledge, HistAuGAN is the first GAN-based color augmentation technique that generates realistic histological color variations.

2 Method

2.1 Model Architecture

We build our model based on a multi-domain GAN using disentangled representations, inspired by DRIT++ [8]. Originally designed for image-to-image translation on natural images using a predefined style, we propose its application on histological images to disentangle the morphological tissue structure from the visual appearance. In contrast to previous cycleGAN-based color normalization methods that use only a single encoder, HistAuGAN is able to separate two essential image properties from each other as visualized in Fig. 1b: the

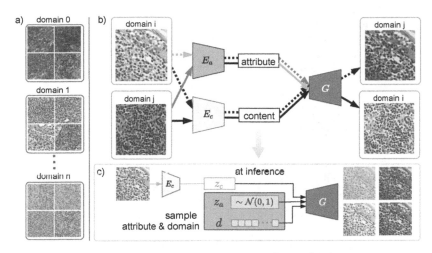

Fig. 1. We propose HistAuGAN for structure-preserving multi-domain stain color augmentation. (a) Histological slides from different laboratories (domains) exhibit color variations. (b) Model architecture. Here, the domain information flow is visualized by colored arrows. (c) At inference, HistAuGAN can be used as an augmentation technique by sampling attribute z_a and domain d. (Color figure online)

domain-invariant content encoder E_c encodes the histopathological structure of the tissue, e.g., size and position of the nuclei, whereas the domain-specific attribute encoder E_a learns the domain-specific color appearance. The model can be trained on data from multiple domains and thereby captures both inter-laboratory variability between multiple domains and intra-laboratory variability within each domain at the same time. Finally, the generator G takes as input a content vector z_c, an attribute vector z_a, and the one-hot-encoded domain vector d and outputs a simulated histological image. The objective function is given by

$$L_{total} = w_{cc}L^{cc} + w_cL^c + w_dL^d + w_{recon}L^{recon} + w_{latent}L^{latent} + w_{KL}L^{KL}, \quad (1)$$

where L^{cc} is the cycle-consistency loss, L^c and L^d are adversarial losses for the content and the attribute encoder, L^{recon} is an L_1-loss for image reconstruction, L^{latent} is an L_1-loss for latent space reconstruction, and L^{KL} enforces the latent attribute space to be distributed according to the standard normal distribution. Please refer to [8] for a detailed explanation of each loss and the precise hyperparameter setting.

At inference, using the fixed content encoding of the input image z_c, we can sample the attribute vector z_a and the one-hot encoded domain vector d as visualized in Fig. 1c. Hence, we can map one image to many different structure-preserving augmentations. More specifically, we sample a random color attribute z_a from a normal distribution that parametrizes the stain color variabilities in one domain. Figure 2b shows randomly sampled outcomes of intra-domain augmentations. Additionally, we can change the one-hot-encoded domain vector d to

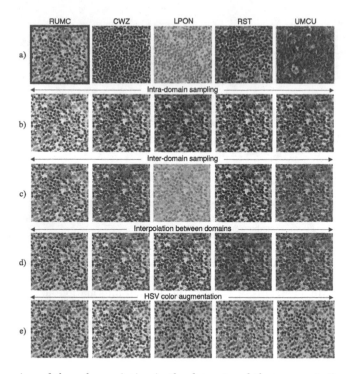

Fig. 2. Overview of the color variation in the dataset and the augmentation techniques used in this paper using the framed image as example tile. (Color figure online)

project the input image into multiple target domains as visualized in Fig. 2c. In addition to sampling from the training domains, we can also interpolate between these domains to obtain an even broader variety of realistic color appearances for histopathological images. Figure 2d demonstrates this by linearly interpolating the domain from domain RUMC to domain UMCU according to

$$d = (1 - t) \cdot d_{\text{RUMC}} + t \cdot d_{\text{UMCU}}, \quad \text{for } t \in [0, 1]. \tag{2}$$

2.2   Competitive Methods for Stain Color Augmentation

Most existing stain color transfer methods are used for stain normalization, i.e., to transfer the stain color of the test domain to that of the training domain. Recently, it has been shown that simple stain color augmentations, such as perturbing the HSV color space of the histological images, perform better and lead to more robust models than traditional and network-based normalization techniques [15]. Therefore, we compare our HistAuGAN to the HSV augmentations used in [15]. Besides HSV augmentation, there is a more complicated augmentation technique based on the Wasserstein distance of different domains [11]. But the method is much slower than HSV and HistAuGAN, thus difficult to be used as an on-the-fly augmentation technique.

For a quantitative evaluation of our augmentation technique, we consider the following augmentation methods:

- *Geometric augmentations*: vertical and horizontal flipping, as well as 90°, 180°, and 270° rotations.
- *HSV color augmentations*: geometric augmentations with Gaussian blur and contrast and brightness perturbations applied with probability 0.25 and 0.5, respectively. We tried both light and strong color augmentations, as suggested in [15]. Strong color augmentations can generate unrealistic color appearances. However, applying hue and saturation jittering with factor 0.5 and probability 0.5, which results in relatively strong color perturbanceas shown in Fig. 2e, performed best for us.
- *HistAuGAN*: geometric augmentations combined with our augmentation technique applied to half of the images during training. For each image, we randomly pick a target domain from the training domains and sample a color attribute vector $z_a \in \mathbb{R}^8$ from the standard normal distribution.

2.3   Evaluation

We evaluate HistAuGAN on three different aspects, in particular, i) whether it can remove batch effects present in histological images collected from multiple medical laboratories, ii) how it affects the out-of-domain generalization of a deep learning model trained for a specific down-stream task, and iii) how HistAu-GAN preserves morphological structure during augmentation. For ii), we choose a binary classification task of classifying WSI tiles into the classes *tumor* versus *non-tumor* as described in more detail in Sect. 3.3. Question iii) is evaluated by asking a pathology expert to check image similarity before and after augmentation. To explore how generalizable our model is, we extend the HistAuGAN training data (lypmh nodes) by tiles from unseen tissue and tumor types, in particular, breast tissue [13].

3   Results and Discussion

3.1   Dataset

For the quantitative evaluation of HistAuGAN, we choose the publicly available Camelyon17 dataset [1] that provides WSIs from five different medical centers (denoted by RUMC, CWZ, UMCU, RST, and LPON) with different scanning properties and stain colors as shown in Fig. 2a. Pixel-wise annotations are given for 50 WSIs in total, 10 from each medical center. To create the training patches, we first threshold the images with naive RGB thresholding combined with Otsu thresholding and then patch the tissue regions of each WSI at the highest resolution based on a grid into tiles of size 512×512 pixels. Each tile is labeled as *tumor* if the ratio of pixels annotated as tumor pixels is larger than 1%,

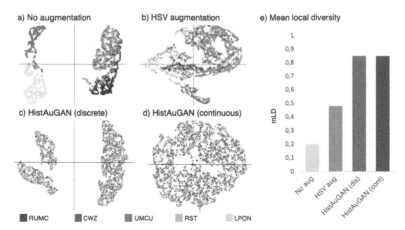

Fig. 3. Effect of color augmentation on batch effects in color statistics. (a-d) UMAP embeddings of color statistics of training data, color-coded by source domains. (e) The quantification of mixing based on mean local diversity (mLD, higher is better) suggests HistAuGAN effectively mitigates batch effects. (Color figure online)

otherwise, it is labelled as *non-tumor*. The tiled dataset has an *imbalanced* class distribution, i.e., overall, 7% of the tiles are labeled as *tumor* and the ratio of tumor tiles is in the same order of magnitude across all medical centers.

3.2 Evaluation of Batch-Effect Removal

To evaluate how color augmentation mitigates batch effects, we quantify the mixing of images from different medical centers with respect to their color statistics. A random set of 1000 image tiles were extracted from the WSIs from each center and analyzed in terms of the average values of each component after transformation to various color spaces (RGB, HSV, LAB, HED, grayscale). To visually observe batch effects, we reduced dimensionality to 2D using UMAP [2] and labeled points according to their domain as shown in Fig. 3a-d. To quantify mixing of different domains, we measured the mean over the local diversity (mLD) for all k-nearest neighborhoods ($k = 10$) in the 2D projection using Shannon's equitability which varies between 0 for non-mixed and 1 for perfectly mixed populations (cf. Figure 3e).

Without color augmentation, we observe a clear batch effect: tiles from different domains form distinct clusters ($mLD = 0.20$, Fig. 3a). HSV augmentations improve data mixing but domain-correlated clusters are still visible ($mLD = 0.48$, Fig. 3b) and single domains, e.g. LPON, are not mixed with other domains. In contrast, HistAuGAN mixes data from multiple domains (Fig. 3c,d) with a high local diversity ($mLD = 0.85$). If HistAuGAN is used to transfer colors to discrete domains, the distinct domain clusters are retained, but each cluster contains well-mixed image samples transferred from all domains (Fig. 3c). When HistAuGAN

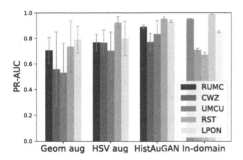 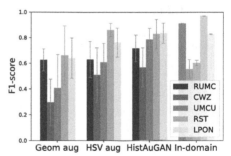

Fig. 4. Precision-recall AUC (left) and F1-score (right) of our binary classification task. The bold bars depict the results on the out-of-domain centers averaged across all runs. The most-right, pale bars denote the in-domain test performance of the classifiers trained with geometric augmentations.

is used to randomly interpolate between domains, a continuous well-mixed color subspace is obtained without any clustering structure (Fig. 3d).

These results show that HistAuGAN is highly effective in removing batch effects present in color statistics of images sampled from different medical centers.

3.3   Evaluation on Down-Stream Classification Task

To evaluate the effect of our proposed augmentation method, we trained a CNN on a binary tumor classification task and compare the performance on different out-of-domain test sets based on the Camelyon17 dataset. Due to the relatively small size of our dataset, in particular the small number of tumor tiles, we choose a small CNN, namely, a pre-trained ResNet18 [7], and fine-tune the last two ResNet-blocks together with the fully-connected layer on our dataset. For training, we use weighted cross-entropy-loss to rebalance the contribution of each class, with a learning rate of 1e-5 and an L_2-regularization of 1e-5 across all runs and for all augmentation techniques. Furthermore, we used random erasing on all augmentation techniques [18]. Since our dataset is highly imbalanced, we report the F1-score of the tumor class in addition to the area under the precision-recall curve (PR-AUC).

Figure 4 shows the results of the quantitative evaluation of different augmentation techniques on the binary tumor-classification task. For each medical center, we trained three classifiers, one for each augmentation type, and aggregated the results evaluated on the test domains. All experiments were repeated three times. On both metrics, HistAuGAN shows better performance on all of the out-of-domain test sets. As visualized in Fig. 2, the appearance of images from medical center UMCU and LPON deviates strongly from the other centers, explaining their lower scores. In comparison to HSV color augmentation, HistAuGAN performs better in handling the stain color discrepancy between training and test domain and is therefore able to generate a more robust classification model that generalizes better to out-of-domain test sets. This can also be

Table 1. Expert evaluation.

Tissue type	High	Moderate	Low	Total
Lymph nodes	10	7	3	20
Breast	14	4	2	20

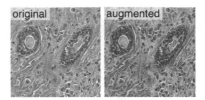

Fig. 5. HistAuGAN on unseen tissue.

measured in the standard deviation of the results across the out-of-domain test sets centers. For our model, the standard deviation of the PR-AUC for the tumor class amounts to 0.08, whereas it higher for geometric (0.22) and color (0.14) augmentations, respectively, which demonstrates that our model is more robust to underlying stain color variations. The right-most group shows the in-domain test results for geometric augmentations. It can be seen as an upper bound for any stain normalization technique, and thus shows that HistAuGAN can even outperform stain normalization techniques on some of the five domains.

3.4　Qualitative Evaluation by an Expert Pathologist

We further check the quality of HistAuGAN by an expert pathologist on the structural similarity of original and augmented WSI tiles from the training set, i.e., the Camelyon17 dataset, and an unseen dataset of breast tissue [13]. We define three levels of similarity: a) "High similarity": a pathologist would find it difficult to distinguish the original tile from the augmented tile. b) "Moderate similarity": some structural variations are observed, but do not affect pathological diagnosis. c) "Low similarity": the augmentated tiles can not be used for diagnostic purposes. As shown in Table 1, most of the augmented images do not have a structural modification that affects diagnosis and over half of them can even *fool* an expert pathologist. It is worth to mention that HistAuGAN is not trained on any of the breast cancer images but is still able to transfer its color in a structure-preserving manner as shown in Fig. 5 on a sample tile.

4　Conclusion

In summary, we propose a novel GAN-based technique, HistAuGAN, for color augmentation of histopathological images. Based on the disentangled representations of content and style, HistAuGAN is able to change the color appearance of an histological image while preserving its morphological structure. Moreover, HistAuGAN captures both intra-domain and inter-domain color variations. It is able to interpolate between domains and can therefore span a continuous color space covering a large variety of realistic stain colors. When applied as an augmentation technique, HistAuGAN yields a robust down-stream classifier that generalizes better to out-of-domain test sets than other color augmentations techniques and, therefore, renders additional stain normalization steps unnecessary. Finally, HistAuGAN can mitigate batch effects present in histopathological data which suggests that it is also able to cover domain shifts beyond color variations, such as noise and artefacts introduced in image compression. The code is publicly available at https://github.com/sophiajw/HistAuGAN together with a model of HistAuGAN trained on the five medical centers of the Camelyon17 dataset.

References

1. Bandi, P., et al.: From detection of individual metastases to classification of lymph node status at the patient level: the CAMELYON17 challenge. IEEE Trans. Med. Imaging **38**(2), 550–560 (2019)
2. Becht, E., et al.: Dimensionality reduction for visualizing single-cell data using UMAP. Nat. Biotechnol. **37**, 38–44 (2018)
3. Bejnordi, D.D., et al.: Stain specific standardization of Whole-Slide histopathological images (2016)
4. de Bel, T., Bokhorst, J.M., van der Laak, J., Litjens, G.: Residual cyclegan for robust domain transformation of histopathological tissue slides. Med. Image Anal. **70**, 102004 (2021)
5. Chan, J.K.C.: The wonderful colors of the Hematoxylin-Eosin stain in diagnostic surgical pathology. Int. J. Surg. Pathol. **22**(1), 12–32 (2014)
6. Cohen, J.P., Luck, M., Honari, S.: Distribution matching losses can Hallucinate features in medical image translation. In: Frangi, A.F., Schnabel, J.A., Davatzikos, C., Alberola-López, C., Fichtinger, G. (eds.) MICCAI 2018. LNCS, vol. 11070, pp. 529–536. Springer, Cham (2018). https://doi.org/10.1007/978-3-030-00928-1_60
7. He, K., Zhang, X., Ren, S., Sun, J.: Deep residual learning for image recognition. In: Proceedings of the IEEE Conference on Computer Vision and Pattern Recognition (CVPR), June 2016
8. Lee, H.Y., et al.: DRIT : diverse Image-to-Image translation via disentangled representations (2020)
9. Liang, H., Plataniotis, K.N., Li, X.: Stain style transfer of histopathology images via structure-preserved generative learning. In: Deeba, F., Johnson, P., Würfl, T., Ye, J.C. (eds.) MLMIR 2020. LNCS, vol. 12450, pp. 153–162. Springer, Cham (2020). https://doi.org/10.1007/978-3-030-61598-7_15
10. Macenko, M., et al.: A method for normalizing histology slides for quantitative analysis. In: 2009 IEEE International Symposium on Biomedical Imaging: From Nano to Macro, pp. 1107–1110. IEEE (2009)
11. Nadeem, S., Hollmann, T., Tannenbaum, A.: Multimarginal Wasserstein barycenter for stain normalization and augmentation. Med. Image Comput. Comput. Assist. Interv. **12265**, 362–371 (2020)
12. Reinhard, E., Adhikhmin, M., Gooch, B., Shirley, P.: Color transfer between images. IEEE Comput. Graph. Appl. **21**(5), 34–41 (2001)
13. Roux, L.: Mitos-atypia-14 grand challenge. https://mitos-atypia-14.grand-challenge.org/. Accessed 03 Mar 2021
14. Shaban, M.T., Tarek Shaban, M., Baur, C., Navab, N., Albarqouni, S.: Staingan: stain style transfer for digital histological images (2019)

15. Tellez, D., et al.: Quantifying the effects of data augmentation and stain color normalization in convolutional neural networks for computational pathology. Med. Image Anal. **58**, 101544 (2019)

16. Tschuchnig, M.E., Oostingh, G.J., Gadermayr, M.: Generative adversarial networks in digital pathology: a survey on trends and future potential. Patterns (N Y) **1**(6), 100089 (2020)

17. Vahadane, A., et al.: Structure-Preserving color normalization and sparse stain separation for histological images. IEEE Trans. Med. Imaging **35**(8), 1962–1971 (2016)

18. Zhong, Z., Zheng, L., Kang, G., Li, S., Yang, Y.: Random erasing data augmentation. In: Proceedings of the AAAI Conference on Artificial Intelligence, vol. 34, no. 07, pp. 13001–13008 (2020)

19. Zhu, J.Y., Park, T., Isola, P., Efros, A.A.: Unpaired image-to-image translation using cycle-consistent adversarial networks. In: Proceedings of the IEEE International Conference on Computer Vision, pp. 2223–2232 (2017)

MetaCon: Meta Contrastive Learning for Microsatellite Instability Detection

Yuqing Liu[1]($\boxtimes$), Weiwen Wang[1], Chuan-Xian Ren[1,2], and Dao-Qing Dai[1]

[1] School of Mathematics, Sun Yat-sen University, Guangzhou, China
`liuyq89@mail2.sysu.edu.cn`
[2] Pazhou Lab, Guangzhou, China

Abstract. Colorectal cancer (CRC) patients who are detected as microsatellite instability (MSI) can receive precise targeted therapies, but existing MSI detection methods are not available to all patients due to various restrictions. The achievements of deep learning in image processing provide the possibility of using pathological images for MSI detection. However, traditional deep networks can not achieve satisfied performance due to discrepancies between MSI patients, which reduces the generalization ability of deep learning models. Noisy labels also hinder the learning of an accurate model. To address these issues, we propose a model in a meta contrastive learning framework (MetaCon) accompanied with an attention-based feature fusion block. In MetaCon, we iteratively train a backbone with a cross entropy loss and a contrastive loss to learn a patient-independent MSI classifier for patches segmented from pathological images. We then blend features of patches from the same patient in an attention-based way, automatically focusing on reliable patches. Finally, we make a patient-level prediction by voting. Experiments on two public datasets from The Cancer Genome Atlas show superiority of our model over previous methods. The patient-level AUC is improved by 8% on average compared to the baseline model. Ablation studies prove effectiveness of each component in our model.

Keywords: Microsatellite instability detection · Meta-learning · Contrastive learning · Pathological images analysis

1 Introduction

Microsatellite instability (MSI) is a specific form of genomic instability caused by the loss of DNA mismatch repair (MMR) activity. MSI accounts for about 15% of patients with colorectal cancer (CRC) and it is related to specific clinic, pathologic, and molecular features of the tumors [1]. CRC patients with MSI benefit from immunotherapy. Hence, precise identification of MSI provides better therapies for patients. Conventionally, MSI detection requires additional genetic or immunohistochemical tests such as immunohistochemistry (IHC) analysis for the MMR proteins and mutation detection in the MMR genes [2], which are not widespread among patients. Inspired by the success of convolutional neural

© Springer Nature Switzerland AG 2021
M. de Bruijne et al. (Eds.): MICCAI 2021, LNCS 12908, pp. 267–276, 2021.
https://doi.org/10.1007/978-3-030-87237-3_26

networks (CNNs) in computer vision [4, 16, 19], therapists believe the ubiquitous biopsy provides opportunities for MSI detection through pathological images.

It was first proposed to use CNNs for MSI detection of gastrointestinal cancer by Kather et al. [5]. They trained a ResNet18 with color-normalized patches for binary classification and then made a majority voting for patient-level prediction. Cao et al. [6] followed Kather's work and combined two traditional machine learning methods to aggregate the patch likelihoods learned by a ResNet18. Under the framework of Multiple Instance Learning (MIL), Chikontwe et al. [7] used a ResNet34 to choose top k patches and defined a center for soft-assignment based inference. All these studies concentrated on the ensemble strategies after patch-level prediction.

However, as microsatellites vary in size between individuals [3], it is supposed to be a great gap between MSI patients, and experience bears this out. Hence, a well-trained model degrades for unseen patients, as shown in [5]. Assigning a patient's label for all patches of his or her pathological images also induces noisy labels in training stage. Previous experiments have shown that a large portion of positive patches are more similar to the negative ones, which results in low probability of a MSI patient being predicted to be MSI. In addition, the general cross entropy loss in classification is considered to be less effective when dealing with migrated data and noisy labels [10, 20, 21]. To address these problems, we propose a meta contrastive learning framework (MetaCon) accompanied with an attention-based feature fusion block. In the spirits of meta-learning for domain generazation [8, 11, 14, 17], we treat patients in training set as multiple source domains and patients in testing set as unseen target domains. By dividing the patients in training set into meta-train and meta-test sets, the meta-learning process simulates the distribution shift between patients. In previous studies, contrastive loss is used to pretrain a backbone network before training with cross entropy loss to enhance the robustness of model [10, 22]. Here, we recast these two steps using patches from disjoint patients into two phases of meta learning procedure, i.e. meta-train and meta-test, to reduce the gap between patients. In meta-train, we train a crude MSI classifier with binary cross entropy loss. A contrastive loss is then applied to learn discriminative representations in the meta-test phase. Finally, the feature fusion block blends features of patches from the same patient for the purpose of weakening the effects of noisy labels and enhancing the effects of reliable patches by reconstructing patches using weighted average. Previous studies simply select top k patches based on prediction scores [7, 12], while our feature fusion block considers all patches making full use of available data. Our major contributions are summarized as follows:

- We develop a new method MetaCon for MSI detection. In MetaCon, we employ a cross entropy loss and a contrastive loss in two phases to learn a patient-independent category-distinguishable feature extractor and an adaptive MSI classifier.
- We propose a feature fusion block combined with a ReLU layer to delete patches with noisy labels and aggregate reliable patches from the same patients in an efficient way.

– We conduct experiments on two public datasets from The Cancer Genome Atlas (TCGA). MetaCon outperforms previous studies on both patch-level accuracy and patient-level AUC. We also demonstrate validity of each component in MetaCon in ablation studies.

2   Methods

Given a dataset of patients $\mathcal{P} = \{(\mathcal{P}_i, y_i)\}_{i=1}^{N}$, where $\mathcal{P}_i$ represents a collection of patches segmented from a patient's pathological image with its label $y_i \in \{0, 1\}$. Patients with microsatellite instability (MSI) are indicated by $y_i = 1$ while the microsatellite stability (MSS) patients are labeled with $y_i = 0$. Patient i contains M_i patches: $\mathcal{P}_i = \{x_j^{(i)}\}_{j=1}^{M_i}$. Patch $x_j^{(i)}$ is labeled according to the corresponding y_i of $\mathcal{P}_i$ by $y_j^{(i)}$, i.e. $y_i = y_j^{(i)}$. The goal is to predict the correct labels of unlabeled patients in the testing stage using their patches.

To this end, we construct a meta contrastive learning framework to eliminate the discrepancies between patients in the patch-level training stage and design an attention-based feature fusion block to alleviate the effect of noisy labels before patient-level prediction. Sketch of the proposed model is presented in Fig. 1. Our model consists of: (1) a framework of meta learning, (2) a contrastive loss to learn discriminative features, (3) a feature fusion block to automatically aggregate features of reliable patches from the same patient, and (4) a majority voting mechanism for patient-level prediction.

Meta-learning Framework. Studies have shown that microsatellite instability varies in sizes from patient to patient [3], so discrepancies between patients leads to the insufficient generalization ability of common deep learning models. In this context, we treat each patient as a separate domain and learn to adapt among patients by drawing on the idea of meta learning.

During the patch-level training stage, we define an iteration of meta-train and meta-test as an epoch. In one epoch, we randomly select n patients $\mathcal{P}_{mtr} = \{\mathcal{P}_i\}_{i=1}^{n}$ for meta-train and n patients $\mathcal{P}_{mte} = \{\mathcal{P}_j\}_{j=1}^{n}$ for meta-test, such that $\mathcal{P}_{mtr} \cap \mathcal{P}_{mte} = \emptyset$. To balance the selection of patch-level classes, we select positive and negative patients in a ratio of 1 to 6.

Meta-train. In the meta-train phase, we randomly select $2\,m$ patches $\hat{\mathcal{P}}_{mtr} \subset \mathcal{P}_{mtr}$ and make positive and negative patches equivalent. We train the parameters of feature extractor F_θ and patch-level classifier C_α using a binary cross entropy loss. In this way, we hope to train a discriminative classifier. Thus, the loss function in meta-train is defined as

$$\mathcal{L}_{BCE} = -\frac{1}{2m} \sum_{x_j^{(i)} \in \hat{\mathcal{P}}_{mtr}} y_j^{(i)} \log(1 - C_\alpha(F_\theta(x_j^{(i)}))) \tag{1}$$

Meta-test. In the meta-test phase, we randomly select $2\,m$ patches $\hat{\mathcal{P}}_{mte} \subset \mathcal{P}_{mte}$ and keep positive and negative patches balance as well. Then, we employ a contrastive loss to update features. The contrastive loss is minimized with patients

(a)

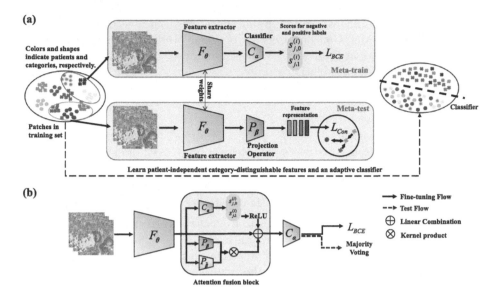

(b)

Fig. 1. The proposed meta contrastive learning framework. (a) We first randomly select two disjoint subsets of patients for two meta-phases, and iteratively do (1) meta-train: optimize $\mathcal{L}_{BCE}$ to update θ and α and (2) meta-test: optimize $\mathcal{L}_{Con}$ to update θ and β. (b) We cascade the well-trained F_θ, P_β, and C_α for inference. Before deploying our model for testing, we fine-tune the concatenated model with fixed F_θ. An attention fusion block is introduced to handle noisy labels.

who are not present during the meta-train phase, so it helps to learn patient-independent category-distinguishable features (see Fig. 2). The loss function in meta-test is defined as

$$\mathcal{L}_{Con} = \frac{1}{2m-1} \sum_{x_j^{(i)} \in \hat{\mathcal{P}}_{mte}} 1\{i \neq q \text{ or } j \neq t\} 1\{\, y_j^{(i)} = y_t^{(q)}\} \log\{\mathcal{L}_{SC}\} \qquad (2)$$

where

$$\mathcal{L}_{SC} = \frac{\exp\{P_\beta(F_\theta(x_j^{(i)}))^T P_\beta(F_\theta(x_t^{(q)}))\}}{\sum_{x_s^{(r)} \in \hat{\mathcal{P}}_{mte}} 1\{i \neq r \text{ or } j \neq s\} \exp\{P_\beta(F_\theta(x_j^{(i)}))^T P_\beta(F_\theta(x_s^{(r)}))\}},$$

and $1\{\cdot\}$ is the indicator function. By increasing the intra-class similarity and decreasing the inter-class similarity, the contrastive loss intends to make features of patches with same labels more compact in a projection space. Previous studies show that projection operator is necessary in contrastive loss [10,13,15].

Feature Fusion Block. Noisy label is another hard nut to crack in this task. The patch-level labels are directly inherited from the patient-level labels. And there is no evidence that all patches from MSI patients express the properties of

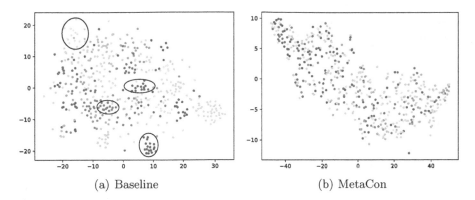

(a) Baseline   (b) MetaCon

Fig. 2. t-SNE [23] visualizations of features extracted by baseline (ResNet18) and MetaCon (ours) from MSI patients in the CRC-DX test set. Colors indicate different patients. (a) Points with same color clusters, which shows high similarity within same patients and low similarity between patients from the MSI category; (b)Points scatters regardless of color, which demonstrates divergence between MSI patients is eliminated. Obviously, MetaCon can obtain patient-independent features.

MSI. Considering the low patch-level probabilities of MSI, we infer that most of the positive patches are actually more similar to the negative ones. The presence of these unreliable patches with noisy labels lowers the patient-level probabilities of true MSI in inference.

Inspired by the Nonlocal Neural Block [9], we design a feature fusion block to reconstruct all the patches in an attention-based way. Through this block, each patch is replaced by a weighted average of other patches from the same patient, i.e., $\hat{f}_j^{(i)} = \sum_{k=1}^{M_i} w_{j,k}^{(i)} f_k^{(i)}$. And the weight are determined by two factors: a response with the patch under reconstruction and a score of MSI probability.

As show in Eq. 3, features are projected into two 128-dimensional spaces, then we use a matrix multiplication to construct a kernel function $K(x_i, x_j) = x_i^T x_j$ to calculate the response between them. The scores are obtained by passing the second dimension of outputs of C_α through a ReLU layer. A *softmax* operator makes the multiplication of responses and scores as normalized weights. The scores are filtered by the ReLU layer so that the patches with negative outputs of the classifier will be deleted in multiplication. And the patches with higher scores will play a more important part during the fusion. It does not require a manually selected the number of patches.

$$w_{j,k}^{(i)} = \text{softmax}\{\text{ReLU}(s_{k,1}^{(i)})K(P_\beta(f_j^{(i)}), P_{\widetilde{\beta}}(f_k^{(i)}))\} \tag{3}$$

Note that P_β is inherited from the meta framework while $P_{\widetilde{\beta}}$ is reinitialized.

Majority Voting Mechanism. At the final decision stage, we apply the majority voting mechanism. Ensemble patch-level decisions are supposed to be more robust than making patient-level decisions directly because of insufficient samples for patient-level training. Moreover, with the feature fusion block, in fact, we have deleted unreliable patches and have maximized the role of reliable patches for each patient. Thus, we believe majority voting mechanism is a good choice to make the patient-level predictions.

3   Experiments and Results

Dataset and Settings. We conducted experiments on two preprocessed colorectal cancer (CRC) WSI datasets from The Cancer Genome Atlas (TCGA): CRC-DX and CRC-KR [5]. For training stage, CRC-DX-TRAIN includes 93,408 paraffin embedded (FFPE) patches from 360 patients; CRC-KR-TRAIN includes 60,894 snap-frozen patches from 378 patients. For testing stage, CRC-DX-TEST includes patches 98904 from 100 patients; CRC-KR-TEST includes 78249 patches from 108 patients. The number of positive and negative patches was balanced, but the ratio of positive and negative patients was 15:85, which was consistent with clinical experience. All the patches were automatically detected of tumor, resized to 224 pixel × 224 pixel.

We also randomly selected 5 MSI patients and 30 MSS patients in training set as a validation set. In all experiments, the patch-level accuracy on the validation set was taken as the criterion for selecting models.

We used ResNet18 as backbone networks. Patch-level classifier C_α and projection operator P_β were constructed by 512 to 2 dimensions and 512 to 128 dimensions of fully connected layers, respectively. The meta-learning framework were trained for 10000 epochs with a learning rate of 1e-4 by Adam optimizer. In feature fusion, with F_θ fixed, the patch-level classifier C_α and the projection operator $P_\beta, P_{\tilde{\beta}}$ were fine-tuned for 20 epochs with learning rate of 1e-4 for CRC-DX and 1e-3 for CRC-KR by Adam optimizer. Batch size was set to 256.

Comparison with Previous Methods. We compared our model with the state-of-the-art models. Kather's study [5] is the first deep-learning based model for this task and we used the same datasets with it. We reported the results of their work directly. Other recent models are under the framework of multiple instance learning (MIL). We evaluated against a two MIL methods [6,12], which we term as CamMIL and BoostMIL. CamMIL involves a two-stage training process. We separately set $k = 1$ and $k = 50$ for the top k patches selection in its second stage. BoostMIL used a dataset sharing same patients and images with CRC-KR, but it was processed manually by selecting regions of interests for training and only about 2/3 of patients in CRC-KR test set were used for testing in [6]. We directly loaded the trained model on their website to predict in our testing set. We used patient-level AUC as an evaluation index. The results were generated by 500 bootstrap sessions, with a 95% confidence interval.

The results are presented in Table 1. In both CRC-DX and CRC-KR, Meta-Con achieved the best performance and had improvement compared to other methods. CamMIL selected top k patches of each patient for training but only

Table 1. Method comparison on patient-level AUC with a 95% confidence interval in parentheses.

Methods	CRC-DX	CRC-KR
Kather's study [5]	0.77 (0.62–0.87)	0.84 (0.73–0.91)
CamMIL(top1) [12]	0.65 (0.53–0.78)	0.47 (0.35–0.59)
CamMIL(top50) [12]	0.74 (0.62–0.85)	0.71 (0.60–0.81)
BoostMIL [6]	0.53 (0.41–0.66)	0.79 (0.67–0.88)
MetaCon	**0.90 (0.80–0.96)**	**0.87 (0.79–0.94)**

used the top 1 patch for patient-level prediction, not making full use of available data while our feature fusion block and majority voting mechanism aggregated all patches. BoostMIL did worse in CRC-KR compared to Kather's study and MetaCon. Since it was originally trained in a dataset similar to CRC-KR, Boost-MIL performed poorly in CRC-DX as expected. Kather's study was the simplest method but its results were second only to MetaCon. Kather's study achieved patient-level AUC around 0.9 when the testing set share same patients with training set, but it got worse for unseen patients. MetaCon adopts the idea of meta-learning to bridge the gap between patients and improve model generalization of unseen patients.

Ablation Study. The key components of our model is the meta contrastive learning framework and the feature fusion block (FB). We designed four ablation studies to verify the validity of them: (1)baseline model by ResNet18; (2) using baseline model with contrastive loss(ConL); (3) using the meta framework with contrastive loss (MetaCon w\o FB); (4)using MetaCon with feature fusion block (MetaCon). The results are shown in Table 2.

Table 2. The performance on ablation studies. Two evaluation indexes are applied: patch-level accuracy (ACC) and patient-level AUC with a 95% confidence interval in parentheses.

Methods	CRC-DX		CRC-KR	
	Test ACC (patch-level)	Test AUC (patient-level)	Test ACC (patch-level)	Test AUC (patient-level)
Baseline	0.66	0.80 (0.68–0.89)	0.68	0.82 (0.71–0.91)
ConL	0.72	0.82 (0.72–0.90)	0.75	0.83 (0.73–0.91)
MetaCon w\o FB	0.75	0.89 (0.79–0.96)	0.74	0.86 (0.76–0.93)
MetaCon	**0.78**	**0.90 (0.80–0.96)**	**0.78**	**0.87 (0.79–0.94)**

The performance of baseline and ConL demonstrates the effectiveness of contrastive loss, especially for patch-level accuracy. From the histogram of the feature similarities on CRC-DX training set (Fig. 3), we find that the contrastive loss helps to learn the category difference between the features. But its performance on unseen patients in testing is not good enough. Figure 2 have shown that the discrepancies between MSI patients can be eliminated by MetaCon, which indicates MetaCon improved generalization ability to new patients. Results on Meta-Con in Table. 2 verifies this again. It has achieved varying degrees of improvement on patch-level accuracy and patient-level AUC compared to baseline and ConL. Finally, the feature fusion block further improves the results.

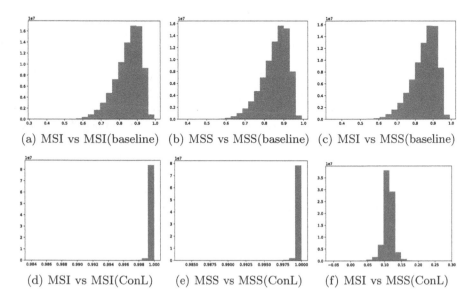

(a) MSI vs MSI(baseline)   (b) MSS vs MSS(baseline)   (c) MSI vs MSS(baseline)

(d) MSI vs MSI(ConL)   (e) MSS vs MSS(ConL)   (f) MSI vs MSS(ConL)

Fig. 3. Histogram of the feature similarities (trained by baseline and ConL) on CRC-DX training set. (a)(b)(c): feature similarities distribute between 0.6 and 1.0 independent of labels, indicating that the features do not have strong categorical identifiability. (d)(e)(f):feature similarities with same labels concentrate around 1.0, which means high intra-class similarity. On the contrary, feature similarities with different labels concentrate around 0.1, which means low inter-class similarity.

4   Conclusion

In this work, we have developed a deep-learning model for MSI detection for patients with colorectal cancer using pathological images. Motivated by the gap between patients and the ubiquity of noisy labels, we propose a meta contrastive learning framework and an attention-based feature fusion block. We eliminate discrepancies between patients by iteratively training with a cross entropy loss and a contrastive loss to get a patient-independent category-distinguishable classifier in meta-learning paradigm. The attention-based feature fusion block automatically focuses on reliable patches for prediction to alleviate the affect of noisy labels. Experiments have shown superiority of our model over the state-of-the-art methods.

Acknowledgement. This work is supported by the National Natural Science Foundation of China (grant numbers 12026601; 61976229; U1611265; 11631015; 61976104).

References

1. Boland, C.R., Goel, A.: Microsatellite instability in colorectal cancer. Gastroenterology **138**(6), 2073–2087 (2010)
2. Niederhuber, J.E., Armitage, J.O., Doroshow, J.H., Kastan, M.B., Tepper, J.E.: Clinical Oncology, 5th edn., pp. 1278–1335. Churchill Livingstone, London (2014)
3. Coleman, W.B., Tsongalis, G.J.: Diagnostic Molecular Pathology 1st edn., pp. 305–320. Academic Press, Cambridge (2017)
4. LeCun, Y., Bengio, Y., Hinton, G.: Deep learning. Nature **521**, 436–444 (2015)
5. Kather, J.N., et al.: Deep learning can predict microsatellite instability directly from histology in gastrointestinal cancer. Nature Med. **25**(7), 1054–1056 (2019)
6. Cao, R., Yang, F., Ma, S.C., et al.: Development and interpretation of a pathomics-based model for the prediction of microsatellite instability in Colorectal Cancer. Theranostics **10**(24), 11080–11091 (2020)
7. Chikontwe, P., Kim, M., Nam, S.J., Go, H., Park, S.H.: Multiple instance learning with center embeddings for histopathology classification. In: Martel, A.L. (ed.) MICCAI 2020. LNCS, vol. 12265, pp. 519–528. Springer, Cham (2020). https://doi.org/10.1007/978-3-030-59722-1_50
8. Balaji, Y., Sankaranarayanan, S., Chellappa, R.: MetaReg: towards domain generalization using meta-regularization. In: NIPS18. Curran Associates Inc., pp. 1006–1016. Red Hook (2018)
9. Wang, X., Girshick, R., Gupta, A., He, K.: Non-local neural networks. in Proceedings IEEE/CVF Conference CVPR2018, pp. 7794–7803. Salt Lake City (2018)
10. Prannay, K., Piotr, T., Chen, W., et al.: Supervised Contrastive Learning (2020)
11. Chen, G., Zhang, T., Lu, J., et al.: Deep meta metric learning. In: IEEE/CVF International Conference on Computer Vision (ICCV). IEEE (2019)
12. Campanella, G.: Clinical-grade computational pathology using weakly supervised deep learning on whole slide images. Nat. Med. **25**(8), 1301–1309 (2019)
13. He, K., Fan, H., Wu, Y., Xie, S., Girshick, R.: Momentum contrast for unsupervised visual representation learning. In: IEEE/CVF Conference on Computer Vision and Pattern Recognition (CVPR2020), Seattle, WA, USA, 2020, pp. 9726–9735. https://doi.org/10.1109/CVPR42600.2020.00975
14. Huisman, M., Rijn, J.N., Plaat, A.: A survey of deep meta-learning. arXiv preprint arXiv:2010.03522v1
15. Chen, T., Kornblith, S., Norouzi, M., Hinton, G.: A simple framework for contrastive learning of visual representations. arXiv preprint arXiv:2002.05709 (2020)
16. Hou, L., Samaras, D., Kurc, T.M., Gao, Y., Davis, J.E., Saltz, J.H.: Patch-based convolutional neural network for whole slide tissue image classification. In: Proceedings of the IEEE Conference on Computer Vision and Pattern Recognition, p. 24242433 (2016)
17. Li, D., Yang, Y., Song, Y.Z., Hospedales, T.M.: Learning to generalize: meta-learning for domain generalization. In: 32nd AAAI Conference on Artificial Intelligence (2018)
18. Andrychowicz, M., et al.: Learning to learn by gradient descent. In: NIPS (2016)
19. Panayides, A.S., et al.: AI in medical imaging informatics: current challenges and future directions. IEEE J. Biomed. Health Inf. **24**(7), 1837–1857 (2020). https://doi.org/10.1109/JBHI.2020.2991043

20. Liu, W., Wen, Y., Yu, Z., Yang, M.: Large-margin softmax loss for convolutional neural networks. In: ICML (2016)
21. Zhang, Z., Sabuncu, M.: Generalized cross entropy loss for training deep neural networks with noisy labels. In: Advances in Neural Information Processing Systems, pp. 8778–8788 (2018)
22. Robinson, J., Chuang, CY., Sra, S., Jegelka, S.: Contrastive learning with hard negative samples, p. 22. arXiv9, USA October 2020
23. Van der Maaten, L., Hinton, G.: Visualizing data using t-SNE[J]. J. Mach. Learn. Res. **9**(85), 2579–2605 (2008)

Generalizing Nucleus Recognition Model in Multi-source Ki67 Immunohistochemistry Stained Images via Domain-Specific Pruning

Jiatong Cai[1,2], Chenglu Zhu[1,2], Can Cui[1,2], Honglin Li[1,2], Tong Wu[1,2], Shichuan Zhang[1,2,3], and Lin Yang[1,2(✉)]

[1] Artificial Intelligence and Biomedical Image Analysis Lab, School of Engineering, Westlake University, Hangzhou, China
[2] Institute of Advanced Technology, Westlake Institute for Advanced Study, Hangzhou, China
yanglin@westlake.edu.cn
[3] College of Computer Science & Technology, Zhejiang University, Hangzhou, China

Abstract. Ki67 is a significant biomarker in the diagnosis and prognosis of cancer, whose index can be evaluated by quantifying its expression in Ki67 immunohistochemistry (IHC) stained images. However, quantitative analysis on multi-source Ki67 images is yet a challenging task in practice due to cross-domain distribution differences, which result from imaging variation, staining styles and lesion types. Many recent studies have made some efforts on domain generalization (DG), whereas there are still some noteworthy limitations. Specifically in the case of Ki67 images, learning invariant representation is at the mercy of the insufficient number of domains and the cell categories mismatching in different domains. In this paper, we propose a novel method to improve DG by searching the domain-agnostic subnetwork in a domain merging scenario. Partial model parameters are iteratively pruned according to the domain gap, which is caused by the data converting from a single domain into merged domains during training. In addition, the model is optimized by fine-tuning on merged domains to eliminate the interference of class mismatching among various domains. Furthermore, an appropriate implementation is attained by applying the pruning method to different parts of the framework. Compared with known DG methods, our method yields excellent performance in multiclass nucleus recognition of Ki67 IHC images, especially in the lost category cases. Moreover, our competitive results are also evaluated on the public dataset over the state-of-the-art DG methods.

Keywords: Ki67 · Nucleus recognition · Domain generalization · Microscopy images · Prune

1 Introduction

In the diagnosis and prognosis of cancer, Ki67 is a significant biomarker [14, 29,32] that can evaluate tumor cell proliferation and growth by quantifying its

© Springer Nature Switzerland AG 2021
M. de Bruijne et al. (Eds.): MICCAI 2021, LNCS 12908, pp. 277–287, 2021.
https://doi.org/10.1007/978-3-030-87237-3_27

expression in Ki67 immunohistochemistry stained images [9,25]. With the increase of data volume, deep learning methods have provided strong advantages in nucleus recognition [26,28]. However, the lack of standardized multicenter data could bring heterogeneous Ki67 interpretations from different stainings, scanners and environments [3,15]. Applying methods trained on a single domain can result in a biased prediction. It is commonly required in practice that the robust model trained on multi-source data should have a reliable prediction on unseen domains. Empirical Risk Minimization (ERM) [23] is a convenient solution, however, the gap still exists due to the complexity of the merged domains.

Methods of cross-domain training can be simply divided into domain adaptation (DA) and domain generalization (DG). Specifically, DA aims to solve the covariate shift between the source domain and target domain. A popular representation learning approach named domain-adversarial neural networks (DANN) was proposed by setting a domain discriminator to confuse domain features in an indiscriminate mechanism [5]. In histopathological image analysis, DANN was applied to organ-level, slide-level [11] and patient-level domains [7]. Similarly, adversarial discriminative domain adaptation (ADDA) [22] is achieved by replacing the weight-shared backbone with exclusive domain-specific encoders, which was introduced into the quality assessment task of fundus images [18]. Besides, some studies implemented unsupervised DA by utilizing generative adversarial networks in liver segmentation [31], microscopy image quantification [27] and diabetic retinopathy detection [30]. Yet, since the model is barely trained on the source domain and target domain, the performance is flawed on unseen domains.

To achieve a desirable generalization performance, data augmentation is an intuitive strategy. For instance, adversarial samples are generated by adaptive data augmentation and deep-stacked transformation in [24] and [33], respectively. Nevertheless, model convergence could be influenced by the generated unrealistic data. Instead, some researchers studied DG with learning domain-agnostic representations. Albuquerque et al. improve generalization by minimizing discrepancies of the pairwise domain [1]. Sikaroudi et al. utilize meta-learning to train a magnification-agnostic histopathology image classification model [19]. Mahajan et al. give a causal interpretation to DG and generalize based on invariant representations [13]. The works above achieved optimistic results on data from unseen domains whereas there are still some non-negligible limitations. First of all, DANN-based methods could not function well with limited data in the source domain. What's more, some studies are not applicable when certain categories do not exist overall training domains.

Based on this, we present a novel DG approach for nucleus recognition in Ki67 immunohistochemistry stained images. The proposed method transforms DG into a domain-agnostic subnetwork searching problem. Invariant representations are learned by iteratively pruning domain-specific model parameters under a domain merging scenario. Moreover, the pruned model is fine-tuned on merged domains, which solves the class mismatch problem to some extent. Furthermore, the appropriate implementation is achieved by applying our pruning method in different modules of the nucleus recognition framework. Compared with the state-of-the-art (SOTA) methods in the Ki67 IHC image and public data set, our method achieves competitive performance in the unseen domains.

2   Methods

2.1   Overview

Motivation. The lottery ticket hypothesis [4] claims only a subset of parameters account for model performance in an over-parameterized neural network. Without any degradation of performance, the subnetwork compression can be still achieved by iteratively pruning trivial parameters. Under some circumstances, the model may not generalize well to unseen domains because of overfitting on domain-specific representations. Consequently, DG could be considered as a domain-agnostic subnetwork searching problem, which keeps domain-agnostic parameters while pruning domain-specific parameters.

Workflow. The proposed prune-based DG framework is illustrated in Fig. 1. Initially, parameters W are obtained by the convergent model (Model-S) trained on a single domain. When training in merged domains, model gradients are collected and sorted globally by their magnitude after the loss backpropagation. Subsequently the subset of W will be achieved by pruning weights with the top $p\%$ gradient magnitude and resetting the remaining parameters without updating in W by iterating n times. Finally, the pruned model (Model-M) will be fine-tuned in merged domains.

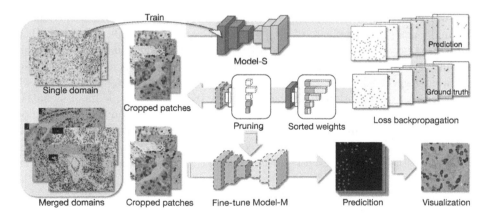

Fig. 1. A workflow of prune-based generalization. We use model-S and model-M to represent the model converged on a single domain and model pruned on merged domains.

2.2   Pruning-Based Algorithm

Our method aims to filter out a fraction of parameters that the remaining parameters W' could preserve the accuracy on the training domains while performing well on the unseen domain(s). To achieve this goal, we construct a domain merging scenario. That is, the model is firstly trained on a single source domain. After it is converged, we replace the training data with merged domains, which contain the source domain and domain(s) never seen before. For the latter, we denote it as invasion domain(s). Under this scenario, the target problem corresponds to the optimization as follows.

$$W^* = \underset{W' \subseteq W}{\arg\min} |C(D_s|W') - C(D_s|W)| + C(D_i|W'), \tag{1}$$

where D_s and D_i are samples from the source domain and invasion domains respectively, W^* is the expected W', and W denotes the parameters trained on D_s. The cost $C(D|W)$ was computed on samples of D under parameters W. Generally, $C(D_s|W')$ of pruned model is larger than $C(D_s|W)$. The Eq. 1 can be simplified as follows:

$$W^* = \underset{W' \subseteq W}{\arg\min} C(D_m|W') - C(D_s|W), \text{ where } D_m = \{D_s, D_i\}, \tag{2}$$

D_m represents a batch of merged samples that consist of D_s and D_i. Subsequently, the second term of Eq. 2 has no contribution to the selection of W thus can be removed, and the optimization of W' can be defined as Eq. 3,

$$W^* = \underset{W' \subseteq W}{\arg\min} C(D_m|W'). \tag{3}$$

The above subnetwork searching problem can be solved by exploring the contribution of each parameter w to $C(D_m|W)$. More concretely, while trained on D_m, model parameters W are updated through loss backpropagation according to the gradient descent. In this procedure, gradients are calculated as derivatives of the cost with respect to W as $g = \partial C(D_m|W)/\partial W$. Correspondingly, the gradient magnitude $|g|$ of the individual parameter $w \in W$ can be regarded as its contribution to $C(D_m|W)$. Intuitively, model convergence depends on the updating of the parameters. Parameters requiring a large variation to fit on merged domains can be considered highly domain-related. The expected remaining parameters W^* can be approximated by preserving parameters with a relatively small $|g|$ as Eq. 4,

$$W_r = \begin{cases} w_i, & \text{if } g_i \leq c_p \\ 0, & \text{otherwise} \end{cases}, \tag{4}$$

where c_p is a scalar related to remaining percentage p of parameters.

Generally, a rather small pruning rate is set for preventing performance degradation by using a large pruning rate. Moreover, the same setting as [4] is adopted through iterative training and pruning followed by resetting the remaining parameters over n steps with each step prunes $p^{\frac{1}{n}}\%$ of the surviving parameters. A few iterations of model pruning is usually enough, therefore a small amount of merged data is enough in the pruning procedure. Although the pruned model suffers degraded performance, it is provided with the potentiality of learning domain-invariant representations. Finally, further fine-tuning is applied to surviving parameters on merged domains for recovering accuracy.

3   Experiments

3.1   Nucleus Recognition

Ki67 Dataset. All Ki67 IHC images were collected under magnification 40× and resolution 1920 × 1080 from 16 domains through data anonymization. Nuclei of each slice were annotated by certified pathologists in seven categories: negative fibroblasts, negative lymphocyte, negative tumor cell, positive fibroblasts, positive lymphocyte, positive tumor cell and other cells. The data set was built under the mismatched categories in different domains as shown in Table.1.

Table 1. Properties of different domains in Ki67 data set

Properties	Merged training domains		Testing unseen domains
	D1	D2	
No. of images	95	51	41
No. of categories	7	5	4,5,7
Neuclei count	35,948	35,948	35,948
Radius of cells	4–6 pixel	7–12 pixel	5–14 pixel
Type of tumor	Breast	Breast	Breast, cervix, pancreas, urethra
Hue	Partial blue	Partial orange	Partial violet, brown red, yellow green

Settings and Implementations. Nucleus recognition was formulated to a structured regression problem by implementing a weakly supervised segmentation [28]. The ground truth mask is a set of continuous-valued proximity maps ranging from 0 to 1, generated by applying a 2D Gaussian filter on the annotations. Image patches are randomly cropped with resolution 512 × 512 and fed into the variant of Albunet (U-Net [16] with ResNet34 [8] pre-trained on ImageNet as the encoder). The model was trained by Adam optimizer under the sum of cross-entropy loss and IOU loss with adjusted hyper-parameters: batch size 8, iterations 500, initial learning rate 5×10^{-4} with gradually decreasing after every 100 epochs. Our base model was pre-trained on D1 and pruned on the merged domain (D1 and D2) with pruning ratio 10^{-4}, prune-reset iterations 4. Besides, an ablation experiment was arranged to observe the effect of pruning, which intervened the encoder, the decoder and all modules under the same pruning rate. In addition, data augmentation was also adopted including random rotation, crop, flip, mirroring and color jitter. The optimal model could be selected if the accuracy no longer improved within 30 epochs. The final prediction was achieved by non-maximum suppression in the probability map.

Table 2. Nucleus Recognition DG results on unseen & merge domains of Ki67

Algorithm	Test (domains)	Detection				Classificaion		
		P	R	F1	$\mu \pm \sigma$	P	R	F1
ERM	merge	**86.86**	**85.70**	**86.28**	5.59 ± 3.17	**86.68**	82.78	83.97
	unseen	89.56	82.92	86.11	5.63 ± 3.02	90.45	87.65	88.35
ERM-F	merge	85.22	83.53	84.37	5.70 ± 3.15	84.43	84.10	84.19
	unseen	88.66	81.75	85.06	5.59 ± 2.99	90.99	88.57	89.38
DANN [5]	merge	75.43	80.90	78.07	5.89 ± 3.36	77.63	72.16	74.09
	unseen	81.73	78.94	80.31	5.76 ± 3.19	86.84	68.31	74.77
Adv-Aug [24]	merge	80.53	60.65	69.19	6.39 ± 3.47	69.45	76.40	72.45
	unseen	**90.88**	61.92	73.66	5.64 ± 3.07	88.17	**90.69**	89.14
Ours-Encoder	merge	85.30	85.76	85.53	5.57 ± 3.17	84.93	84.24	84.39
	unseen	89.26	83.11	86.08	5.51 ± 3.01	**91.81**	89.03	89.72
Ours-Decoder	merge	84.86	84.96	84.91	**5.53 ± 3.17**	84.85	82.81	83.52
	unseen	87.99	83.01	85.43	**5.45 ± 3.02**	91.37	87.82	88.89
Ours-All	merge	85.95	85.19	85.57	5.57 ± 3.15	86.43	**85.25**	**85.70**
	unseen	88.83	**84.67**	**86.46**	5.54 ± 3.02	91.04	89.42	**89.91**

Evaluation. The results were evaluated on precision, recall and F1-score under the two tasks as follows. The final score is averaged over 41 cases.

- Detection. Hungarian matching algorithm [10] was applied to the predictions and annotations under the valid area with a radius of 16 pixels to calculate true positive (TP), false positive (FP) and false negative (FN). The average distance μ and standard deviation σ of paired results were computed as an additional indicator.
- Classification. The pair-wise results in detection were further assessed according to whether their categories are matched using metrics in [20].

The competitive methods and results were shown in Table 2. We take ERM-F(trained and fine-tuned the same as our method but without pruning) as a reference to guarantee the improvement is not gained from fine-tuning. Moreover, DANN[5] was implemented by embedding a domain discriminator following the model encoder. Adv-Aug[24] was adjusted with the adversarial learning rate ranging from 0 to 10^5, step 10.

Results and Discussions. Nucleus Recognition results are shown in Table 2. 'Merge' and 'unseen' represent domains participating in training and never involved in training, respectively. 'Ours-Encoder' and 'Ours-Decoder' denote applying the pruning method only on the 'encoder' and 'decoder' modules. Our method exhibits the best comprehensive performance on merged domains and unseen domains. Considering the performance on unseen domains, metrics of recall and F1-score show competitive results of our method on both nucleus detection and classification. Particularly, the proposed method improve the detection F1-score by 0.35% for ERM and 1.40% for ERM-F and for nuclues classification our method outperforms ERM and ERM-F in terms of F1-score by 1.56% and 0.53%, respectively. On merge domains, the proposed method slightly under-performs the ERM algorithm in nucleus detection. Such performance degradation is reasonable. Because ERM, with limited generalization, tends to over-fit on domain-specific features which may help with the accuracy of merge domains. Even so, our methods surpass ERM and ERM-F by a non-trivial margin of 1.73% and 1.51%(F1-score), respectively on merge domains in classification.

It is worth noting that DANN shows rather worse metrics than ERM in our experiment, which indicates its vulnerability in coping with the class mismatching problem both on merged domains and the generalization on unseen domains. The expected effect of Adv-Aug is marginal on unseen domains because of the complexity of histopathological images. It is observed that model training interferes with the generated unrealistic images. The above two methods utilize adversarial mechanisms for the expansion of available domains, whose limitation appears when only a small number of domains is available for training. On the contrary, our pruning method attempts to learn the domain-agnostic representations by preventing the model's over-fitting on training domains.

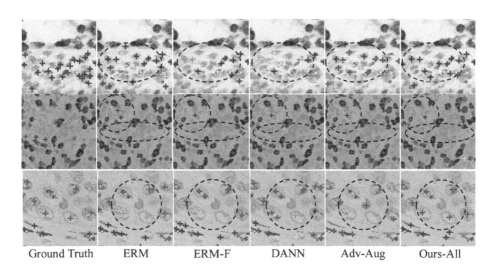

| Ground Truth | ERM | ERM-F | DANN | Adv-Aug | Ours-All |

Fig. 2. Comparison of nuclei detection and classification with different methods (Color figure online)

Figure 2 shows representative Ki67 recognition results of the above methods in three distinct domains for comparison. Blue, yellow, green, red and violet represent negative fibroblasts, negative lymphocytes, negative tumor cells, positive tumor cells and other cells. The remaining two categories do not show up in these cases. Areas with a significant difference among methods are highlighted with black dash ellipses. Compared with other approaches, the proposed method produces relatively better results in classification (case 1, 3 in row 1 and 3) and detection (case 2 in row 2). To be specific, in case 1, our method shows competitive classification results given the mixture of negative tumors, negative fibroblasts and other cells. The improvements of detection are also noticeable in case 2 even though the color of negative tumor cells is too shallow to be figured out. Case 3 further shows the robustness of our method on hollow cells.

The ablation experiment explores the pruning availability in different modules. Generally, pruning on all modules achieves the best performance. This can be caused by the remaining percentage of parameters within each layer. It was observed that the proportion of remaining parameters has a wide variance in different network depths although pruned with a tiny rate. The Decoder-only approach prunes the final layer to a large sparsity (70% − 80%) and Encoder-only reserves 30% − 50% parameters for shallow layers. By contrast, pruning on all modules preserves 40% − 50% parameters for the final layer and 40% − 60% parameters for the shallow layers. All evaluations illustrate the importance of allocating parameters to prune in a balanced manner.

3.2 PACS Classificaion

Table 3. Domain generalization on PACS, Model selection: oracle

Algorithm	Art	Cartoon	Photo	Sketch	Average
ERM [23]	**87.42** ± 0.4	82.56 ± 0.6	96.73 ± 0.4	80.02 ± 0.6	86.68
IRM [2]	86.37 ± 0.8	80.12 ± 1.2	97.24 ± 0.4	76.38 ± 1.1	85.02
DRO [17]	87.53 ± 0.7	81.74 ± 0.7	**97.61** ± 0.2	79.80 ± 0.8	86.67
MLDG [12]	87.17 ± 0.8	81.35 ± 1.4	97.36 ± 0.4	80.94 ± 1.0	86.71
DANN [5]	86.52 ± 1.2	80.25 ± 1.1	97.58 ± 0.2	77.26 ± 1.2	85.40
CORAL [21]	87.21 ± 0.6	82.16 ± 0.4	97.52 ± 0.1	80.01 ± 0.3	86.77
Ours	85.33 ± 0.5	**84.83** ± 0.6	96.11 ± 0.4	**83.95** ± 0.2	**87.56**

PACS (photo, art painting, cartoon, sketches) classification benchmark was also introduced to evaluate our method with ResNet50 backbone on test domains validation set (oracle) [6]. The results are shown in Table. 3. is the maximum value over 3 experiments, and within each experiment, the source domain and the invasion domain are arranged alternately in a ratio of 1:2. It is observed that our method boosts the performance on the sketches domain, outperforming the SOTA methods by 3.01%. The proposed method also surpasses other approaches on the domain of cartoon by a margin of 2.27%. Note that skeletons in sketches and contours in cartoons are cross-domain structural information. Therefore, the above results could well demonstrate the effectiveness of our approach in learning domain-agnostic representations. The potential reason for our mediocre results on the photos might be the pruning method is applied on the model pre-trained on the photo domain (ImageNet). Consequently, the corresponding results are biased and have limited reference value. In addition, the factor that leads to our imperfect performance is probably the huge variance between the art painting domain and other domains. Even so, our method still achieves the best performance in the average accuracy.

4 Conclusion

In this paper, we propose a novel DG method based on subnetwork searching, which generalizes the model by discarding the domain-specific representations and reserving the invariant representations in a domain merging scenario. Our method attempts to solve practical limitations of DG including the insufficient number of domains and the class mismatching problem cross domains. Competitive results demonstrate our method's superiority and robustness on multi-class nucleus recognition in Ki67 IHC images. In addition, the proposed method achieves good performance by effectively learning generic representations the on PACS classification benchmark.

References

1. Albuquerque, I., Monteiro, J., Darvishi, M., Falk, T.H., Mitliagkas, I.: Generalizing to unseen domains via distribution matching. arXiv preprint arXiv:1911.00804 (2019)
2. Arjovsky, M., Bottou, L., Gulrajani, I., Lopez-Paz, D.: Invariant risk minimization. arXiv preprint arXiv:1907.02893 (2019)
3. Focke, C.M., et al.: Interlaboratory variability of ki67 staining in breast cancer. Eur. J. Cancer **84**, 219–227 (2017)
4. Frankle, J., Carbin, M.: The lottery ticket hypothesis: finding sparse, trainable neural networks. arXiv preprint arXiv:1803.03635 (2018)
5. Ganin, Y., et al.: Domain-adversarial training of neural networks. J. Mach. Learn. Res. **17**(1), 2030–2096 (2016)
6. Gulrajani, I., Lopez-Paz, D.: In search of lost domain generalization. arXiv preprint arXiv:2007.01434 (2020)
7. Hashimoto, N., et al.: Multi-scale domain-adversarial multiple-instance CNN for cancer subtype classification with unannotated histopathological images. In: Proceedings of the IEEE/CVF Conference on Computer Vision and Pattern Recognition, pp. 3852–3861 (2020)
8. He, K., Zhang, X., Ren, S., Sun, J.: Deep residual learning for image recognition. In: Proceedings of the IEEE Conference on Computer Vision and Pattern Recognition, pp. 770–778 (2016)
9. Klöppel, G., La Rosa, S.: Ki67 labeling index: assessment and prognostic role in gastroenteropancreatic neuroendocrine neoplasms. Virchows Arch. **472**(3), 341–349 (2018)
10. Kuhn, H.W.: The hungarian method for the assignment problem. Naval Res. Logistics Q. **2**(1–2), 83–97 (1955)
11. Lafarge, M.W., Pluim, J.P., Eppenhof, K.A., Veta, M.: Learning domain-invariant representations of histological images. Front. Med. **6**, 162 (2019)

12. Li, D., Yang, Y., Song, Y.Z., Hospedales, T.: Learning to generalize: meta-learning for domain generalization. In: Proceedings of the AAAI Conference on Artificial Intelligence, vol. 32 (2018)
13. Mahajan, D., Tople, S., Sharma, A.: Domain generalization using causal matching. arXiv preprint arXiv:2006.07500 (2020)
14. Reis-Filho, J.S., Davidson, N.E.: Ki67 assessment in breast cancer: are we there yet?. JNCI: J. Natl. Cancer Inst. (2020)
15. Rimm, D.L., et al.: An international multicenter study to evaluate reproducibility of automated scoring for assessment of ki67 in breast cancer. Mod. Pathol. **32**(1), 59–69 (2019)
16. Ronneberger, O., Fischer, P., Brox, T.: U-Net: convolutional networks for biomedical image segmentation. In: Navab, N., Hornegger, J., Wells, W.M., Frangi, A.F. (eds.) MICCAI 2015. LNCS, vol. 9351, pp. 234–241. Springer, Cham (2015). https://doi.org/10.1007/978-3-319-24574-4_28
17. Sagawa, S., Koh, P.W., Hashimoto, T.B., Liang, P.: Distributionally robust neural networks for group shifts: On the importance of regularization for worst-case generalization. arXiv preprint arXiv:1911.08731 (2019)
18. Shem, Y., et al.: Domain-invariant interpretable fundus image quality assessment. Med. Image Anal. **61**, 101654 (2020)
19. Sikaroudi, M., Ghojogh, B., Karray, F., Crowley, M., Tizhoosh, H.: Magnification generalization for histopathology image embedding. arXiv preprint arXiv:2101.07757 (2021)
20. Sirinukunwattana, K., Raza, S.E.A., Tsang, Y.W., Snead, D.R., Cree, I.A., Rajpoot, N.M.: Locality sensitive deep learning for detection and classification of nuclei in routine colon cancer histology images. IEEE Trans. Med. Imaging **35**(5), 1196–1206 (2016)
21. Sun, B., Saenko, K.: Deep CORAL: correlation alignment for deep domain adaptation. In: Hua, G., Jégou, H. (eds.) ECCV 2016. LNCS, vol. 9915, pp. 443–450. Springer, Cham (2016). https://doi.org/10.1007/978-3-319-49409-8_35
22. Tzeng, E., Hoffman, J., Saenko, K., Darrell, T.: Adversarial discriminative domain adaptation. In: Proceedings of the IEEE Conference on Computer Vision and Pattern Recognition, pp. 7167–7176 (2017)
23. Vapnik, V.N.: An overview of statistical learning theory. IEEE Trans. Neural Netw. **10**(5), 988–999 (1999)
24. Volpi, R., Namkoong, H., Sener, O., Duchi, J., Murino, V., Savarese, S.: Generalizing to unseen domains via adversarial data augmentation. arXiv preprint arXiv:1805.12018 (2018)
25. Volynskaya, Z., Mete, O., Pakbaz, S., Al-Ghamdi, D., Asa, S.L.: Ki67 quantitative interpretation: insights using image analysis. J. Pathol. Inf. **10** (2019)
26. Xie, Y., Xing, F., Shi, X., Kong, X., Su, H., Yang, L.: Efficient and robust cell detection: a structured regression approach. Med. Image Anal. **44**, 245–254 (2018)
27. Xing, F., Bennett, T., Ghosh, D.: Adversarial domain adaptation and pseudo-labeling for cross-modality microscopy image quantification. In: Shen, D. (ed.) MICCAI 2019. LNCS, vol. 11764, pp. 740–749. Springer, Cham (2019). https://doi.org/10.1007/978-3-030-32239-7_82
28. Xing, F., Cornish, T.C., Bennett, T., Ghosh, D., Yang, L.: Pixel-to-pixel learning with weak supervision for single-stage nucleus recognition in ki67 images. IEEE Trans. Biomed. Eng. **66**(11), 3088–3097 (2019)
29. Yang, C., et al.: Ki67 targeted strategies for cancer therapy. Clin. Transl. Oncol. **20**(5), 570–575 (2018)

30. Yang, D., Yang, Y., Huang, T., Wu, B., Wang, L., Xu, Yanwu: Residual-cyclegan based camera adaptation for robust diabetic retinopathy screening. In: Martel, A.L. (ed.) MICCAI 2020. LNCS, vol. 12262, pp. 464–474. Springer, Cham (2020). https://doi.org/10.1007/978-3-030-59713-9_45

31. Yang, J., Dvornek, N.C., Zhang, F., Chapiro, J., Lin, M., Duncan, J.S.: Unsupervised domain adaptation via disentangled representations: application to cross-modality liver segmentation. In: Shen, D. (ed.) MICCAI 2019. LNCS, vol. 11765, pp. 255–263. Springer, Cham (2019). https://doi.org/10.1007/978-3-030-32245-8_29

32. Yerushalmi, R., Woods, R., Ravdin, P.M., Hayes, M.M., Gelmon, K.A.: Ki67 in breast cancer: prognostic and predictive potential. Lancet Oncol. **11**(2), 174–183 (2010)

33. Zhang, L., et al.: Generalizing deep learning for medical image segmentation to unseen domains via deep stacked transformation. IEEE Trans. Med. Imaging **39**(7), 2531–2540 (2020)

Cells are Actors: Social Network Analysis with Classical ML for SOTA Histology Image Classification

Neda Zamanitajeddin[(✉)], Mostafa Jahanifar, and Nasir Rajpoot

Tissue Image Analytics Centre, Department of Computer Science, University of Warwick, Coventry, UK
neda.zamanitajeddin@warwick.ac.uk

Abstract. Digitization of histology images and the advent of new computational methods, like deep learning, have helped the automatic grading of colorectal adenocarcinoma cancer (CRA). Present automated CRA grading methods, however, usually use tiny image patches and thus fail to integrate the entire tissue micro-architecture for grading purposes. To tackle these challenges, we propose to use a statistical network analysis method to describe the complex structure of the tissue micro-environment by modelling nuclei and their connections as a network. We show that by analyzing only the interactions between the cells in a network, we can extract highly discriminative statistical features for CRA grading. Unlike other deep learning or convolutional graph-based approaches, our method is highly scalable (can be used for cell networks consist of millions of nodes), completely explainable, and computationally inexpensive. We create cell networks on a broad CRC histology image dataset, experiment with our method, and report state-of-the-art performance for the prediction of three-class CRA grading.

Keywords: Social network analysis · Computational pathology · Histopathological graph · Colorectal cancer grading

1 Introduction

With the advances of digital pathology and the advent of sophisticated computerized methods (like deep learning), achieving reliable computer-assisted diagnostic systems for pathology applications has become conceivable. Many automatic approaches have been introduced in the literature to work with large histology images also known as the Whole Slide Images (or WSIs) for automatic cancer diagnosis or patient prognosis [1–5], most of which rely on convolutional neural networks (CNN) [6]. Most existing methods are unable to handle large WSI and often follow a patch prediction paradigm, where the WSI is divided into small patches for CNN based prediction and finally all predictions are aggregated to achieve the final decision. In this paradigm, critical contextual information from the larger field of view (FOV) in WSIs can be lost. Recent works on context-aware CNNs have aimed at addressing that problem by processing multi-scale fields of view (FOVs) [7, 8]. However, those methods are still bounded by the GPU memory limitation.

© Springer Nature Switzerland AG 2021
M. de Bruijne et al. (Eds.): MICCAI 2021, LNCS 12908, pp. 288–298, 2021.
https://doi.org/10.1007/978-3-030-87237-3_28

Lack of interpretability is another limitation faced by deep CNN features. In particular, the connection of deep CNN features with tissue morphology or structure of pathology primitives in a histology image is unknown. To avoid these shortcomings, methods based on graph theory have been proposed in the area of computational pathology where the histology primitives (nuclei, glands, etc.) and their interactions are modelled as a graph [9–12]. For example, Javed et al. [11, 13] showed that constructing graphs of histology image patches and finding cell communities in the graphs can be used to classify tissue phenotypes. However, in these works, it is unclear how to choose and integrate graph-level features to better reflect the diverse arrangement of cells in various tissue components. Zhou et al. [14] proposed a sophisticated Graph Convolutional Network (GCN) based approach, called CGC-Net, for histology image classification which can automatically extract features from histology graphs, classify them, and achieve state-of-the-art performance. Although CGC-Net can accept larger contextual patches than CNNs, it is a computationally expensive method, the GCN features lack interpretability and are still restricted by the GPU memory size.

In this paper, we propose to tackle these problems and approach the classification of histology images using a novel social network analysis (SNA) paradigm [15]. Cell graphs from WSIs may contain millions of nodes, edges (connections) and cellular communities which contain diagnostically relevant information about tissue micro-environment that may be difficult to quantify by visual inspection. In this work, we incorporate SNA measures to translate the raw information of cell-to-cell connections in cell graphs into perceivable and interpretable features that can help distinguishing tissue phenotypes or highlight the biological significance of tissue regions. We propose three different approaches to utilize SNA measures as features in a classical machine learning setting for automatic image-level Colorectal Adenocarcinoma (CRA) grading from patch-level cell graphs, achieving state-of-the-art performance. Our approach does not rely on precise nuclei segmentation or feature extraction as it extracts information from the cell network by investigating only cell-cell connections and encoding spatial relationships between cells. It is computationally efficient and is not bounded by GPU memory, which makes it easily scalable.

To the best of our knowledge, this is the first study that proposes the analysis of histology images using SNA measures for automatic CRA grading, demonstrating the role of cells and cellular communities as actors. The rest of the paper is organized as follows. In Sect. 2, we describe details of the proposed methodology, afterwards, results of applying our method on a CRA grading dataset are reported and discussed in Sect. 3. Finally, we conclude the paper with a summary of our findings and future directions.

2   Materials and Methods

In this section, we will describe our proposed method of using social network analysis techniques for the classification of colorectal cancer (CRC) into three CRA degrees. First, we will describe the cell social networks construction. Then, utilized social network analysis (SNA) measures are introduced. Afterwards, statistical tools are employed to abstract the representation of SNA measures into relatively low-dimensional feature vectors. Finally, three different scenarios are proposed to aggregate patch-level information into the image-level prediction of CRA grade. A schematic overview of these steps is shown in Fig. 1. The following subsections describe these steps in more detail.

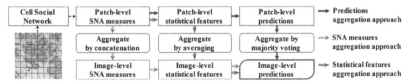

Fig. 1. Overview of the proposed SNA paradigm for image-level prediction.

2.1 Data

The proposed method is tested on the CRC dataset [16], consisting of 139 images with an average size of 4548×7520 taken from WSIs captured at $20\times$ magnification related to 38 patients. Two experienced pathologists classified all images into normal (#71 Grade 1), low-grade (#33 Grade 2), and high-grade (#35 Grade 3) categories for CRA grading based on glandular morphology. To fairly compare the performance of the proposed SNA based features with CNN and CGC based features, like [7, 14], we split the dataset into three folds and extract large patches of 1792×1792 pixels to be used for cell network construction.

2.2 Cell Social Network

Our approach relies on building a meaningful network (graph) from a histology image that represents the possible cell-to-cell interactions. For such a graph $G = (V, E)$, we can consider nuclei as network nodes (V) and their potential interactions as network edges (E). Therefore, we follow these two steps to construct cell networks for each patch in the dataset: 1) node identification by nuclear instance segmentation and 2) finding the network's edge configuration.

Node Identification. For the sake of comparison fairness, we utilize CIA-Net [17] for nuclei instance segmentation similar to Zhou et al. [14]. However, unlike [14], our approach does not need precise nuclei segmentation because we do not include nuclear appearance features in our cell network. Therefore, detecting the centroid position of each nucleus [18] would suffice. Also, there is no need for nuclei sampling because our approach is not restricted to computationally extensive CGNs.

Edge Configuration. Hypothesizing that close cells in a histology sample are more likely to interact with each other, we consider an edge between two nuclei if their Euclidean distance is smaller than a specific radius. Also, we bound the number of edges to the k-nearest neighbours to avoid over-connecting a node. In other words, the adjacency matrix for nodes i, j is $A_{ij} = 1$ if their Euclidean distance is smaller than a radius $D(i, j) < r$, and if j belongs to the k-nearest neighbours of node i.

2.3 SNA Measures

Raw data from a large cell network is not easily understandable. Assuming that cells are social actors in the tumour micro-environment, we extract several measures from the social network analysis (SNA) discipline [15, 19], as listed below.

Node Degree (NDe). Node degree $\deg(v_i)$ of node v_i in graph $G = (V, E)$ is simply the number of edges connected to that node. For instance, in a cell social network, a cell's degree is the number of cells it is directly connected to.

Clustering Coefficient (CCo). This is defined as the fraction of the possible triangles that occur across a node: $CCo_v = 2\mathrm{Tri}(v)/(\deg(v)(\deg(v)-1))$ which quantifies the density of triangles $\mathrm{Tri}(v)$ in a network. In a social network of cells, the clustering coefficient measures how many cells in the graph tend to cluster together.

Closeness Centrality (CC). In a network with N nodes, the closeness centrality of a node v_i is reciprocal of the average of the shortest-path distances, $d(.,.)$ between node v_i and all other nodes in the network: $CC(v_i) = (N - 1)/\sum_{j, j \neq i} d(v_i, v_j)$. Closeness centrality highlights nodes that can easily access other nodes. In cell social network analogy, a cell with higher closeness centrality is closer to all other cells.

Degree Centrality (DC). This is the simplest centrality defined for a network which is calculated by normalizing the node degree: $DC(v_i) = \sum_{j=1}^{N} A_{ij}/(N - 1)$. In comparison to node degree, network size information is embedded in this measure.

Betweenness Centrality (BC). For node v, $BC(v) = \sum_{s,t \in V} \sigma(s, t|v)/\sigma(s, t)$ is the betweenness centrality in which $\sigma(s, t)$ is the total number of shortest paths from node s to node t and $\sigma(s, t|v)$ is the number of those paths that pass through v. BC can highlight nodes that act as bridges connecting two parts of a network. Interpretation of this measure in cell social network depends on the clinical application, however, in some cell graphs, BC does not show significant importance [20].

Eigen Vector Centrality (EVC). This centrality measures the influence of a node in the network. EVC is an extension of degree centrality in which the score of each node is calculated based on the scores of its neighbouring nodes. Therefore, a node in the network can have a high EVC score if it is connected to either many nodes or some nodes with high degrees. The eigenvector centrality for node i is x_i, $x_i = \lambda^{-1} \sum_j A_{ij} x_j$ where A is network adjacency matrix with eigenvalue of λ [15]. EVC in cell social network highlights the cells which hold wide-reaching influence in the network.

Katz Centrality (KC). Similar to EVC, Katz centrality is a generalization of degree centrality where all connected neighbouring nodes, immediate or distant, are taken into consideration when calculating each node's centrality score [21]. In KC every neighbouring node will be assigned an initial constant centrality β, and contributions of distant nodes are penalized with attenuation factor α, as in $x_i = \alpha \sum_j A_{ij} x_j + \beta_i$.

2.4 SNA-Based Statistical Features

We extract statistical features from each SNA measure of a cell network to represent that network with a relatively low-dimensional fixed-size feature vector. For each cell social network, we find the distribution of values of every SNA measure by calculating their histogram and then concatenate the resulting histogram counts and bins alongside with maximum, mean, and standard deviation of those values to build the feature vector. In total, we extract 180 features from all SNA measures for each cell network.

2.5 Generating Image-Level Prediction

We propose three approaches to aggregate patch-level information for image-level predictions. A schematic overview of these three approaches is shown in Fig. 1.

Predictions Aggregation. We train an SVM [22] on statistical feature vectors extracted from patch-level cell networks. Having patch-level predictions, majority voting is utilized to aggregate them into the final image-level label.

Network Measure Aggregation. In this approach, we aggregate SNA measures for all patches of an image by simply concatenating them to form the image-level SNA measures. Having these, we extract statistical features for each image as described in Sect. 2.4 and they can be used to train an SVM model for image-level classification.

Statistical Feature Aggregation. Here, we average patch-level statistical features of the patch-level SNA measures over patches belonging to each image.

To avoid overfitting and choosing the optimal subset of features, we incorporated sequential features selection (SFS) [23]. In all experiments, we used an SVM classifier [22] with an RBF kernel. Also, SVM training and evaluation are done in a 3-fold cross-validation framework similar to [7, 14] for a fair comparison.

3 Results and Discussions

3.1 Feature Selection for CRA Grade Prediction

In this section, we report the image-level accuracy of classifying the CRC dataset [16] in three CRA grades. In Table 1, the results of cross-validation experiments using different methods are reported in which the last three rows correspond to proposed methods in the current work. Utilizing social network analysis techniques, we achieve an image-level accuracy of 96.27%, 97.8%, and 99.24% using patch-level predictions, network measures, and statistical features aggregation approaches, respectively, outperforming all other approaches in the literature by a large margin. Keep in mind that these values

Table 1. Performance comparison of different CRA grading methods.

Method	Acc %
BAM-entropy	90.66 ± 2.45
Context-G	89.96 ± 3.54
ResNet50	92.08 ± 2.08
CA-CNN	95.70 ± 3.04
CGC-Net	97.00 ± 1.10
Predictions agg.	96.27 ± 2.82
SNA measures agg.	97.80 ± 2.17
Statistical features agg.	**99.24 ± 1.31**

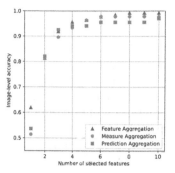

Fig. 2. Feature selection experiments for different aggregation approaches.

are achieved using only a handful of selected features from sequential feature selection experiments as illustrated in Fig. 2 for different aggregation scenarios. Furthermore, we observed that using a Random Forest classifier instead of SVM in the proposed framework would cause a decrease in performance, achieving the accuracy of 95.2%, 95.5%, 96.3% for patch prediction aggregation, SNA measures aggregation, and statistical features aggregation scenarios, respectively.

Some of the top-performing selected features are the number of nodes whose clustering coefficient attribute is in the range (0.4, 0.5) and range (0.9, 1), the number of nodes with node degree of 10 and 12, the number of nodes that have eigenvector centrality attribute less than 0.005, and the number of nodes that their closeness centrality attribute is less than 0.001. Our feature selection experiments show that there are always statistical features derived from clustering coefficient measures in the selected set in all scenarios whereas none of them has features related to Betweenness centrality. Having said that, discussing specific ranges from the distribution of SNA measures can be more intuitive and explain the biological significance of these measures (refer to Sects. 3.2 and 3.3).

In comparison with the baseline method, BAM [16], which is based on glandular morphology analysis, our best performing method gains over 8.52% accuracy. By comparing the results of predictions aggregation scenario with other methods that similarly use majority voting over patch-level predictions (Context-G [8], C A-CNN [7], and ResNet50 [24]), one can infer that patch-level statistical features extracted from SNA measures are very discriminative for CRA grading. On the other hand, using statistical feature aggregation can lead to better image-level performance (2.24% better than CGC-Net in accuracy). Moreover, our method can be easily scaled up to work directly on WSI-based cell networks, while methods like CGC-Net [14], CA-CNN [7] or any other deep learning-based models cannot abide by such tasks due to hardware limitation. This shows the effectiveness and efficiency of the proposed SNA based method.

We trained and tested the patch classifier model (in the first aggregation scenario) based on the labels of the large images whereas there are some regions (patches) in Grade 2, 3 samples that look normal and should be labelled as Grade 1. This noise in patch prediction refrains the model to learn optimal weights for image-level prediction. On the other hand, image-level classifiers in the other two aggregation methods are using information over the whole image area to predict a single label per image. The aggregation of information obviate the mentioned noise effect and leads to better results. Also, Table 1 suggests that local statistics of SNA measures are more important than statistics of global aggregation of SNA measures, as the statistical feature aggregation method performs better.

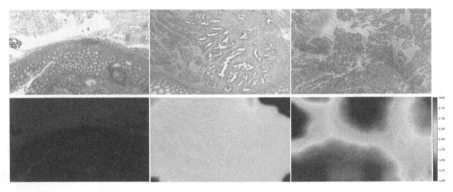

Fig. 3. Image-level prediction heatmap overlayed on images of three CRA grades (left to right: Grades 1, 2, and 3). The color bar indicates the estimated CRA grade score for regions.

The qualitative performance of the selected statistical features for identifying different tissue phenotypes in large histology images is also illustrated in Fig. 3. These saliency maps are generated by predicting labels for overlapping image patches. Although selected features are chosen based on image-level classification performance, samples in Fig. 3 show that these features can perform very well on patch-level classification and meaningfully detect different tissue phenotypes present in the image.

Table 2. Results of statistical comparison (*t*-test) experiments on SNA measure distributions.

CRA types	*p*-value						
	ND	*CCo*	*DC*	*BC*	*CC*	*EVC*	*KC*
Grade 1 vs. Grade 2	**0.01**	**0.003**	**0.0007**	0.1	**<1e-23**	**<7e-5**	**<4e-26**
Grade 1 vs. Grade 3	0.05	**0.006**	**<8e-5**	0.2	**<5e-9**	**0.0003**	1e-25
Grade 2 vs. Grade 3	0.2	**0.04**	**0.04**	0.3	**0.001**	**0.01**	**<8e-11**

3.2 Distributions of SNA Measures

To better represent the discriminative power of the proposed SNA-based statistical features, we investigate the difference in average distributions of various SNA measures over each CRA grade using the student's t-test. For each SNA measure, the t-test is done in a pairwise manner between three different grades (Grade 1 vs. Grade 2, Grade 1 vs. Grade 3, and Grade 2 vs. Grade 3) and results are summarized in Table 2. Values in Table 2 indicate that pairwise differences in distributions of most SNA measures over three grades are significantly different (p-value < 0.05), except for Betweenness Centrality (BC). This observation acknowledges that extracted statistical features from SNA measures are powerful enough for CRA grade discrimination. This is also visually verified by plotting the average distributions for "Katz Centrality", "Clustering Coefficient" and "Closeness Centrality" SNA measures in Fig. 4.

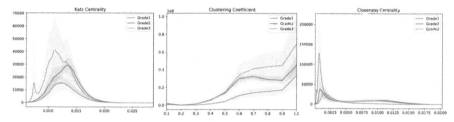

Fig. 4. Average distribution of three SNA measures from CRA samples in different grades.

3.3 Understanding the Biological Significance of SNA Measures

As mentioned above, high values of node clustering coefficient indicate that there is a more significant intra-cell interaction present in the network and nodes tend to create tightly knit groups which are usually due to hyper aggregation of nuclei in tumour regions. Therefore, the high number of nodes with a high value of clustering coefficient can indicate the presence of a high-grade CRA community in the tissue. This phenomenon is easily observable in Fig. 4 and the fourth row of Fig. 5, where nodes coloured based on the values of the SNA measure represented in that row.

Closeness centrality operates the exact opposite, where cells that are in a close-knit and dense community would be assigned smaller values because the average short-path distance increases throughout the network with the increased number of cells. Therefore, in Grade 3 phenotypes we would have a large number of cells with low closeness centrality and we expect that distribution of this SNA measure for high-grade cases be higher around small closeness values, as depicted in Fig. 4 and the third row and last column of Fig. 5. Stroma and non-mucosa regions are visibly differentiable in Grade 1 samples, based on closeness centrality in Fig. 5 while in Grade 3, the ***tumour-stromal interface*** seems segmentable based on this measure. Also, it is obvious in the second row of Fig. 5 that Katz centrality can assign values to every node in the network by considering the degrees of all nodes, resulting in a visible difference in node measure values for different CRA grades. These examples show the power of SNA measures in highlighting the biological significance of every node in the cell network.

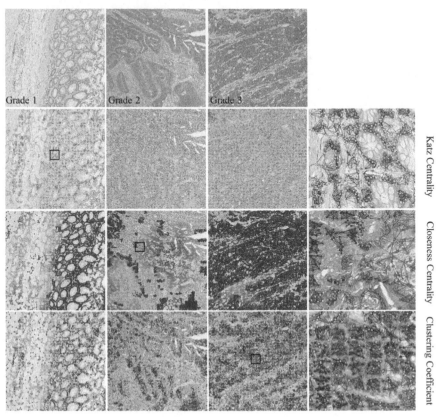

Fig. 5. Sample images from three CRA grades and their corresponding cell graphs overlaid on the original images. Color of each node is based on the values of 3 specific SNA measures with their minimum and maximum values shown in blue and red, respectively. Final column shows zoomed-in regions (shown as black squares) in one of the images for each of the grades. (Color figure online)

4   Conclusion

In this paper, we proposed to use social network analysis for histology image classification which relies only on the locations and interactions of cells. We showed how SNA measures can highlight the biological importance of cells and tissue regions in the histology image while their statistics significantly segregate between different types of CRA grades. We were able to achieve SOTA accuracy (99.24%) in CRA grading using only a handful of statistical features extracted from SNA measures. Being highly performant and non-reliant on GPUs (intensive computation), we believe that SNA based approaches hold promise for analyzing large cell networks and deserve further investigation for other cancer diagnosis or prognosis applications.

References

1. Bilal, M., et al.: Novel deep learning algorithm predicts the status of molecular pathways and key mutations in colorectal cancer from routine histology images. medRxiv (2021)
2. Koohbanani, N.A., et al.: NuClick: a deep learning framework for interactive segmentation of microscopic images. Med. Image Anal. **65**, 101771 (2020)
3. Koohbanani, N.A., et al.: Self-path: self-supervision for classification of pathology images with limited annotations (2020). https://arxiv.org/abs/2008.05571
4. Shapcott, M., Hewitt, K.J., Rajpoot, N.: Deep learning with sampling in colon cancer histology. Front. Bioeng. Biotechnol. **7**, 52 (2019)
5. Srinidhi, C.L., Ciga, O., Martel, A.L.: Deep neural network models for computational histopathology: a survey. Med. Image Anal. **67**, 101813 (2020)
6. LeCun, Y., Bengio, Y., Hinton, G.: Deep learning. Nature **521**(7553), 436–444 (2015)
7. Shaban, M., et al.: Context-aware convolutional neural network for grading of colorectal cancer histology images. IEEE Trans. Med. Imaging **39**(7), 2395–2405 (2020)
8. Sirinukunwattana, K., Alham, N.K., Verrill, C., Rittscher, J.: Improving whole slide segmentation through visual context - a systematic study. In: Frangi, A.F., Schnabel, J.A., Davatzikos, C., Alberola-López, C., Fichtinger, G. (eds.) MICCAI 2018. LNCS, vol. 11071, pp. 192–200. Springer, Cham (2018). https://doi.org/10.1007/978-3-030-00934-2_22
9. Bilgin, C.C., et al.: ECM-aware cell-graph mining for bone tissue modeling and classification. Data Min. Knowl. Disc. **20**(3), 416–438 (2010)
10. Demir, C., Gultekin, S.H., Yener, B.: Augmented cell-graphs for automated cancer diagnosis. Bioinformatics **21**(Suppl_2), ii7–ii12 (2005)
11. Javed, S., et al.: Cellular community detection for tissue phenotyping in colorectal cancer histology images. Med. Image Anal. **63**, 101696 (2020)
12. Sirinukunwattana, K., et al.: Novel digital signatures of tissue phenotypes for predicting distant metastasis in colorectal cancer. Sci. Rep. **8**(1), 1–13 (2018)
13. Javed, S., et al.: Multiplex cellular communities in multi-gigapixel colorectal cancer histology images for tissue phenotyping. IEEE Trans. Image Process. **29**, 9204–9219 (2020)
14. Zhou, Y., et al.: Cgc-net: Cell graph convolutional network for grading of colorectal cancer histology images. In: Proceedings of the IEEE/CVF International Conference on Computer Vision Workshops (2019)
15. Newman, M.: Networks. Oxford University Press, Oxford (2018)
16. Awan, R., et al.: Glandular morphometrics for objective grading of colorectal adenocarcinoma histology images. Sci. Rep. **7**(1), 1–12 (2017)
17. Zhou, Y., Onder, O.F., Dou, Q., Tsougenis, E., Chen, H., Heng, P.-A.: Cia-net: robust nuclei instance segmentation with contour-aware information aggregation. In: Chung, A.C.S., Gee, J.C., Yushkevich, P.A., Bao, S. (eds.) IPMI 2019. LNCS, vol. 11492, pp. 682–693. Springer, Cham (2019). https://doi.org/10.1007/978-3-030-20351-1_53
18. Raza, S.E.A., et al.: Deconvolving convolutional neural network for cell detection. In: 2019 IEEE 16th International Symposium on Biomedical Imaging (ISBI 2019). IEEE (2019)
19. Scott, J.: Social network analysis. Sociology **22**(1), 109–127 (1988)
20. Failmezger, H., et al.: Topological Tumor Graphs: a graph-based spatial model to infer stromal recruitment for immunosuppression in melanoma histology. Can. Res. **80**(5), 1199–1209 (2020)
21. Katz, L.: A new status index derived from sociometric analysis. Psychometrika **18**(1), 39–43 (1953)
22. Bishop, C.M.: Pattern Recognition and Machine Learning. Springer, New York (2006)

23. Jahanifar, M., Hasani, M., Khaleghi, S.J.: Automatic zone identification in blood smear images using optimal set of features. In: 2016 23rd Iranian Conference on Biomedical Engineering and 2016 1st International Iranian Conference on Biomedical Engineering (ICBME). IEEE (2016)
24. He, K., et al.: Deep residual learning for image recognition. In: Proceedings of the IEEE Conference on Computer Vision and Pattern Recognition (2016)

Instance-Based Vision Transformer for Subtyping of Papillary Renal Cell Carcinoma in Histopathological Image

Zeyu Gao[1,2], Bangyang Hong[1,2], Xianli Zhang[1,2], Yang Li[1,2], Chang Jia[1,2], Jialun Wu[1,2], Chunbao Wang[3], Deyu Meng[2,4], and Chen Li[1,2(✉)]

[1] School of Computer Science and Technology, Xi'an Jiaotong University, Xi'an 710049, Shaanxi, China
[2] National Engineering Lab for Big Data Analytics, Xi'an Jiaotong University, Xi'an 710049, Shaanxi, China
[3] Department of Pathology, The First Affiliated Hospital of Xi'an Jiaotong University, Xi'an 710061, China
[4] School of Mathematics and Statistics, Xi'an Jiaotong University, Xi'an 710049, Shaanxi, China

Abstract. Histological subtype of papillary (p) renal cellular and cell-layer level patterns almost cannot be captured by existing CNN-based models in large-size histopathological images, which brings obstacles to directly applying these models to such a fine-grained classification task. This paper proposes a novel instance-based Vision Transformer (i-ViT) to learn robust representations of histopathological images for the pRCC subtyping task by extracting finer features from instance patches (by cropping around segmented nuclei and assigning predicted grades). The proposed i-ViT takes top-K instances as the inputs and aggregates them for capturing both the cellular and cell-layer level patterns by a position-embedding layer, a grade-embedding layer, and a multi-head multi-layer self-attention module. To evaluate the performance of the proposed framework, experienced pathologists select 1162 regions of interest from 171 whole slide images of type 1 and type 2 pRCC. Experimental results show that the proposed method achieves better performance than existing CNN-based models with a significant margin.

Keywords: Fine-grained classification · Transformer · Histopathology

1 Introduction

Papillary renal cell carcinoma (pRCC) is the second common type of RCC, which accounts for 10% to 20% of all RCC cases [1]. The International Society of Urological Pathology (ISUP) system [2] and other researches [3–5] indicate that pRCC subtyping can provide valuable prognostic information. For example, according to different subtypes, different treatment strategies that aim to improve the patients' survival rate can be precisely conducted. Based on the

© Springer Nature Switzerland AG 2021
M. de Bruijne et al. (Eds.): MICCAI 2021, LNCS 12908, pp. 299–308, 2021.
https://doi.org/10.1007/978-3-030-87237-3_29

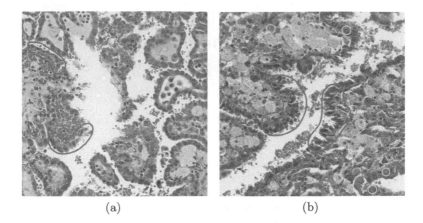

(a)   (b)

Fig. 1. An illustration of papillary renal cell carcinoma (a) type 1 and (b) type 2. Red outlines highlight the different papillary structures: (a) a single layer, and (b) pseudostratified cell layers. Green circles in (b) indicate some high-grade nuclei that exclusively exist in type 2. Note that all the areas marked by red outlines and green circles are relatively small and randomly distributed. (Color figure online)

histologic features, pRCC can be classified into two subtypes: type 1 and type 2 [6]. Type 1 composes of papillae covered with a single layer of small cells with low ISUP grade containing basophilic cytoplasm, while type 2 tumors have pseudostratified cells with high ISUP grade containing eosinophilic cytoplasm. However, subtyping of pRCC has poor clinical consistency, the diagnostic difference between experienced pathologists and TCGA is more than 35%, so it is necessary to design an automated subtyping model for pRCC.

As a fundamental task in digital pathology analysis, cancer subtyping has attracted much attention from researchers in the computer vision domain. Recently, several convolutional neural network (CNN)-based models have been proposed for cancers in different body locations, *e.g.*, breast [7], lung [8] and kidney [9]. The key point of these models is to identify the subtypes of these cancers according to certain histological features that can be easily extracted by CNN, such as the architectural pattern of tumors. In contrast, pRCC subtyping is a fine-grained classification task because type 1 and type 2 pRCC have similar architectural patterns (*i.e.*, papillary structure), which bring obstacle to apply existing models directly to the pRCC subtyping task.

In the pRCC pathology analysis routine, pathologists distinguish type 1 and type 2 pRCC mainly based on two fine features: the *cellular level* and the *cell-layer level* patterns (see Fig. 1 for detail). Unfortunately, it is almost impossible for traditional CNN-based models devised for small images or patches to capture these two small but essential characteristics from large-size histopathological images. In the term of *cell-layer level* patterns, existing CNN-based models cannot percept the relative position patterns between cells (which with papillary structures) and layers composed by their surrounding cells. Moreover, both *cellular level* and *cell-layer level* patterns are relatively small and randomly distributed in different locations of a pRCC histopathological image, thus making it challenging to highlight such patterns in the extracted features of a traditional CNN. Recently, some works attempt to construct features manually, based on the predicted results generated by the nuclei segmentation and classification model, to capture the *cellular level* patterns [10,11]. However, these hand-craft features are task-specific that hard to generalize to different digital pathology tasks.

To tackle the aforementioned challenges, in this paper, we propose a novel two-stage framework based on Transformer [12], namely instance-based Vision Transformer (i-ViT), for the pRCC subtyping. The first stage is the nuclei segmentation and classification, where tumor nuclei patches with the corresponding position and grade information are extracted. Then these patches are further aggregated together with their positions and grades in i-ViT (the second stage) to represent the key patterns for the final classification. The main difference between our i-ViT and existing vision Transformer models, such as vision Transformer (ViT) [13], is that i-ViT only uses instance-level patches, to learn the key features with a relatively low computational complexity, while ViT takes all split image patches into account. Meanwhile, we propose to leverage the nuclei grade features by applying the nuclei label embeddings. Extensive experiments are conducted on a dataset derived initially from the kidney renal papillary cell carcinoma project of The Cancer Genome Atlas (TCGA-KIRP) database. The experimental results demonstrate that i-ViT achieves better performance than other comparison methods.

2   Method

The central idea of the proposed i-ViT is to extract and select instance features from instance-level patches first, then aggregate these features for further capturing the *cellular level* and *cell-layer level* features, at last encode both of the fine-gained features into the final image-level representation. Specifically, each instance-level patch of a histopathological image includes a nucleus with part of the surrounding background, is a graded nuclei segment extracted and classified by a segmentation network with additional classification channels (the classification target is the grade of a nucleus). We select the top-K instance-level patches according to the grades and sizes of their nuclei. Then, use a CNN to embed each selected instance-level patch into instance-embedding. Considering the importance of the relative position between nuclei and the grade of nuclei, we encode the position and grade information into the instance-embedding through a position embedding layer and a grade embedding layer, respectively. Finally, we use the multi-head multi-layer self-attention to integrate the instance-embeddings with position and grade encodings.

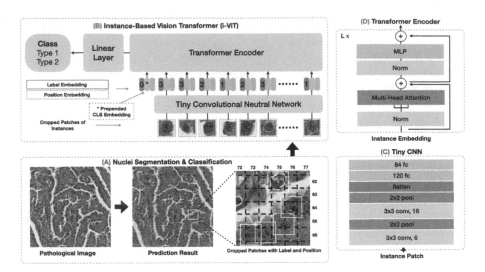

Fig. 2. The proposed framework for papillary renal cell carcinoma subtyping. It include two stages: (A) for obtaining instances features, (B) for pRCC subtyping via extracting and aggregating instance-level features.

An overview of our proposed framework for pRCC subtyping is depicted in Fig. 2. The pipeline can be briefly described as follows: (1) Training a nuclei segmentation and classification model for segmenting nuclei and predicting their grades in an input histopathological image. (2) Extracting patches with assigned grades as instances according to the predicted results of step (1). (3) Select top-K instances and input them into the proposed i-VIT for predicting the subtype of the input image. As shown in Fig. 2(B), the proposed i-ViT consists of a tiny CNN and a Transformer encoder. The corresponding architectures of the tiny CNN and the Transformer encoder are shown in Fig. 2(C) and (D).

2.1 Nuclei Segmentation and Classification

To capture the fine features of pRCC subtypes, we need to segment out nuclei from the original image to avoid redundant information in a large-size histopathological image and highlight the critical information for the downstream subtyping network. Considering that nuclei grades are an essential basis for subtyping, we predict each segmented nucleus's grade as well. The deep neural network has been widely used for medical image segmentation [14,15]. To this end, we train a deep neural network for jointly learning the nuclei segmentation and classification (grading) tasks.

We adopt the nuclei grading dataset introduced in [16] to train the segmentation and classification model. This dataset contains 1000 region of interests (ROIs) that are selected from histopathological images of clear cell RCC (ccRCC) and pRCC. All the tumor nuclei with grades 1, 2, 3, and endothelial nuclei are labeled in these ROIs. Although this dataset is originally proposed for ccRCC, the nuclei grading system (ISUP) used in the annotation is recommended and validated on both ccRCC and pRCC. We only use the images of pRCC from the testing set to evaluate the model performance. Several deep learning models, such as U-Net, HoVer-Net [17], and Micro-Net [18] have been assessed. As Micro-Net achieves higher accuracy and faster inference speed than other models, we adopt it as the nuclei segmentation and classification network in our framework.

2.2 Instance-Based Vision Transformer

After training the nuclei segmentation and classification model, we crop instance-level patches from the original image according to the segmentation results as shown in Fig. 2 (A). Each patch is in a size of $P \times P, P = 64$ and centered by a nucleus point, in which a whole nucleus and part of the surrounding background are included. Therefore, the cropped patches carry the cellular and location (whether the cells locate on the papillary structure or not) features.

The standard Transformer [12] is restrict to only take the sequences of 1D embeddings as input by its architecture. To extract 1D feature embeddings $S \in \mathbb{R}^{N \times D}$ from a sequence of 2D instance-level patches $X \in \mathbb{R}^{N \times P \times P \times C}$ (Eq. 1), we construct a tiny CNN model which consists of two convolution and two fully-connection layers as the trainable patch embedding projection $\mathcal{L}$. D denotes the patch embedding dimension and serves as the latent vector size for all the Transformer layers, C is the number of input channels. Note that, different images contain different number of nuclei, similar to the standard processing approach of NLP, we set a hyper-parameter N which is the number of instances, also as the input sequence length of Transformer to handle this variation. Due to the importance of nucleus grade and size for subtyping, we remove the endothelial nuclei and sort other nuclei instances (tumor nuclei) by grade and size, which are easily obtained from nuclei segmentation and classification results, then the top N of nuclei instances are selected as the input of tiny CNN.

Following the similar idea of ViT [13], we assign a learnable class embedding $s_{cls}^0 \in \mathbb{R}^{1 \times D}$ to learn the image representation that can be regarded as an aggregation of all the selected instance embeddings. During the training and testing process, a single linear layer classification head s_{cls}^L is attached (Eq. 4). L is the number of Transformer layer.

The nuclei positional information, which is the coordinates of each nucleus in the image, reflects the relative position between nuclei and is related with the *cell-layer level* patterns. Since the histopathological image size is large and meaningless to learn the redundant position embedding, we grid the image coordinates into 1/20 of the original size and use the grid's position where the center of a nucleus is located to be the position of the nucleus, as shown in Fig. 2(A). Thereby, the position embeddings $s_X, s_Y \in \mathbb{R}^{(N+1) \times D/2}$ are learned from the nuclei position with two axes. Then we concatenate the X and Y embeddings to form the final position embeddings of the nuclei. To encode the nuclei grades information, we employ a grade embedding to integrate the ISUP nucleolar grade features as $s_{grade} \in \mathbb{R}^{(N+1) \times D}$. Finally, the position embeddings and grade embeddings are added to instance embeddings (Eq. 1).

The architecture of our Transformer encoder is similar to ViT. It consists of repeated stacked multi-head self-attention (MSA) and multilayer perceptron (MLP) blocks (Eq. 2,3). The MLP consists of two hidden layers with GELU activation. Layernorm (LN) and residual connection are applied in every block.

$$S_0 = \left[s_{cls}^0; \mathcal{L}(x_1); \mathcal{L}(x_2); ...; \mathcal{L}(x_N) \right] + [s_X, s_Y] + s_{grade} \qquad (1)$$

$$\hat{S}_l = \text{MSA}\left(\text{LN}\left(S_{l-1}\right)\right) + S_{l-1} \qquad l = \{1...L\} \qquad (2)$$

$$S_l = \text{MLP}\left(\text{LN}\left(\hat{S}_l\right)\right) + \hat{S}_l \qquad l = \{1...L\} \qquad (3)$$

$$y = \text{Linear}\left(s_{cls}^L\right) \qquad (4)$$

where y is the output vector of i-ViT, it can be transformed as predicted probabilities via a softmax function.

3　Experiment

3.1　Dataset

The pRCC subtyping dataset comprised 171 diagnostic whole slide images (WSI) from 171 patients (scanned at 40x), 62 are type 1, and 109 are type 2. These WSIs are downloaded from KIRP project of TCGA and re-diagnosed by two experienced pathologists. The pathologists have selected a total of 1162 (613 vs. 549) ROIs in 2000×2000 size, approximately 10 ROIs for every type 1 case, 5 for type 2. We randomly divide the dataset into three subsets in patient-level, training (60%), validation (20%), and testing (20%) set. This dataset and source code of our work are available at: https://dataset.chenli.group/home/prcc-subtyping and https://github.com/ZeyuGaoAi/Instance_based_Vision_Transformer.

3.2　Implementation Details

Nuclei Segmentation and Classification. To avoid bias from different staining conditions, we perform the staining normalization and image augmentations (flip, rotate, blur) on all images. For the training process, the batch size is 8, and the learning rate is $1.0e-4$ at the beginning, then decreases to $1.0e-5$ after 25 epochs. Adam optimizer is adopted, and the total training epochs is 50. The weighted panoptic quality (wPQ) used in the MoNuSAC challenge [19] is adopted for evaluation in which the weight of each class is 1. The wPQ of Micro-Net is up to 0.5, which is an acceptable performance for pRCC nuclei segmentation and classification.

Subtyping of pRCC. Four methods are adopted for performance comparison. 1. A CNN model (ResNet-34) without considering nuclei features, the model's input are the original ROIs, denoted by CNN-ORI. 2. The traditional classifier (Decision Tree) with the grade distribution of each ROI, denoted by DT-G. 3. The gradient boosting decision tree (GBDT) with the grade distribution and hand-craft cellular features aggregation, denoted by GBDT-GH. 4. The single Transformer encoder with hand-craft cellular features, denoted by i-ViT-H.

The grade distribution is obtained from the nuclei classification result of each ROI. We normalize the number of nuclei in each grade (1,2 and 3) to get the corresponding rate for DT-G. For hand-craft cellular feature extraction, four types of features, which are size, shape, color, and distance to neighbors, are extracted for each nucleus. We select ten cellular features: the area of nucleus, the major and minor axes lengths of a nucleus and the ratio between these two lengths, the mean pixel values in three color channels (RGB) of a nucleus, three distances (maximum, minimum, mean) to neighbors in the Delaunay triangulation. Similar to [11], we adopt five distribution statistics, *i.e.*, mean, std, skewness, kurtosis, entropy, and a 10-bin histogram to integrate the selected cellular features into one image-level feature. Finally, 150-dimensional hand-craft features and three grade-distribution features are generated for the third method GBDT-GH. The fourth model i-ViT-H only takes the ten cellular features of each nucleus as the input of the Transformer encoder. The grade embedding and the prepend class token are also adopted.

We implement all the methods in experiments with the open-source library Pytorch 1.6 and scikit-learn 0.24.0 on a work-station with four NVIDIA 2080Ti GPUs. For traditional classifiers (DT, GBDT), we use the default parameters from scikit-learn. Except for the image-net pre-trained ResNet-34 is used in the first comparison method, we do not use any other pre-trained models. For deep models, the adam optimizer is adopted for training, and the maximum epochs are 50. The learning rate is $1.0e-3$ initially and decreases to $1.0e-4$ after 30 epochs for CNN-ORI and i-ViT, and is $1.0e-2$ ($1.0e-3$ after 30 epochs) for i-ViT-H. Due to the low-dimensional embeddings of i-ViT-H, the number of heads, layers, and hidden dimensions are set to 2, 1, and 32, respectively. For i-ViT, the number of heads, layers, and hidden dimensions are set to 12, 12, and 128, respectively. The input sequence length N is set to 500 for i-ViT-H and i-ViT. A linear warm-up learning rate schedule is used in i-ViT and i-ViT-H for 10 epochs.

3.3   Results

The overall accuracy, precision, recall, and F1-scores of each class are applied to evaluate the performance of subtyping models, and the classification results are shown in Table 1. As we expected, CNN-ORI shows the worst performance because traditional convolution structures can hardly capture the small and randomly distributed features. GBDT-GH outperforms DT-G by about 8% in ACC, which benefits from the rich hand-craft cellular features. The i-ViT-H achieves better performance than GBDT-GH, where the improvements are due to the

Table 1. The comparison results, overall-accuracy (Acc), precision (Prec), recall (Rec), F1-score (F1) for pRCC subtyping.

Model	All	Type 1			Type 2		
	Acc%	Prec%	Rec%	F1%	Prec%	Rec%	F1%
CNN-ORI	75.11	77.39	74.17	75.74	72.81	76.15	74.44
DT-G	80.35	85.05	75.83	80.18	76.23	85.32	80.52
GBDT-GH	88.21	**94.29**	82.50	88.00	83.06	**94.50**	88.41
i-ViT-H	89.18	91.30	87.50	89.36	86.84	90.83	88.79
i-ViT	**93.01**	90.00	**97.50**	**93.60**	**96.97**	88.07	**92.31**

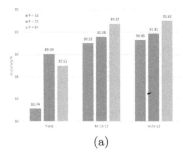 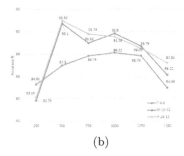

(a)   (b)

Fig. 3. The i-ViT performance under various parameters. The T-6-6, M-12-12, and H-24-12 indicate three Transformers (tiny, middle, and huge), the first and second digits are the number of layers and heads, and all hidden dimensions are 128. (a) Different sizes of instance patches with the input sequence length $N = 500$. (b) Different input sequence lengths with the size of instance patches $P = 64$.

self-attention-based architecture. Moreover, our proposed i-ViT significantly outperforms other methods, which proves that the instance level features (nucleus patch, position, and grade embeddings) and the learning schema (learning with instance) we designed are effective for this fine-grained classification task.

Sensitivity Analysis. Because our proposed subtyping framework relies on parameters of the i-ViT model, three main parameters are analyzed: 1) The size of instance patches P for tiny CNN, P=16, 32, and 64. 2) The input sequence length N of the Transformer encoder, from 250 to 1500 at an interval of 250. 3) Three Transformer encoders with different scales (*i.e.*, T-6-6, M-12-12, and H-24-12).

From Fig. 3, we can observe that the performance of the i-ViT is related to these three parameters. The performances of the middle and huge scale models (M-12-12, H-24-12) are competitive in most of the parameter settings, and the tiny scale model has the worst performance due to the under-fitting problem. The smallest size patches ($P = 16$) lead to worse performance because these patches only contain part of nuclei, see Fig. 3(a). Also, in Fig. 3(b), the performances are worse with $N = 250$. We consider that the models cannot extract discriminate features from limited instances, and these models are relatively stable with input sequence lengths (from 500 to 1000). Note that the model performances decrease rapidly from 1000 to 1500 because most of the tumor nuclei numbers extracted from the images are less than 1250.

4 Conclusion

Subtyping of pRCC is a critical diagnostic task with poor clinical consistency. In digital pathology, this task is a fine-grained image classification task based on some detailed features and hard to solve by traditional CNN models. In this paper, we introduced a new learning schema, "learning with instances," for this particular task. Unlike the standard ViT that considers every pixel of each image, we integrated the instance information extracted from the nuclei segmentation and classification results with the ViT to form the i-ViT. The i-ViT only takes pixels of each instance into account, making the model ignore useless background information and pay more attention to learning useful features.

Acknowledgements. This work has been supported by the National Key Research and Development Program of China (2018YFC0910404); This work has been supported by National Natural Science Foundation of China (61772409); The consulting research project of the Chinese Academy of Engineering (The Online and Offline Mixed Educational Service System for "The Belt and Road" Training in MOOC China); Project of China Knowledge Centre for Engineering Science and Technology; The innovation team from the Ministry of Education (IRT_17R86); and the Innovative Research Group of the National Natural Science Foundation of China (61721002). The results shown here are in whole or part based upon data generated by the TCGA Research Network: https://www.cancer.gov/tcga.

References

1. Incidence and long-term prognosis of papillary compared to clear cell renal cell carcinoma - a multicentre study. Eur. J. Cancer **48**(15), 2347–2352 (2012). https://doi.org/10.1016/j.ejca.2012.05.002
2. Delahunt, B., et al.: The international society of urological pathology (isup) grading system for renal cell carcinoma and other prognostic parameters. Am. J. Surg. Pathol. **37**(10), 1490–1504 (2013)
3. Wong, E.C., et al.: Morphologic subtyping as a prognostic predictor for survival in papillary renal cell carcinoma: type 1 vs. type 2. Urol. Oncol. Semin. Original Invest. **37**(10), 721–726 (2019). https://doi.org/10.1016/j.urolonc.2019.05.009
4. Leroy, X., et al.: Morphologic subtyping of papillary renal cell carcinoma: correlation with prognosis and differential expression of muc1 between the two subtypes. Mod. Pathol. **15**(11), 1126–1130 (2002)
5. Pan, H., Ye, L., Zhu, Q., Yang, Z., Hu, M.: The effect of the papillary renal cell carcinoma subtype on oncological outcomes. Sci. Rep. **10**(1), 1–7 (2020). https://doi.org/10.1038/s41598-020-78174-9

6. Moch, H., Cubilla, A.L., Humphrey, P.A., Reuter, V.E., Ulbright, T.M.: The 2016 who classification of tumours of the urinary system and male genital organs–part a: Renal, penile, and testicular tumours. Eur. Urol. **70**(1), 93–105 (2016). https://doi.org/10.1016/j.eururo.2016.02.029

7. Zhang, X., et al.: Classifying breast cancer histopathological images using a robust artificial neural network architecture. In: Rojas, I., Valenzuela, O., Rojas, F., Ortuño, F. (eds.) IWBBIO 2019. LNCS, vol. 11465, pp. 204–215. Springer, Cham (2019). https://doi.org/10.1007/978-3-030-17938-0_19

8. Coudray, N., et al.: Classification and mutation prediction from non-small cell lung cancer histopathology images using deep learning. Nature Med. **24**(10), 1559–1567 (2018). https://doi.org/10.1038/s41591-018-0177-5

9. Gao, Z., Puttapirat, P., Shi, J., Li, C.: Renal cell carcinoma detection and subtyping with minimal point-based annotation in whole-slide images. In: Martel, A.L. (ed.) MICCAI 2020. LNCS, vol. 12265, pp. 439–448. Springer, Cham (2020). https://doi.org/10.1007/978-3-030-59722-1_42

10. Wang, S., et al.: Computational staining of pathology images to study the tumor microenvironment in lung cancer. Cancer Res. **80**(10), 2056–2066 (2020). https://doi.org/10.1158/0008-5472.CAN-19-1629

11. Cheng, J., et al.: Integrative analysis of histopathological images and genomic data predicts clear cell renal cell carcinoma prognosis. Cancer Res. **77**(21), e91–e100 (2017). https://doi.org/10.1158/0008-5472.CAN-17-0313

12. Vaswani, A., et al.: Attention is all you need. In: Guyon, I. (eds.) et al. Advances in Neural Information Processing Systems, vol. 30. Curran Associates, Inc. (2017)

13. Dosovitskiy, A., et al.: An image is worth 16x16 words: transformers for image recognition at scale (2020)

14. Zhao, R., et al.: Rethinking dice loss for medical image segmentation. In: 2020 IEEE International Conference on Data Mining (ICDM), pp. 851–860 (2020). https://doi.org/10.1109/ICDM50108.2020.00094

15. Xie, C., et al.: Recist-net: Lesion detection via grouping keypoints on recist-based annotation. In: 2021 IEEE 18th International Symposium on Biomedical Imaging (ISBI), pp. 921–924 (2021). https://doi.org/10.1109/ISBI48211.2021.9433794

16. Gao, Z., et al.: Nuclei grading of clear cell renal cell carcinoma in histopathological image by composite high-resolution network (2021)

17. Graham, S., et al.: Hover-net: simultaneous segmentation and classification of nuclei in multi-tissue histology images. Med. Image Anal. **58**, 101563 (2019). https://doi.org/10.1016/j.media.2019.101563

18. Raza, S.E.A., et al.: Micro-net: a unified model for segmentation of various objects in microscopy images. Med. Image Anal. **52**, 160–173 (2019). https://doi.org/10.1016/j.media.2018.12.003

19. Verma, R., Kumar, N., Patil, A., Kurian, N., Rane, S., Sethi, A.: Multi-organ nuclei segmentation and classification challenge 2020 (2020). https://doi.org/10.13140/RG.2.2.12290.02244/1

Hybrid Supervision Learning for Pathology Whole Slide Image Classification

Jiahui Li[1], Wen Chen[1], Xiaodi Huang[1], Shuang Yang[1], Zhiqiang Hu[1],
Qi Duan[1], Dimitris N. Metaxas[2], Hongsheng Li[3,4], and Shaoting Zhang[1,4(✉)]

[1] SenseTime Research, Shanghai, China
{lijiahui,chenwen,huangxiaodi,yangshuang1,huzhiqiang,duanqi,
zhangshaoting}@sensetime.com
[2] Rutgers University, New Jersey, USA
dnm@cs.rutgers.edu
[3] The Chinese University of Hong Kong, Hong Kong, China
hsli@ee.cuhk.edu.hk
[4] Centre for Perceptual and Interactive Intelligence (CPII) Ltd, Hong Kong, China

Abstract. Weak supervision learning on classification labels has demonstrated high performance in various tasks, while a few pixel-level fine annotations are also affordable. Naturally a question comes to us that whether the combination of pixel-level (e.g., segmentation) and image level (e.g., classification) annotation can introduce further improvement. However in computational pathology this is a difficult task for this reason: High resolution of whole slide images makes it difficult to do end-to-end classification model training, which is challenging to research of weak or hybrid supervision learning in the past. To handle this problem, we propose a hybrid supervision learning framework for this kind of high resolution images with sufficient image-level coarse annotations and a few pixel-level fine labels. This framework, when applied in training patch model, can carefully make use of coarse image-level labels to refine generated pixel-level pseudo labels. Complete strategy is proposed to suppress pixel-level false positives and false negatives. A large hybrid annotated dataset is used to evaluate the effectiveness of hybrid supervision learning. By extracting pixel-level pseudo labels in initially image-level labeled samples, we achieve 5.2% higher specificity than purely training on existing labels while retaining 100% sensitivity, in the task of image-level classification to be positive or negative.

Keywords: Computational pathology · Hybrid and Weak supervision learning

This study has been financially supported by fund of Science and Technology Commission Shanghai Municipality (19511121400), also partially supported by the Centre for Perceptual and Interactive Intelligence (CPII) Ltd under the Innovation and Technology Fund. Code of this paper is available at https://github.com/JarveeLee/HybridSupervisionLearning_Pathology.

M. de Bruijne et al. (Eds.): MICCAI 2021, LNCS 12908, pp. 309–318, 2021.
https://doi.org/10.1007/978-3-030-87237-3_30

1   Introduction

Hybrid supervision learning on various levels of annotations has shown its effectiveness in various machine learning applications [8,11,12] . However, we find those tasks in computational pathology is more challenging as high resolution (over $100{,}000 \times 100{,}000$ pixels) of whole slide images makes it difficult to conduct end-to-end training of deep learning models, which is challenging to perform weak or hybrid supervision learning research in the past [3,4,11,12,16,17,19].

To handle aforementioned challenges, a novel hybrid supervision learning framework is proposed for whole slide images classification to distinguish positive or negative. Due to high resolution we can only train deep learning model on patches, and propose a well-designed strategy to modify pixel-level pseudo labels on patches, according to image-level labels: A positive image is guaranteed to contain at least one positive patch, while a negative image shall be entirely pixelwisely negative. Secondly pixel-level errors, false negatives and false positives, are gathered during pseudo labels generation. We perform re-weighting on pixel-level pseudo labels of patches from positive images, converting false negatives to true positives and false positives. We use hard negatives patches from negative images with a higher sampling ratio to train model, to further convert false positives to true negatives. Because noise tolerant deep learning model can discriminate a pattern as negative if during training it is mostly labeled as negative. As for the few pixel-level annotations, we use them to initialize pre-trained model and to mix a constant ratio in each training batch with pixel-level pseudo labels to regularize training. With such strategy, without end-to-end training, we can make best use of image-level labels, pixel-level fine-grained labels and pseudo labels on unlabeled areas.

The main contributions of our hybrid supervision learning framework is to utilize both the limited amount of pixel-level annotations and the large number of image-level labels. Without end-to-end image-level training, image-level labels are used to refine pseudo labels on the entire training dataset, with well-designed strategy to control false positives and false negatives. We evaluated the framework on a large whole slide images dataset of histopathology. According to experiments results, the hybrid supervision learning shows specificity 8.92% better than image-level training and 5.2% better than pixel-level training, while retaining 100% sensitivity.

2   Related Work

For hybrid supervision learning: In most medical image tasks, hybrid supervision is a common data situation, with large amount of clinical reports and small group of segmentation annotations shown in Fig. 1. However focus was mostly given to semi and weak supervision learning [5,7,10,22,24], defined on single format then to make use of unlabeled images. There exists some achievements related to our framework [8,11,12]. Our framework is different from theirs because end-to-end classification training with entire image input is difficult in whole slide images.

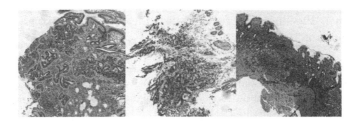

Fig. 1. Illustration of hybrid supervision data, containing 2 types of label. The first expensive and rare type is pixel-level fine-grained labels, contoured by green lines. The second type is image-level labeled images. The rest two images are image-level positive and negative. (Color figure online)

Instead only patches are involved in our total pipeline, image-level labels are not directly related to loss calculation. As for computational pathology: Usually the size of one whole slide image is 100,000 × 100,000 pixels, which is too big to run directly on GPU, therefore most of previous contributions process images in a two-stage manner [1,6,9,13,18,20,21,25]. In **the first stage**, discriminative patches are extracted from whole slide image by specific patch models, in the second stage a whole slide image classifier is trained by the selected patches from first stage.

3   Hybrid Supervision Learning for Whole Slide Image Classification

The main objective of hybrid supervision learning is to use image-level labels to refine pixel-level pseudo labels on patches, without the entire huge image input. Pipeline is shown in Fig. 2 and Algorithm. 1, which involves two stages: patch segmentation, whole slide image classification.

A clinically effective system can tolerate false positives for further recheck by pathologists, while false negatives are vital faults for patients. Thus we need to locate the positive patterns in positive images as much as possible, while precluding more negative images. Our goal is to maintaining 100% sensitivity and pursue higher specificity to reduce workloads. Under this consideration, comparing positive images and negative images, patterns that only exist in positive images shall all be suspicious and at least one patch is responsible for image-level positive diagnosis. Also, negative patterns that exist in negative images, can certainly be regarded as true negative patterns, and positive predictions in negative images can be regarded as hard negative patches. At the same time, it is the fact that collecting negative images is much easier than positive images. With sufficient suppression of various hard negative patches, we give a positive growing tendency to patterns in positive images. Only the confidence of those true positive patterns, not covered by negative patches, will be able to gradually

---

Algorithm 1: Pipeline of hybrid supervision learning. y_p is pixel-level fine-grained label from pathologists.

Data:

y_p: pixel-level fine-grained label from pathologists.

$\hat{y_p}, \hat{y_{p+}}, \hat{y_{p-}}$: pixel-level pseudo label, from positive and negative images, created by models and image-level labels guided re-weighting.

y_i: image-level label from clinical reports.

θ_1: patch segmentation model initially trained by y_p, outputs the probability that each pixel of input patch is positive.

θ_2: whole slide image classifier, outputs the probability that input whole slide image is positive.

I: high resolution whole slide image.

x: image patches.

T: patch removing threshold.

V: re-weighting constant.

R: sampling ratio of y_p, $\hat{y_{p+}}$ and $\hat{y_{p-}}$.

K: select top K patches as input to train whole slide image classifier.

while *the model do not converge* **do**

    Stage 1: patch segmentation ;

    E-step: $\hat{y_p} \leftarrow P(y_p|\text{x}, \theta_1)$

    Remove those x whose maximum $\hat{y_p}$ is less than T ;

    if $y_i == 1$ **then**

        $\hat{y_{p+}} \leftarrow \hat{y_p} \times \text{V}$ (pseudo labels re-weighting for patches in positive images, V >1.0);

        $\hat{y_{p+}} \leftarrow 1.0$ if $\hat{y_{p+}} > 1.0$ (clip within 1.0);

        $\hat{y_{p+}} \leftarrow 0.0$ if $\hat{y_{p+}} < 0.01$ (clip to 0.0 if lower than 0.01, to remain true negative which was slightly scaled up by V);

    else

        $\hat{y_{p-}} \leftarrow \hat{y_p} \times 0$ (hard negative labels);

    M-step: Retrain patch segmentation model θ_1 at proper sampling ratio of R in each training batch, and by Loss $= -\frac{1}{N}$ $\sum_N \sum_{y=y_p, \hat{y_{p+}}, \hat{y_{p-}}} y \times logP(y_p|x, \theta_1) + (1.0 - y) \times log(1.0 - P(y_p|x, \theta_1))$

    Stage 2: whole slide image classification ;

    Select K patches for each whole slide image according to pixel-wise maximum $P(y_p|x, \theta_1)$;

    $P(y_i|I, \theta_2) = \frac{1}{K} \sum_K P(y_i|x, \theta_2)$

    Train classification model θ_2 by Loss $= -\frac{1}{N}$ $\sum_N y_i \times logP(y_i|I, \theta_2) + (1.0 - y_i) \times log(1.0 - P(y_i|I, \theta_2))$

    Convergence criteria: For each round of stage1, perform stage2 training. Select the round whose stage2 training loss is the lowest, which means the top K patches selected in that round by stage1 is the optimal to fit image-level annotations.

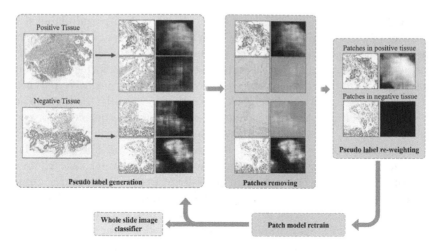

Fig. 2. The overall pipeline of our hybrid supervision learning for whole slide image. The image-level label guided pixel-level pseudo label generation is iterated in this manner. The gray scale map is the predicted probability map of patch model.

grow up and reach 1.0 eventually. Those noisy false positive introduced by growing tendency will be suppressed by various hard negative patches and higher sampling ratio during deep learning model training.

As for pixel-level fine-grained labels y_p, the best performance is certain if we perform all the pixel-level fine-grained labels for all the positive images, however with limited budget we could just afford a few, whose quantity is significantly smaller than the image-level labels. To involve pixel-level fine-grained labels y_p into training, firstly it is used to initialize a pre-trained model θ_1, to minimize false positives and false negatives at the beginning. Secondly it consists of a large ratio in each training batch.

To implement our intuition, shown in Fig. 2, we separate large size of whole slide images into patches, then develop an *Expectation-Maximization (EM)*-like method to make full use of three types of annotation: image-level labels y_i, pixel-level fine-grained labels y_p and pixel-level pseudo labels $\hat{y}_p$. In the E-step, pixel-level pseudo labels $\hat{y}_p$ are firstly created from segmentation confidence map of patches from both positive and negative images. We remove all the patches from both positive and negative images whose maximum pixel-level positive confidence is less than a threshold T, to reduce the number of training patches. Provided with image-level labels, we obtain hard negative patches $\hat{y_{p-}}$ from negative images and noisy pseudo labeled positive patches from positive images. Then we multiply a weight V $(V > 1)$ on noisy pseudo labels in positive patches and clipped withing 1.0, assigning them as $\hat{y_{p+}}$, which transforms false negatives to true positives and false positives, while keeping true positives as the same. In the M-step, patch segmentation model is then trained on a sampling ratio of pixel-level fine-grained labels y_p, pseudo labeled positive patches $\hat{y_{p+}}$ and hard negative patches $\hat{y_{p-}}$. For sampling ratio of y_p, $\hat{y_{p+}}$ and $\hat{y_{p-}}$ in each training batch, hard negative patches $\hat{y_{p-}}$ shall be much more than pseudo labeled positive patches $\hat{y_{p+}}$ so that if one pattern is both labeled as negative in hard negative patches and positive in pseudo labeled patches, model can still regard such pattern as negative for much higher sampling ratio, which transforms false positives to true negatives. Only those patterns not suppressed by negative patches are possible to be eventually discriminated as positive by models. Such procedure is iterated for several rounds and we evaluate sensitivity and specificity for each to decide when to stop. Loss function in patch segmentation stage is pixel-level soft-label cross entropy loss to deal with both soft pseudo and fine-grained labels. During whole slide image classification stage, for each super size whole slide image, top K patches with maximum pixel-level probability are the input to image classifier θ_2. Average probability is the final image-level confidence to calculate loss with image-level labels. Stage2 training also decides the convergence criteria. We perform stage2 training for each round of stage1 and select that round whose stage2 training loss is the lowest. That means the top K patches selected in this round by stage1 is the optimal to fit image-level annotations in stage2.

4   Experiments

4.1   Experimental Setting

To verify the effectiveness of hybrid supervision learning,we design three experiments of different supervision for comparison: **image-level**, **pixel-level** and **hybrid**. **Image-level** experiment is applied with source code from Campanella et al. [1], whose method relies only on image-level labels and searches top K responsible patches for image-level labels. Patch classification model predicts every patch's confidence to be positive, then top K patches are further trained by image-level labels. It is $K = 1$ in the released code [1]. **Pixel-level** experiment uses all of existing pixel-level fine-grained labels to train patch segmentation model and image-level labels to train whole slide image classification model, without extracting hidden pixel-level pseudo labels. We modified code from Khened et al. [9] as our pixel-level baseline. **Hybrid** experiment makes use of image-level labels, pixel-level fine-grained labels, and pseudo labels which are generated from the first two, as described above. We use normal classification task's evaluation metrics to evaluate the performance including Sensitivity, Specificity, ROC curve and AUC. Higher specificity while retaining 100% sensitivity is our eventual preference.

4.2   Implementation Details

Deep learning algorithms are developed by Pytorch1.0 [15] along with Openslide [2]. Otsu's [14] method is performed to quickly extract valid patches that contain tissue. DLA34up and DLA34 [23] are the patch segmentation and whole slide image classification models θ_1, θ_2 . Re-weighting constant is $V = 4.0$ for all the experiments. This value only influences the training time, the lower V is, the longer time it will take. V bigger than 4.0 shows no significant improvement in speed. The pixel-wise maximum confidence patch selection threshold T is 0.4. Higher threshold T can exclude some positive images, thus degrades sensitivity. Lower threshold T involves too much patches during training, leading to longer convergence time but nearly the same final performance. Patch size for both of patch segmentation and whole slide image classification is H = 512, W = 512, overlapped 128. For classification top K patches, here we set K as 16. During patch segmentation model training, R, sampling ratio of pixel-level fine-grained labels y_p, pseudo labels y_{p+} and hard negative patches $\hat{y_{p-}}$ is 2:1:7, to allow hard negative patches to overwhelm wrong patterns in noisy positive pseudo labels and keep pixel-level fine-grained labels participating in training procedure. For multi-round iteration, patch model initializes the weights from previous round, not from scratch. For whole slide image classifier, sampling ratio of positive and negative images is 1:1. Finally, the framework iterates to round 2 during experiments. During training each round, patch model is trained 30 epochs while whole slide image classifier is trained 15 epochs.

Table 1. Data distribution and train/test separation of gastric cancer dataset.

Distribution	Pixel-level train	Images train	Images train	Total images	Total patients
Positive	200 patches	585	499	1,084	724
Negative	0	4,096	5,714	9,810	5941
Total	200 patches	4,681	6,213	10,894	6,665

4.3 Dataset

The dataset is especially developed for the commonly seen gastric cancer with 10,894 whole slide images in total. Data distribution of pixel-level fine-grained labeled patches, positive and negative whole slides, train/test separation are shown in Table 1, this ratio 1:9 of positive and negative is approximately the same distribution of clinical daily works. All the slides are automatically scanned by digital pathology scanner Leica Aperio AT2 at 20X magnification (0.50 μm/pixel). The image-level annotation is either 'Positive', which refers to low-grade intraepithelial neoplasia, high-grade intraepithelial neoplasia, adenocarcinoma, signet ring cell carcinoma, and poorly cohesive carcinoma, or 'Negative', including chronic atrophic gastritis, chronic non-atrophic gastritis, intestinal metaplasia, gastric polyps, gastric mucosal erosion, etc.

4.4 Results

Released source code from Campanella et al. [1] running on our data is the compared image-level baseline for our hybrid supervision learning, which only uses

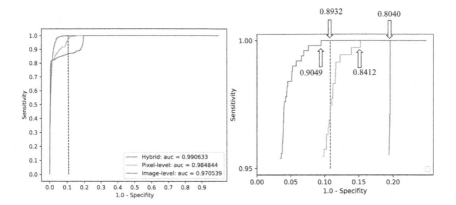

Fig. 3. ROC curve detail of the three setting. In fact hybrid supervision learning can finally achieve specificity 0.9049 at probability threshold 0.1421.

the image-level label for training. This code can produce patch-level classification probability, not pixel-level. Statistically their weak supervision learning on our data achieve 80.40% specificity while retaining 100% sensitivity at threshold $P = 0.0012$. At the same time our hybrid supervision framework can achieve 89.32% specificity with 100% sensitivity at threshold $P = 0.1000$, 8.92% far more than image-level annotation. These are summarized in Fig. 3.

The reason for this phenomenon is that with image-level labels only, Campanella et al. [1] searches the minimum representative patches responsible for image-level labels, without covering the most positive regions. At the same time our hybrid supervision learning framework is trained on most of positive patches in each positive whole slide image. More positive training samples establish more clear boundary between positive and negative patches, leading to higher specificity and area under curve.

Table 2. Statistics results of gastric cancer dataset.

Metrics	Hybrid	Pixel-level [9]	Image-level [1]
Sensitivity	1.0000	1.0000	1.0000
Specificity	0.8932	0.8412	0.8040
AUC	0.9906	0.9848	0.9705
Threshold	0.1000	0.0041	0.0012

In pixel-level training, 200 pixel-level fine-grained labeled big patches are used to train the initial patch segmentation model then select top patches for whole slide images classifier training, without image-level labels guided pixel-level pseudo labels generation. This procedure can be regarded as backbone shared hybrid supervision learning, using existing annotations without extracting pixel-level pseudo labels in image-level positive images. This configuration provided us 84.12% specificity, 5.2% lower than hybrid supervision learning, indicating the proposed hybrid supervision learning is better than simple backbones sharing manner. As for thresholds, in test data hybrid supervision learning could reach 0.9049 specificity at threshold = 0.1421, while Pixel-level and Image-level have to use extremely low threshold for 100% sensitivity, due to less supervision information.

5   Conclusions

In this paper we propose a novel hybrid supervision framework especially for whole slide images classification. Without entire image input to do end-to-end classification training. Pixel-level false negatives is prevented by re-weighting on pseudo labels of selected patches from positive images. False positives is suppressed by high training sampling ratio of hard negative patches. With this framework and a few pixel-level fine-grained labeled data, we can properly utilize large amount of image-level labeled whole slide images, train models in segmentation manner, and get much higher performance compared to using single format of annotation only, or just the existing pixel-level fine-grained labels.

References

1. Campanella, G., et al.: Clinical-grade computational pathology using weakly supervised deep learning on whole slide images. Nature Med. **25**(8), 1301–1309 (2019)
2. Goode, A., Gilbert, B., Harkes, J., Jukic, D., Satyanarayanan, M.: Openslide: a vendor-neutral software foundation for digital pathology. J. Pathol. Inf. **4** (2013)
3. He, X., Zemel, R.S.: Learning hybrid models for image annotation with partially labeled data. In: Advances in Neural Information Processing Systems, pp. 625–632 (2009)
4. Heng, Z., Dipu, M., Yap, K.H.: Hybrid supervised deep learning for ethnicity classification using face images. In: 2018 IEEE International Symposium on Circuits and Systems (ISCAS), pp. 1–5. IEEE (2018)
5. Hosang, A.K.R.B.J., Schiele, M.H.B.: Weakly supervised semantic labelling and instance segmentation. arXiv preprint arXiv:1603.07485 (2016)
6. Hou, L., Samaras, D., Kurc, T.M., Gao, Y., Davis, J.E., Saltz, J.H.: Patch-based convolutional neural network for whole slide tissue image classification. In: Proceedings of the IEEE Conference on Computer Vision and Pattern Recognition, pp. 2424–2433 (2016)
7. Hu, R., Dollár, P., He, K., Darrell, T., Girshick, R.: Learning to segment every thing. In: Proceedings of the IEEE Conference on Computer Vision and Pattern Recognition, pp. 4233–4241 (2018)
8. Huang, Y.J., et al.: Rectifying supporting regions with mixed and active supervision for rib fracture recognition. IEEE Trans. Med. Imaging (2020)
9. Khened, M., Kori, A., Rajkumar, H., Srinivasan, B., Krishnamurthi, G.: A generalized deep learning framework for whole-slide image segmentation and analysis. arXiv preprint arXiv:2001.00258 (2020)

10. Li, J., et al.: Signet ring cell detection with a semi-supervised learning framework. In: Chung, A.C.S., Gee, J.C., Yushkevich, P.A., Bao, S. (eds.) IPMI 2019. LNCS, vol. 11492, pp. 842–854. Springer, Cham (2019). https://doi.org/10.1007/978-3-030-20351-1_66

11. Li, Z., et al.: Thoracic disease identification and localization with limited supervision. In: Proceedings of the IEEE Conference on Computer Vision and Pattern Recognition, pp. 8290–8299 (2018)

12. Mlynarski, P., Delingette, H., Criminisi, A., Ayache, N.: Deep learning with mixed supervision for brain tumor segmentation. J. Med. Imaging 6(3), 034002 (2019)

13. Nagpal, K., et al.: Development and validation of a deep learning algorithm for improving gleason scoring of prostate cancer. NPJ Digit. Med. 2(1), 1–10 (2019)

14. Otsu, N.: A threshold selection method from gray-level histograms. IEEE Trans. Syst. Man Cybern. 9(1), 62–66 (1979)

15. Paszke, A.,et al.: Automatic differentiation in pytorch. In: NIPS-W (2017)

16. Pei, L., Vidyaratne, L., Monibor Rahman, M., Shboul, Z.A., Iftekharuddin, K.M.: Multimodal brain tumor segmentation and survival prediction using hybrid machine learning. In: Crimi, A., Bakas, S. (eds.) BrainLes 2019. LNCS, vol. 11993, pp. 73–81. Springer, Cham (2020). https://doi.org/10.1007/978-3-030-46643-5_7

17. Robert, T., Thome, N., Cord, M.: Hybridnet: classification and reconstruction cooperation for semi-supervised learning. In: Proceedings of the European Conference on Computer Vision (ECCV), pp. 153–169 (2018)

18. Shaban, M., Awan, R., Fraz, M.M., Azam, A., Snead, D., Rajpoot, N.M.: Context-aware convolutional neural network for grading of colorectal cancer histology images. arXiv preprint arXiv:1907.09478 (2019)

19. Shah, M.P., Merchant, S.N., Awate, S.P.: MS-Net: mixed-supervision fully-convolutional networks for full-resolution segmentation. In: Frangi, A.F., Schnabel, J.A., Davatzikos, C., Alberola-López, C., Fichtinger, G. (eds.) MICCAI 2018. LNCS, vol. 11073, pp. 379–387. Springer, Cham (2018). https://doi.org/10.1007/978-3-030-00937-3_44

20. Ström, P., et al.: Pathologist-level grading of prostate biopsies with artificial intelligence. arXiv preprint arXiv:1907.01368 (2019)

21. Takahama, S., et al.: Multi-stage pathological image classification using semantic segmentation. In: Proceedings of the IEEE International Conference on Computer Vision, pp. 10702–10711 (2019)

22. Xie, Q., Hovy, E., Luong, M.T., Le, Q.V.: Self-training with noisy student improves imagenet classification. arXiv preprint arXiv:1911.04252 (2019)

23. Yu, F., Wang, D., Shelhamer, E., Darrell, T.: Deep layer aggregation. In: Proceedings of the IEEE Conference on Computer Vision and Pattern Recognition, pp. 2403–2412 (2018)

24. Zhao, X., Liang, S., Wei, Y.: Pseudo mask augmented object detection. In: Proceedings of the IEEE Conference on Computer Vision and Pattern Recognition, pp. 4061–4070 (2018)

25. Zhou, Y., Graham, S., Alemi Koohbanani, N., Shaban, M., Heng, P.A., Rajpoot, N.: CGC-Net: Cell graph convolutional network for grading of colorectal cancer histology images. In: Proceedings of the IEEE International Conference on Computer Vision Workshops (2019)

MorphSet: Improving Renal Histopathology Case Assessment Through Learned Prognostic Vectors

Pietro Antonio Cicalese[1(✉)], Syed Asad Rizvi[1], Victor Wang[1], Sai Patibandla[1],
Pengyu Yuan[1], Samira Zare[1], Katharina Moos[2], Ibrahim Batal[3],
Marian Clahsen-van Groningen[4], Candice Roufosse[5], Jan Becker[2], Chandra Mohan[1],
and Hien Van Nguyen[1]

[1] University of Houston, Houston, TX, USA
pcicalese@uh.edu
[2] Institute of Pathology, University Hospital of Cologne, Cologne, Germany
[3] Columbia University College of Physicians and Surgeons, New York, NY, USA
[4] Department of Pathology, Erasmus MC, Rotterdam, The Netherlands
[5] Department of Medicine, Imperial College, London, UK

Abstract. Computer Aided Diagnosis (CAD) systems for renal histopathology applications aim to understand and replicate nephropathologists' assessments of individual morphological compartments (e.g. glomeruli) to render case-level histological diagnoses. Deep neural networks (DNNs) hold great promise in addressing the poor intra- and interobserver agreement between pathologists. This being said, the generalization ability of DNNs heavily depends on the quality and quantity of training labels. Current "consensus" labeling strategies require multiple pathologists to evaluate every compartment unit over thousands of crops, resulting in enormous annotative costs. Additionally, these techniques fail to address the underlying reproducibility issues we observe across various diagnostic feature assessment tasks. To address both of these limitations, we introduce MorphSet, an end-to-end architecture inspired by Set Transformers which maps the combined encoded representations of Monte Carlo (MC) sampled glomerular compartment crops to produce Whole Slide Image (WSI) predictions on a case basis without the need for expensive fine-grained morphological feature labels. To evaluate performance, we use a kidney transplant Antibody Mediated Rejection (AMR) dataset, and show that we are able to achieve 98.9% case level accuracy, outperforming the consensus label baseline. Finally, we generate a visualization of prediction confidence derived from our MC evaluation experiments, which provides physicians with valuable feedback.

Keywords: Self attention · Antibody Mediated Rejection · Morphology

1 Introduction

Histopathology is on the verge of transforming into a highly quantitative and computational discipline. Within the next decade, Deep Neural Network (DNN) based Computer Aided Diagnosis (CAD) systems are expected to become indispensable for

© Springer Nature Switzerland AG 2021
M. de Bruijne et al. (Eds.): MICCAI 2021, LNCS 12908, pp. 319–328, 2021.
https://doi.org/10.1007/978-3-030-87237-3_31

histopathologists in their daily routine diagnostics, improving reproducibility and accuracy at considerably lower costs and with better transparency than molecular tests. Nephropathology is a subspecialty of histopathology that integrates paraffin histology, immunohistology and transmission electron microscopy observations into a single diagnosis for non-tumor diseases in native and transplant kidneys. In nephropathology, the diagnosis of disease entities like glomerulonephritis (as either present or absent) is highly reproducible. On the other hand, the assistance of such CADs is much more urgently needed for fine-grained prognostic details and disease entities with discriminative, gradual biology, such as Antibody-Mediated Rejection (AMR). For diagnostic simplicity, AMR is diagnosed as present (chronic active, chronic, or active) or absent according to the Banff Classification of histopathological and clinical parameters [11]. To address the limitations observed in existing classification methods for diseases with gradual manifestation, several research groups have developed supervised Convolutional Neural Network (CNN) classification architectures that can approximate the scoring criteria developed for several renal pathologies with variable success. They do not, however, solve the issues underlying pathologists' scores of individual compartment units.

Various research groups have opted to have multiple renal pathologists annotate the same images independently, treating their assessments as votes that can be used to approximate the general concepts underlying the given scoring criteria. This allows the CNN to generalize well to new cases, but it introduces significant annotative cost. In addition, consensus voting schemes aim to reflect the general opinion of the pathologists, but the fact that the minority votes are discarded may be harmful to performance since these discarded votes may still be informative for a disease with a gradual manifestation [12]. While other approaches may attempt to make use of all annotations, these processes still depend on votes generated with scoring criteria that lack reproducibility and undergo frequent revision [10]. We were interested in bypassing the scoring process for individual compartments entirely, leveraging the ability of DNNs to learn prognostic features in order to achieve reliable case-level accuracy. This could bypass the need for standardized nephropathology descriptors, as recently defined by Haas *et al.* [5], which have unknown underlying biology and uncertain reproducibility. Moreover, it would obviate the need for pre-analytical standardization of laboratory procedures as proposed by Barisoni *et al.* [3]. Thus, we introduce MorphSet, an architecture capable of attributing prognostic features to individual morphological compartments through a mechanism inspired by Set Transformers [9]. Our contributions are as follows:

– We propose a novel Monte Carlo (MC) glomeruli sampling method for generating unique subsets of available images for a given case, which we use to produce case-level predictions while improving regularization.
– We introduce two case-level architectures; the first architecture uses convolutional layers to process the input images for a given case, while the second architecture, which we call MorphSet, utilizes a multi-head self attention mechanism to compare embeddings of input images to various learned prognostic vectors.
– We repeat the MC sampling step which allows us to produce an aggregate prediction that is more representative of the input case. We subsequently use these MC predictions to generate model confidence visualizations, which provide meaningful feedback to the pathologist.

Related Works. Much of the recent DNN-based classification work in renal histopathology has been centered around the prediction of pathological findings in individual morphological compartments, particularly in glomeruli due to its diagnostic or prognostic relevance. Uchino *et al.* developed glomerular classifiers for seven pathological findings by fine-tuning an InceptionV3 network and using a majority decision approach to predict consensus labels on glomerular image crops [14]. While promising, we note that several important pathological findings could not be accurately classified, meaning that performance across the full spectrum of renal diseases remains elusive. Possible reasons for this are data scarcity and interobserver disagreement for the compartment unit labels, even with consensus descriptors. Overcoming scarcity problems and correcting for annotative disagreements in available nephropathology datasets will be a critical step for the further digitization of histopathology.

Other techniques for case-level classification of renal diseases have focused on resisting label noise and non-descriptive images in renal datasets, as well as patch-evaluation methods for WSI prediction. Cicalese *et al.* proposed an uncertainty guided CAD system for kidney-level case prediction that assigned case-level labels to individual morphological compartments in images and allowed the classifier to filter out non-descriptive images in its predictions [4]. Xu *et al.* used a Multiple-Instance Learning (MIL) framework to classify high resolution colon histopathology images, aggregating patch predictions by a voting criterion in which a WSI is predicted positive if it contains a patch that is predicted positive [16]. While promising, the vote aggregating criterion used is not robust, potentially giving single patches disproportionate influence over the final WSI prediction. Hou *et al.* addressed this by training a decision fusion model to aggregate high-resolution patch predictions into WSI-level predictions, outperforming both max-pooling and voting aggregation mechanisms on glioma and Non-Small-Cell Lung Carcinoma WSI cases [6]. This technique, however, relies on the automated extraction of discriminative crops from WSIs through the use of an Expectation Maximum (EM) based CNN method, which risks rejecting patches that are hard to classify but still biologically relevant. We were interested in explicitly learning prognostic features which we could use to produce unique embeddings corresponding to individual discriminative concepts with prognostic relevance. To accomplish this, we took inspiration from the Set Transformer architecture, which computes pixel-wise interactions with respect to a series of learned concepts for an input set [9]. We could then use these learned concepts to map a set of glomerular images to its relevant disease diagnosis, thus circumventing the need for fine-grained glomerular labels.

2   Methodology

2.1   AMR Dataset Generation and Annotation

To evaluate the effectiveness of our method with respect to a fine-grained annotation scheme, we used an Antibody Mediated Rejection (AMR) glomerular crop dataset. We chose this dataset given that we knew the case-level ground truths prior to data processing (i.e. we knew which transplants were positive for AMR through other criteria as donor-specific antibodies or C4d positive on immunohistology). We randomly selected a total of 89 (51 chronic active, chronic, or active AMR and 38 Non-AMR) blood group

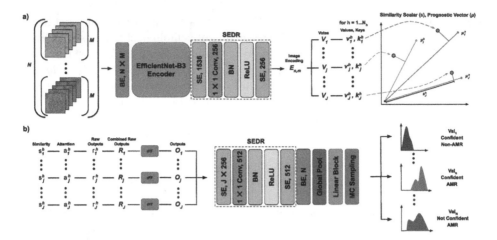

Fig. 1. The overall MorphSet architecture. **a)** We begin by sampling our M images across N cases, and encode each image as an individual batch element. After passing our encoded images through our Squeeze-Excitation Dimensionality Reduction (SEDR) block, we compare each image to a set of J parametrized Prognostic Vectors (PVs). **b)** Once we have computed our similarity scores, we proceed to produce unique embeddings for each μ_j, thus generating image-level assessments for each PV. We then pass our outputs through a second SEDR block, and concatenate the M encoded image embeddings together, yielding a batch size of N. After our global pooling and linear classification blocks, we can then perform Monte Carlo (MC) sampling during the evaluation phase to generate probability density curves, providing valuable feedback to the physician.

ABO- compatible, paraffin embedded kidney transplant biopsies, all of which satisfied the minimum sample criteria (≥ 7 glomeruli, ≥ 1 artery) [11]. All sections were cut to $2\,\mu m$ and were Periodic acid-Schiff (PAS) stained in the same pathology lab over a two year time frame. Micrographs were taken from all non-globally sclerosed glomeruli that were at least four levels apart at a resolution of 1024×768, yielding a total of 1,655 glomerular crops. Each of these images were then labeled by any combination of three experienced nephropathologists (from a group of four) using the LabelBox platform, with choices being AMR, non-AMR, or inconclusive [1]. In the event of a three way disagreement, the fourth pathologist would break the tie (54 tiebreakers, yielding a total of 5,019 annotations). Each image was then manually segmented by a single experienced pathologist using QuPath, a digital pathology software, to produce fine-grained masks for the biologically relevant glomerular compartment unit which were then used to extract the glomerular information prior to classification [2].

2.2 MorphSet

Given the variable number of glomerular crops that we see for any of our given N cases, we chose to pursue a MC sampling scheme; this allows us to sample M unique images at each iteration of training for a given case n. By doing this, we ensure that the architecture sees a new combination of images for each pass through the network, allowing it to account for the variability we see between glomerular crops and entire cases. In the event that there are fewer than M images available for a given case, we simply use online augmentation on the available set to produce the remaining images. We then pass these images through a CNN encoder to produce our initial feature embeddings. Once this is done, we then pass the outputs of our encoder network through a Squeeze-Excitation Dimensionality Reduction (SEDR) block (see Fig. 1), which consists of Squeeze-Excitation (SE) attention, followed by a linear layer, batch normalization, a ReLU activation function, and another SE attention operation [7].

A key component of our architecture lies in its ability to generate output representations for each image with respect to every encoded Prognostic Vector (PV), which we refer to as the MorphSet operation. We define PVs as learned discriminative feature embeddings that can be used to interpret individual images with respect to a specified number of key concepts (i.e. the number of PVs). Let $E^{m,n} \in \mathbb{R}^{p \times p}$ represent the encoded representation of the mth image from the nth case, with $p \times p$ features. These embeddings are then transformed to yield our votes $V_j^{m,n} \in \mathbb{R}^{p \times p}$, where j repre sents a particular PV that we wish to learn. We generate our votes using shared learned transformation matrices $W_j \in \mathbb{R}^{p \times p}$, following

$$V_j^{m,n} = W_j E^{m,n} \tag{1}$$

The vote generation process can be interpreted as a preparatory step which we will use to learn to compare each discriminative feature separately, mimicking how pathologists assess tissue morphology with respect to each relevant scoring task.

We chose to use an attention mechanism similar to that described in the Set Transformer architecture to compute the similarity between a set of votes V_j and their respective parametrized PVs μ_j, which were Kaiming initialized [9]. We accomplish this by generating a similarity measure between each vote and its parametrized PV, thus biasing the network to information that is representative of the given discriminative marker. Using this set operation also allows our comparison mechanism to retain linear time complexity $\mathcal{O}(J)$, where J is the number of learned PVs. To describe our comparison mechanism, we adopt the following naming conventions: the number of attention heads is denoted by N_h, while the number of dimensions for the key and value vectors are given by d_k and d_v, respectively. We define multi-head attention as evenly dividing the features in d_k and d_v into N_h pairs of output vectors such that d_k^h and d_v^h represent the key and value vectors of head h. We will omit the image indices m and n for the sake of simplicity while describing this mechanism.

We begin by flattening our vote matrices V_j to then generate N_h different d_k^h and d_v^h dimensional key (k_j^h) and value (v_j^h) vectors, using a set of learnable transformation matrices $\Lambda = \{W_k^h, W_v^h\}_{h=1}^{N_h}$, where $W_k^h \in \mathbb{R}^{p^2 \times d_k^h}$ and $W_v^h \in \mathbb{R}^{p^2 \times d_v^h}$. To simplify our presentation, we will set $d = d_v^h = d_k^h$ throughout the remainder of the paper. We parametrize our PV as μ^h and compute each element of our similarity matrix $S \in \mathbb{R}^{N_h \times J}$ following

$$s_j^h = k_j^h \cdot \mu_j^h \tag{2}$$

We can now generate our output using our computed similarity matrix with

$$r_j^h = \mu_j^h + a_j^h \cdot v_j^h \quad \text{where} \quad a^h = \texttt{softmax}(s^h/\sqrt{d}) \tag{3}$$

We scale the similarity vectors s^h by a factor of $1/\sqrt{d}$ to avoid the vanishing gradient problem described in [15], and then softmax the result to generate our final attention coefficients a^h. We can think of each PV μ_j^h as a static memory component, encoding the typical appearance of some discriminative feature, while the dynamic component $a_j^h \cdot v_j^h$ represents the degree to which a given input image deviates from the static concept. We then transform our concatenated outputs following

$$R = \texttt{Norm}[\texttt{concat}(r^1, ..., r^{N_h})W_o] \tag{4}$$

using Batch-Normalization (BN) for our $\texttt{Norm}$ computation [8]. Finally, the fully processed output representation is given by

$$O = \texttt{Norm}[R + \texttt{rFF}(R)] \tag{5}$$

with $\texttt{rFF}$ corresponding to a linear transformation that processes the inputs identically.

We then pass our feature embeddings through another SEDR dimensionality reduction block to facilitate our case-level computations. At this point, we edit the batch size to be of size N, where each stack of M image embeddings correspond to a single batch element n. Once this is done, we perform global pooling and pass our model through three linear layers to generate our case-level predictions. Another advantage of this architecture lies in its MC sampling protocol, which allows us to construct confidence metrics during evaluation. We may chose to sample multiple times in order to construct a probability density curve, which provides the operating physician with valuable feedback about the model's confidence in its assessment.

3   Results and Discussion

Training Settings. Throughout our experiments, we used an EfficientNet-B3 encoder that was pre-trained on ImageNet, given its computational efficiency and high performance [13]. To analyze the benefits of treating each case as an unlabeled set during classification, we also trained an EfficientNet-B3 AMR/Non-AMR glomerulus level classifier using a consensus labeling scheme (pre-trained on ImageNet, all inconclusive glomeruli removed). To analyze the impact of our PV embeddings, we trained a separate model that replaced the MorphSet operation with a simple convolution with the same output dimensionality, yielding our convolutional baseline model. All models were trained using a Binary Cross Entropy loss function with the Adam optimizer for 400 epochs with a learning rate of 1×10^{-4}, a β_1 value of 0.9, β_2 value of 0.999, and L2 coefficient of 0.01. For all of our experiments, we used a five-fold cross validation scheme, and all images were resized to 256×256 before being passed through each model. During training of both the convolutional baseline model and MorphSet, a batch size of three cases was used, with 12 glomerular crops being sampled from each case, yielding 36 input images per batch. To ensure that our comparisons were fair, we trained the EfficientNet-B3 glomerulus level classifier using a batch size of 36.

All images were ImageNet normalized, and were augmented during training using standard online transformations, where each image had a 50% chance of being horizontally flipped, vertically flipped, cropped to 70%–100% of its input size, and rotated between 0–90°, in that order.

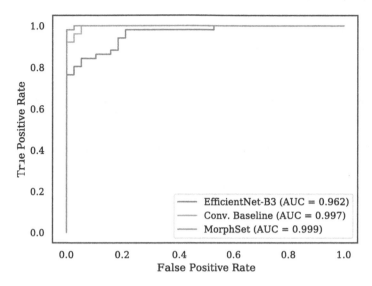

Fig. 2. ROC case-level curves for our three experimental models. The EfficientNet-B3 model's ROC curve was computed using the percentage of glomeruli classified as AMR for each case to avoid introducing a threshold bias. The models trained using the MC sampling scheme yielded higher AUC scores when compared to the EfficientNet-B3 baseline model.

MorphSet Performance. After encoding each of our input images with our EfficientNet-B3 encoder, we then reduce the dimensionality of the output from $[36, 1536, 8, 8]$ to $[36, 256, 8, 8]$ using our SEDR block (as shown in Fig. 1a). We train our architecture using eight parametrized PVs with one attention head ($k = 3$, $s = 2$, $p = 1$), resulting in an output dimensionality of $[32, 2048, 4, 4]$. We then pass the resulting outputs through our second SEDR block, concatenate the image embeddings for each case, and perform global pooling, producing an output dimensionality of $[3, 6144]$ (as shown in Fig. 1b). Our linear block consists of three linear layers, two of which reduce the dimensionality by a factor of two with batch normalization, followed by an output layer. We then perform MC sampling 100 times on each validation set, taking the average of our sigmoid activation outputs to produce our final predictions. To compare our EfficientNet-B3 baseline to both MC architecture's case-level scores, we chose to assign the percentage of glomeruli classified as AMR by the EfficientNet-B3 architecture for each case as it's respective case-level score. We then used an ROC curve to compare the performance between the three models (as shown in Fig. 2). We did this as opposed to fixing some classification threshold for EfficientNet-B3 AMR case level predictions (i.e. >50% of glomeruli classified as AMR constitutes an AMR case prediction) because pathologists do not generate case level diagnoses by using a hard set threshold on their glomerular assessments. Reporting case level accuracy in this way would therefore not be particularly meaningful from a medical standpoint, whereas reporting our results using an ROC curve allows us to avoid introducing a threshold bias, thus allowing us to compare the models fairly. Our resulting ROC curve highlights the performance improvements that we can attribute to our MC sampling set approach, with AUC increases in both the MorphSet and convolutional baseline models when compared to the glomerular level classifier. The convolutional baseline and MorphSet models achieve a case-level validation accuracy of 97.8% and 98.9%, respectively.

Probability Density Curves. To better understand the differences between MorphSet and the convolutional baseline model, we produced probability density curves using the 100 sigmoid activation outputs generated for each case during the MC sampling step. We found that MorphSet tended to produce higher probability point estimates for each AMR case, while also remaining more confident than the convolutional baseline model, as determined by our standard deviation (STD) computation, illustrated in Fig. 3. This result implies that MorphSet was better suited to learning the glomerular characteristics of AMR, and highlights the potential of our PV approach.

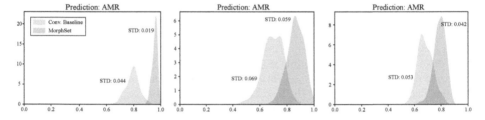

Fig. 3. Density versus probability point estimate curves generated using the convolutional baseline architecture (green) and MorphSet (red) for three AMR examples. We note that higher prediction densities at higher probability point estimate values imply that a model is more confident in its case level AMR prediction. MorphSet tended to produce AMR predictions with higher confidence, suggesting that MorphSet achieved a better understanding of glomerular AMR characteristics. (Color figure online)

4   Conclusion

In this work, we present an MC sampling approach for the case-level assessment of AMR in PAS stained renal histopathology glomerular crops, relieving the need for fine-grained structural annotation. We introduce both a convolutional case-level classifier and MorphSet, which learns unique Prognostic Vectors (PVs) meant to represent the discriminative concepts used by a pathologist when assessing tissue biopsies. We show that both of our proposed models outperform our fine-grained glomerulus classifier without having to remove inconclusive images or rely on using glomerular-level annotations. We also show that MorphSet was more confident in its AMR predictions while producing higher probability point estimates, suggesting it achieved a stronger understanding of the disease characteristics. Future works should aim to investigate the performance of MorphSet with larger datasets and multiple disease cases to improve our understanding of its generalization ability and how well it adapts to an increased number of discriminative concepts. The ability of the architecture to identify discriminative images for cases is another potential area of further study, as is the possibility of scaling up learning sets through reference pathologist cases without the need for fine-grained annotation.

References

1. Labelbox, labelbox, online (2020). https://labelbox.com
2. Bankhead, P., et al.: QuPath: open source software for digital pathology image analysis. bioRxiv (2017). https://doi.org/10.1101/099796, https://www.biorxiv.org/content/early/2017/03/06/099796
3. Barisoni, L., et al.: Digital pathology imaging as a novel platform for standardization and globalization of quantitative nephropathology. Clin. Kidney J. **10**(2), 176–187 (2017). https://doi.org/10.1093/ckj/sfw129
4. Cicalese, P.A., Mobiny, A., Shahmoradi, Z., Yi, X., Mohan, C., Van Nguyen, H.: Kidney level lupus nephritis classification using uncertainty guided Bayesian convolutional neural networks. IEEE J. Biomed. Health Inform. **25**(2), 315–324 (2021). https://doi.org/10.1109/JBHI.2020.3039162
5. Haas, M., et al.: Consensus definitions for glomerular lesions by light and electron microscopy: recommendations from a working group of the Renal Pathology Society. Kidney Int. **98**(5), 1120–1134 (2020). https://doi.org/10.1016/j.kint.2020.08.006
6. Hou, L., Samaras, D., Kurc, T.M., Gao, Y., Davis, J.E., Saltz, J.H.: Patch-based convolutional neural network for whole slide tissue image classification (2016)
7. Hu, J., Shen, L., Sun, G.: Squeeze-and-excitation networks. In: Proceedings of the IEEE Conference on Computer Vision and Pattern Recognition, pp. 7132–7141 (2018)
8. Ioffe, S., Szegedy, C.: Batch normalization: Accelerating deep network training by reducing internal covariate shift. CoRR arXiv:1502.03167 (2015)
9. Lee, J., Lee, Y., Kim, J., Kosiorek, A., Choi, S., Teh, Y.W.: Set transformer: a framework for attention-based permutation-invariant neural networks. In: International Conference on Machine Learning, pp. 3744–3753. PMLR (2019)
10. Liapis, G., Singh, H.K., Derebail, V.K., Gasim, A.M.H., Kozlowski, T., Nickeleit, V.: Diagnostic significance of peritubular capillary basement membrane multilaminations in kidney allografts: old concepts revisited. Transplantation **94**(6), 620–629 (2012)
11. Roufosse, C., et al.: A 2018 reference guide to the Banff classification of renal allograft pathology. Transplantation **102**(11), 1795–1814 (2018)
12. Smith, B., et al.: A method to reduce variability in scoring antibody-mediated rejection in renal allografts: implications for clinical trials - a retrospective study. Transpl. Int. **32**(2), 173–183 (2019). https://doi.org/10.1111/tri.13340
13. Tan, M., Le, Q.: EfficientNet: rethinking model scaling for convolutional neural networks. In: Chaudhuri, K., Salakhutdinov, R. (eds.) Proceedings of the 36th International Conference on Machine Learning. Proceedings of Machine Learning Research, vol. 97, pp. 6105–6114. PMLR, June 2019. http://proceedings.mlr.press/v97/tan19a.html
14. Uchino, E., et al.: Classification of glomerular pathological findings using deep learning and nephrologist-AI collective intelligence approach. Int. J. Med. Inform. **141**, 104231 (2020)

328   P. A. Cicalese et al.

15. Vaswani, A., et al.: Attention is all you need (2017)
16. Xu, Y., Mo, T., Feng, Q., Zhong, P., Lai, M., Chang, E.I.: Deep learning of feature representation with multiple instance learning for medical image analysis. In: 2014 IEEE International Conference on Acoustics, Speech and Signal Processing (ICASSP), pp. 1626–1630 (2014). https://doi.org/10.1109/ICASSP.2014.6853873

Accounting for Dependencies in Deep Learning Based Multiple Instance Learning for Whole Slide Imaging

Andriy Myronenko$^{(\boxtimes)}$, Ziyue Xu , Dong Yang , Holger R. Roth ,
and Daguang Xu

NVIDIA, Santa Clara, CA, USA
amyronenko@nvidia.com

Abstract. Multiple instance learning (MIL) is a key algorithm for classification of whole slide images (WSI). Histology WSIs can have billions of pixels, which create enormous computational and annotation challenges. Typically, such images are divided into a set of patches (a bag of instances), where only bag-level class labels are provided. Deep learning based MIL methods calculate instance features using convolutional neural network (CNN). Our proposed approach is also deep learning based, with the following two contributions: Firstly, we propose to explicitly account for dependencies between instances during training by embedding self-attention Transformer blocks to capture dependencies between instances. For example, a tumor grade may depend on the presence of several particular patterns at different locations in WSI, which requires to account for dependencies between patches. Secondly, we propose an instance-wise loss function based on instance pseudo-labels. We compare the proposed algorithm to multiple baseline methods, evaluate it on the PANDA challenge dataset, the largest publicly available WSI dataset with over 11K images, and demonstrate state-of-the-art results.

Keywords: Multiple instance learning · Histopathology · Transformer · Whole slide imaging · Self-attention

1 Introduction

Whole slide images (WSI) are digitizing histology slides often analysed for diagnosis of cancer [3]. WSI can contain several billions pixels, and are commonly tiled into smaller patches for processing to reduce the computational burden (Fig. 1). Another reason to use patches is because the area of interest (tumor cells) occupies only a tiny fraction of the image, which impedes the performance of conventional classifiers, most of which assume that the class object occupies a large central part of the image. Unfortunately, patch-wise labels are usually not available, since the detailed annotations are too costly and time-consuming.

Electronic supplementary material The online version of this chapter (https://doi.org/10.1007/978-3-030-87237-3_32) contains supplementary material, which is available to authorized users.

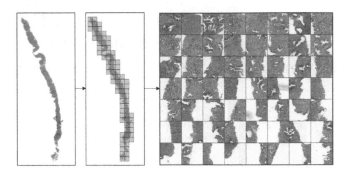

Fig. 1. An example of patch extraction from WSI from the PANDA challenge dataset [2]. We tile the image and retain only the foreground patches, out of which we take a random subset to form a bag.

An alternative to supervised learning is weakly-supervised learning, where only a single label per WSI is available.

Multiple Instance Learning (MIL) is a weakly supervised learning algorithms, which aims to train a model using a set of weakly labeled data [5,13]. Usually a single class label is provided for a bag of many unlabeled instances, indicating that at least one instance has the provided class label. It has many applications in computer vision and language processing [4], however learning from bags raises important challenges that are unique to MIL. In context of histopathology, a WSI represents a bag, and the extracted patches (or their features) represent instances (we often use these notations interchangeably).

With the advent of convolutional neural networks (CNN), deep learning based MIL has become the mainstream methodological choice for WSI [10]. Campanella et al. [3] was one of the first works to conduct a large study on over 44K WSI, laying the foundation for MIL applications in clinical practise. Since the instance labels are not known, classical MIL algorithm usually selects only one (or a few) instances based on the maximum of the prediction probability at the current iteration. Such approach is very time consuming, as all patches need to be inferenced, but only a single patch contributes to the training of CNNs at each iteration. Ilse et al. [14] proposed to use an attention mechanism (a learnable weights per instance) to utilize all image patches, which we also adopt.

More recent MIL methods include works by Zhao et al. [18], who proposed to pre-train a feature extractor based on the variational auto-encoder, and use a graph convolutional network for final classification. Hashimoto et al. [7] proposed to combine MIL with domain adversarial normalization and multiple scale learning. Lu et al. [11] precomputed patch-level features (using pretrained CNN) offline to speed up training, and proposed an additional clustering-based loss to improve generalization during MIL training. Maksoud et al. [12] proposed to use a hierarchical approach to process the down-scaled WSI first, followed by high resolution processing when necessary. Such approach demonstrated significant reduction in processing time, while maintaining the baseline accuracy.

We observed that most MIL methods assume no dependencies among instances, which is seldom true especially in histopathology [10]. Furthermore, a lack of instance-level loss supervision creates more opportunities for CNNs to overfit. In this work, we propose a deep learning based MIL algorithm for WSI classification with the following contributions:

- we propose to explicitly account for dependencies between instances during training. We embed transformer encoder [15] blocks into the classification CNN to capture the dependencies between instances.
- we propose an instance-wise loss supervision based on instance pseudo-labels. The pseudo-labels are computed based on the ensemble of several models, by aggregating the attention weights and instance-level predictions.

We evaluate the proposed method on PANDA challenge [2] dataset, which is currently the largest publicly available WSI dataset with over 11000 images, against the baseline methods as well as against the Kaggle challenge leaderboard with over 1000 competing teams, and demonstrate state-of-the-art (SOTA) classification results.

2   Method

MIL aims to classify a bag of instances $\mathbf{H} = \{\mathbf{h}_1, \ldots, \mathbf{h}_K\}$ as positive if at least one of the instances $\mathbf{h}_k$ is positive. The number of instances K could vary between the bags. Individual instance labels are unknown, and only the bag level label $Y = [0, 1]$ is provided:

$$Y = \begin{cases} 0, & \text{iff all } y_k = 0, \\ 1, & \text{iff any } y_k = 1. \end{cases} \tag{1}$$

which is equivalent to $Y = \max_k\{y_k\}$ definition using a Max operator. Training a model whose loss is based on the maximum over instance labels is problematic due to vanishing gradients [14], and the training process becomes slow since only a single patch contributes to the optimization. Ilse et al. [14] proposed to use all image patches as linear combination weighted by attention weights. Consider $\mathbf{H} \in \mathbb{R}^{M \times K}$ to be instance embeddings, e.g. features of a CNN final layer after average pooling. Then a linear combination of patch embeddings is

$$\mathbf{z} = \sum_{k=1}^{K} a_k \mathbf{h}_k = \mathbf{Ha} \tag{2}$$

where the attention weights of patch embeddings are $\mathbf{a} = softmax(\tanh(\mathbf{HV})\mathbf{w})$ where $\mathbf{w} \in \mathbb{R}^{L \times 1}$ and $\mathbf{V} \in \mathbb{R}^{M \times L}$ are parameters. The attention weights are computed using a multilayer perceptron (MLP) network with a single hidden layer.

2.1   Dependency Between Instances

The assumption of no dependency between the bag instances often does not hold. For example, for grading the severity of prostate cancer, pathologists need to find

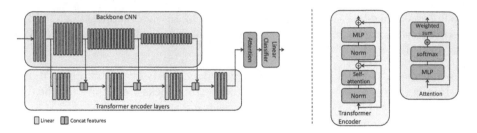

Fig. 2. Model architecture overview. The backbone CNN (blue) extracts features at different scales, which are spatially averaged-pooled before feeding into the transformer encoder layers (green), to account for dependencies between instances. The input to the network is $B \times N \times 3 \times W \times H$. Where B is the batch size, N is the number of instances (patches extracted from a single whole slide image), and $3 \times W \times H$ is the spatial patch size. (Color figure online)

two distinct tumor growth patterns in the image and assign Gleason scores to each [1]. Then the International Society of Urological Pathology (ISUP) grade is calculated, based on the combination of major and minor Gleason patterns. ISUP grade indicates a severity of the tumor and plays a crucial role in treatment planning. Here, we propose to use the self-attention to account for dependencies between instances. In particular, we adopt the transformer, which was initially introduced to capture long range dependencies between words in sentences [15] and later applied to vision [6]. Whereas traditional convolutions are local operation, the self-attention block of Transformers computes attention between all combinations of tokens at a larger range directly.

A key component of transformer blocks is a scaled dot product self-attention which is defined as $softmax(QK^T/\sqrt{d})V$, where queries Q, keys K, and values V matrices are all derived as linear transformations of the input (in our case the instance features space **H**). The self-attention is performed several times with different, learned linear projections in parallel (multi-head attention). In addition to self-attention, each of the transformer encoder layers also contains a fully connected feed-forward network and layer normalization (see Fig. 2) [6,15].

We propose two variants of utilizing transformers. In the simplest case we attach a transformer encoder block only to the end of the backbone classification CNN after avg pooling. The idea is similar to the approach proposed in Visual transformers, but before avg pooling [6]. The difference here is that in Visual transformers, the goal was to account for dependencies between the spatial regions (16px × 16px) of the same patch. Whereas we want to account for the dependencies among the patches. Another relevant work was proposed by Wang et al. [16] to utilize self-attention within MIL, but for text-based disease symptoms classification. We maintain the dimensionality of encoded data, so that the input, output and hidden dimensionality of the transformer encoder are the same. We call it Transformer MIL.

We also consider a variant of a deeper integration of the transformer with the backbone CNN. We attach separate transformer encoder blocks after each of the main ResNet blocks [8] to capture the patch encodings at different levels of its feature pyramid. The output of the first transformer encoder is concatenated with next feature scale space of ResNet (after average pooling), and is fed into the next level transformer encoder, up until the final encoder layer, followed by the attention layer. We want to capture dependencies between patches at multiple scales, since different level of CNN output features include different semantic information. Such a Pyramid Transformer MIL network is shown in Fig. 2 (Fig. 3).

2.2 Instance Level Semi-supervision and Pseudo-labeling

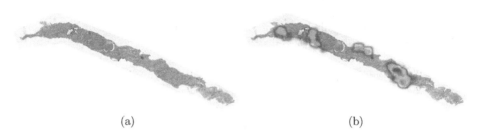

(a)   (b)

Fig. 3. An example ISUP grade 5 prostate cancer WSI. (a) Green mask overlay shows ground truth location of cancer regions (provided in the PANDA dataset [2]). (b) an additional heat map overlay visualizes our pseudo-labels of ISUP 5 (weighted by attention), achieved from training on weak (bag-level) labels only. Notice the close agreement between the dense pseudo-labels and the ground truth. In practice, pseudo-labels are computed per patch; here we used a sliding-window approach for dense visualization. (Color figure online)

One of the challenges of MIL training is the lack of instance labels to guide the optimization process. A somewhat similar issue is encountered in semi-supervised learning [17], where pseudo-labels are used either offline or on the fly based on some intermediate estimates or another network's predictions. Here, we propose to generate pseudo-labels for each image patch and use the additional patch-wise loss to assist the optimization process.

$$L = L_{bag} + \lambda \sum_k L_{patch} \tag{3}$$

where the total loss L includes a bag-level loss L_{bag} (based on the ground truth labels) and a patch level loss L_{patch} (based on the pseudo-labels). We use cross-entropy loss function for both bag-level and patch-level losses.

We opt for a simple approach to generate pseudo-labels based on ensembling of several identical models trained from random initialization. The final ensembled labels are hard label (rounded to the nearest classes). Consider a trained network, its bag-level prediction output is based on the final output vector z (see Eq. 2), followed by a linear projection onto the number of output classes:

$$\mathbf{c} = sigm(\mathbf{W}\mathbf{z}) = sigm(\mathbf{W}\mathbf{H}\mathbf{a}) \tag{4}$$

Pseudocode 1: Pseudo-labels assignment

Train N MIL models (N=5)
for *all patches in the bag* **do**
   Run inference on patches for each image
   Ensemble predictions of attention weights **a** and instance classes c_k
   if *bag label is not zero* **then**
      for patches with top 10% of highest attention **a** weights, assign the ensembled labels as pseudo-label
      for patches with top 10% of lowest attention **a** weights, assign the zero labels as the pseudo-label
      otherwise flag the patch as unknown pseudo-label
   else
      assign zero pseudo-labels for all patches, since here we know that all patches must have zero labels
   end
end

---

here we assumed a final sigmoid function (but the same holds with softmax). We approximate the individual instance level prediction as

$$c_k = sigm(\mathbf{W}\mathbf{h}_k) \tag{5}$$

Pseudocode 1 shows the algorithm to compute the pseudo-labels. For some patches, whose ensembled attention weights are neither small nor large (defined by 10% threshold), we do not assign any pseudo-labels, and mark then and unknown to exclude from the L_{patch} loss. Given the pseudo-labels we re-optimize the model using the additional patch-wise loss. The 10% heuristic was chosen to retain only most confident patches, that contribute the most to the final bag-level classification. A relevant approach was recently proposed by Lerousseau et al. [9]. However the goal of their work is a dense segmentation map, and not the improvements to the global classification accuracy, and the pseudo-labels are calculated differently, through thresholding of current prediction probability estimates on the fly.

3   Experiments

We implemented our method in PyTorch[1] and trained it on 4 NVIDIA Tesla V100 16 GB GPUs, batch size of 16. For the classification backbone, we use ResNet50 pretrained on ImageNet [8]. For the transformer layers, we keep a similar config-uration as in [15], with 4 stacked transformer encoder blocks. The lower pyramid level transformer has dimensionality of 256 for both input and hidden. The final transformer encoder has input dimension of 2308 (a concatenation of ResNet50 output features and the previous transformer outputs). We use Adam optimizer

---

[1] https://pytorch.org/.

with initial learning rate of $\alpha_0 = 3e-4$ for CNN parameters, and $3e-5$ for transformer parameters, then gradually decrease it using cosine learning rate scheduler for 50 epochs. We use 5-fold cross validations to tune the parameters. For transformer layers only, we use weight decay of 0.1 and no dropout.

PANDA Dataset. Prostate cANcer graDe Assessment (PANDA) challenge dataset consists of 11K whole-slide images from two centers [2]. Currently, this is the largest public WSI dataset available. The grading process consisted of finding and classifying cancer tissue into Gleason patterns based on the architectural growth patterns of the tumor [1]. Consequently, it is converted into an ISUP grade on a 1–5 scale, based on the presence of two distinct Gleason patterns. The dataset was provided as part of the Panda kaggle challenge, which attracted more than 1000 teams, with the goal to predict the most accurate ISUP grades. Each individual image on average is about 25,000px × 25,000px RGB. The challenge also includes a hidden dataset, whose images were graded by multiple pathologists. The private dataset labels are not publicly available, but can be used to asses your model blindly via Kaggle website (invisible to the public as the challenge is closed now). In our experiments, we use a medium resolution input images (4× smaller than the highest resolution).

Patch Selection. To extract patches from WSI, we tile the image into a grid of 224px × 224px patches. At each iteration, the grid has a random offset from the top left corner, to ensure randomness of the patches. We then retain only the foreground patches. From the remaining patches, we maintain only a random subset (K = 56), which is a trade-off between covering the tissue content and GPU memory limits (see Fig. 1). We use batch size 16, which makes the data input size $16 \times K \times 3 \times 224 \times 224$ at each iteration. During testing, inference is done using all foreground patches.

3.1 Results

Transformer MIL. We evaluate and compare our method to the Attention MIL and its Gated Attention MIL [14], as well as to a classical MIL with Max operator [3]. For evaluation metrics we use Accuracy, Area Under Curve (AUC) and Quadratic Weighted Kappa (QWK) of ISUP grade prediction (see Table 1). QWK metric measures the similarity between the predictions and targets, with a maximum value of 1. QWK was chosen as the main metric during the PANDA challenge [2], since it is more appropriate for the tasks with predicted classes being severity grades/levels. All metrics are computed using our 5-fold (80%/20% training/validation) splits, except for the *Leaderboard* column results, which come from the evaluation on kaggle challenge hidden private test-set. Even though the challenge is closed now, it allows for blind submission of the code snippet, which runs on the PANDA hidden set and outputs the final QWK number. These results are not added to the kaggle leaderboard, and are allowed only for post-challenge evaluations. Table 1 shows that the proposed two transforms based approaches outperform other methods both in our validation sets, and on the challenge hidden set.

We have also inspected the self-attention matrices and found that for many cases, they have distinct off-diagonal high value elements. In particular, instances with WSI tumor cells of different Gleason scores have higher off-diagonal values, indicating that such a combination is valuable for the final classification, which was captured by the transformer self-attention.

Patch-Wise Pseudo-labels. We train 5 models and ensemble their patch-level predictions. We use $\lambda = 100$. We show the performance of adding the pseudo-labels supervision in Table 2. In all cases the performance has improved compared to the baselines shown in Table 1 by $\sim$1%. Table 2 also shows the QWK results of the winners (top 3 places) of the PANDA kaggle challenge. Notice that our single model results are on par with the winners of the challenge (who all use ensembling of several models). We also experimented with ensembling, and the ensemble of our 10 models, achieves the leaderboard QWK of 0.94136, which would have been the first place in the leaderboard.

We have also tried but found no benefit of repeating pseudo-labeling several rounds, because the pseudo-label values almost do not change after the 1st round.

Table 1. Evaluations results on PANDA dataset. The Leaderboard column shows the QWK results of the private leaderboard of Kaggle's challenge, which allows direct comparison to more then 1000 participants.

	Accuracy	AUC	QWK	Leaderboard
Attention MIL [14]	0.793 ± 0.035	0.983 ± 0.021	0.948 ± 0.036	0.915 ± 0.086
Gated attention MIL [14]	0.795 ± 0.037	0.981 ± 0.011	0.936 ± 0.042	0.914 ± 0.069
Max MIL [3]	0.770 ± 0.055	0.973 ± 0.048	0.910 ± 0.053	0.868 ± 0.091
Transformer MIL	0.801 ± 0.014	0.988 ± 0.015	0.960 ± 0.034	0.930 ± 0.012
Pyramid Transformer MIL	$\mathbf{0.805 \pm 0.011}$	$\mathbf{0.989 \pm 0.018}$	$\mathbf{0.961 \pm 0.032}$	$\mathbf{0.932 \pm 0.015}$

Table 2. Evaluation results of adding pseudo-labels to our baseline transformer MIL approaches. We also include the results of the top three places of this challenge[a] (who all use ensembling of several models). Our results indicate that pseudo-labeling further improves the performance, with our single model providing results on par with the top winning teams.

	QWK (val)	QWK (Leaderboard)
Attention MIL [14] + Pseudo-labels	0.9502 ± 0.0319	0.9304 ± 0.0542
Transformer MIL + Pseudo-labels	0.9614 ± 0.0367	0.9347 ± 0.0353
Pyramid Transformer MIL + Pseudo-labels	$\mathbf{0.9652 \pm 0.0168}$	$\mathbf{0.9365 \pm 0.0513}$
First place - Panda kaggle challenge [2]	–	0.94085
Second place - Panda kaggle challenge [2]	–	0.93768
Third place - Panda kaggle challenge [2]	–	0.93480
Pyramid Transformer MIL (ours, ensemble of 10)	–	**0.94136**

[a] https://www.kaggle.com/c/prostate-cancer-grade-assessment/leaderboard

4   Discussion and Conclusion

We proposed a new deep learning based MIL approach for WSI classification with the following two main contributions: the addition of the transformer module to account for dependencies among instances and the instance-level supervision loss using pseudo-labels. We evaluated the method on PANDA challenge prostate WSI dataset, which includes over 11000 images. To put in perspective, most recently published SOTA methods evaluated their performance on datasets with the order of only several hundred images [7,11,12,18]. Furthermore, we compared our results directly to the leaderboard of the PANDA kaggle challenge with over 1000 participating teams, and demonstrated that our single model performance is on par with the top three winning teams, as evaluated blindly on the same hidden private test-set. Finally, recently proposed visual transformers [6] have shown a capability to replace the classification CNN completely, allowing for the possibility to create deep learning based MIL model solely based on the transformer blocks; we leave these investigations for future research.

References

1. Bulten, W., et al.: Artificial intelligence assistance significantly improves Gleason grading of prostate biopsies by pathologists. Mod. Pathol. **34**, 660–671 (2021)
2. Bulten, W., et al.: The panda challenge: Prostate cancer grade assessment using the Gleason grading system. In: MICCAI challenge (2020). https://panda.grand-challenge.org/home/
3. Campanella, G., et al.: Clinical-grade computational pathology using weakly supervised deep learning on whole slide images. Nat. Med. **25**, 1301–1309 (2019)
4. Carbonneau, M.A., Cheplygina, V., Granger, E., Gagnon, G.: Multiple instance learning: a survey of problem characteristics and applications. Pattern Recogn. **77**, 329–353 (2018)
5. Dietterich, T.G., Lathrop, R.H., Lozano-Perez, T.: Solving the multiple instance problem with axis-parallel rectangles. Artif. Intell. **89**, 31–71 (1997)
6. Dosovitskiy, A., et al.: An image is worth 16 × 16 words: transformers for image recognition at scale. In: ICLR (2021)
7. Hashimoto, N., et al.: Multi-scale domain-adversarial multiple-instance CNN for cancer subtype classification with unannotated histopathological images. In: CVPR (2020)
8. He, K., Zhang, X., Ren, S., Sun, J.: Identity mappings in deep residual networks. In: Leibe, B., Matas, J., Sebe, N., Welling, M. (eds.) ECCV 2016. LNCS, vol. 9908, pp. 630–645. Springer, Cham (2016). https://doi.org/10.1007/978-3-319-46493-0_38
9. Lerousseau, M., et al.: Weakly supervised multiple instance learning histopathological tumor segmentation. In: Martel, A.L., et al. (eds.) MICCAI 2020. LNCS, vol. 12265, pp. 470–479. Springer, Cham (2020). https://doi.org/10.1007/978-3-030-59722-1_45
10. Srinidhi, C.L., Ciga, O., Martel, A.L.: Deep neural network models for computational histopathology: a survey. Med. Image Anal. **67**, 329–353 (2021)
11. Lu, M.Y., Williamson, D.F.K., Chen, T.Y., Chen, R.J., Barbieri, M., Mahmood, F.: Data efficient and weakly supervised computational pathologyon whole slide images. Nat. Biomed. Eng. **19**, 555–570 (2021)

12. Maksoud, S., Zhao, K., Hobson, P., Jennings, A., Lovell, B.C.: SOS: selective objective switch for rapid immunofluorescence whole slide image classification. In: CVPR (2020)
13. Maron, O., Lozano-Perez, T.: A framework for multiple-instance learning. In: NIPS, pp. 570–576 (1998)
14. Ilse, M., Jakub, M., Tomczak, M.W.: Attention-based deep multiple instance learning. In: ICML, pp. 2127–2136 (2018)
15. Vaswani, A., et al.: Attention is all you need. In: NIPS, vol. 30 (2017)
16. Wang, Z., Poon, J., Poon, S.K.: AMI-net+: a novel multi-instance neural network for medical diagnosis from incomplete and imbalanced data. Aust. J. Intell. Inf. Process. Syst. 15(3), 8–15 (2019)
17. Xie, Q., Luong, M.T., Hovy, E., Le, Q.V.: Self-training with noisy student improves ImageNet classification. In: CVPR, pp. 10687–10698 (2020)
18. Zhao, Y., et al.: Predicting lymph node metastasis using histopathological images based on multiple instance learning with deep graph convolution. In: CVPR (2020)

Whole Slide Images are 2D Point Clouds: Context-Aware Survival Prediction Using Patch-Based Graph Convolutional Networks

Richard J. Chen[1,2,3,4(✉)], Ming Y. Lu[1,2,3,4], Muhammad Shaban[1,2,3,4], Chengkuan Chen[1,2,3,4], Tiffany Y. Chen[1,2,3,4], Drew F. K. Williamson[1,2,3,4], and Faisal Mahmood[1,2,3,4]

[1] Department of Pathology, Brigham and Women's Hospital, Boston, USA
faisalmahmood@bwh.harvard.edu
[2] Department of Biomedical Informatics, Harvard Medical School, Boston, USA
richardchen@g.harvard.edu
[3] Cancer Data Science Program, Dana Farber Cancer Institute, Boston, USA
[4] Cancer Program, Broad Institute of Harvard and MIT, Cambridge, USA

Abstract. Cancer prognostication is a challenging task in computational pathology that requires context-aware representations of histology features to adequately infer patient survival. Despite the advancements made in weakly-supervised deep learning, many approaches are not context-aware and are unable to model important morphological feature interactions between cell identities and tissue types that are prognostic for patient survival. In this work, we present Patch-GCN, a context-aware, spatially-resolved patch-based graph convolutional network that hierarchically aggregates instance-level histology features to model local- and global-level topological structures in the tumor microenvironment. We validate Patch-GCN with 4,370 gigapixel WSIs across five different cancer types from the Cancer Genome Atlas (TCGA), and demonstrate that Patch-GCN outperforms all prior weakly-supervised approaches by 3.58–9.46%. Our code and corresponding models are publicly available at https://github.com/mahmoodlab/Patch-GCN.

Keywords: Computer vision · Computational pathology · Weakly-supervised learning · Graph convolutional networks · Interpretability

1 Introduction

Weakly-supervised deep learning has made remarkable progress in computational pathology in using whole slide images (WSIs) for cancer diagnosis and prognosis [1–5]. Due to the computational complexities in training with WSIs, many

Electronic supplementary material The online version of this chapter (https://doi.org/10.1007/978-3-030-87237-3_33) contains supplementary material, which is available to authorized users.

© Springer Nature Switzerland AG 2021
M. de Bruijne et al. (Eds.): MICCAI 2021, LNCS 12908, pp. 339–349, 2021.
https://doi.org/10.1007/978-3-030-87237-3_33

weakly-supervised methods have approached WSIs using multiple instance learning (MIL), in which: 1) small image patches from the WSI are extracted as independent instances, and then 2) pooled using a global aggregation operator over the bag of unordered instances. Despite not being context-aware and without needing detailed clinical annotation, many of these MIL-based approaches are able to still solve difficult tasks such as cancer grading and subtyping using only slide-level labels, as the distinction between morphological phenotypes such as tumor vs. non-tumor tissue may only depend on instance-level patch-based features [6].

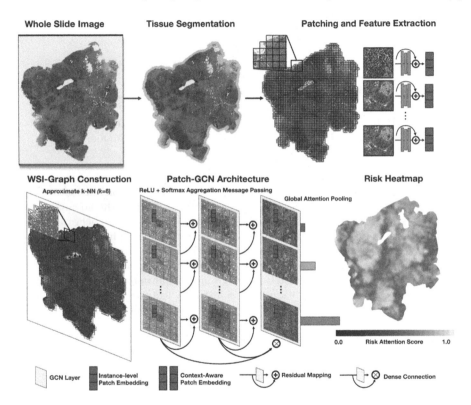

Fig. 1. Patch-GCN framework for context-aware survival outcome prediction in WSIs. Non-overlapping 256×256 patches are patched as used as input into a ResNet-50 CNN to construct the node feature matrix, with edges drawn between adjacent image patches in the WSI. A ReLU + Softmax Message Passing scheme is used to aggregate instance-level embeddings in local neighborhoods, with residual mappings and skip connections used to construct context-aware embeddings, followed by global attention-based pooling.

In contrast with cancer grading and subtyping, cancer prognostication is a challenging task that requires considering both instance- and global-level features in the tumor and surrounding tissues for assessing patient risk of mortality [7,8]. In adapting the MIL framework to WSIs, many approaches follow the standard multiple instance (SMI) assumption for solving clinical tasks in computational pathology, *e.g.* - if a bag contains at least one positive instance, it is labeled positive, else negative [9]. This assumption holds when the clinical task is solving binary instance-level feature discrimination problems such as tumor vs. non-tumor tissue. However, in tasks such as survival outcome prediction in cancer pathology, MIL-based approaches are unable to capture important contextual and hierarchical information that have known prognostic significance in cancer survival [10,11]. For example, though MIL would be able to learn instance-level features that discriminate image patches of lymphocytes and tumor cells, it is unable to distinguish whether those immune cells are tumor-infiltrating lymphocytes (TILs) or from an adjacent inflammatory response, which depends on the lymphocytes' apposition to tumor cells or normal stroma respectively [8,12].

In this work, we propose a context-aware, spatially-resolved patch-based graph convolutional network (Patch-GCN) for survival prediction in patients with multiple WSIs (Fig. 1). One of the key contributions of our work is that we formulate WSIs as a graph-based data structure in the Euclidean space similar to a point cloud in which: 1) nodes correspond to histology image patches, and 2) edges are connected between adjacent image patches from the true spatial coordinates of the WSI. As a result, message passing in Patch-GCN generalizes the standard convolutional operator in CNNs, in which node features are hierarchically aggregated from local to global structures in the WSI. Compared to other weakly-supervised learning approaches such as MIL, Patch-GCN is context-aware and is able to build hierarchical representations of morphological image patch features in context with their surrounding environment. To robustly validate Patch-GCN, we quantitatively assessed our model on five different cancer datasets from The Cancer Genome Atlas (TCGA) in survival outcome prediction against several state-of-the-art methods in weakly-supervised learning for WSIs, and evaluated the interpretability of Patch-GCN through attention heatmaps in low and high risk patients (Fig. 2). Our code is made available at https://github.com/mahmoodlab/Patch-GCN.

2   Related Work

2.1   Survival Analysis in WSIs

In recent years, deep learning methods using CNNs and MIL-based approaches have been proposed for survival analysis in WSIs [13–15]. Due to the large image sizes of WSIs, many of these methods rely on selective sampling of small image ROIs for tractable training and inference, which are then used matched with patient-level outcome labels. Mobadersany et al. [13] proposed one of the first methods for end-to-end training with 1024 × 1024 image ROIs using CNNs supervised with the Partial Cox Proportional Hazard loss. Zhu et al. [14] developed a two-step-based approach for WSI-level survival outcome prediction, in which patches are clustered using K-Means groups using K-Means clustering method then used as inputs into a CNN. Yao et al. [16] similarly proposed patch-based sampling K-Means clustering to identify morphological phenotypes in WSIs.

2.2   Graph-Based Analysis in Computational Pathology

In addition to CNNs and MIL-based approaches, GCNs and other graph-based methods have received attention in computational pathology, solving problems such as cancer classification [9,17–20], cancer grading [21–23], and survival analysis [24,25]. Many of these approaches, however, consider only cell identities as graph nodes, which ignores important prognostic tissue features such as stroma and are confined again to small image regions [10]. In survival analysis, Chen *et al.* [25] constructed a cell-based graph for small image ROIs followed by spectral convolutions. Alternatively, Li *et al.* [24] proposed sampling patches in a WSI as nodes, followed by constructing edges between patches via feature similarity on the embedding space and using spectral convolutions. However, we argue that in using this approach for graph construction, GCNs are unable to learn context-aware features as message passing as feature interactions between adjacent image patches are not modeled.

3   Method

3.1   WSI-Graph Construction

For a given sample, let patient P, overall survival time T and censorship status C be a single triplet observation in a dataset $\{P_i, T_i, C_i\}_{i=1}^N$. In addition, let $\{W_j\}_{j=1}^K \in P$ be the set of all WSIs for P, as there may exist multiple WSIs collected for a single patient. To construct graph G for P, we first perform automatic tissue segmentation for all W_j by: 1) transforming a low-downsampled version of W_j into HSV colorspace, and then 2) using Otsu's Binarization on the saturation channel to separate H&E-stained tissue from the background. Then, non-overlapping 256×256 instance-level image regions at $20\times$ magnification are patched and used as input for a truncated ResNet-50 model pretrained on ImageNet, which extracts a 1024-dimensional feature vector $h \in \mathbb{R}^{1024}$ via spatial average pooling after the 3rd residual block and is then packed into a node feature matrix $X_j \in \mathbb{R}^{m \times 1024}$ for M_j total patches in W_j. For each patch, we save (x,y)-coordinates from the tissue segmentation, from which we use to build an adjacency matrix A_j for each W_j via fast approximate k-NN ($k = 8$) that models a 3×3 image receptive field in CNN convolutions. Finally, we build a subgraph $G_j = (X_j, A_j)$, with the patient-level graph across all WSIs constructed as $G = \{G_j\}_{j=1}$ which we denote as a WSI-Graph.

  In comparison to previous graph-based approaches that build neighborhoods using nearest neighbors in the embedding space, our approach is distinct in that graphs are constructed in the Euclidean space. As a result, WSI-Graphs are effectively 2D point clouds (e.g. nodes/points connected to other proximal points in a 2D planar grid), which allows us to leverage spatial convolutions that perform local neighborhood aggregation functions similar to CNNs. In comparison to CNNs, however, Path-GCN is able to tractably perform CNN-like convolution operations on thousands on extracted instance-level image features.

3.2 Patch-GCN Architecture

Message Passing: For a WSI-Graph G with M instances, we learn a differentiable function $\mathcal{F}_{GCN} : \mathbb{R}^{M \times d_{in}} \rightarrow \mathbb{R}^{M \times d_{out}}$ parameterized using a GCN that iteratively aggregates and combines node features in their spatial neighborhoods across different hidden layers via message passing. For instance, for the message passing of vertex v (that has node feature $\mathbf{h}_v$) with its neighboring vertices $u \in \mathcal{N}(v)$ in hidden layer $G^{(l)}$, we use the graph convolution layer $\mathcal{F}_{GCN}^{(l)}(G^{(l)}; \phi^{(l)}, \rho^{(l)}, \zeta^{(l)})$ that implement the following functions:

$$
\begin{aligned}
\mathbf{m}_v^{(l)} &= \rho^{(l)} \left(\left\{ \phi^{(l)} \left(\mathbf{h}_v^{(l)}, \mathbf{h}_u^{(l)}, \mathbf{h}_{e_{vu}}^{(l)} \right) \rightarrow \mathbf{m}_{vu}^{(l)} : u \in \mathcal{N}(v) \right\} \right) \\
\mathbf{h}_v^{(l+1)} &= \zeta^{(l)} \left(\mathbf{h}_v^{(l)}, \mathbf{m}_v^{(l)} \right)
\end{aligned}
\tag{1}
$$

where $\phi^{(l)}$ is a message construction function that calculates a message $\mathbf{m}_{vu}^{(l)}$ between $\mathbf{h}_v$ and its neighbor $\mathbf{h}_u$ (with edge feature $\mathbf{h}_{e_{vu}}^{(l)}$), $\rho^{(l)}$ is a permutation invariant aggregation function that aggregates all messages passed to $\mathbf{h}_v$, and $\zeta^{(l)}$ is an update function that updates the existing node feature at v with the aggregated message $\mathbf{h}_v^{(l+1)}$. Note that the $\phi^{(l)}, \rho^{(l)}$ in Eq. 1 use similar instance-level and bag-level functions in MIL [26], in which GCN layers can be considered as performing multiple MIL operations in local graph neighborhoods, with $\zeta^{(l)}$ used as an additional differentiable function for propagating bag-level features across hidden layers in a neural network. In viewing neighborhood aggregation in GCNs has a formulation of MIL with structural neighborhood constraints, we adapt the message passing functions from DeepGCN [27] which implement $\phi^{(l)}, \rho^{(l)}, \zeta^{(l)}$ as:

$$
\begin{aligned}
\phi^{(l)} \left(\mathbf{h}_v^{(l)}, \mathbf{h}_u^{(l)}, \mathbf{h}_{e_{vu}}^{(l)} \right) &= \mathrm{ReLU} \left(\mathbf{h}_u^{(l)} + \mathbf{1} \left(\mathbf{h}_{e_{vu}}^{(l)} \right) \cdot \mathbf{h}_{e_{vu}}^{(l)} \right) + \epsilon \rightarrow \mathbf{m}_{vu}^{(l)} \\
\rho^{(l)} \left(\left\{ \mathbf{m}_{vu}^{(l)} : \forall u \in \mathcal{N}(v) \right\} \right) &= \sum_{u \in \mathcal{N}(v)} \frac{\exp\left(\beta \mathbf{m}_{vu}^{(l)} \right)}{\sum_{u \in \mathcal{N}(v)} \exp\left(\beta \mathbf{m}_{vu}^{(l)} \right)} \cdot \mathbf{m}_{vu}^{(l)} \rightarrow \mathbf{m}_v^{(l)} \\
\zeta^{(l)} \left(\mathbf{h}_v^{(l)}, \mathbf{m}_v^{(l)} \right) &= \mathrm{MLP} \left(\mathbf{h}_v^{(l)} + \mathbf{m}_v^{(l)} \right) \rightarrow \mathbf{h}_v^{(l+1)}
\end{aligned}
\tag{2}
$$

in which $\phi^{(l)}$ is the additively combines node and edge features followed by ReLU activation, $\rho^{(l)}$ is a Softmax Aggregation scheme similar to Ilse et al. [28] that computes an attention weight $a_{vu}^{(l)}$ that weights how much $\mathbf{m}_{vu}^{(l)}$ should contribute to the aggregated message $\mathbf{m}_v^{(l)}$, and $\zeta^{(l)}$ additive combines the current node feature and aggregated message followed by a multilayer perceptron. Additionally, $\mathbf{1}(\cdot)$ is an indicator function when an edge feature $\mathbf{h}_{e_{vu}}^{(l)}$ exists, ϵ is a positive constant for numerical stability (set to 10^{-7}), and β is a hyperparameter for the inverse temperature in Softmax (set to 1). We argue that $\rho^{(l)}$ can be viewed as a formulation of attention pooling operation in Ilse et al. [28] with structural neighborhood constraints, in which attention pooling of instance-level features is performed in local graph neighborhoods instead of across the entire bag.

Learning Hierarchical Features: To learn global-level morphological features in WSIs, following [27], we make $\mathcal{F}_{\mathrm{GCN}}^{(l)}$ a residual mapping and stack multiple layers of $\mathcal{F}_{\mathrm{GCN}}^{(l)}$ where the output of $\mathcal{F}_{\mathrm{GCN}}^{(l)}$ additively combines with its input.

$$G^{(l+1)} = \mathcal{F}_{\mathrm{GCN}}^{(l)}(G^{(l)}; \phi^{(l)}, \rho^{(l)}, \zeta^{(l)}) + G^{(l)} \tag{3}$$

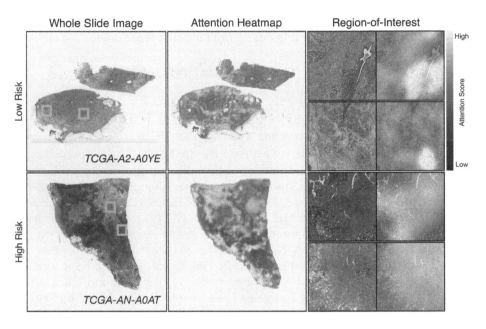

Fig. 2. Patch-GCN interpretability in BRCA survival prediction. In low risk patients, high attention regions corresponded to aggregates of lymphocytes near tumor cells, whereas in high risk patients, high attention regions corresponded to areas of tumor-associated stroma and necrosis.

We implement the spatial neighborhood aggregation backbone of Patch-GCN using $L = 4$ graph convolutional layers. As a result, each patch-based histology image feature aggregates features from other nodes in a 4-hop neighborhood, which results in an effective image receptive field size of 2302×2302 for 256×256 patches connected to its 8 nearest neighbors (Fig. 3, Supplementary Material). Furthermore, we also implement dense connections from the output of every GCN Layer to the last hidden layer of $\mathcal{F}_{\mathrm{GCN}}$, so that the representation of each histology patch would be an amalgamation of its instance-level embedding and its learned surrounding context, written as $\mathbf{H}^{(L)} = [X^{(1)}, \ldots, X^{(L)}]$.

Global Neighborhood Aggregation and Supervision: From the penultimate node feature matrix $\mathbf{H}^{(L)}$, following [28], we learn a global attention-based pooling layer $\mathcal{F}_{\mathrm{AttnMIL}}(\mathbf{H}^{(L)}; \phi^{(L)}, \rho^{(L)})$ that adaptively computes a weighted sum of all node features in the graph, which generalizes aggregation function in Eq. 2 to function on all nodes in the graph, in which the node feature matrix for the last hidden layer $\mathbf{H}^{(L)} \in \mathbb{R}^{m \times d_{out}}$ is pooled to a WSI-level embedding $\mathbf{h}_m^{(L)} \in \mathbb{R}^{1 \times d_{out}}$, which is subsequently supervised using the cross entropy-based Cox proportional loss function following [29] for survival analysis.

Implementation Details: To train Patch-GCN, we used Adam optimization with a default learning rate of 2×10^{-4}, weight decay of 1×10^{-5}, using a ResNet-50 CNN backbone pretrained on ImageNet, and trained for 20 epochs. To train with large graphs, we used 4 NVIDIA 2080 Ti GPUs with a batch size of 1 with 32 steps for gradient accumulation.

4 Experimental Setup

For this study, we used 4,370 diagnostic gigapixel WSIs across five different cancer types from The Cancer Genome Atlas: Bladder Urothelial Carcinoma (BLCA) ($n = 437$), Breast Invasive Carcinoma (BRCA) ($n = 1022$), Glioblastoma & Lower Grade Glioma (GBMLGG) ($n = 1011$), Lung Adenocarcinoma (LUAD) ($n = 515$), and Uterine Corpus Endometrial Carcinoma (UCEC) ($n = 538$). Our selection criterion in choosing these cancer types for training and evaluation were defined by: 1) dataset size, and 2) balanced distribution of uncensored-to-censored patients. On average, each WSI contained approximately 13487 256×256 image patches at $20\times$ magnification, with some patients having graph sizes as large as 100000 instances.

To evaluate Patch-GCN, we trained our proposed model using 5-fold cross-validation for each cancer type, in which each dataset was split into 5 80/20 partitions for training and validation. The cross-validated concordance index (c-Index) across the validation splits was used to measure the predictive performance in correctly ranking the survival times of each patient. As qualitative assessment, we used Kaplan-Meier curves to visualize the quality of patient stratification in stratifying low and high risk patients as two different survival distributions, as well as attention-based heatmaps using the weights computed by $\mathcal{F}_{\text{AttnMIL}}$ (Fig. 2 and 4). In addition, we compared Patch-GCN against several other weakly-supervised deep learning approaches for processing in WSIs in computational pathology. As a fair comparison, we used the same survival loss function, ResNet-50 feature embeddings, and training hyperparameters in Patch-GCN.

5 Results and Discussion

5.1 Quantitative Results

In comparing our approach to other weakly-supervised learning methods for WSIs in computational pathology, Patch-GCN outperforms all prior approaches on 4 out of 5 cancer types in head-to-head comparisons, achieving an overall c-Index of **0.636** (Table 1). For cancer types such as GBMLGG which has known intertumoral and intratumoral heterogeneity, Patch-GCN achieves a c-Index of

0.824 using WSIs and shows patient stratification into distinct survival groups (Fig. 4, Supplementary Material), which empirically suggests that Patch-GCN is able to learn context-aware features via hierarchical feature aggregation in local spatial neighborhoods. In comparing Patch-GCN to permutation-invariant/MIL-based approaches, we observe that Patch-GCN improves over all methods on all 5 cancer types (9.46% performance increase over DeepAttnMISL and 3.58% performance increase over Attention MIL), which further suggests that context matters in survival outcome prediction in WSIs. In comparison to DeepGraph-Conv which samples random patch features from WSIs as nodes and connects these nodes on the embedding space, Patch-GCN improves on all cancer types except UCEC (2.58% performance increase), which suggests the importance of building graphs via adjacent patches rather than feature similarity in the embedding space. Though DeepGraphConv has higher c-Index on UCEC, we note that in comparison to other cancer types, cancer prognosis in UCEC correlates with global-level morphological determinants such as tumor size and depth of tumor invasion in the myometrium, rather than cell-to-cell mediated interactions between tumor cells and other cell types. BLCA is a similar cancer type to UCEC that also depends on the depth of invasion into the bladder wall, but because the bladder wall is thinner than the myometrium, the invasion may be adequately captured via a limited receptive field, hence better Patch-GCN performance on that cancer type.

Table 1. c-Index performance comparisons of Patch-GCN against prior state-of-the-art weakly-supervised approaches on 5 cancer types in the TCGA.

Models	BLCA	BRCA	GBMLGG
MIL (Deep Sets) [26]	0.500 ± 0.000	0.500 ± 0.000	0.498 ± 0.014
Attention MIL [28]	0.536 ± 0.038	0.564 ± 0.050	0.787 ± 0.028
DeepAttnMISL [16]	0.504 ± 0.042	0.524 ± 0.043	0.734 ± 0.029
DeepGraphConv [24]	0.499 ± 0.057	0.574 ± 0.044	0.816 ± 0.025
Patch-GCN (Ours)	**0.560 ± 0.034**	**0.580 ± 0.025**	**0.824 ± 0.024**
	LUAD	UCEC	Overall
MIL (Deep Sets) [26]	0.496 ± 0.008	0.500 ± 0.000	0.499
Attention MIL [28]	0.559 ± 0.060	0.625 ± 0.057	0.614
DeepAttnMISL [16]	0.548 ± 0.050	0.597 ± 0.059	0.581
DeepGraphConv [24]	0.552 ± 0.058	**0.659 ± 0.056**	0.620
Patch-GCN (Ours)	**0.585 ± 0.012**	0.629 ± 0.052	**0.636**

5.2 Attention Visualization

To understand how Patch-GCN uses morphological features to predict risk, we visualized heatmaps using the attention weights from the attention pooling layer and utilized two trained pathologists to assess high-attention image regions. Across all cancers, we observed that in high risk patients, the network assigned high attention to necrosis, dense tumor aggregates, and regions of desmoplastic stroma containing tumor infiltrates, which are indicative of tumor invasion and proliferation (Fig. 2). In low risk patients, we observe that lymphocyte aggregates and normal stroma were frequently assigned high attention, which corroborates with the prognostic significance of stroma [10]. Figure 2 shows exemplar low and high risk cases in BRCA, with lymphocytes adjacent to tumor cells and infiltrating normal stroma given high attention in low risk patients, while necrosis and desmoplastic stroma were given high attention in high risk patients.

5.3   Conclusion

Despite the progress made in weakly-supervised deep learning in computational pathology, many current approaches are not context-aware in modeling important local- and global-level morphological features in the tumor microenvironment. In this work, we present Patch-GCN, a context-aware, attention-based graph convolutional network for survival analysis using WSIs. In comparing Patch-GCN to permutation-invariant network architectures that learn only instance-level morphological features, we observe that Patch-GCN outperforms all prior approaches on 5 cancer types in the TCGA. Moreover, we demonstrate the improvement in connecting nodes via adjacent image patches, which allows node aggregation in GCNs to learn such coarse-grained to fine-grained topological structures in the tumor microenvironment. Our approach is adaptable to any weakly-supervised learning task in computational pathology that uses slide-level or patient-level labels, and contributes towards a more holistic view of representation learning in the tumor microenvironment.

Acknowledgements. Funding: This work was supported in part by internal funds from BWH Pathology, Google Cloud Research Grant, Nvidia GPU Grant Program, and NIGMS R35GM138216 (F.M.). R.J.C. was additionally supported by the NSF Graduate Fellowship. The content is solely the responsibility of the authors and does not reflect the official views of the National Institutes of Health, National Institute of General Medical Sciences or the National Science Foundation.

References

1. Yu, K.H., et al.: Predicting non-small cell lung cancer prognosis by fully automated microscopic pathology image features. Nat. Commun. **7**(1), 1–10 (2016)
2. Campanella, G., et al.: Clinical-grade computational pathology using weakly supervised deep learning on whole slide images. Nat. Med. **25**(8), 1301–1309 (2019)
3. Courtiol, P., et al.: Deep learning-based classification of mesothelioma improves prediction of patient outcome. Nat. Med. **25**(10), 1519–1525 (2019)
4. Wulczyn, E., et al.: Interpretable survival prediction for colorectal cancer using deep learning. NPJ Digit. Med. **4**(1), 1–13 (2021)
5. Lu, M.Y., Williamson, D.F., Chen, T.Y., Chen, R.J., Barbieri, M., Mahmood, F.: Data efficient and weakly supervised computational pathology on whole slide images. Nat. Biomed. Eng. **5**, 555–570 (2020)

6. Bandi, P., et al.: From detection of individual metastases to classification of lymph node status at the patient level: the CAMELYON17 challenge. IEEE Trans. Med. Imaging **38**(2), 550–560 (2018)
7. Balkwill, F.R., Capasso, M., Hagemann, T.: The tumor microenvironment at a glance. J. Cell Sci. **125**(23), 5591–5596 (2012)
8. Saltz, J., et al.: Spatial organization and molecular correlation of tumor-infiltrating lymphocytes using deep learning on pathology images. Cell Rep. **23**(1), 181–193 (2018)
9. Zhao, Y., et al.: Predicting lymph node metastasis using histopathological images based on multiple instance learning with deep graph convolution. In: Proceedings of the IEEE/CVF Conference on Computer Vision and Pattern Recognition (CVPR), pp. 4837–4846 (2020)
10. Beck, A.H., et al.: Systematic analysis of breast cancer morphology uncovers stromal features associated with survival. Sci. Transl. Med. **3**(108), 108ra113 (2011)
11. Abdul Jabbar, K., et al.: Geospatial immune variability illuminates differential evolution of lung adenocarcinoma. Nat. Med. **26**(7), 1054–1062 (2020)
12. Shaban, M., et al.: A novel digital score for abundance of tumour infiltrating lymphocytes predicts disease free survival in oral squamous cell carcinoma. Sci. Rep. **9**(1), 1–13 (2019)
13. Mobadersany, P., et al.: Predicting cancer outcomes from histology and genomics using convolutional networks. Proc. Natl. Acad. Sci. **115**(13), E2970–E2979 (2018)
14. Zhu, X., Yao, J., Zhu, F., Huang, J.: WSISA: making survival prediction from whole slide histopathological images. In: Proceedings of the IEEE/CVF Conference on Computer Vision and Pattern Recognition (CVPR), pp. 7234–7242 (2017)
15. Lu, M.Y., Williamson, D.F., Chen, T.Y., Chen, R.J., Barbieri, M., Mahmood, F.: Data-efficient and weakly supervised computational pathology on whole-slide images. Nat. Biomed. Eng. **5**(6), 555–570 (2021)
16. Yao, J., Zhu, X., Jonnagaddala, J., Hawkins, N., Huang, J.: Whole slide images based cancer survival prediction using attention guided deep multiple instance learning networks. Med. Image Anal. **65**, 101789 (2020)
17. Anand, D., Gadiya, S., Sethi, A.: Histographs: graphs in histopathology. In: Medical Imaging 2020: Digital Pathology, vol. 11320, p. 113200O. International Society for Optics and Photonics (2020)
18. Raju, A., Yao, J., Haq, M.M.H., Jonnagaddala, J., Huang, J.: Graph attention multi-instance learning for accurate colorectal cancer staging. In: Martel, A.L., et al. (eds.) MICCAI 2020. LNCS, vol. 12265, pp. 529–539. Springer, Cham (2020). https://doi.org/10.1007/978-3-030-59722-1_51
19. Ding, K., Liu, Q., Lee, E., Zhou, M., Lu, A., Zhang, S.: Feature-enhanced graph networks for genetic mutational prediction using histopathological images in colon cancer. In: Martel, A.L., et al. (eds.) MICCAI 2020. LNCS, vol. 12262, pp. 294–304. Springer, Cham (2020). https://doi.org/10.1007/978-3-030-59713-9_29
20. Pati, P., et al.: Hierarchical cell-to-tissue graph representations for breast cancer subtyping in digital pathology. arXiv e-prints arXiv-2102 (2021)
21. Zhou, Y., Graham, S., Alemi Koohbanani, N., Shaban, M., Heng, P.A., Rajpoot, N.: CGC-Net: cell graph convolutional network for grading of colorectal cancer histology images. In: Proceedings of the IEEE/CVF International Conference on Computer Vision Workshops (2019)
22. Wang, J., Chen, R.J., Lu, M.Y., Baras, A., Mahmood, F.: Weakly supervised prostate TMA classification via graph convolutional networks. In: 2020 IEEE 17th International Symposium on Biomedical Imaging (ISBI), pp. 239–243. IEEE (2020)

23. Javed, S., Mahmood, A., Werghi, N., Benes, K., Rajpoot, N.: Multiplex cellular communities in multi-gigapixel colorectal cancer histology images for tissue phenotyping. IEEE Trans. Image Process. **29**, 9204–9219 (2020)
24. Li, R., Yao, J., Zhu, X., Li, Y., Huang, J.: Graph CNN for survival analysis on whole slide pathological images. In: Frangi, A.F., Schnabel, J.A., Davatzikos, C., Alberola-López, C., Fichtinger, G. (eds.) MICCAI 2018. LNCS, vol. 11071, pp. 174–182. Springer, Cham (2018). https://doi.org/10.1007/978-3-030-00934-2_20
25. Chen, R.J., et al.: Pathomic fusion: an integrated framework for fusing histopathology and genomic features for cancer diagnosis and prognosis. IEEE Trans. Med. Imaging (2020)
26. Zaheer, M., Kottur, S., Ravanbakhsh, S., Poczos, B., Salakhutdinov, R., Smola, A.: Deep sets. In: Advances in Neural Information Processing Systems (NeurIPS) (2017)
27. Li, G., Muller, M., Thabet, A., Ghanem, B.: DeepGCNs: can GCNs go as deep as CNNs? In: Proceedings of the IEEE/CVF International Conference on Computer Vision (ICCV), pp. 9267–9276 (2019)
28. Ilse, M., Tomczak, J., Welling, M.: Attention-based deep multiple instance learning. In: Proceedings of the 35th International Conference on Machine Learning (ICML), pp. 2132–2141 (2018)
29. Zadeh, S.G., Schmid, M.: Bias in cross-entropy-based training of deep survival networks. IEEE Trans. Pattern Anal. Mach. Intell. **43**, 3126–3137 (2020)

Pay Attention with Focus: A Novel Learning Scheme for Classification of Whole Slide Images

Shivam Kalra[1,2(✉)], Mohammed Adnan[1,2], Sobhan Hemati[1],
Taher Dehkharghanian[3], Shahryar Rahnamayan[3], and Hamid R. Tizhoosh[1,2]

[1] Kimia Lab, University of Waterloo, Waterloo, Canada
`shivam.kalra@uwaterloo.ca`
[2] Vector Institute, MaRS Centre, Toronto, Canada
[3] NICI Lab, Ontario Tech University, Oshawa, Canada

Abstract. Deep learning methods such as convolutional neural networks (CNNs) are difficult to directly utilize to analyze whole slide images (WSIs) due to the large image dimensions. We overcome this limitation by proposing a novel two-stage approach. First, we extract a set of representative patches (called mosaic) from a WSI. Each patch of a mosaic is encoded to a feature vector using a deep network. The feature extractor model is fine-tuned using hierarchical target labels of WSIs, i.e., anatomic site and primary diagnosis. In the second stage, a set of encoded patch-level features from a WSI is used to compute the primary diagnosis probability through the proposed *Pay Attention with Focus* scheme, an attention-weighted averaging of predicted probabilities for all patches of a mosaic modulated by a trainable focal factor. Experimental results show that the proposed model can be robust, and effective for the classification of WSIs.

Keywords: Whole slide image · Classification · Multi-instance learning

1 Introduction

The success of deep learning has opened promising horizons for digital pathology. AI experts and pathologists are now working together to design novel image analysis algorithms. The last decade has witnessed the widespread adoption of digital pathology, leading to the emergence of machine learning (ML) models for analyzing whole slide images (WSIs). The major applications of ML in digital pathology include (i) reducing the workload on pathologists, and (ii) improving cancer treatment procedures [17]. The computational analysis of WSIs offers various challenges in terms of image size and complexity. These challenges necessitate the inquiry into more effective ways of analyzing WSIs. CNNs are at the forefront of computer vision, showcasing significant improvements over conventional methodologies for visual understanding [14]. However, CNNs can not be directly utilized for processing WSIs due to their large image dimensions. The majority of the recent work analyzes WSIs at the patch level that requires manual delineations from experts. These manual delineations reduce the feasibility

© Springer Nature Switzerland AG 2021
M. de Bruijne et al. (Eds.): MICCAI 2021, LNCS 12908, pp. 350–359, 2021.
https://doi.org/10.1007/978-3-030-87237-3_34

of such approaches for real-world scenarios. Moreover, most of the time, labels are available for an entire WSI and not for individual patches [2]. Therefore, to learn a WSI representation, it is necessary to leverage the information present in all patches. Hence, multiple instance learning (MIL) is a promising venue for vision-related tasks for WSIs.

The paper's contribution is three-fold (i) we propose a novel attention-based MIL approach for the classification of WSIs, (ii) we fine-tune a feature extractor model using multiple and hierarchically arranged target labels of WSIs, and (iii) we present insights of the model's decision making by visualizing attention values. The method is tested on two large-scale datasets derived from The Cancer Genomic Atlas (TCGA) repository provided by NIH [23].

2   Background

CNN based methods for analyzing histopathological images is well represented in the literature [4–6,18]. Deep learning methods generalize well across patients, disease conditions, and are robust to the vendor or human-induced variations, especially when a large amount of training data is available [5].

A WSI usually contains at least two target labels, anatomic site, and primary diagnosis that are arranged in a hierarchy. The simplest way to deal with multi-label classification with k labels is to treat this as k independent binary classification. Although this approach may be helpful, it does not capture label dependencies. This limitation can degrade the performance in many applications where there is strong dependency among labels, for example, in WSI classification. To address this limitation, two different approaches, i.e., transformation and algorithm adaption methods, have been proposed [27]. In transformation-based methods, multi-label data is converted to new single label data to apply regular single-label classification. On the other hand, in the adaptation-based category, this is attempted to modify the basic single-label algorithm to handle multi-label data [21].

There are two main methods for characterizing WSIs [3]. The first method is called sub-setting, which considers a small section of a large WSI as an essential region for analysis. On the other hand, the tiling method, segments a WSI into smaller and controllable patches (i.e., tiles) [8]. The tiling or patch-based methods can benefit from MIL [11]. Isle et al. used MIL for digital pathology and introduces a different variety of MIL pooling functions [10]. Sudarshan et al. used MIL for histopathological breast cancer image classification [20]. Permutation invariant operator for MIL was introduced by Tomczak et al. for WSIs processing [22]. Graph neural networks (GNNs) have also been used for MIL applications because of their permutation invariant characteristics [2].

3   Method

There are two stages in the proposed method (i) bag preparation, and (ii) multi-instance learning with FocAtt-MIL. In the first stage, representative patches

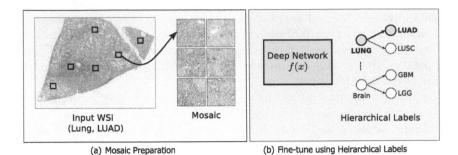

(a) Mosaic Preparation　　　　　　　　(b) Fine-tune using Heirarchical Labels

Fig. 1. Training a Feature Extractor. A feature extractor is trained with hierarchical target labels of a WSI. (a) A set of representative WSI patches (called mosaic) is extracted [13]. (b) The patches are used to fine-tune a deep network; each patch is assigned the parent WSI's labels, i.e., anatomic site and primary diagnosis.

(called mosaic) are extracted from a WSI. The mosaic's patches are encoded to a set of feature vectors (called bag) using a deep network. The feature extraction model can be a pre-trained network, or can be fined-tuned to increase its effectiveness as shown in Fig. 1. In the second stage, the proposed MIL technique (called FocAtt-MIL) is trained to predict the primary diagnosis for a given bag (a WSI). The schematic for the second stage is shown in Fig. 2.

Bag Preparation. A patch selection method proposed by Kalra et al. [13] is used to extract the representative patches from a WSI. We removed non-tissue regions using colour threshold. The remaining tissue-containing patches are grouped into a pre-set number of categories through a clustering algorithm. A portion of all clustered patches (e.g., 10%) are randomly selected within each cluster, yielding a *mosaic*. The mosaic is transformed into a bag $X = \{x_1, \ldots, x_n\}$, where x_i is the feature vector of ith patch, obtained through a deep network (a feature extractor). The Fig. 2 shows the bag preparation stage, the frozen network $f(x)$ represents a non-trainable deep network used as a feature extractor.

Fine-tune a Feature Extractor using Hierarchical Labels. In MIL, robust features enable weak learners to make better predictions thus improving the final aggregated prediction. A WSI is generally associated with the following two labels—anatomic site and primary diagnosis. These two labels are arranged in hierarchy as shown in Fig. 1. Consider, y_{as} and y_{pd} represent anatomic site and primary diagnosis respectively. Then, instead of predicting these labels independently, we predict $P(y_{as})$, and $P(y_{pd}|y_{as})$. The conditional probability $P(y_{pd}|y_{as})$ helps in modelling the dependent relationship. Using Bayes theorem, we get, $P(y_{as}|y_{pd}) = P(y_{pd}|y_{as})P(y_{as})/P(y_{pd})$, where $P(y_{as}|y_{pd}) = 1$, because of the dependence. We simplify $P(y_{pd}) = P(y_{pd}|y_{as})P(y_{as})$, and compute cross entropy losses for the predictions of both y_{as} and y_{pd}. We equally weight both the losses towards the final loss of the network.

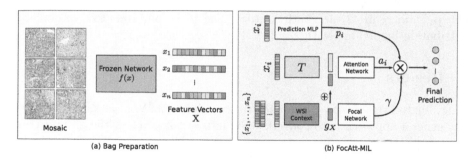

(a) Bag Preparation   (b) FocAtt-MIL

Fig. 2. Classification of WSIs with FocAtt-MIL. The two-stage method for the classification of WSI. (a) The mosaic of a WSI is converted to a bag X containing a set of feature vectors $\{x_1, \ldots, x_n\}$. (b) The feature vectors in a bag X are transformed to the primary diagnosis probability through FocAtt-MIL. The prediction probability p_i is computed for an individual feature vector x_i. A WSI context g_X is computed for the entire bag X using (1). The WSI context g_X is used to compute the attention value a_i and the focal factor γ. The final prediction is computed using (2).

WSI Context Learning. A single vector representation of a WSI (or a bag X) is computed as,

$$g_X = \phi(\theta(x_1), \ldots, \theta(x_n)), \tag{1}$$

where, θ is a neural network and ϕ is a pooling function, such as sum, mean, and max. It has been proven in [25] that (1) can approximate any set function. The vector g_X is used by the attention module and the focal network.

The FocAtt-MIL Approach. The FocAtt-MIL is a permutation-invariant model that learns to predict a target label (primary diagnosis) y_{pd} from a bag X (a WSI). The approach is composed of four major components (Fig. 2):

1. *Prediction MLP.* A prediction p_i is computed for each item x_i in the bag X, using a trainable deep network called Prediction MLP.
2. *WSI Context.* It a deep network that computes a single vector representing an entire bag X using (1).
3. *Attention Module.* The attention module is composed of two networks, a transformation network T, and the Attention Network. The attention module takes the ith patch $x_i \in X$, and the WSI context g_X to compute an attention value $a_i \in [0, 1]$ for that patch.
4. *Focal Network.* Another deep network that uses WSI context g_X to compute a focal factor γ (a vector) that modulates the final prediction. The length of γ is same as the number of discrete values in the target label, thus allowing the per dimension modulation.

The Final Prediction. The final output from the FocAtt-MIL is computed by aggregating individual attention-weighted predictions modulated by the learned focal factor, as follows

$$y(j) = \sum_{i=1}^{n} \mathbf{p_i}(j)^{\gamma(j)} a_i. \tag{2}$$

The $\mathbf{p_i}$, and $\boldsymbol{\gamma}$ in (2) are both vectors. The y is converted to a probability distribution by dividing with $sum(y)$.

4   Results

We evaluated the proposed approach for two different WSI classification tasks. The general approach is to convert WSIs into set of patches. the ground truth for each set is the label for the associated WSI. All experiments are conducted with 4 Nvidia V100 GPUs (32 GB vRAM each). The code has been written using the Tensorflow library [1].

For the LUAD/LUSC dataset, we have mixed 20x and 40x slides, and for the second experiment, we have used 40x slides only. We did not down-sample patches for the first experiment. However, for the second experiment, we down-sampled patches to 256 × 256, which corresponds to the 5x magnification. Based on [1], computer-aided diagnosis prediction can be reliably conducted at 5x and it performs at par (or better) than 20x magnification.

LUAD vs LUSC Classification – Lung Adenocarcinoma (LUAD) and Lung Squamous Cell Carcinoma (LUSC) are two main subtypes of non-small cell lung cancer (NSCLC) that account for 65–70% of all lung cancers [26]. An automated classification of these two main sub-types of NSCLC is a crucial step to assist pathologists [7,26]. For this task, we obtained 2,580 hematoxylin and eosin (H&E) stained WSIs of lung cancer from TCGA repository [23] with magnification of 20x and 40x. The dataset is approximately 2 TB and split into 1,806 training, and 774 testing WSIs [11]. We obtained mosaic for each WSI using the approach in [13] with patches of 1000 × 1000 pixels at 20x. We converted the mosaic to a bag X of features using a pre-trained DenseNet [9] without fine-tuning the deep network for the fair comparison against other approaches. We trained the FocAtt-MIL to classify bags between the two sub-types of lung cancer. We achieved the accuracy of 88% on test WSIs (AUC of 0.92). The accuracy has been reported in Table 1.

We conducted an **ablation study** to understand the effect of different model parameters. Removing the WSI context g_X from the attention module, resulted in 4% reduction of the accuracy. Excluding the focal factor γ and the global

Table 1. Performance comparison for LUAD/LUSC classification via transfer learning.

Algorithm	Accuracy
Coudray et al. [4]	0.85
Kalra & Adnan et al. [11]	0.85
Khosravi et al. [15]	0.83
Yu et al. [24]	0.75
FocAtt-MIL (proposed method)	**0.88**

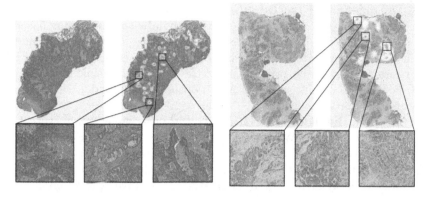

Fig. 3. Attention Visualization. The attention values augmented on the two exemplar WSIs. **Left Image (LUAD):** Regions of the highest importance come from the cancerous regions while sparing normal lung tissue, fibrosis, and mucin deposition. Additionally, by inspecting important regions at a higher magnification, it is noticeable that the malignant glandular formations border with non-malignant areas. **Right Image (LUSC):** Regions that are considered to be important for classification are composed of malignant squamous cells. However, unlike LUAD, the attention model seems to be responsive to regions with solid malignant structures.

context g_X from the final prediction, resulted in 6% reduction in the accuracy. The ablation suggests that the model's performance is the most optimal by (i) incorporating the WSI context g_X in the attention computation, and (ii) allowing the focal factor to modulate the final aggregated prediction.

We used the attention module of the trained model to **visualize the attention heat-map** on the unseen WSIs (Fig. 3). Due to unavailability of unavailability of regional annotations for WSIs, we showed these attention map to an expert medical professional for the validation. The visual inspection reveals that the model made its decision based on regions containing malignant tissue and ignored non-cancerous regions (see caption page 6).

Pan-cancer Analysis – In the second experiment series, we evaluated the approach against a large-scale pan-cancer classification of WSIs. The **dataset** used for this task has been proposed by Riasatian et al. [19]. It comprises more than 7 TB data, consisting of 7,097 training, and 744 test WSIs, distributed across 24 different anatomic sites, and 30 different primary diagnoses. All WSIs in the dataset are taken from a public repository of WSIs, TCGA [23]. We obtained a mosaic for each WSI, and then applied a cellularity filter [19] to further reduce the number of patches in each mosaic. Subsequently, we obtained 242,202 patches for training WSIs and 116,088 patches for testing WSIs. Each patch is of the size 1000 × 1000, but we resized them to 256 × 256 pixels.

We used three different **feature extractors** to validate the FocAtt-MIL. We prepared a separate "bag" for each feature extractor. These three feature extractors are: DenseNet (DN) [9], KimiaNet [19], and the fine-tuned DenseNet

(FDN). We fined-tuned the DenseNet on training patches using weak labels obtained from their respective WSIs. The weakly labelled fine-tuning has shown to be effective [19]. In our case, the weak labels are anatomic site, and primary diagnosis, arranged in a hierarchy. This hierarchical arrangement of labels is incorporated during the training using the approach outlined earlier in the Sect. 3. For the fine-tuning, we used Adam optimizer [16] and a learning rate of 10^{-5} were used for 20 epochs.

We **trained the FocAtt-MIL** model with the same architecture for all the three different bags. We tested three different configurations of FocAtt-MIL, i.e., FocAtt-MIL-DN, FocAtt-MIL-KimiaNet, and FocAtt-MIL-FDN. For all the three configurations, we used the SGD optimizer with a learning rate of 0.01, weight decay of 10^{-6}, and momentum of 0.9. We applied *gradient clipping* of 0.01 and dropout between layers to prevent the exploding gradients. We trained models for 45 epochs. Figure 4 shows the validation loss and accuracy while training the three different configurations. It is evident that FocAtt-MIL-FDN is outperforming from the very early epochs. It is interesting to note that, both FocAtt-MIL-FDN, and FocAtt-MIL-KimiaNet (feature extractors specialized for histopathology) seems to have converged to an optimal validation accuracy around 20–25 epochs.

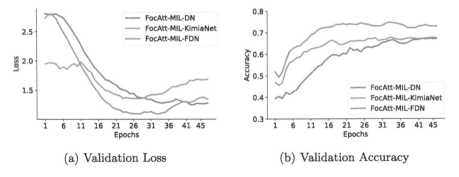

(a) Validation Loss　　　　　　　　(b) Validation Accuracy

Fig. 4. FocAtt-MIL Training. The loss and accuracy on validation dataset during the training of three different configurations of FocAtt-MIL, i.e. FocAtt-MIL-DN, FocAtt-MIL-KimiaNet, and FocAtt-MIL-FDN.

The 30 unique primary diagnoses in the dataset can be further grouped into 13 tumor types. The type of tumour is generally known at the inference time, and the objective is to predict the cancer sub-type. To **validate the efficacy of our model**, we computed the cancer sub-type classification (i.e., primary diagnosis) accuracy for the given tumour type. This type of classification is called *vertical classification*. The vertical classification results are reported in Table 2[1]. The results show that FocAtt-MIL can elevate the accuracy of pre-trained features; DenseNet features have shown to under-perform compared to KimiaNet

---

[1] For abbreviations GBM, LGG, ACC,..., see *wiki.cancerimagingarchive.net*.

Table 2. Pan-cancer vertical classification accuracy of FocAtt-MIL for features from regular DenseNet (FocAtt-MIL-DN), KimiaNet (FocAtt-MIL-KimiaNet), and DenseNet fine-tuned with hierarchical labels (FocAtt-MIL-FDN).

Tumor Type	Primary Diagnosis	FocatAtt-MIL-DN	FocAtt-MIL-KimiaNet	FocAtt-MIL-FDN
Brain	GBM	**0.9714**	0.9429	0.8571
	LGG	0.6410	0.7692	**0.8205**
Endocrine	ACC	0.6667	0.6667	0.6667
	PCPG	1.0000	1.0000	1.0000
	THCA	0.9608	1.0000	1.0000
Gastrointestinal tract	COAD	**0.6875**	0.4375	0.5000
	ESCA	0.5000	**0.8571**	0.5714
	READ	0.0833	0.5000	**0.6667**
	STAD	**0.8333**	0.7333	**0.8333**
Gynaecological	CESC	0.8824	**0.9412**	0.7647
	OV	0.5000	0.8000	1.0000
	UCS	0.6667	**1.0000**	0.3333
Liver, pancreaticobiliary	CHOL	0.2500	0.0000	**0.5000**
	LIHC	0.8857	**0.9143**	0.8571
	PAAD	1.0000	0.7500	0.8333
Melanocytic malignancies	SKCM	**0.9167**	0.8750	**0.9167**
	UVM	1.0000	0.2500	1.0000
Prostate/testis	PRAD	1.0000	0.9500	1.0000
	TGCT	1.0000	1.0000	1.0000
Pulmonary	LUAD	0.5789	0.8158	**0.8947**
	LUSC	**0.9302**	0.6977	0.7442
	MESO	0.6000	1.0000	1.0000
Urinary tract	BLCA	0.9118	1.0000	0.8529
	KICH	0.5455	0.6364	**0.7273**
	KIRC	0.9200	0.9000	**0.9600**
	KIRP	0.5714	0.6786	**0.7143**

features [12,19]. However, within the proposed FocAtt-MIL scheme, DenseNet features become quite competitive. This applies to the fine-tuned DenseNet (FocAtt-MIL-FDN) as well, whose results are on par with the highly customized KimiaNet features when used within the FocAtt-MIL framework.

5   Conclusions

The accelerated adoption of digital pathology offers a historic opportunity to find novel solutions for major challenges in diagnostic histopathology. In this study, we proposed a novel attention-based MIL technique for the classification of WSIs. We introduced a focal factor, computed using a global representation of WSI for modulating the individual patch-level prediction, thus promoting more accurate aggregated final prediction. We also proposed a novel fine-tuning approach to extract more robust features from WSI patches. We fine-tune a feature extraction model using patches and the hierarchical weak labels from their respective WSIs. We validated the proposed framework on two large datasets derived from

TCGA repository [23]. The results suggest competitive performance on both the datasets. Furthermore, the proposed method is explainable and transparent as we utilized the attention values to visualize important regions.

References

1. Abadi, M., et al.: Tensorflow: a system for large-scale machine learning. In: 12th {USENIX} Symposium on Operating Systems Design and Implementation ({OSDI} 16), pp. 265–283 (2016)
2. Adnan, M., Kalra, S., Tizhoosh, H.R.: Representation learning of histopathology images using graph neural networks. In: Proceedings of the IEEE/CVF Conference on Computer Vision and Pattern Recognition Workshops, pp. 988–989 (2020)
3. Barker, J., Hoogi, A., Depeursinge, A., Rubin, D.L.: Automated classification of brain tumor type in whole-slide digital pathology images using local representative tiles. Med. Image Anal. **30**, 60–71 (2016)
4. Coudray, N., et al.: Classification and mutation prediction from non-small cell lung cancer histopathology images using deep learning. Nat. Med. **24**(10), 1559–1567 (2018)
5. Dimitriou, N., Arandjelović, O., Caie, P.D.: Deep learning for whole slide image analysis: an overview. Front. Med. **6**, 264 (2019)
6. Gao, F., et al.: Sd-cnn: a shallow-deep cnn for improved breast cancer diagnosis. Comput. Med. Imaging Graph. **70**, 53–62 (2018)
7. Graham, S., Shaban, M., Qaiser, T., Koohbanani, N.A., Khurram, S.A., Rajpoot, N.: Classification of lung cancer histology images using patch-level summary statistics. In: Medical Imaging 2018: Digital Pathology, vol. 10581, p. 1058119. International Society for Optics and Photonics (2018)
8. Gutman, D.A., et al.: Cancer digital slide archive: an informatics resource to support integrated in silico analysis of tcga pathology data. J. Am. Med. Inform. Assoc. **20**(6), 1091–1098 (2013)
9. Huang, G., Liu, Z., Van Der Maaten, L., Weinberger, K.Q.: Densely connected convolutional networks. In: Proceedings of the IEEE Conference on Computer Vision and Pattern Recognition, pp. 4700–4708 (2017)
10. Ilse, M., Tomczak, J.M., Welling, M.: Deep multiple instance learning for digital histopathology. In: Handbook of Medical Image Computing and Computer Assisted Intervention, pp. 521–546. Elsevier (2020)
11. Kalra, S., Adnan, M., Taylor, G., Tizhoosh, H.R.: Learning permutation invariant representations using memory networks. In: Vedaldi, A., Bischof, H., Brox, T., Frahm, J.-M. (eds.) ECCV 2020. LNCS, vol. 12374, pp. 677–693. Springer, Cham (2020). https://doi.org/10.1007/978-3-030-58526-6_40
12. Kalra, S., et al.: Pan-cancer diagnostic consensus through searching archival histopathology images using artificial intelligence. NPJ Digit. Med. **3**(1), 1–15 (2020)
13. Kalra, S., Tizhoosh, H., Choi, C., Shah, S., Diamandis, P., Campbell, C.J., Pantanowitz, L.: Yottixel-an image search engine for large archives of histopathology whole slide images. Med. Image Anal. **65**, 101757 (2020)
14. Khan, A., Sohail, A., Zahoora, U., Qureshi, A.S.: A survey of the recent architectures of deep convolutional neural networks. Artif. Intell. Rev. **53**(8), 5455–5516 (2020). https://doi.org/10.1007/s10462-020-09825-6

15. Khosravi, P., Kazemi, E., Imielinski, M., Elemento, O., Hajirasouliha, I.: Deep convolutional neural networks enable discrimination of heterogeneous digital pathology images. EBioMedicine **27**, 317–328 (2018)
16. Kingma, D.P., Ba, J.: Adam: A method for stochastic optimization. arXiv preprint arXiv:1412.6980 (2014)
17. Madabhushi, A., Lee, G.: Image analysis and machine learning in digital pathology: challenges and opportunities. Med. Image Anal. **33**, 170–175 (2016)
18. Mahmood, T., Arsalan, M., Owais, M., Lee, M.B., Park, K.R.: Artificial intelligence-based mitosis detection in breast cancer histopathology images using faster r-cnn and deep cnns. J. Clin. Med. **9**(3), 749 (2020)
19. Riasatian, A., et al.: Fine-tuning and training of densenet for histopathology image representation using tcga diagnostic slides. arXiv preprint arXiv:2101.07903 (2021)
20. Sudharshan, P., Petitjean, C., Spanhol, F., Oliveira, L.E., Heutte, L., Honeine, P.: Multiple instance learning for histopathological breast cancer image classification. Expert Syst. Appl. **117**, 103–111 (2019)
21. Tidake, V.S., Sane, S.S.: Multi-label classification: a survey. Int. J. Eng. Technol. **7**, 1045 (2018)
22. Tomczak, J.M., Ilse, M., Welling, M.: Deep learning with permutation-invariant operator for multi-instance histopathology classification. arXiv preprint arXiv:1712.00310 (2017)
23. Tomczak, K., Czerwińska, P., Wiznerowicz, M.: The cancer genome atlas (tcga): an immeasurable source of knowledge. Contemp. Oncol. **19**(1A), A68 (2015)
24. Yu, K.H., et al.: Predicting non-small cell lung cancer prognosis by fully automated microscopic pathology image features. Nat. Commun. **7**, 12474 (2016)
25. Zaheer, M., Kottur, S., Ravanbakhsh, S., Poczos, B., Salakhutdinov, R., Smola, A.: Deep sets. arXiv preprint arXiv:1703.06114 (2017)
26. Zappa, C., Mousa, S.A.: Non-small cell lung cancer: current treatment and future advances. Trans. Lung Cancer Res. **5**(3), 288 (2016)
27. Zhang, M.L., Zhou, Z.H.: A review on multi-label learning algorithms. IEEE Trans. Knowl. Data Eng. **26**(8), 1819–1837 (2013)

Modalities - Microscopy

Developmental Stage Classification of Embryos Using Two-Stream Neural Network with Linear-Chain Conditional Random Field

Stanislav Lukyanenko[1]($\boxtimes$), Won-Dong Jang[2], Donglai Wei[2],
Robbert Struyven[2,5], Yoon Kim[6], Brian Leahy[2,3], Helen Yang[3,4],
Alexander Rush[7], Dalit Ben-Yosef[9,10], Daniel Needleman[2,3,8],
and Hanspeter Pfister[2]

[1] Department of Informatics, Technical University of Munich, Munich, Germany
stanislav.lukyanenko@tum.de
[2] School of Engineering and Applied Sciences, Harvard University, Cambridge, USA
[3] Department of Molecular and Cellular Biology,
Harvard University, Cambridge, USA
[4] Graduate Program in Biophysics, Harvard University, Cambridge, USA
[5] University College London, London, UK
[6] MIT, Cambridge, USA
[7] Cornell University, Ithaca, USA
[8] Center for Computational Biology, Flatiron Institute, New York, USA
[9] Lis Maternity Hospital, Tel-Aviv Sourasky Medical Center, Tel Aviv-Yafo, Israel
[10] Cell and Developmental Biology, Tel-Aviv University, Tel Aviv, Israel

Abstract. The developmental process of embryos follows a monotonic order. An embryo can progressively cleave from one cell to multiple cells and finally transform to morula and blastocyst. For time-lapse videos of embryos, most existing developmental stage classification methods conduct per-frame predictions using an image frame at each time step. However, classification using only images suffers from overlapping between cells and imbalance between stages. Temporal information can be valuable in addressing this problem by capturing movements between neighboring frames. In this work, we propose a two-stream model for developmental stage classification. Unlike previous methods, our two-stream model accepts both *temporal* and *image* information. We develop a linear-chain conditional random field (CRF) on top of neural network features extracted from the temporal and image streams to make use of both modalities. The linear-chain CRF formulation enables tractable training of global sequential models over multiple frames while also making it possible to inject monotonic development order constraints into the learning process explicitly. We demonstrate our algorithm on two time-lapse embryo video datasets: i) mouse and ii) human embryo datasets. Our method achieves 98.1% and 80.6% for mouse and human embryo stage classification, respectively. Our approach will enable more profound clinical and biological studies and suggests a new direction for developmental stage classification by utilizing temporal information.

S. Lukyanenko—Works were done during the internship at Harvard University.

M. de Bruijne et al. (Eds.): MICCAI 2021, LNCS 12908, pp. 363–372, 2021.
https://doi.org/10.1007/978-3-030-87237-3_35

Keywords: Developmental stage classification · Linear-chain conditional random field · Time-lapse video · Dynamic programming

1   Introduction

Biological developments often follow a monotonic order. A mammalian embryo's developmental process is a typical example of the monotonic constraint, which develops through cell cleavages (from 1 cell to multiple cells), morula, and blastocyst. This monotonic constraint does not allow transitions to previous developmental stages, *e.g.*, a transition from 2 cells to 1 cell. Automated developmental stage classification can advance studying an embryo's cellular function, a basic but hard biological problem. Besides, developmental stage classification of embryos is important for *in vitro* fertilization (IVF). To achieve a pregnancy, clinicians select embryos with the highest viability and transfer them to a patient. Division timing is one of the main biomarkers to assess an embryo's viability [11]. The current standard of choosing the most promising embryos is a manual examination by clinicians via a microscope. However, manual inspection is time-consuming and prone to inter-person variability. As such, it is essential to develop a model for automated developmental stage classification.

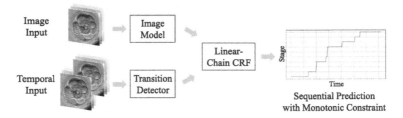

Fig. 1. Developmental Stage Classification of Embryo Time-Lapse Videos. Our two-stream model accepts the current and the previous frames as the input. We feed the current frame into the image model. For the transition detector, we input the concatenation of the current and the previous frames to capture motion information between them. We apply the two-stream model to all the frames in a video and obtain sequential predictions using a linear-chain CRF.

In automated developmental stage classification for time-lapse videos, difficulties mainly come from overlaps between cells and imbalance between stages. Even though cells are transparent, their overlaps confuse a classifier when identifying their developmental stage. Also, a few developmental stages (*e.g.*, 1, 2 cells) dominate most of the frames in time-lapse videos, which can induce class imbalance in learning. Temporal information is valuable for addressing these two challenges. It can differentiate overlapping cells based on their movements and transitions between stages regardless of their frequencies. Existing developmental stage classification methods [9,11,12] usually classify per-frame stages and apply dynamic programming to make use of the monotonic constraints. However, they do not incorporate temporal information, potentially solving the overlap and imbalance problems. Besides, they do not include dynamic programming in the learning process, making classification models may not learn to maximize the accuracy of dynamic programming.

In this work, we propose a two-stream model for the developmental stage classification of embryos as displayed in Fig. 1. We first introduce a two-stream convolutional neural network (CNN) model, which consists of an image model and a transition detector. While the image model identifies a stage of the current frame, the transition detector returns a high value when the current frame has a different label compared to the previous frame. Unlike the previous methods, we exploit temporal information in our transition detector, which can better suppress the overlap and stage imbalance issues. We build a linear-chain conditional random field (CRF) [16] upon our two-stream model for the monotonic constraints. Unlike conventional methods, our method effectively combines two-stream outputs using linear-chain CRF and enables learning of sequential predictions while constraining the monotonic order. We demonstrate our algorithm's efficacy by comparing it with existing stage classification approaches on two time-lapse video datasets: i) mouse and ii) human embryos.

We have two main contributions. First, our method improves the performance for rare cell stages by combining image and temporal information in a two-stream model. Second, we inject the monotonic constraint into the learning process using linear-chain CRF to optimize the sequential predictions. Our code will be publicly available upon acceptance.

2   Related Work

Developmental Stage Classification of Embryos. Researchers have proposed many stage classification methods due to their importance for IVF. With the emergence of deep learning methods, most state-of-the-art methods rely on CNN. Khan et al. [9] adopt CNN for human embryonic cell counting over the first five cell stages. Ng et al. [12] introduce late fusion nets, where multiple images are input for CNN, and additionally exploit dynamic programming to ensure a monotonical progression over time. Lau et al. [10] detects a region of interest and uses LSTM [5] for sequential classification. Rad et al. [13] use CNN to parse centroids of each cell from embryo images. Recently, Leahy et al. [11] develop computer vision models that extract five key morphological features from time-lapse videos, including stage classification. They improve a baseline by using multiple focuses, a soft loss, and dynamic programming.

However, most previous methods focus on improving a per-frame prediction and utilize dynamic programming during testing to incorporate the monotonic development order constraint. In this work, we make use of temporal information and directly inject the monotonic condition into the learning process with CRFs for sequential stage prediction.

Two-Stream Models. Researchers widely use two-stream models for action recognition. Two-stream 2D CNN [15] classifies an action by averaging predictions from image and motion branches. 3D-fused two-stream [4] blends features from image and motion information using 3D convolution. I3D [1] replaces 2D

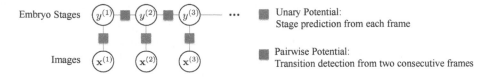

Fig. 2. Linear-Chain CRF Model. For each image, we compute the unary potential using a image model. For pairwise ones, we use predictions from a transition detector.

convolutions in the two-stream 2D CNN to 3D convolutions to incorporate temporal information better.

In their two-stream models, image and motion branches' objectives are the same; predicting an action from the input video. However, the embryo's temporal information could be useful for detecting stage transition timing rather than stage classification. Besides, their architectural designs are for action recognition, which outputs a per-video prediction. Since embryo stage classification requires per-frame classification, the previous two-stream models may not fit sequential prediction. For sequential prediction, one may use recurrent neural networks, *e.g.*, long short-term memory [5]. However, it is hard to incorporate the monotonic constraint of embryo development. Instead, we adopt a linear-chain CRF [16] to encode the constraints.

3   Model

We construct a two-stream approach for the developmental stage classification of embryos. The input is a sequence of frames $X = [\mathbf{x}^{(1)}, \ldots, \mathbf{x}^{(T)}]$, and the output is a sequence of stage predictions $Y = [y^{(1)}, \ldots, y^{(T)}]$. As depicted in Fig. 2, we use features extracted from the two-stream model as input to a linear-chain conditional random field, where the unary potentials are from the image stream, and the pairwise potentials are from the temporal stream. Our parameterization of the pairwise potentials (to be explained below) makes it possible to incorporate the monotonic constraint into the learning process. The entire model is trained end-to-end.

3.1   Two-Stream Feature Encoding

Our model uses temporal information in addition to image data to address the problems of overlapping cells and imbalance between stages, in contrast to many prior works, which often only use image information [9–11]. While the temporal information may not be valid for stage classification, it can be useful when there is a stage transition between two frames. To make use of this, we adopt a two-stream approach, which consists of an *image model* and a *transition detector*. While the image model outputs scores (*i.e.*, unary potentials) for each frame's stage, the transition detector outputs transition scores (*i.e.*, pairwise potentials) that recognize the existence of a stage transition between two consecutive frames.

The image model infers a stage from an input frame using ResNet50 [6] pretrained on the ImageNet dataset [3]. Concretely, the unary potential for class $c \in \{1, \ldots, C\}$ (*i.e.*, there are C possible stages) at time step t is given by,

$$\Phi_{\mathrm{I}}(\mathbf{x}^{(t)}; \theta_{\mathrm{I}})_c = \mathsf{softmax}\left(\mathbf{W}_{\mathrm{I}}\, \mathsf{ResNet}(\mathbf{x}^{(t)}) + \mathbf{b}_{\mathrm{I}}\right)_c,$$

where $\mathbf{W}_{\mathrm{I}}, \mathbf{b}_{\mathrm{I}}$ are the parameters of the linear layer that outputs class scores from ResNet features, and the $\mathsf{softmax}(\cdot)$ function normalizes the output to turn them into probabilities.[1]

Our transition detector outputs a score for whether the current frame is in a different stage compared to the previous frame. Even though many two-stream methods [1,4,15] exploit optical flow [7] as temporal information, it cannot distinguish stage transition from cell movements. Hence, we feed two consecutive frames into the detector instead. For the transition detector, we use ResNet50 [6] also pretrained on the ImageNet dataset [3], but we modify the first convolution layer to make it accept two consecutive frames as the input, $\mathbf{x}^{(t-1)}$ and $\mathbf{x}^{(t)}$. The detector returns a probability of stage change existence defined as,

$$\rho_{\mathrm{M}}(\mathbf{x}^{(t-1)}, \mathbf{x}^{(t)}; \theta_{\mathrm{M}})_k = \mathsf{softmax}\left(\mathbf{W}_{\mathrm{M}}\, \mathsf{ResNet}(\mathbf{x}^{(t-1)}, \mathbf{x}^{(t)}) + \mathbf{b}_{\mathrm{M}}\right)_k,$$

where $k \in \{0, 1\}$ indicates whether there was a stage change between $\mathbf{x}^{(t-1)}$ and $\mathbf{x}^{(t)}$. The detector also implicitly parameterizes the pairwise potentials via,

$$\Phi_{\mathrm{M}}(\mathbf{x}^{(t-1)}, \mathbf{x}^{(t)}; \theta_{\mathrm{M}})_{(c,c')} = \begin{cases} \rho_{\mathrm{M}}(\mathbf{x}^{(t-1)}, \mathbf{x}^{(t)}; \theta_{\mathrm{M}})_0, & \text{if } c = c' \\ \rho_{\mathrm{M}}(\mathbf{x}^{(t-1)}, \mathbf{x}^{(t)}; \theta_{\mathrm{M}})_1, & \text{if } c < c' \\ -\infty, & \text{otherwise,} \end{cases}$$

where we penalize inverse transitions with $-\infty$ to incorporate the monotonic constraint. We use these potentials as input to the linear-chain CRF, which enables sequential classification of the input sequences taking into account the pairwise correlations that exist among the output labels.

3.2   Linear-Chain Conditional Random Field

We define a probability distribution over the output sequence Y given the input sequence X with a linear-chain CRF

$$p(Y|X; \theta_{\mathrm{I}}, \theta_{\mathrm{M}}) = \frac{1}{Z(X)} \prod_{t=1}^{T} \exp\left\{\Phi(y^{(t-1)}, y^{(t)}, \mathbf{x}^{(t)}; \theta_{\mathrm{I}}, \theta_{\mathrm{M}})\right\},$$

---

[1] Since the potentials in a CRF do not need to be probabilities, normalization via the softmax function is not strictly necessary. However, we found the normalization to be helpful for stable training. Note that if the unary potential is defined to be the output of a *log*-softmax function (which is not the case in our approach), the model will reduce to a Maximum Entropy Markov Model.

where Φ is a score for transitioning from $y^{(t-1)}$ to $y^{(t)}$, which is given by combining the unary and pairwise potentials from above,

$$\Phi(y^{(t-1)}, y^{(t)}, \mathbf{x}^{(t)}; \theta_I, \theta_M) = \Phi_I(\mathbf{x}^{(t)}; \theta_I)_{y^{(t)}} + \Phi_M(\mathbf{x}^{(t-1)}, \mathbf{x}^{(t)}; \theta_M)_{(y^{(t-1)}, y^{(t)})}.$$

Here $Z(X)$ is a normalizing constant,

$$Z(X) = \sum_{y^{(1)}=1}^{C} \cdots \sum_{y^{(T)}=1}^{C} \prod_{t=1}^{T} \exp\left\{\Phi(y^{(t-1)}, y^{(t)}, \mathbf{x}^{(t)}; \theta_I, \theta_M)\right\},$$

which can be calculated in $O(TC^2)$ with dynamic programming.

Training. During training, we also found it helpful to minimize the CRF negative log likelihood along with single-model losses derive from the image and transition models. The single-model loss for the image model is defined as,

$$\mathcal{L}_I = \sum_{c=1}^{C} -q_c^{(t)} \log \Phi_I(\mathbf{x}^{(t)}; \theta_I)_c,$$

where $\mathbf{q}^{(t)}$ is the one-hot representation of the ground truth stage at frame t, and the single-model loss for the transition detector is defined as,

$$\mathcal{L}_M = \sum_{k=0}^{1} -(1 - \mathbf{q}^{(t-1)^T} \mathbf{q}^{(t)}) \log \rho_M(\mathbf{x}^{(t-1)}, \mathbf{x}^{(t)}; \theta_M)_c.$$

Thus the final loss is given by,

$$-\log p(Y|X; \theta_I, \theta_M) + \mathcal{L}_I + \mathcal{L}_M,$$

and we perform end-to-end training with gradient-based optimization using the Torch-struct library [14].[2] We use a batch size of four and a learning rate of 0.0001 with the Adam optimizer. To construct a batch, we randomly sample 50 frames from each video and then sort them in a consecutive order. We also perform data augmentation by random resized cropping, rotation, and flipping.

Inference. For prediction, our aim is in obtaining the most likely sequence of labels given a new test video X, *i.e.*,

$$\hat{Y} = \underset{Y}{\operatorname{argmax}}\, p(Y|X; \theta_I, \theta_M).$$

We obtain this maximum a posteriori sequence with standard dynamic programming (*i.e.*, the Viterbi algorithm). At inference time only, we also smooth the unary potentials from the image model by modifying the potential for class c,

$$\frac{1}{13} \cdot \Phi_I[c-2] + \frac{3}{13} \cdot \Phi_I[c-1] + \frac{5}{13} \cdot \Phi_I[c] + \frac{3}{13} \cdot \Phi_I[c+1] + \frac{1}{13} \cdot \Phi_I[c+2],$$

and using the above weighted average as the input to the Viterbi algorithm. This reweighting values, which were found via a search on the validation set, take into account the ordinal nature of the output space (boundaries are zero-padded).

---

[2] The single-model losses and the CRF negative log likelihood are complementary each other by taking into account local and global predictions, respectively.

Table 1. Accuracies (%) of stage classification methods on the test mouse embryos [2].

Method	Global	Per-Stage	1	2	3	4	5	6	7	8
A. Per-Image Classification Model										
ResNet50 [6]	90.9 ± 0.6	59.4 ± 1.2	99.0	98.3	89.1	90.7	25.1	15.8	26.5	30.4
AutoIVF [11]	96.4 ± 0.1	60.9 ± 3.1	99.8	**99.9**	92.3	**99.9**	4.3	33.5	50.8	6.2
B. Spatiotemporal Classification Model										
Early Fusion [8]	91.9 ± 0.1	57.1 ± 0.2	98.8	**99.9**	74.0	93.2	0.0	14.9	37.9	**37.6**
LSTM [10]	98.0 ± 0.1	45.0 ± 1.7	96.9	98.7	22.9	42.2	0.0	9.2	**90.1**	0.0
Ours	**98.1 ± 0.3**	**76.8 ± 5.4**	**99.9**	**99.9**	**94.9**	**99.9**	**35.1**	**84.6**	71.4	29

4   Experimental Results

We evaluate our method's performance, demonstrating each design choice's effect in the models with ablation studies. We evaluate stage classification algorithms on two embryo datasets: i) mouse and ii) human embryo datasets.

Compared Methods. We compare our method with a general classification model, ResNet50 [6], one state-of-the-art embryo stage classification method, AutoIVF [11], an early fusion method [8] that leverages temporal information, and a sequential model [10] based on LSTM. For a fair comparison, we re-implement AutoIVF using a single focus and the same backbone as ours. The early fusion takes five successive frames as input and learns to predict the middle frame's stage. We adopt the PyTorch 1.7 library to implement all the methods.

Evaluation Metric. We evaluate classification accuracy as the number of correct predictions over the number of data (Global). Since the majority stages, such as 1 cell and 2 cells, can dominate the average accuracy, we calculate the per-stage accuracies and the mean of them (Per-Stage). We train all methods for five seeds and report their average performances with standard deviations.

4.1   Developmental Stage Classification of Mouse Embryos

Dataset. We use the NYU Mouse Embryo dataset consisting of 100 videos of developing mouse embryos [2]. The videos contain 480 × 480 resolution images taken every seven seconds, with a median of 314 frames per embryo, totaling an average length of 36.6 min per embryo. The videos have frames with up to 8 cells, *i.e.*, eight developmental stages. For training and evaluation, we randomly split the data 80/10/10 into train, validation, and test videos, respectively. We use the validation set to select hyper-parameters and models for evaluation.

Result. In Table 1, we list overall and per-stage classification performances of the embryo stage classification methods. Our method outperforms all other methods on average for various stages. The frequency imbalance between the stages allows LSTM to achieve comparable results on average over all the data.

Table 2. Scores (%) of stage classification methods on the test human embryos [11].

Method	Global	Per-Stage	1	2	3	4	5	6	7	8	9+	M	B
A. Per-Image Classification Model													
ResNet50 [6]	74.6 ± 1.0	58.2 ± 1.6	97.6	93.8	24.3	80.8	24.1	16.2	19.8	55.2	63.5	70.7	93.9
AutoIVF [11]	77.8 ± 1.2	60.9 ± 2.2	98.2	**96.6**	22.9	88.2	26.5	15.6	22.4	59.3	67.3	77.0	96.1
B. Spatiotemporal Classification Model													
Early Fusion [8]	75.1 ± 0.6	55.7 ± 0.7	97.5	93.4	10.2	84.5	11.5	7.9	12.8	63.5	65.7	72.5	93.7
LSTM [10]	77.1 ± 0.9	61.8 ± 0.9	97.8	92.7	31.4	79.9	21.4	25.4	**28.8**	58.3	**67.6**	**79.3**	**97.0**
Ours	**80.6 ± 0.7**	**66.3 ± 1.9**	**99.4**	96.2	**41.2**	**89.4**	**43.3**	**27.6**	19.7	**69.8**	67.0	78.7	96.7

4.2   Developmental Stage Classification of Human Embryos

Dataset. We evaluate the stage classification methods on the human embryo dataset [11]. There are 13 stage labels: empty well, 1 cell to 9+ cells, morula (M), blastocyst (B), and degenerate embryo. To focus on the embryo development's monotonicity, we only use 11 stages, excluding frames with the empty well and degenerate embryo labels. The dataset includes 341 training, 73 validation, and 73 test time-lapse videos of embryos. Each video consists of 325 frames on average. As the network input, we crop zona-centered patches from each frame to exclude outside regions of interest and resize the frames to 112 × 112 resolution.

Result. Table 2 benchmarks the developmental stage classification methods. Overall, our approach surpasses the other classification methods. In terms of the mean per-stage accuracy, the performance gain over the existing methods is much higher, which indicates our method notably performs better for rare developmental stages. Since we incorporate the transition detector and use it to force the predictions of our model to be monotonic, our method outperforms the two spatiotemporal methods; Early Fusion and LSTM. Unlike AutoIVF, our model learns the features for the stage change detection, which are helpful for the monotonic predictions.

Our method runs in 268 frames per second on a single TITAN X GPU. Our model has 47M parameters and requires up to 4 GB GPU memory in the inference phase. Figure 3 visually compares our method with AutoIVF [11]. Our method is better at detecting cell division timings. As one example of failure cases, our model fails to detect the transition between 9+ cells and morula in Fig. 3 (b) since it takes two consecutive frames as the input, which visually have no major difference in this example.

4.3   Ablation Study

We analyze our method's efficacy by conducting an ablation study on the human embryo dataset. To this end, we add one of our components to the baseline at a time. By performing dynamic programming without pairwise potentials, our model improves the baseline's accuracy from 76.7% to 80.0%. Using both unary and pairwise terms in linear-chain CRF, our two-stream model yields 80.6% score, which performs the best. In conclusion, our full setting enables the maximum performance for developmental stage classification.

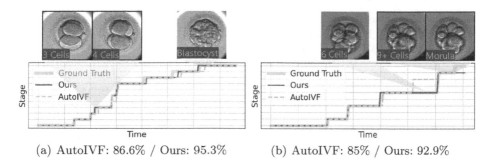

(a) AutoIVF: 86.6% / Ours: 95.3%   (b) AutoIVF: 85% / Ours: 92.9%

Fig. 3. Qualitative Stage Classification Results. We visualize frames with ground truths (lower left corner), where our method and AutoIVF [11] predict different stages.

5   Conclusion and Future Work

Our method will enable better clinical and embryological studies by improving the accuracies on rare stages, which are infrequent in videos but equally important as frequent stages when analyzing embryos. Since we measure stage transition probabilities, cell division timings predicted by our method are highly interpretable, which will allow tractable inspection in clinical practice. Our future work includes further improving performance on rare stages by combining a stage classifier and a cell detector, developing sequential models for other developmental features of embryos, and experimenting with different ways of acquiring unary and pairwise potentials, e.g., calculating the transition probability over longer sliding windows of frames.

Acknowledgements. This work was funded in part by NIH grants 5U54CA225088 and R01HD104969, NSF Grant NCS-FO 1835231, the NSF-Simons Center for Mathematical and Statistical Analysis of Biology at Harvard (award number 1764269), the Harvard Quantitative Biology Initiative, and Sagol fund for studying embryos and stem cells; Perelson Fund.

References

1. Carreira, J., Zisserman, A.: Quo vadis, action recognition? a new model and the kinetics dataset. In: proceedings of the IEEE Conference on Computer Vision and Pattern Recognition, pp. 6299–6308 (2017)
2. Cicconet, M., Gutwein, M., Gunsalus, K.C., Geiger, D.: Label free cell-tracking and division detection based on 2D time-lapse images for lineage analysis of early embryo development. Comput. Biol. Med. **51**, 24–34 (2014)
3. Deng, J., Dong, W., Socher, R., Li, L.J., Li, K., Fei-Fei, L.: Imagenet: a large-scale hierarchical image database. In: 2009 IEEE Conference on Computer Vision and Pattern Recognition, pp. 248–255. IEEE (2009)
4. Feichtenhofer, C., Pinz, A., Zisserman, A.: Convolutional two-stream network fusion for video action recognition. In: Proceedings of the IEEE Conference on Computer Vision and Pattern Recognition, pp. 1933–1941 (2016)

5. Gers, F.A., Schmidhuber, J., Cummins, F.: Learning to forget: Continual prediction with LSTM. IET (1999)
6. He, K., Zhang, X., Ren, S., Sun, J.: Deep residual learning for image recognition. In: Proceedings of the IEEE Conference on Computer Vision and Pattern Recognition, pp. 770–778 (2016)
7. Horn, B.K., Schunck, B.G.: Determining optical flow. Artif. Intell. **17**(1–3), 185–203 (1981)
8. Karpathy, A., Toderici, G., Shetty, S., Leung, T., Sukthankar, R., Fei-Fei, L.: Large-scale video classification with convolutional neural networks. In: Proceedings of the IEEE Conference on Computer Vision and Pattern Recognition, pp. 1725–1732 (2014)
9. Khan, A., Gould, S., Salzmann, M.: Deep convolutional neural networks for human embryonic cell counting. In: Hua, G., Jégou, H. (eds.) ECCV 2016. LNCS, vol. 9913, pp. 339–348. Springer, Cham (2016). https://doi.org/10.1007/978-3-319-46604-0_25
10. Lau, T., Ng, N., Gingold, J., Desai, N., McAuley, J., Lipton, Z.C.: Embryo staging with weakly-supervised region selection and dynamically-decoded predictions. In: Machine Learning for Healthcare Conference, pp. 663–679. PMLR (2019)
11. Leahy, B.D., et al.: Automated measurements of key morphological features of human embryos for IVF. In: Martel, A.L., et al. (eds.) MICCAI 2020. LNCS, vol. 12265, pp. 25–35. Springer, Cham (2020). https://doi.org/10.1007/978-3-030-59722-1_3
12. Ng, N.H., McAuley, J.J., Gingold, J., Desai, N., Lipton, Z.C.: Predicting embryo morphokinetics in videos with late fusion nets & dynamic decoders. In: ICLR (Workshop) (2018)
13. Rad, R.M., Saeedi, P., Au, J., Havelock, J.: Cell-Net: embryonic cell counting and centroid localization via residual incremental atrous pyramid and progressive upsampling convolution. IEEE Access **7**, 81945–81955 (2019)
14. Rush, A.M.: Torch-struct: Deep structured prediction library. arXiv preprint arXiv:2002.00876 (2020)
15. Simonyan, K., Zisserman, A.: Two-stream convolutional networks for action recognition in videos. In: Neural Information Processing Systems (2014)
16. Sutton, O.: Introduction to k nearest neighbour classification and condensed nearest neighbour data reduction. University lectures, University of Leicester, vol. 1 (2012)

Semi-supervised Cell Detection in Time-Lapse Images Using Temporal Consistency

Kazuya Nishimura$^{(\boxtimes)}$, Hyeonwoo Cho, and Ryoma Bise

Kyushu University, Fukuoka, Japan
kazuya.nishimura@humna.ait.kyushu-u.ac.jp , bise@ait.kyushu-u.ac.jp

Abstract. Cell detection is the task of detecting the approximate positions of cell centroids from microscopy images. Recently, convolutional neural network-based approaches have achieved promising performance. However, these methods require a certain amount of annotation for each imaging condition. This annotation is a time-consuming and labor-intensive task. To overcome this problem, we propose a semi-supervised cell-detection method that effectively uses a time-lapse sequence with one labeled image and the other images unlabeled. First, we train a cell-detection network with a one-labeled image and estimate the unlabeled images with the trained network. We then select high-confidence positions from the estimations by tracking the detected cells from the labeled frame to those far from it. Next, we generate pseudo-labels from the tracking results and train the network by using pseudo-labels. We evaluated our method for seven conditions of public datasets, and we achieved the best results relative to other semi-supervised methods. Our code is available at https://github.com/naivete5656/SCDTC.

Keywords: Semi-supervised learning · Cell detection · Microscopy image

1 Introduction

Non-invasive imaging techniques such as phase-contrast and differential interference contrast microscopy can capture images of cells without staining them. These techniques have been widely used for the long-term monitoring of living cells, in which hundreds of cells are captured as time-lapse images at short time intervals over days. Cell detection that detects the approximate positions of cell centroids from such microscopy images is a fundamental task for biomedical research [2,4,5,8,8,15,17,19,20,32]. Time-lapse images include hundreds of cells, so manual analysis is time consuming. Therefore, there is significant demand for automated cell-detection tools.

Traditionally, image processing-based methods such as thresholding [16], level sets [24] have been proposed for cell detection [2,3,26,27,31]. Recently, convolutional neural network-based detection methods have performed well with a large amount of labeled data [4,5,15,17,20,32]. For cell detection, heatmap-based methods have achieved promising results [15,17,20]. However, these methods

© Springer Nature Switzerland AG 2021
M. de Bruijne et al. (Eds.): MICCAI 2021, LNCS 12908, pp. 373–383, 2021.
https://doi.org/10.1007/978-3-030-87237-3_36

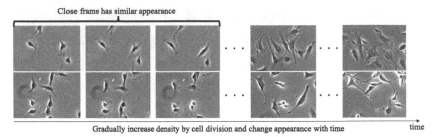

Fig. 1. Appearance of sequence images.

require a certain amount of annotation for each imaging condition (*e.g.*, type of microscopy, type of cell, and growth conditions). Preparing the necessary amount of annotation for each condition is a time-consuming and labor-intensive task.

To address this annotation problem, semi-supervised object-detection methods have been proposed mainly for bounding-box-based detection [1,7,11,13, 13,21,22,28,29], and a few methods have been proposed based-on consistency learning [6,14]. For example, Moskvyak *et al.* have proposed a consistency loss to train the network so that it consistently estimates the heatmap for data augmented by shifting or rotating [14]. These consistency-based methods assume that the labeled data are randomly sampled, *i.e.* labeled and unlabeled data have a similar distribution. However, this assumption often does not hold for time-lapse images of cell. In the time-lapse images, the cell density changes due to cell division, or the characteristics of cells may change due to the cultured condition (Fig. 1). As a result, the appearances of cells are different between the early frames and the later frames. Using consistency loss with an image as the label and the entire sequence as unlabeled data shows that the loss has an adversarial effect on training and does not work for the test data.

In this paper, we propose a semi-supervised cell-detection method that utilizes one time-lapse sequence, in which one image is labeled data and the other images are unlabeled data. Our method can improve the performance of the detection network by finding reliable detection positions from the unlabeled data using the labeled image as a clue. First, we train a detection network f_d with a labeled image. As shown in Fig. 1, if we capture time-lapse images with short intervals, cells in frames close to the labeled frame have a similar appearance to the labeled-frame cells because the appearances of cells change gradually. Thus, the trained network can perform an accurate estimation for these frames close to the labeled image. In contrast, the estimation for the later frames often does not perform well since the cell appearance changes from the labeled frame due to the increase of the density, and stimulation from culture conditions. On the basis of this observation, we track cells using estimated results from the labeled frame to the further frames, and the consistently tracked cells are considered to be the reliable estimations. We use tracking results as pseudo-labels for retraining the detection CNN. By iteratively performing this process, our method can improve the detection CNN. Our main contributions are summarized as follows:

- We propose a semi-supervised cell-detection method that can effectively train a detection network using a time-lapse sequence that contains one labeled image with the remaining images unlabeled. We improve the network by gradually adding pseudo-labels from the nearby frames.
- We propose a pseudo labeling method for heat map-based cell detection by using tracking. We generate pseudo-heatmaps from high-confidence detection results that selected by tracking.
- We demonstrated the effectiveness of our method for seven different conditions and demonstrated that our method can improve the detection network with one labeled image for various conditions.

Related Work: To address this annotation problem, semi-supervised object-detection methods have been proposed for mainly general images [1,6,7,13,13, 21,22,28,29]. These methods can be divided into two groups.

The first group is consistency-based semi-supervised object detection [6,7,14, 22]. As mentioned in the introduction, the consistency-based methods assume that the labeled image is randomly sampling. Therefore, it does not work in our setting.

The second group is pseudo-labeling-based semi-supervised method [1,12,13, 28–30]. The main approach of pseudo-labeling first trains the model on a small amount of data, and samples with high confidence are selected from the estimation results. Next, the model is trained using the selected samples. The performance of the model is improved by iterative labeling and learning. However, these methods have proposed a semi-supervised object detection method for a bounding box-based detection model. The cost of annotating a bounding box of a cell is expensive since a cell has a deformed shape with blurry boundaries. Therefore, the heatmap prediction is more suitable for cell detection tasks. As semi-supervised learning for heatmap prediction, Gberta *et al.* [1] have proposed video pose propagation for sparsely annotated sequence. By warping a heatmap from a labeled image to an unlabeled image, the method generates a pseudo label. However, this method requires a certain pair of labeled and unlabeled images for training of the warping network, *i.e.*, it requires a certain labeled images in a sequence.

Unlike these methods, our method improves the detection performance with a single labeled image by gradually increasing the number of reliable pseudo-labels with tracking.

2   Semi-supervised Cell Detection

An overview of the proposed method is shown in Fig. 2. Given one sequence $\mathcal{X} = \{x_t\}_{t=1}^{T}$, in which there is one labeled image $\mathcal{X}_l = \{(x_l, y_l)\}$ and the other images are unlabeled, our method improves the detection network f_d. T is the

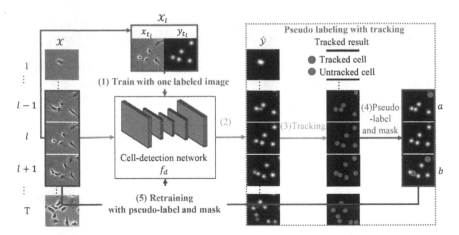

Fig. 2. Overview of proposed method. First, we train a cell-detection network with one labeled image $\mathcal{X}_l$ and predict unlabeled sequence $\mathcal{X}_u$. Then, we generate pseudo-labels and masks from high-confidence detected results that is selected by the tracking. Finally, we retrain the detection CNN with selected pseudo-labels. In this process, we train the network f_d, ignoring the cell regions that are not tracked by the mask. The red region of the right images indicates the masked region. (Color figure online)

number of frames in the sequence. (1) The cell-detection network f_d is trained with a labeled image $\mathcal{X}_l$. (2) The prediction results $\hat{\mathcal{Y}}$ are obtained by the trained detection network f_d from the whole sequence $\mathcal{X}$. (3) The detection results are tracked from the labeled frame l to the frames far from it. (4) We generate pseudo-heatmaps y_t^p and masks M_t for each frame based-on the tracking result, and we get pseudo labeled images $\mathcal{X}_p = \{(x_t, y_t^p, m_t)\}_{t=1}^b$. The mask M_t is used on the next training step for mitigating the effect of untracked cells and mitosis cells. (5) The network f_d is trained with generated pseudo labels $\mathcal{X}_p$. We improve performance by iteratively performing pseudo-labeling and learning.

Cell Detection: For cell detection, we use the heatmap-based detection method [15]. Given an input image x_t, the network output a heatmap $\hat{y}_t$ that is generated by blurring the approximate cell centroids. The network is trained by the mean squared error loss between the output $\hat{y}_l$ and the ground-truth of the heatmap y_l. After training, the cell position can be determined by finding the peak of the estimated heatmap. The detected positions for each frame $\mathcal{P} = \{\vec{p}_t\}_{t=1}^T$ are determined by detecting the peaks of the network output $\hat{\mathcal{Y}} = \{\hat{y}_t\}_{t=1}^T$, where $\hat{y}_t = f_d(x_t)$.

Pseudo-labeling with Tracking: Next, we select high-confidence positions from detected positions $\mathcal{P}$ based on tracking, and generate pseudo-heatmaps using the selected high-confidence positions. Our key assumption is that reliable estimations can be found by tracking. If detected positions in unlabeled frames can be continuously tracked from the labeled frame, we consider these as reliable estimations. The other assumption is that the additional training using reliable pseudo-labels can improve f_d, and the reliable estimations increase in the next iteration by the re-trained network, which can be used as the additional pseudo-labels for further re-training. The network gradually improves by iterating this process.

The detection points of successive frames are associated by using a one-by-one matching [9], which optimizes the assignment among detected points in successive frames. The association is performed bi-directions, from the labeled frame to far frames. To avoid selecting the unconfident results, if the distance between the associated positions is small enough, we associate these. The right images in Fig. 2 show the examples of the estimated heat-maps $\hat{y}$ and the tracking results. We can observe that the heat-maps of frames close to the frame l, were more accurately estimated compared to the results of later frames. Thus, the number of successfully tracked cells from l gradually decreases with far from l. If the pseudo-heatmaps contain many unreliable regions, which may be cell regions or background, these affect re-training. Therefore, we generate pseudo-heatmaps at the frames that the ratio of the tracked positions is larger than a threshold α. The range of the tracked frames is defined as $[a, b]$.

Next, we generate the pseudo-heatmaps from the tracking results in $[a, b]$. We generate the set of the pseudo-heat-maps $\{y_t^p\}_{t=a}^b$ using the positions of the tracked cells $\{\vec{p}_t^{tr}\}_{t=a}^b$ in the same manner to the supervised heatmap generation [15]. These frames still contain few unreliable regions, $i.e.$, the regions on untracked cells. To mitigate the affect from the un-tracked cell regions, we re-train the detection network using the masked loss that ignores the masked regions in training. There are two types of unreliable regions.

The first is a region that is detected but is not tracked. Most of this type's region is the region of a daughter cell that newly appears by cell mitosis after frame l. Since cells monotonically increase with time by mitosis, we only consider this type of unreliable region at $t > l$. These regions can be easily defined using an unassociated detected positions $\{\vec{p}_t^o\}$. We define this region as $R(\vec{p}_t^o)$ that is a set of pixels within radius β from $\{\vec{p}_t^o\}$.

The second is a region that is not detected but there is a cell (miss detection). If detected points in a certain region are continuously tracked from frame l until the previous frame t_{ut} $i.e.$, it is possible that miss-detection occurred at $t_{ut} + 1$. To define the second regions, we use the position and timing when a track was terminated based on the tracking results, in which a terminate point and the frame are denoted as $\{\vec{p}_{t_{ut}}^{ut}\}$. Since cells move slowly, the positions of the un-tracked cell in the later/earlier frames can be roughly predicted by random work from the terminated position and time. A region at t is defined as $R(\vec{p}_{t_{ut}}^{ut}, t)$ that is a set of pixels within radius $\beta + ||t^{ut} - t||$. The mask is defined using these unreliable regions as follows:

$$M_t(\vec{p}) = \begin{cases} 0 & if \ (\vec{p} \in R(\vec{p}_t^{ut}, t) \\ 0 & if \ (\vec{p} \in R(\vec{p}_t^o)) and(t > l) \\ 1 & otherwise. \end{cases} \tag{1}$$

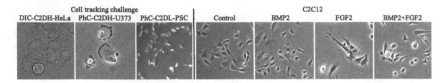

Fig. 3. Example of image on each dataset.

We train f_d with $\mathcal{X}_p = \{(x_t, y_t, M_t)\}_{t=a}^{b}$. When we train f_d with $\mathcal{X}_p$, we use following loss function:

$$L = \frac{1}{N} \sum_N \left(\frac{1}{\sum M_t} M_t * (y_t^p - \hat{y}_t)^2 \right), \tag{2}$$

where $\vec{i}$ is a coordinate, and N is the number of pseudo-labels. We repeat Pseudo-labeling and re-training the network are iteratively performed until we reach γ iterations.

3   Experiments

Implementation Details: The detection network is trained for 10000 iterations using the Adam optimizer with a learning rate of 0.001 in each step. We set the hyperparameter α, which is the error rate for terminating tracking, to 0.8, β, which is the radius of the region, to 18 or 27 according to cell size, and γ, which is the number of iterations of our pseudo-labelings, to 3.

Metrics: To evaluate detection performance, we used F1-score $= \frac{2 \cdot Precision \cdot Recall}{Recall + Precision}$, in which TP, FP, and FN are true positive, false positive, and false negative, respectively (Precision $= \frac{TP}{TP+FP}$, Recall $= \frac{TP}{TP+FN}$). We associate detected positions with ground-truth positions. We define true positive as the number of associated positions. We define the number of unassociated detected positions and ground-truth positions as false positive, and false-negative, respectively.

Evaluation on Cell Tracking Challenge Datasets: To evaluate our method, we used Cell Tracking Challenge [18,25], which are well-known cell image datasets. In this dataset, the cell were captured in various conditions as time-lapse images. We use three type of conditions: DIC-C2DH-HeLa, PhC-C2DH-U373, and PhC-C2DL-PSC. Two sequences that include 83 to 113 frames were fully annotated at a resolution ranging from 512×512 to 720×576 pixels. Since the magnification of the images (the size of cells) are different, we resized the images. The examples of the images are shown in Fig. 3 Please to refer to [18,25] for the detailed information of this dataset. We used one image at the 20th frame as labeled frames and the rest frames as unlabeled sequence on all datasets, and we performed two fold cross validation. We used the twentieth frame as the labeled frame and the other frames as unlabeled sequences on all datasets, and we performed twofold cross-validation.

Table 1. Quantitative evaluation results for Cell Tracking Challenge datasets on F1-score.

Method	Label	HeLa	U373	PSC	Ave.
Vicar [27]	U	0.597	0.387	0.597	0.527
Baseline [15]	O	0.748	0.879	0.933	0.853
Moskvyak [14]	O	0.266	0.475	0.820	0.520
Ours	O	**0.778**	**0.914**	**0.948**	**0.881**
Moskvyak half [14]	H	0.714	0.910	0.834	0.819
Supervised [15]	F	0.908	0.925	0.972	0.935

HeLa: DIC-C2DH-HeLa, U373: PhC-C2DH-U373, PSC: PhC-C2DL-PSC, U: unsupervised, O: use one labeled image, H: use 50 % labeled images for the first half of the sequence, F: fully supervised label.

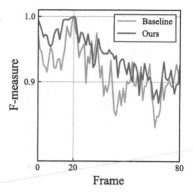

Fig. 4. F1 score for each frame of training data on cell tracking challenge.

We compared our method with 3 conventional methods using one labeled image or unlabeled: Baseline, in which Nishimura's method [15] was trained by one labeled image; Vicar [27], which is an image processing-based method by combining preconditioning of Yin [33] and distance transform [23]; Moskvyak [14], which is a consistency based semi-supervised detection method. In addition, to clarify how the number of the labeled data affect to the detection performance, we also compared several methods using additional labeled data: Supervised, in which Nishimura's method [15] was trained by fully labeled image; Moskvyak half, in which the first half of the sequence was additionally labeled and used for training.

Table 1 shows a quantitative evaluation of the F1 score on Cell Tracking Challenge. Our method achieves the best performance among the methods that trained with one labeled image. Since the time-lapse images gradually change the appearance of the image, Moskvyak's performance worsens performance. Even if Moskvyak used 50% of labeled data, the performance decreases from the baseline on DIC-C2DH-HeLa and PhC-C2DL-PSC. It indicates that the previous method that assumes the labeled images are randomly sampled can not work on our target setting. In contrast, our method can improve the performance with one labeled image. It can observe that our method is suitable for time-lapse sequences and effectively improves performance in a semi-supervised manner.

Figure 4 shows the average F1 score of the three datasets for each frame in the training data. The horizontal axis indicates the F1 score, and the vertical axis indicates the frame. The performance of the F1 score is gradually decreasing from the twentieth frame. We observe that the performance of our method is improved compared to baseline by adding pseudo-labels from the close frames. Figure 5 shows the example of result for iteration on DIC-C2DH-HeLa. As shown in Fig. 5, the heatmaps of our method become more clear than the baseline even in frames away from the labeled frame.

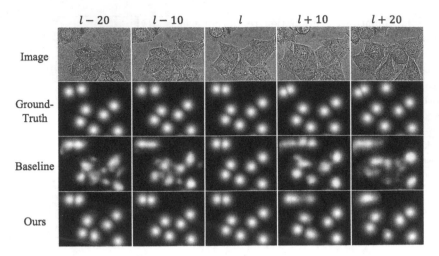

Fig. 5. Example of estimation on training data. l is the labeled frame.

Evaluation on C2C12: To further evaluate our method on a more challenging case, we used a public dataset [10] (C2C12), which consists of 48 sequences with 1,013 images respectively. C2C12 cell is captured by phase-contrast microscopy under four different media conditions (Control, FGF2, BMP2, FGF2+BMP2) at a resolution of 1040×1392 pixels. An example of the images is shown in Fig. 3. The appearance of the image changed depend on cultured media conditions. Since only one sequence is fully annotated (BMP2), we additionally annotated three conditions (FGF2, Control, and BMP2 and BMP2+FGF2) to evaluate our method on various media conditions. We annotated 100 frames for the test data between the 600th and 700th frames: the total number of cells of is 27723, 85518, 7764, and 15082 for Control, FGF2, BMP2, and BMP2+FGF2, respectively. We annotated the 400th frame for all conditions to a different sequence of test data as training data: the total number of cells are 116, 28, 99, and 99 for respective conditions. Because cell type changes rapidly on FGF2 in the latter frames, we annotated frames 300 to 400 for test data and the 100th frame as training data in FGF2. Our model is trained on a sequence that includes 1 labeled image while the other 1,012 images are unlabeled. We compared our method with semi-supervised and unsupervised methods that are used in previous experiments.

Table 2 shows the quantitative evaluation results with the F1 score on four cultured conditions. Our method achieves the best performance on whole-culture conditions. Even if the cell shape slightly changes depending on the culture condition, the detection performance can be improved by this method. It indicate that the proposed method is effective for various time-lapse images.

Table 2. Quantitative evaluation results for C2C12 on F1-score

Method	Control	BMP2	FGF2	BMP2+FGF2	Ave.
Vicar [27]	0.731	0.607	0.676	0.820	0.709
Baseline [15]	0.740	0.844	0.651	0.824	0.765
Moskvyak [14]	0.598	0.170	0.478	0.520	0.442
Ours	**0.756**	**0.886**	**0.830**	**0.901**	**0.843**

4 Conclusion

We proposed a semi-supervised cell detection method for time-lapse images in which there is one labeled image and the other images are unlabeled. Our method can improve detection network by adding pseudo labels that is selected by tracking from detection results. We demonstrated our method's effectiveness on seven different conditions, and we demonstrated that our method can improve detection performance on various conditions.

Acknowledgment. This work was supported by JSPS KAKENHI Grant Number JP20H04211.

References

1. Bertasius, G., Feichtenhofer, C., Tran, D., Shi, J., Torresani, L.: Learning temporal pose estimation from sparsely labeled videos. In: NeurIPS (2019)
2. Bise, R., Sato, Y.: Cell detection from redundant candidate regions under nonoverlapping constraints. IEEE Trans. Med. Imaging **34**(7), 1417–1427 (2015)
3. Cosatto, E., Miller, M., Graf, H.P., Meyer, J.S.: Grading nuclear pleomorphism on histological micrographs. In: ICPR, pp. 1–4 (2008)
4. Cruz-Roa, A.A., Arevalo Ovalle, J.E., Madabhushi, A., González Osorio, F.A.: A deep learning architecture for image representation, visual interpretability and automated basal-cell carcinoma cancer detection. In: Mori, K., Sakuma, I., Sato, Y., Barillot, C., Navab, N. (eds.) MICCAI 2013. LNCS, vol. 8150, pp. 403–410. Springer, Heidelberg (2013). https://doi.org/10.1007/978-3-642-40763-5_50
5. Fujita, S., Han, X.-H.: Cell detection and segmentation in microscopy images with improved mask R-CNN. In: Sato, I., Han, B. (eds.) ACCV 2020. LNCS, vol. 12628, pp. 58–70. Springer, Cham (2021). https://doi.org/10.1007/978-3-030-69756-3_5
6. Honari, S., Molchanov, P., Tyree, S., Vincent, P., Pal, C., Kautz, J.: Improving landmark localization with semi-supervised learning. In: CVPR, pp. 1546–1555 (2018)
7. Jeong, J., Lee, S., Kim, J., Kwak, N.: Consistency-based semi-supervised learning for object detection. In: NeurIPS, vol. 32 (2019)
8. Kainz, P., Urschler, M., Schulter, S., Wohlhart, P., Lepetit, V.: You should use regression to detect cells. In: Navab, N., Hornegger, J., Wells, W.M., Frangi, A.F. (eds.) MICCAI 2015. LNCS, vol. 9351, pp. 276–283. Springer, Cham (2015). https://doi.org/10.1007/978-3-319-24574-4_33

9. Kanade, T., et al.: Cell image analysis: Algorithms, system and applications. In: WACV, pp. 374–381 (2011)
10. Ker, D.F.E., et al.: Phase contrast time-lapse microscopy datasets with automated and manual cell tracking annotations. Sci. Data **5**(1), 1–12 (2018)
11. Kikkawa, R., Sekiguchi, H., Tsuge, I., Saito, S., Bise, R.: Semi-supervised learning with structured knowledge for body hair detection in photoacoustic image. In: ISBI, pp. 1411–1415 (2019)
12. Li, J., et al.: Signet ring cell detection with a semi-supervised learning framework. In: Chung, A.C.S., Gee, J.C., Yushkevich, P.A., Bao, S. (eds.) IPMI 2019. LNCS, vol. 11492, pp. 842–854. Springer, Cham (2019). https://doi.org/10.1007/978-3-030-20351-1_66
13. Misra, I., Shrivastava, A., Hebert, M.: Watch and learn: Semi-supervised learning for object detectors from video. In: CVPR, pp. 3593–3602 (2015)
14. Moskvyak, O., Maire, F., Dayoub, F., Baktashmotlagh, M.: Semi-supervised keypoint localization. In: ICLR (2021)
15. Nishimura, K., Ker, D.F.E., Bise, R.: Weakly supervised cell instance segmentation by propagating from detection response. In: Shen, D., et al. (eds.) MICCAI 2019. LNCS, vol. 11764, pp. 649–657. Springer, Cham (2019). https://doi.org/10.1007/978-3-030-32239-7_72
16. Otsu, N.: A threshold selection method from gray-level histograms. IEEE Trans. Syst. Man Cybern. **9**(1), 62–66 (1979)
17. Raza, S.E.A., et al.: Deconvolving convolutional neural network for cell detection. In: ISBI, pp. 891–894 (2019)
18. Redmon, J., Divvala, S., Girshick, R., Farhadi, A.: You only look once: unified, real-time object detection. In: CVPR, pp. 779–788 (2016)
19. Ren, S., He, K., Girshick, R., Sun, J.: Faster R-CNN: towards real-time object detection with region proposal networks. In: NeurIPS, pp. 91–99 (2015)
20. Sirinukunwattana, K., Raza, S.E.A., Tsang, Y., Snead, D.R.J., Cree, I.A., Rajpoot, N.M.: Locality sensitive deep learning for detection and classification of nuclei in routine colon cancer histology images. IEEE Trans. Med. Imaging **35**(5), 1196–1206 (2016)
21. Sohn, K., Zhang, Z., Li, C.L., Zhang, H., Lee, C.Y., Pfister, T.: A simple semi-supervised learning framework for object detection. arXiv:2005.04757 (2020)
22. Tang, P., Ramaiah, C., Wang, Y., Xu, R., Xiong, C.: Proposal learning for semi-supervised object detection. In: WACV, pp. 2291–2301 (2021)
23. Thirusittampalam, K., Hossain, M.J., Ghita, O., Whelan, P.F.: A novel framework for cellular tracking and mitosis detection in dense phase contrast microscopy images. IEEE J. Biomed. Health Inf. **17**(3), 642–653 (2013)
24. Tse, S., Bradbury, L., Wan, J.W., Djambazian, H., Sladek, R., Hudson, T.: A combined watershed and level set method for segmentation of brightfield cell images. In: Medical Imaging 2009: Image Processing, vol. 7259, p. 72593G (2009)
25. Ulman, V., et al.: An objective comparison of cell-tracking algorithms. Nat. Methods **14**(12), 1141–1152 (2017)
26. Veta, M., Van Diest, P.J., Kornegoor, R., Huisman, A., Viergever, M.A., Pluim, J.P.: Automatic nuclei segmentation in H&E stained breast cancer histopathology images. PloS one **8**(7), e70221 (2013)
27. Vicar, T., et al.: Cell segmentation methods for label-free contrast microscopy: review and comprehensive comparison. BMC Bioinf. **20**(1), 360 (2019)
28. Wang, K., Lin, L., Yan, X., Chen, Z., Zhang, D., Zhang, L.: Cost-effective object detection: Active sample mining with switchable selection criteria. IEEE Trans. Neural Netw. Learn. Syst. **30**(3), 834–850 (2018)

29. Wang, K., Yan, X., Zhang, D., Zhang, L., Lin, L.: Towards human-machine cooperation: self-supervised sample mining for object detection. In: CVPR, pp. 1605–1613 (2018)
30. Wang, T., Yang, T., Cao, J., Zhang, X.: Co-mining: Self-supervised learning for sparsely annotated object detection. In: AAAI (2020)
31. Xu, H., Lu, C., Berendt, R., Jha, N., Mandal, M.: Automatic nuclei detection based on generalized Laplacian of gaussian filters. IEEE J. Biomed. Health Inf. **21**(3), 826–837 (2016)
32. Xu, J., et al.: Stacked sparse autoencoder (SSAE) for nuclei detection on breast cancer histopathology images. IEEE Trans. Med. Imaging **35**(1), 119–130 (2015)
33. Yin, Z., Kanade, T., Chen, M.: Understanding the phase contrast optics to restore artifact-free microscopy images for segmentation. Med. Image Anal. **16**(5), 1047–1062 (2012)

Cell Detection in Domain Shift Problem Using Pseudo-Cell-Position Heatmap

Hyeonwoo Cho[1(✉)], Kazuya Nishimura[1], Kazuhide Watanabe[2], and Ryoma Bise[1]

[1] Kyushu University, Fukuoka, Japan
hyeonwoo.cho@human.ait.kyushu-u.ac.jp
[2] RIKEN Center for Integrative Medical Sciences, Yokohama, Japan

Abstract. The domain shift problem is an important issue in automatic cell detection. A detection network trained with training data under a specific condition (source domain) may not work well in data under other conditions (target domain). We propose an unsupervised domain adaptation method for cell detection using the pseudo-cell-position heatmap, where a cell centroid becomes a peak with a Gaussian distribution in the map. In the prediction result for the target domain, even if a peak location is correct, the signal distribution around the peak often has a non-Gaussian shape. The pseudo-cell-position heatmap is re-generated using the peak positions in the predicted heatmap to have a clear Gaussian shape. Our method selects confident pseudo-cell-position heatmaps using a Bayesian network and adds them to the training data in the next iteration. The method can incrementally extend the domain from the source domain to the target domain in a semi-supervised manner. In the experiments using 8 combinations of domains, the proposed method outperformed the existing domain adaptation methods.

Keywords: Cell detection · Domain adaptation · Pseudo labeling

1 Introduction

Cell detection has an important role in quantification in bio-medical research. Automatic cell-detection methods can be classified as traditional image-processing-based methods and deep-learning-based methods. Image-processing-based methods are generally designed based on the image characteristics of the target images. For example, methods using thresholding [23,32], image filters [3], region growing [34], watershed [32], and graph cuts [1] use the intensity or edge information. These methods work under the specific conditions used for developing them but often not under others.

Deep-learning-based methods have recently achieved very promising results in cell-detection problems [6,16,19,22,30]. However, a network trained with training data under a specific condition (source domain), *e.g.*, culture conditions, may not work well in data under other conditions (target domain) since the image features differ among different domains (domain shift problem).

© Springer Nature Switzerland AG 2021
M. de Bruijne et al. (Eds.): MICCAI 2021, LNCS 12908, pp. 384–394, 2021.
https://doi.org/10.1007/978-3-030-87237-3_37

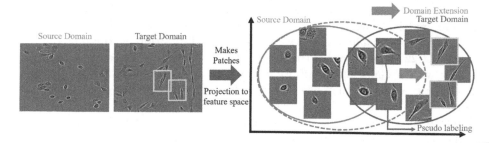

Fig. 1. Left shows examples of cell images on source and target domain and red and yellow rectangles show cells in target with similar and different shape to those in source, respectively. **Right** shows illustration of feature space of patches cut from left images, where orange arrow indicates domain extension. (Color figure online)

For example in Fig. 1, although both the source and target domains are the same cell type, the shapes of cells in the target domain cultured under different conditions are elongated compared with those in the source domain (the F-score decreased from 0.941 (source) to 0.768 (target) in our experiments). This indicates that it is necessary to prepare training data for not only cell types but also the different culture conditions, even though the condition often changes depending on the purpose of biological research.

To address the domain shift problem, unsupervised domain adaptation (UDA) methods, which use only data on the source domain without data on the target domain, have been proposed [9, 10, 12, 13, 15, 25–27]. Most are designed for classification tasks but not for detection tasks. A major approach of UDA method uses adversarial learning that transfers the distribution of the target to the source's in the same feature [4, 9, 13, 27]. Haq *et al.* [13] extended this to the cell-segmentation task by introducing an auto-encoder. This method transfers the feature distribution of an entire image, in which it is implicitly assumed that the characteristics, such as illumination, and color, of the entire image differ between the source and target domains. However, our target has a deference difficulty from entire image adaptation, where an image contains many cells with various appearances (*e.g.*, shapes, density), as shown in the red and yellow boxes in Fig. 1. It is important to consider the different appearances of cells in an image for further improvement. Another type of domain adaptation method uses semi-supervised learning for selecting pseudo labels from data in the target domain, and the network is re-trained using those pseudo labels [11, 14, 17, 18, 24, 29, 33], in which our method is categorized to this approach. The main idea of pseudo labeling is that some samples in the target domain can be correctly classified, and if we can select correctly predicted samples as the additional training data, the performance improves. However, such methods were designed for classification tasks.

In this paper, we propose a cell-detection method that addresses the domain shift problem and also improves detection performance in the same domain in a semi-supervised manner. To handle various cell appearances in an image, our method first separates an image into patches. Some patch images in the target are often similar to some in the source, $i.e.$, the image feature distributions between domains partially overlap, as shown in Fig. 1, which is assumed in most UDA methods. In our preliminary study, we used the cell-position-heatmap prediction method [2,22], which is one of the state-of-the-arts, where a cell centroid becomes a peak with a Gaussian distribution in the map. The key observation is that it could detect a cell that has a similar but slightly different shape from the source's even the prediction map is a non-Gaussian shape as shown in Fig. 2. Moreover, the detection performance improved using the correctly detected cells with clear Gaussian maps (pseudo-cell-position heatmaps) as training data in our preliminary study. Since it is important to select the confident patches as pseudo labels, we introduce a Bayesian discriminator that can estimate the uncertainty for each patch. We then use the selected patches with the clear Gaussian maps as pseudo-cell-position heatmaps for re-training the detector. These processes are iteratively performed. Since this process incrementally adds the confident pseudo labels, as shown in Fig. 1 (called domain extension), this can improve detection performance both on the source and target domains. The main contributions of this paper are as follows:

- We propose the unsupervised domain adaptation method for cell detection using the pseudo-cell-position heatmap that can incrementally extend the domain from the source to the target in a semi-supervised manner.
- We introduce a Bayesian discriminator that can estimate the uncertainty of each patch for selecting confident pseudo labels with high certainty under a self-training framework.
- The proposed method is applicable not only to the same domain but also to different domains with a small amount of training data. We confirmed the effectiveness of the method regarding detection performance through experiments involving 8 combinations of domains.

2   Domain Extension in Cell Detection

Figure 2 shows an overview of our method. Initially, the entire images are separated to patch images that may contain several cells (1 to 10 cells). We denote I_s, O_s as the set of the original patch images and the ground truth of the cell-position heatmap on the source domain, and I_t as the unlabeled images on the target domain. The proposed method consists of five steps. In step 1, using I_s and O_s, we train the detection network D that estimates the cell-position heatmap [22] and the Bayesian discriminator B that estimates the uncertainty of the estimated cell-position heatmap. In step 2, D estimates this heatmap for I_t, in which the predicted cell-position heatmap O_t may have a distorted shape (non-Gaussian) even if the peak position is correct, as shown in Fig. 2. In step 3, the pseudo cell position heatmaps (pseudo-ground-truth) P_t with clear Gaussian shapes are generated on the basis of O_t. In step 4, given pairs of the original I_t and its P_t as inputs, B estimates the uncertainty score if the inputted pseudo label is correct. In step 5, the method selects confident pseudo-position heatmaps SP_t with high certainty, which are used as the additional training data for D and B. This process is iteratively performed on I_t.

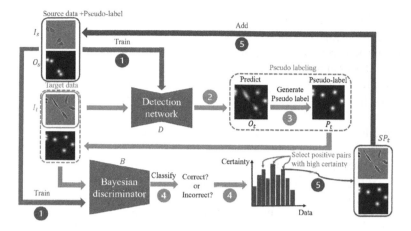

Fig. 2. Overview of proposed method. Blue arrows represent training detection network and Bayesian discriminator with source data and pseudo labels. Orange arrows represent predicting heatmap of unlabeled data on target domain and generating pseudo-cell-position heatmap. Green and purple arrows represent selecting positive pseudo-cell-position heatmaps with high certainty by Bayesian discriminator, and adding selected patches as pseudo heatmap. This flow is iteratively performed. (Color figure online)

Cell Detection with Cell-Position Heatmap (Steps 1 and 2): Object-detection tasks often use a bounding box as the ground truth for localizing objects. However, the bounding box is not suitable for cell detection due to its complex shape and high density since it may often contain other cells. Instead, we use a cell-position heatmap that has produced a good performance [22]. Given the set of annotated cell centroid positions for an image, a ground truth of the cell-position heatmap is generated so that a cell centroid becomes a peak with a Gaussian distribution in the map, as shown in Fig. 2. To train D, we use the mean squared error (MSE) loss function between the estimated image and ground-truth heatmap.

Pseudo Labeling for Cell Detection (Step 3): The predicted cell-position heatmap O_t in the target domain may have a distorted Gaussian distribution, even if the peak position is correct. We generate the pseudo-cell-position heatmaps P_t on the basis of O_t so that detected positions C_t in the predicted cell-position heatmap becomes a peak with a clear Gaussian distribution in the same manner as in step 1. Here, if the peak of O_t is higher than a threshold th_d, the position C_t is detected. Examples of predicted and pseudo-cell-position heatmaps are shown in the red dotted box in Fig. 2. The pseudo-cell-position heatmap will be used for training D and B. Even if the signals of a cell in the initially estimated cell-position heatmap have a non-Gaussian shape, cells that have a similar appearance to the pseudo labels can be detected with a clear Gaussian shape by the re-trained D using the pseudo-cell-position heatmap. The D will incrementally improve from the iteration of this pseudo-labeling process.

Bayesian Discriminator (Steps 4 and 5): If a pseudo-cell-position heatmap contains many incorrect labels, detection performance may be affected. To select confident pseudo-cell-position heatmaps SP_t, we introduce a Bayesian CNN to D that estimates uncertainty in whether the estimated detection result is correct. To represent model uncertainty, we leverage a dropout-based approximate uncertainty inference [7,8], in which the variance of the estimation of samples from the posterior distribution can be considered as an uncertainty measure.

The model with dropout learns the distribution of weights at training. We then sample the posterior weights of the model by using the dropout at test to find the predictive distribution over output from the model [7,8]. In practice, at test, the averaging stochastic forward passes through the model with dropout and averaging results are identical to the variance to model uncertainty [7,8]. We use this as a measure of model uncertainty. Model uncertainty is defined as

$$Uncertainty \approx \frac{1}{T} \sum_{t=1}^{T} p(\widehat{y}^* \mid \widehat{x}^*, \widehat{w}_t), \tag{1}$$

where $\widehat{w}_t$ are weights sampled from the distribution over the model's weights and T is the number of sampling (the number of networks with dropout), $\widehat{x}^*$ and $\widehat{y}^*$ are input and output from the model. This model is referred to as MC dropout [8].

In our model, the input of the network in inference is a pair of the original image and generated pseudo-cell-position heatmap $\mathbf{X}^{(k)} = \{I_t^{(k)}, P_t^{(k)}\}$, and the output is the label $Y = \{0, 1\}$ with $Uncertainty$, where k is the data index. If $P_t^{(k)}$ looks like a correct label for the original image $I_t^{(k)}$, Y takes 0; otherwise, 1. If the estimated label is confident, it produces lower uncertainty; otherwise, higher uncertainty. To train B in the initial iteration, we deliberately make the incorrect ground truth from the ground truth of I_s as negative samples by adding or removing and shifting the Gaussian in the ground truth of I_s. In inference, we T times apply the network for a single input with the different dropout and obtain the predicted labels with uncertainties for all image pairs of $\{I_t, P_t\}$ based on the T results. We then select SP_t that have with th_u lowest uncertainty and add them as training data for D and B in the next step.

3   Experiment

We evaluated the effectiveness of our method by using 8 combinations of domains. The baseline (Sup.) of the proposed method is a supervised method [22] that uses training data on the source only. We also compared the proposed method with four other methods; an unsupervised image-processing-based method proposed by Vicar [28] that combined Yin [31] and distance transform, a semi-supervised learning method proposed by Moskvyak [20] using consistency of prediction and is not for domain adaptation, a method (Haq w/o AE) [13] that simply introduces adversarial domain adaptation for cell segmentation, and

Table 1. Performance of proposed methods on same and target domains

Data	S to T	Sup. on S	Ours on S	Sup. on T	Vicar [28]	Moskvyak [20]	Haq w/o AE [13]	Haq [13]	Ours on T
C2C12	F → C	0.800	**0.833**	0.684	0.700	0.642	0.766	0.771	**0.845**
	B → C	0.885	**0.941**	0.756	0.700	0.775	0.843	0.848	**0.860**
	C → F	0.850	**0.867**	0.705	0.612	0.642	0.755	0.767	**0.807**
	B → F	0.885	**0.899**	0.632	0.612	0.648	0.766	0.771	**0.798**
	C → B	0.850	**0.862**	0.709	0.584	0.761	0.779	0.795	**0.820**
	F → B	0.800	**0.835**	0.742	0.584	0.721	0.761	0.757	**0.817**
HMEC	C → E	0.941	**0.962**	0.768	0.797	0.798	0.851	0.849	**0.875**
	E → C	0.941	**0.971**	0.939	0.857	0.835	0.924	0.921	**0.959**
	Average	0.869	**0.896**	0.742	0.681	0.728	0.806	0.810	**0.848**

Table 2. Performance when proposed method was used as semi-supervised learning using additional data in same domain.

Data	Cond	Sup.	Vicar [28]	Moskvyak [20]	Ours
C2C12	C	0.850	0.700	0.851	**0.888**
	B	0.885	0.584	0.899	**0.924**
	F	0.800	0.612	**0.859**	0.842
HMEC	C	0.941	0.857	**0.963**	0.961
	E	0.941	0.797	0.958	**0.961**
	Average	0.883	0.710	0.906	**0.915**

a domain adaptation method proposed by Haq [13] that introduced auto-encoder to adversarial learning for cell segmentation.

Implementation Details: In this experiment, We employed U-Net as the detection network and Resnet18 as the discriminator, and the four iterations (Iters 0 to 3) were performed in all experiments. We used Adam to optimize our model and set the learning rate is 1.0×10^{-3} and all datasets are normalized between 0 and 255. Hyperparameters to the proposed method are th_d, th_u and T which are 100, 10 and 10 in all experiments.

Datasets and Evaluation Metric: To determine how our method performs regarding domain shift, we evaluated two datasets. The first is C2C12 [5] consisting of myoblast cells captured by phase contrast microscopy at a resolution of 1040 × 1392 pixels and cultured under three different conditions; 1) Control (no growth factor), 2) FGF2 (fibroblast growth factor), 3) BMP2 (bone morphogenetic protein). The second dataset is Human mammary epithelial cells (HMEC), consisting of cells captured by phase-contrast microscopy at a resolution of 1272 × 952 and cultured under two conditions; 1) Control (no stimulus) and 2) EMT (epithelial-mesenchymal transition) [21]. As shown in Fig. 3 (a), the cell appearance under each condition is different. We made patches of 128 × 128 pixels from full images of all datasets, and the ground truth was given for only 24 patches (approximately a quarter of one entire image) under each condition.

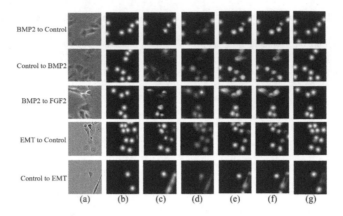

Fig. 3. (a) Original image, (b) Ground-truth, (c)Sup., (d)Moskvyak, (e) Haq w/o AE, (f) Haq, (g) Ours

In the evaluation of domain adaptation, we used a sequence as unlabeled data (100 entire images), and the other sequence as test data (100 entire images) under different conditions from the training data. We used F-score as the performance metric, which is measured by solving a one-by-one matching based on proximity of the estimated cell positions and the ground truth. The cell location is defined as the peak position of each Gaussian distribution. If the detected result is close enough to the given ground truth, it is counted as True Positive. When there is no ground truth around the detected location, it is counted as False Positive, and when there is no detected result around the ground-truth location, it is counted as False Negative.

Evaluation: Table 1 shows the detection performances (F-score) in the target domain and source domain. The source and target are denoted as S and T and each culture condition (Cond.) is denoted by the first letter of the condition name. 'Sup. on S' indicates the performance of the baseline method when evaluated on the other sequences in the same domain. The performances of the baseline (Sup. on T) significantly decreased from those (Sup. on S) evaluated on the same domain (average: −0.127). Although Haq w/o AE and Haq's methods improved in performance in the target domain, our method outperformed these methods for all combinations. The columns (Sup. on S), (Ours. on S) in Table 1 shows the performances in the additional test data on the source domain after applying our method. In all data, our method also improved in performance not only in the target domain but also in the source domain. We consider that the pseudo-cell-position heatmaps for cells that have similar appearances to those in the source domain improved the detection performance of the proposed method. Figure 3 shows example detection results of the test data on the target domains. As shown in Fig. 3(c), the supervised method did not effectively predict cell-position heatmaps, but the peaks in some were correctly detected. In contrast,

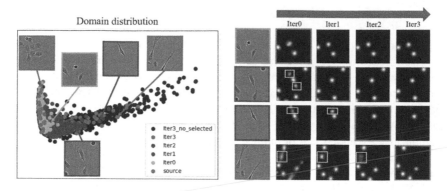

Fig. 4. Left is feature distribution of source and target domains (Iteration 0 to 3-no-selected). **Right** represents cell shape and detection result at each iteration. Green prediction cell-position map signifies correct detection results and yellow boxes represent False Positive. (Color figure online)

our method could predict these maps with a clear Gaussian shape. These results support the idea of the proposed method.

Next, we evaluated the effectiveness of the proposed method as semi-supervised learning to confirm that it can improve detection performance from the few labeled and many unlabeled data. In this experiment, 24 patch images were used as labeled data, and 8000 patch images (100 entire images) were used as unlabeled data for each condition. The evaluation was then conducted in which all the images were in the same domain. Since Haq w/o AE and Haq's methods are not for semi-supervised learning, we did not evaluate them. Table 2 shows that our method performed better for all domains compared with the baseline, and the average was slightly better than Moskvyak's method [20], which was developed for semi-supervised learning.

Visualization of Domain-Extension Process: The left image in Fig. 4 shows the feature distribution of the source (control of HMEC) and the target domain (EMT), where each iteration is marked with a different color. In this map, the cells in the source domain are round (red) and distributed on the left side, and the cells in the target domain have various shapes (orange, purple, blue, magenta, and black) and distributed from the left to right. The colored box images are the samples from this distribution. We can observe that the proposed method incrementally increased the pseudo patches from left to right in the feature map with iteration. The right image in Fig. 4 shows examples of estimated cell-position heatmaps in each iteration. In iteration 0, the elongated cell, which is located on the right side of the feature map, was mistakenly detected as several cells. Such cells far from the source images in the map were not selected in the early iterations, but the prediction results of the heatmap improved in the later iterations, which were finally selected when the prediction was successful. These results indicate that the discriminator performed well in finding the correct pseudo-position heatmap, and the proposed method incrementally extended the domains from the source to target.

4   Conclusion

We proposed a domain adaptation method for cell detection based on semi-supervised learning by selecting pseudo-cell-position heatmaps using model uncertainty. The experiment results using various combinations of domains demonstrated the effectiveness of our method, which improved the performance of detection on unannotated cells on not only different domains but also source domains. Also, the analysis of each iteration demonstrated that the method incrementally extended the domain from the source and target.

Acknowledgment. This work was supported by JSPS KAKENHI Grant Number JP20H04211 and JP21K19829.

References

1. Al-Kofahi, Y., Lassoued, W., Lee, W., Roysam, B.: Improved automatic detection and segmentation of cell nuclei in histopathology images. IEEE Trans. Biomed. Eng. **57**(4), 841–852 (2009)
2. Cao, Z., Hidalgo, G., Simon, T., Wei, S.E., Sheikh, Y.: Openpose: realtime multi-person 2D pose estimation using part affinity fields. IEEE Trans. Pattern Anal. Mach. Intell. **43**(1), 172–186 (2019)
3. Cosatto, E., Miller, M., Graf, H.P., Meyer, J.S.: Grading nuclear pleomorphism on histological micrographs. In: ICPR (2008)
4. Cui, S., Wang, S., Zhuo, J., Su, C., Huang, Q., Tian, Q.: Gradually vanishing bridge for adversarial domain adaptation. In: CVPR (2020)
5. Eom, S., et al.: Phase contrast time-lapse microscopy datasets with automated and manual cell tracking annotations. Sci. Data **5**(1), 1–12 (2018)
6. Fujita, S., Han, X.-H.: Cell detection and segmentation in microscopy images with improved mask R-CNN. In: Sato, I., Han, B. (eds.) ACCV 2020. LNCS, vol. 12628, pp. 58–70. Springer, Cham (2021). https://doi.org/10.1007/978-3-030-69756-3_5
7. Gal, Y., Ghahramani, Z.: Bayesian convolutional neural networks with Bernoulli approximate variational inference. arXiv preprint arXiv:1506.02158 (2015)
8. Gal, Y., Ghahramani, Z.: Dropout as a Bayesian approximation: representing model uncertainty in deep learning. In: ICML (2016)
9. Ganin, Y., Lempitsky, V.: Unsupervised domain adaptation by backpropagation. In: ICML (2015)
10. Ge, P., Ren, C.X., Dai, D.Q., Yan, H.: Domain adaptation and image classification via deep conditional adaptation network. arXiv preprint arXiv:2006.07776 (2020)
11. Ge, Y., Chen, D., Li, H.: Mutual mean-teaching: Pseudo label refinery for unsupervised domain adaptation on person re-identification. In: ICLR (2020)
12. Ghifary, M., Kleijn, W.B., Zhang, M., Balduzzi, D., Li, W.: Deep reconstruction-classification networks for unsupervised domain adaptation. In: Leibe, B., Matas, J., Sebe, N., Welling, M. (eds.) ECCV 2016. LNCS, vol. 9908, pp. 597–613. Springer, Cham (2016). https://doi.org/10.1007/978-3-319-46493-0_36
13. Haq, M.M., Huang, J.: Adversarial domain adaptation for cell segmentation. In: MIDL (2020)

14. Jiang, P., Wu, A., Han, Y., Shao, Y., Qi, M., Li, B.: Bidirectional adversarial training for semi-supervised domain adaptation. In: IJCAI (2020)

15. Jin, S.Y., et al.: Unsupervised hard example mining from videos for improved object detection. In: Ferrari, V., Hebert, M., Sminchisescu, C., Weiss, Y. (eds.) ECCV 2018. LNCS, vol. 11217, pp. 316–333. Springer, Cham (2018). https://doi.org/10.1007/978-3-030-01261-8_19

16. Kainz, P., Urschler, M., Schulter, S., Wohlhart, P., Lepetit, V.: You should use regression to detect cells. In: Navab, N., Hornegger, J., Wells, W.M., Frangi, A.F. (eds.) MICCAI 2015. LNCS, vol. 9351, pp. 276–283. Springer, Cham (2015). https://doi.org/10.1007/978-3-319-24574-4_33

17. Kim, T., Kim, C.: Attract, perturb, and explore: learning a feature alignment network for semi-supervised domain adaptation. In: Vedaldi, A., Bischof, H., Brox, T., Frahm, J.-M. (eds.) ECCV 2020. LNCS, vol. 12359, pp. 591–607. Springer, Cham (2020). https://doi.org/10.1007/978-3-030-58568-6_35

18. Li, D., Hospedales, T.: Online meta-learning for multi-source and semi-supervised domain adaptation. In: Vedaldi, A., Bischof, H., Brox, T., Frahm, J.-M. (eds.) ECCV 2020. LNCS, vol. 12361, pp. 382–403. Springer, Cham (2020). https://doi.org/10.1007/978-3-030-58517-4_23

19. Li, J., et al.: Signet ring cell detection with a semi-supervised learning framework. In: Chung, A.C.S., Gee, J.C., Yushkevich, P.A., Bao, S. (eds.) IPMI 2019. LNCS, vol. 11492, pp. 842–854. Springer, Cham (2019). https://doi.org/10.1007/978-3-030-20351-1_66

20. Moskvyak, O., Maire, F., Dayoub, F., Baktashmotlagh, M.: Semi-supervised keypoint localization. arXiv preprint arXiv:2101.07988 (2021)

21. Nieto, M.A., Huang, R.Y.J., Jackson, R.A., Thiery, J.P.: EMT: 2016. Cell **166**(1), 21–45 (2016)

22. Nishimura, K., Ker, D.F.E., Bise, R.: Weakly supervised cell instance segmentation by propagating from detection response. In: Shen, D., et al. (eds.) MICCAI 2019. LNCS, vol. 11764, pp. 649–657. Springer, Cham (2019). https://doi.org/10.1007/978-3-030-32239-7_72

23. Otsu, N.: A threshold selection method from gray-level histograms. IEEE Trans. Syst. Man Cybern. **9**(1), 62–66 (1979)

24. Saito, K., Kim, D., Sclaroff, S., Darrell, T., Saenko, K.: Semi-supervised domain adaptation via minimax entropy. In: CVPR (2019)

25. Saito, K., Ushiku, Y., Harada, T., Saenko, K.: Strong-weak distribution alignment for adaptive object detection. In: CVPR (2019)

26. Tsai, Y.H., Sohn, K., Schulter, S., Chandraker, M.: Domain adaptation for structured output via disentangled patch representations. In: ICCV (2018)

27. Tzeng, E., Hoffman, J., Saenko, K., Darrell, T.: Adversarial discriminative domain adaptation. In: CVPR (2017)

28. Vicar, T., et al.: Cell segmentation methods for label-free contrast microscopy: review and comprehensive comparison. BMC Bioinf. **20**(1), 1–25 (2019)

29. Wang, Q., Breckon, T.: Unsupervised domain adaptation via structured prediction based selective pseudo-labeling. In: AAAI (2020)

30. Yi, J., et al.: Multi-scale cell instance segmentation with keypoint graph based bounding boxes. In: Shen, D., et al. (eds.) MICCAI 2019. LNCS, vol. 11764, pp. 369–377. Springer, Cham (2019). https://doi.org/10.1007/978-3-030-32239-7_41

31. Yin, Z., Kanade, T., Chen, M.: Understanding the phase contrast optics to restore artifact-free microscopy images for segmentation. Med. Image Anal. **16**(5), 1047–1062 (2012)

32. Yuan, Y., et al.: Quantitative image analysis of cellular heterogeneity in breast tumors complements genomic profiling. Sci. Transl. Med. **4**(157), 157ra143 (2012)
33. Zheng, Z., Yang, Y.: Rectifying pseudo label learning via uncertainty estimation for domain adaptive semantic segmentation. Int. J. Comput. Vis. **129**, 1106–1120 (2020)
34. Zhou, Y., Starkey, J., Mansinha, L.: Segmentation of petrographic images by integrating edge detection and region growing. Comput. Geosci. **30**(8), 817–831 (2004)

2D Histology Meets 3D Topology: Cytoarchitectonic Brain Mapping with Graph Neural Networks

Christian Schiffer[1,2]([📧]) [iD], Stefan Harmeling[3], Katrin Amunts[1,4] [iD], and Timo Dickscheid[1,2] [iD]

[1] Institute of Neuroscience and Medicine (INM-1),
Research Centre Jülich, Jülich, Germany
{c.schiffer,k.amunts,t.dickscheid}@fz-juelich.de
[2] Helmholtz AI, Research Centre Jülich, Jülich, Germany
[3] Heinrich Heine University, Düsseldorf, Germany
harmeling@hhu.de
[4] Cécile and Oskar Vogt Institute for Brain Research,
University Hospital Düsseldorf, Düsseldorf, Germany

Abstract. Cytoarchitecture describes the spatial organization of neuronal cells in the brain, including their arrangement into layers and columns with respect to cell density, orientation, or presence of certain cell types. It allows to segregate the brain into cortical areas and subcortical nuclei, links structure with connectivity and function, and provides a microstructural reference for human brain atlases. Mapping boundaries between areas requires to scan histological sections at microscopic resolution. While recent high-throughput scanners allow to scan a complete human brain in the order of a year, it is practically impossible to delineate regions at the same pace using the established gold standard method. Researchers have recently addressed cytoarchitectonic mapping of cortical regions with deep neural networks, relying on image patches from individual 2D sections for classification. However, the 3D context, which is needed to disambiguate complex or obliquely cut brain regions, is not taken into account. In this work, we combine 2D histology with 3D topology by reformulating the mapping task as a node classification problem on an approximate 3D midsurface mesh through the isocortex. We extract deep features from cortical patches in 2D histological sections which are descriptive of cytoarchitecture, and assign them to the corresponding nodes on the 3D mesh to construct a large attributed graph. By solving the brain mapping problem on this graph using graph neural networks, we obtain significantly improved classification results. The proposed framework lends itself nicely to integration of additional neuroanatomical priors for mapping.

Keywords: Graph neural networks · Deep learning · Contrastive learning · Histology · Cytoarchitecture · Brain mapping · Human brain

© Springer Nature Switzerland AG 2021
M. de Bruijne et al. (Eds.): MICCAI 2021, LNCS 12908, pp. 395–404, 2021.
https://doi.org/10.1007/978-3-030-87237-3_38

1   Introduction

Cytoarchitectonic areas are characterized by a distinct spatial organization of neuronal cells in the brain, including their arrangement into layers and columns, as well as density, orientation, or presence of certain types of cells. As indicators for connectivity and functional modules, they provide an important microstructural reference for human brain atlases [2]. Mapping the borders of cytoarchitectonic areas requires to analyze brain sections at microscopic resolution. To capture the human brain's considerable variability, it needs to be performed in many different brain samples. [2] created a comprehensive probabilistic cytoarchitectonic atlas based on delineations in serial histological sections stained for cell bodies in a sample of ten brains, using image analysis and statistical tools to identify architectonic borders [22]. These resulting maps are aggregated in a 3D reference space at the millimeter scale. Although today's high-throughput scanners allow to digitize complete human brains at micrometer resolution, it is practically impossible to scale this approach for doing delineations in all sections of a human brain, which may have, in dependence of the size, approx. 6000–8000 sections. This motivates the development of automatic mapping algorithms.

Recent work formulated cytoarchitectonic mapping of cortical regions as an image segmentation [23, 24] or classification [21] problem, which can be approached with deep convolutional networks. These methods process each 2D section individually, responding to the lack of routine workflows for computing a precise 3D reconstruction from histology en par with high throughput imaging. In fact, as of today only one 3D reconstruction of a whole human brain from histology is available [1], with a spatial resolution of $20\,\mu$m isotropic. The 3D topology of a brain is thus not used by these models, although it is key to disambiguate complex or obliquely cut brain regions. Other authors suggested to incorporate inter-slice information using 3D convolutions [19] or recurrent networks [3], which again requires a precise 3D reconstruction.

Here we present a novel paradigm for cytoarchitectonic brain mapping which overcomes the above restrictions. The basic idea is to reformulate the mapping task as a node classification problem on the approximate 3D midsurface mesh through the isocortex. Since the mesh is not assumed to be precise, it can be derived from a simple linear reconstruction which is straightforward to compute from a histological image stack, and can handle a significant amount of missing sections. Building on [21], we extract deep features from 2D cortical patches at microscopic resolution using convolutional neural networks (CNNs) that were trained with a contrastive learning task to encode cytoarchitectonic characteristics. These features are then assigned to the corresponding nodes on the reconstructed surface mesh to construct a large, attributed graph. The brain mapping problem is solved on this graph using graph neural networks (GNNs) [8, 11].

We make the following contributions: 1) We introduce a novel deep learning approach for cytoarchitecture classification in large stacks of whole brain sections which integrates high-resolution 2D texture features with global 3D topology. 2) The approach outperforms the state of the art on DL-based cytoarchitectonic mapping on a dataset of histological sections from eight postmortem human

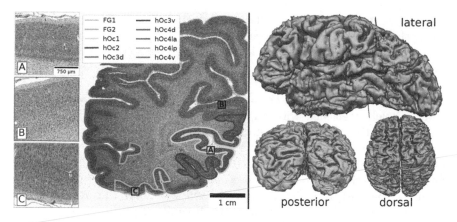

Fig. 1. Left: Histological brain section from brain B01 (see also Fig. 2, left) with expert annotations of cytoarchitectonic areas shown in different colors. **Right:** Approximate midsurface through the isocortex extracted from a linear reconstruction of the histological stack. Points on the surface corresponding to points in the image on the left are shown in red. (Color figure online)

brains. 3) The approach allows flexible integration of neuroanatomical priors into the mapping problem, which further boosts classification performance.

2   Methods

The proposed framework consists of three components: 1) A linear 3D reconstruction of the histological stack to compute an approximate midsurface mesh of the isocortex, which is interpreted as a graph. 2) A CNN trained with contrastive learning which extracts cortical features from the histological sections, serving as node attributes in the graph. 3) A GNN to label each graph node with a cytoarchitectonic area, exploiting both high-resolution texture and approximate 3D topology encoded in the graph.

Construction of the Approximate Midsurface Graph. A coarse segmentation of each section into background, white matter and cortical gray matter is performed using morphological active contours [17]. Histological brain sections (Fig. 1, left) are 3D reconstructed by rigid alignment of adjacent sections using feature based registration as described in [6]. From the segmented linear 3D reconstruction, a 3D cortical midsurface mesh is extracted by solving Laplace's equation inside the cortical mantle [13] using the *highres-cortex* package[1] and extracting the 0.5 isosurface from the resulting volumetric Laplacian fields using marching cubes [14]. In a manual postprocessing stage, hemispheres are split, and small disconnected components as well as cerebellum and brainstem are removed from the mesh. Finally, isotropic explicit remeshing is applied using *meshlab*[4] to unify edge

---

[1] https://github.com/neurospin/highres-cortex.

lengths in the mesh to $\approx 300\,\mu\text{m}$, thereby reducing the number of triangles and ensuring that connections between vertices represent comparable distances. Each resulting mesh (Fig. 1, right) is then interpreted as a graph $\mathcal{G} = (\mathcal{V}, \mathcal{E})$ with nodes $\mathcal{V}$ and edges $\mathcal{E}$.

Computing Node Level Texture Features. Each node $u \in \mathcal{V}$ in the resulting graph can be uniquely identified with an image coordinate p_u in a 2D histological section by inverting the rigid transformation applied for 3D reconstruction. We apply an encoder CNN f to extract a cytoarchitectonic feature embedding h_u from an image patch x centered at each coordinate p_u. The encoder f is trained using the contrastive approach proposed in [21] to produce an embedding that maps image patches from the same brain area to similar feature vectors, and image patches from different brain areas to dissimilar feature vectors. Given an image patch x, f produces a lower dimensional vector $h = f(x) \in \mathbb{R}^{D_e}$, which is passed through a projection network $g(h) = \tilde{z} \in \mathbb{R}^{D_p}$ and normalized as $z_i = \tilde{z}_i / \|\tilde{z}_i\|_2$. Given a minibatch of N image patches x_i with corresponding labels y_i ($i = 1, \ldots, N$), the contrastive loss

$$\mathcal{L} = \frac{1}{N} \sum_{i=1}^{N} \mathcal{L}_i \tag{1}$$

$$\mathcal{L}_i = -\frac{1}{N_{y_i}} \sum_{j=1}^{N} \mathbb{I}_{i \neq j} \mathbb{I}_{y_i = y_j} \log \frac{e^{\langle z_i, z_j \rangle / \tau}}{\sum_{k=1}^{N} \mathbb{I}_{i \neq k} e^{\langle z_i, z_k \rangle / \tau}} \tag{2}$$

is optimized during training, where $\mathbb{I}$ is the indicator function, $\tau \in \mathbb{R}$ is a temperature scaling parameter and N_{y_i} is the number of batch elements with the same label as x_i. The projection network g is discarded after training.

Graph Neural Networks. We consider two GNN architectures to integrate spatial relationships of image patches into the classification model: GraphSAGE [8] and Graph Attention Network (GAT) [25]. Both architectures are suitable for inductive tasks, so that trained networks can be applied to previously unseen nodes or graphs. Due to common memory constraints, training on full graphs is not possible given the level of detail of our models. We therefore adapt the neighborhood sampling scheme proposed in [8]: Given a node $u \in \mathcal{V}$ and a GNN with K layers, we sample its K-hop neighborhood $\mathcal{N}_K(u)$ and use the resulting subgraph as input for the GNN. This way, information from the immediate neighborhood of u can be propagated through the GNN to classify u.

Integrating Anatomical Priors. Previous work [23] showed that the integration of prior anatomical knowledge - there given in the form of probabilistic cytoarchitectonic maps [2] - can improve classification performance. Inspired by this finding, we adapt the registration workflow from [2] to project probabilistic maps of 152 brain areas from the MNI Colin27 reference space onto the histological sections, and assign an additional vector h_u^P to each node u. Each dimension of h_u^P encodes the probability to belong to a particular region of the Julich-Brain atlas [2]. We further consider spatial locations in Colin27 space as another anatomical prior by assigning a 3D coordinate vector h_u^C to each node u, again using the workflow from [2].

Implementation Details. Models were implemented using *pytorch* [20] and *pytorch-geometric* [7]. Training was performed on the HPC clusters JURECA [12] (NVidia K80, 12 GB) and JURECA-DC (NVidia A100, 40 GB) using 4 to 32 GPUs. Code will be made publicly available[2].

3   Experiments and Results

We systematically evaluate all components of the proposed approach: 1) We compare different encoder architectures for contrastive feature learning from images patches. 2) Using the best performing encoder architecture, we compare the performance of GNNs with SAGE and GAT architectures. 3) We investigate the additional benefit of adding neuroanatomical priors for classification.

Dataset. We use an in-house dataset containing images of 1860 histological sections from 7 human postmortem brains acquired from the body donor programs of the Anatomical Institute of the University of Düsseldorf (Germany), and corresponding annotations of 113 cytoarchitectonic cortical areas. Sections have an approximate thickness of 20 μm, were marked for neuronal cell bodies using a modified Merker stain [18], and imaged at a resolution of 1 μm with a light-microscopic scanner (TissueScope, Huron Digital Pathology Inc.). 80% of the sections are used for training ($\mathcal{X}_{tr}$), remaining sections for testing ($\mathcal{X}_{te}$). Transferability to unseen brains is evaluated on 325 sections from an 8th brain ($\mathcal{X}_{un}$). Graph nodes $\mathcal{V}$ are split into $\mathcal{V}_{tr}$, $\mathcal{V}_{te}$ and $\mathcal{V}_{un}$, containing nodes with corresponding points p_u in $\mathcal{X}_{tr}$, $\mathcal{X}_{te}$ and $\mathcal{X}_{un}$, respectively. Performance is evaluated using macro-F1 score on nodes $\mathcal{V}_{te}$ and $\mathcal{V}_{un}$. The study requires no ethical approvals.

Performance of Different Feature Encoders. The encoder network f is trained on 1200 image patches per class sampled from $\mathcal{X}_{tr}$, oversampling small areas for class balancing. Data augmentation steps include random pixel intensity augmentation, rotation, mirroring, translation, blurring and sharpening with parameters detailed in [21]. Training is performed for 150 epochs using LARS optimizer [26] with constant learning rate $0.01 * N/128$, batch size $N = 4096$ ($N = 2048$ for res[w,l] due to memory constraints) and $\tau = 0.07$. We consider the two network architectures listed in Table 1: base is the architecture presented in [21,23,24] which we include as baseline. res uses pre-activation residual building blocks [9] and is based on ResNet18. For both architectures, we also consider wider variants with twice as many channels per layer (base[w], res[w]). For res, we further investigate larger input image patches (res[l], res[w,l]). The following image patch sizes are used (2 μm/pixel): 1129^2 pixel for base/base[w], 1024^2 pixel for

---

[2] https://jugit.fz-juelich.de/c.schiffer/miccai2021_2d_histology_meets_3d_topology.

Table 1. Network architecture of **base** and **res** models. **res** uses pre-activation residual connections as in ResNet18 [9]. **base** uses no padding, **res** uses zero-padding ($\mathtt{CONV}(k, c, s)$: c-channel $k \times k$ stride s convolutional layer, $\mathtt{MP}(k, s)$: $k \times k$ stride s maxpooling, $\mathtt{FC}(d)$: d-dimensional fully connected layer, $\mathtt{GAP}$: global average pooling).

Layer name	base	res
conv_1_x	$\mathtt{CONV}(5, 16, 4)$, $\mathtt{CONV}(3, 16, 1)$, $\mathtt{MP}(2, 2)$	
conv_2_x	$\mathtt{CONV}(3, 32, 1) \times 2$, $\mathtt{MP}(2, 2)$	$\mathtt{CONV}(3, 32, 1) \times 4$
conv_3_x	$\mathtt{CONV}(3, 64, 1) \times 2$, $\mathtt{MP}(2, 2)$	$\mathtt{CONV}(3, 64, 2)$, $\mathtt{CONV}(3, 64, 1) \times 3$
conv_4_x	$\mathtt{CONV}(3, 64, 1) \times 2$, $\mathtt{MP}(2, 2)$	$\mathtt{CONV}(3, 64, 2)$, $\mathtt{CONV}(3, 64, 1) \times 3$
conv_5_x	$\mathtt{CONV}(3, 128, 1) \times 2$, $\mathtt{MP}(2, 2)$	$\mathtt{CONV}(3, 128, 2)$, $\mathtt{CONV}(3, 128, 1) \times 3$
conv_6_x	$\mathtt{CONV}(3, 128, 1) \times 2$	–
Projection	$\mathtt{GAP}$, $\mathtt{FC}(128)$, $\mathtt{FC}(128)$	

Table 2. Macro-F1 scores (average across three runs) obtained on $\mathcal{V}_{te}$ and $\mathcal{V}_{un}$. *Left:* Independent patch classification based on features extracted using different encoder architectures. *Center:* Node level classification on graphs using different GNN architectures and features extracted with **res[w,l]** (MLP performance for comparison). *Right:* Node level classification exploiting prior knowledge using **SAGE[5+r]**, features from **res[w,l]** and different combinations of cytoarchitectonic features (**CY**), probabilistic maps (**PM**) and canonical coordinates (**CO**).

model	$\mathcal{V}_{te}$	$\mathcal{V}_{un}$
base [21]	30.62	11.14
base[w]	36.94	10.40
res	35.17	13.47
res[l]	44.67	17.82
res[w]	44.08	13.72
res[w,l]	**50.57**	**18.99**

model	$\mathcal{V}_{te}$	$\mathcal{V}_{un}$
MLP	50.57	18.99
SAGE[3]	66.48	**20.75**
SAGE[3+r]	68.64	19.84
SAGE[5+r]	**70.18**	20.22
GAT[3]	66.40	20.17
GAT[3+r]	61.98	20.02
GAT[5+r]	63.46	20.06

model	$\mathcal{V}_{te}$	$\mathcal{V}_{un}$
CY	70.18	20.22
CY/PM	77.06	30.90
CY/CO	79.28	33.40
CY/PM/CO	**79.93**	32.67
PM	47.39	30.43
CO	56.30	**34.19**
PM/CO	56.03	32.30

res/res[w], 2048^2 pixel for res[l]/res[w,l]. Performance is evaluated on $\mathcal{V}_{te}$ and $\mathcal{V}_{un}$ by training a multi-layer perceptron (MLP) (three layers à 256 hidden units, batch normalization (BN) [10], ReLU) to classify brain areas from features extracted by each considered model f for all nodes in $\mathcal{V}_{tr}$. MLP is trained for 100 epochs using SGD with Nesterov momentum 0.9, constant learning rate $0.001 * N/4096$, batch size $N = 16384$ and cross-entropy loss. We apply dropout with probability 0.5 and 0.25 to the input and hidden layers, respectively.

We found that **res** models perform better than **base** models (Table 2 left). Wider networks and a larger input size improve performance on $\mathcal{V}_{te}$. On $\mathcal{V}_{un}$, increased input size (res[l]) outperforms wider networks (res[w]). Best results are obtained by combining both (res[w,l]).

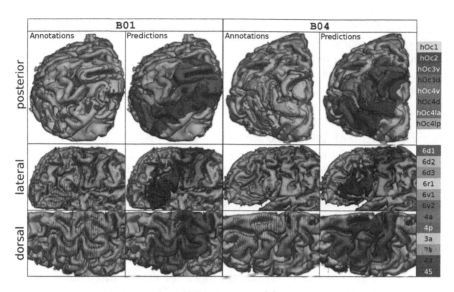

Fig. 2 Visualization of available expert annotations and predictions by `SAGE[5+r]` for the left hemisphere of two brains (`B01` and `B04`). The model was trained using features from `res[w,1]` (`CY`) as well as anatomical priors in the form of probabilistic maps (`PM`) and canonical coordinates (`CO`). Annotations include both training and test labels. Since they are only available for a subset of sections, they appear as stripes.

Graph Neural Networks. We create one graph per brain hemisphere, resulting in 16 graphs overall (1.2 million nodes with node degree 6, on average). Training nodes are sampled from $\mathcal{V}_{tr}$, inversely proportional to their class frequency to account for class imbalance. Node features are computed using `res[w,1]`. Node labels are assigned using annotations of cytoarchitectonic areas. We consider two basic GNN architectures: `SAGE[3]` consists of three GraphSAGE layers with mean aggregation [8], while `GAT[3]` consists of three GAT layers [25]. Following [15,16], we further investigate variants with pre-activation residual connections (`SAGE[3+r]`, `GAT[3+r]`) and five layers (`SAGE[5+r]`, `GAT[5+r]`). All layers use 256 hidden units, BN and ReLU activation. GAT layers use 8 attention heads with 32 units each (256 units in total). Remaining training parameters are identical to those used for `MLP`. For `SAGE` models, we adapt fixed-size neighborhood sampling from [8] with a neighborhood size of three. For `GAT` models, we sample full neighborhoods, but apply dropout with probability 0.5 to attention coefficients as proposed in [25]. Both sampling methods aim to make models robust against missing nodes or edges.

All GNN architectures obtain significantly higher scores than `MLP` on both $\mathcal{V}_{te}$ and $\mathcal{V}_{un}$ (Table 2, center). `SAGE[5+r]` achieves overall best scores, with an increase by 19.61 points and 1.23 points on $\mathcal{V}_{te}$ and $\mathcal{V}_{un}$ compared to `MLP`, respectively. Using the same number of layers and residual connections, `SAGE` outperforms `GAT` in almost all cases.

Incorporating Prior Knowledge. We examine classification performance under all possible combinations of using cytoarchitectonic features extracted from images (CY), weights from probabilistic cytoarchitectonic maps (PM) [2], and canonical 3D locations (CO) at each node. Dropout with probability 0.5 and additive Gaussian white noise with standard deviation 0.05 is applied to h_u^P and h_u^C, respectively. h_u^P and h_u^C are each projected by a fully connected layer (256 units, BN, ReLU) before concatenation.

Incorporating both PM and CO with the texture features CY improves scores by 9.75 points on $\mathcal{V}_{te}$ and 12.45 points on $\mathcal{V}_{un}$ (Table 2, right; Fig. 2). Using them in isolation, CO leads to slightly better performance than PM. Scores on $\mathcal{V}_{te}$ drop significantly when removing texture features CY. Best scores on $\mathcal{V}_{un}$ are obtained using only canonical coordinates, without texture features.

4   Discussion and Conclusion

We presented a graph neural network approach for cytoarchitectonic classification of cortical image patches in microscopic scans of human brain sections, which combines 2D texture features with topological information from an approximate 3D surface reconstruction. While [5] employed GNNs for surface parcellation of Broca's areas 44 and 45 using MRI-based features, the present work is the first to our knowledge that integrates deep texture features from histology with 3D topology in a graph framework to label a large number of highly different brain areas across several brains. The proposed method significantly outperforms previous methods that operate only on individual 2D sections: The best trained model increases classification scores by 161%/193% on $\mathcal{V}_{te}/\mathcal{V}_{un}$ wrt. the recent baseline model base representing the work from [21]. Our experiments further suggest that deeper and wider architectures for the CNN encoder f benefit performance, motivating more systematic architecture search in the future. Larger input sizes in the encoders res[l] and res[w,l] showed additional positive impact by enabling models to capture the entire width of the isocortex (2 mm–4 mm). SAGE outperformed GAT, suggesting that mean aggregation (SAGE) might be better suited than self-attention (GAT) for our use case. The presented framework allows straightforward integration of anatomical priors, and the results indicate that this might be a crucial strategy for optimizing cytoarchitectonic mapping with deep networks. Unfortunately, transferability of learned features to completely unseen brains still seems to be limited, as indicated by the performance gaps between $\mathcal{V}_{te}$ and $\mathcal{V}_{un}$ and thus confirming observations in [21]. In the future, we plan to perform more rigorous architecture search for the encoders, study more anatomical priors, and investigate the reasons underlying the reduced performance on unseen brain samples.

Acknowledgements. This project received funding from the European Union's Horizon 2020 Research and Innovation Programme, grant agreement 945539 (HBP SGA3), and from the Helmholtz Association's Initiative and Networking Fund through the Helmholtz International BigBrain Analytics and Learning Laboratory (HIBALL) under the Helmholtz International Lab grant agreement InterLabs-0015. Computing time was granted through JARA on the supercomputer JURECA at Jülich Supercomputing Centre (JSC).

References

1. Amunts, K., et al.: BigBrain: an ultrahigh-resolution 3D human brain model. Science **340**(6139), 1472–1475 (2013). https://doi.org/10.1126/science.1235381
2. Amunts, K., Mohlberg, H., Bludau, S., Zilles, K.: Julich-Brain: a 3D probabilistic atlas of the human brain's cytoarchitecture. Science **369**(6506), 988 (2020). https://doi.org/10.1126/science.abb4588
3. Chen, J., Yang, L., Zhang, Y., Alber, M., Chen, D.Z.: Combining fully convolutional and recurrent neural networks for 3D biomedical image segmentation. In: Advances in Neural Information Processing Systems, pp. 3036–3044 (2016)
4. Cignoni, P., Callieri, M., Corsini, M., Dellepiane, M., Ganovelli, F., Ranzuglia, G.: MeshLab: an open-source mesh processing tool. In: Scarano, V., Chiara, R.D., Erra, U. (eds.) Eurographics Italian Chapter Conference. The Eurographics Association, Salerno (2008)
5. Cucurull, G., et al.: Convolutional neural networks for mesh-based parcellation of the cerebral cortex. In: Medical Imaging with Deep Learning (2018)
6. Dickscheid, T., Haas, S., Bludau, S., Glock, P., Huysegoms, M., Amunts, K.: Towards 3D reconstruction of neuronal cell distributions from histological human brain sections. Future Trends HPC Disruptive Scenario **34**, 223 (2019)
7. Fey, M., Lenssen, J.E.: Fast graph representation learning with PyTorch geometric. In: ICLR Workshop on Representation Learning on Graphs and Manifolds (2019)
8. Hamilton, W.L., Ying, R., Leskovec, J.: Inductive representation learning on large graphs. In: Proceedings of the 31st International Conference on Neural Information Processing Systems, pp. 1025–1035 (2017)
9. He, K., Zhang, X., Ren, S., Sun, J.: Deep residual learning for image recognition. In: Proceedings of the IEEE Conference on Computer Vision and Pattern Recognition, pp. 770–778 (2016)
10. Ioffe, S., Szegedy, C.: Batch normalization: accelerating deep network training by reducing internal covariate shift. In: International Conference on Machine Learning, pp. 448–456 (2015)
11. Kipf, T.N., Welling, M.: Semi-supervised classification with graph convolutional networks. arXiv:1609.02907 [cs, stat] (2017)
12. Krause, D., Thörnig, P.: JURECA: modular supercomputer at Jülich supercomputing centre. J. Large-Scale Res. Facil. JLSRF **4**, A132 (2018). https://doi.org/10.17815/jlsrf-4-121-1
13. Leprince, Y., Poupon, F., Delzescaux, T., Hasboun, D., Poupon, C., Rivière, D.: Combined Laplacian-equivolumic model for studying cortical lamination with ultra high field MRI (7 T). In: IEEE International Symposium on Biomedical Imaging, pp. 580–583 (2015). https://doi.org/10.1109/ISBI.2015.7163940
14. Lewiner, T., Lopes, H., Vieira, A.W., Tavares, G.: Efficient implementation of marching cubes' cases with topological guarantees. J. Graph. Tools **8**(2), 1–15 (2003). https://doi.org/10.1080/10867651.2003.10487582

15. Li, G., Muller, M., Thabet, A., Ghanem, B.: DeepGCNs: can GCNs go as deep as CNNs? In: Proceedings of the IEEE/CVF International Conference on Computer Vision, pp. 9267–9276 (2019)
16. Li, G., Xiong, C., Thabet, A., Ghanem, B.: DeeperGCN: all you need to train deeper GCNs. arXiv:2006.07739 [cs, stat] (2020)
17. Márquez-Neila, P., Baumela, L., Alvarez, L.: A morphological approach to curvature-based evolution of curves and surfaces. IEEE Trans. Pattern Anal. Mach. Intell. **36**(1), 2–17 (2014). https://doi.org/10.1109/TPAMI.2013.106
18. Merker, B.: Silver staining of cell bodies by means of physical development. J. Neurosci. Methods **9**(3), 235–241 (1983). https://doi.org/10.1016/0165-0270(83)90086-9
19. Milletari, F., Navab, N., Ahmadi, S.A.: V-Net: fully convolutional neural networks for volumetric medical image segmentation. In: 2016 Fourth International Conference on 3D Vision (3DV), pp. 565–571 (2016)
20. Paszke, A., et al.: PyTorch: an imperative style, high-performance deep learning library. arXiv:1912.01703 [cs, stat] (2019)
21. Schiffer, C., Amunts, K., Harmeling, S., Dickscheid, T.: Contrastive representation learning for whole brain cytoarchitectonic mapping in histological human brain sections. In: 2021 IEEE 18th International Symposium on Biomedical Imaging (ISBI), pp. 603–606. IEEE, April 2021. https://doi.org/10.1109/ISBI48211.2021.9433986
22. Schleicher, A., Amunts, K., Geyer, S., Morosan, P., Zilles, K.: Observer-independent method for microstructural parcellation of cerebral cortex: a quantitative approach to cytoarchitectonics. NeuroImage **9**(1), 165–177 (1999). https://doi.org/10.1006/nimg.1998.0385
23. Spitzer, H., Amunts, K., Harmeling, S., Dickscheid, T.: Parcellation of visual cortex on high-resolution histological brain sections using convolutional neural networks. In: 2017 IEEE 14th International Symposium on Biomedical Imaging (ISBI 2017), pp. 920–923 (2017). https://doi.org/10.1109/ISBI.2017.7950666
24. Spitzer, H., Kiwitz, K., Amunts, K., Harmeling, S., Dickscheid, T.: Improving cytoarchitectonic segmentation of human brain areas with self-supervised Siamese networks. In: Frangi, A.F., Schnabel, J.A., Davatzikos, C., Alberola-López, C., Fichtinger, G. (eds.) MICCAI 2018. LNCS, vol. 11072, pp. 663–671. Springer, Cham (2018). https://doi.org/10.1007/978-3-030-00931-1_76
25. Veličković, P., Cucurull, G., Casanova, A., Romero, A., Liò, P., Bengio, Y.: Graph attention networks. arXiv:1710.10903 [cs, stat] (2018)
26. You, Y., Gitman, I., Ginsburg, B.: Large batch training of convolutional networks. arXiv:1708.03888 [cs] (2017)

Annotation-Efficient Cell Counting

Zuhui Wang and Zhaozheng Yin[✉]

Stony Brook University, Stony Brook, NY, USA
{zuwang,zyin}@cs.stonybrook.edu

Abstract. Recent advances in deep learning have achieved impressive results on microscopy cell counting tasks. The success of deep learning models usually needs sufficient training data with manual annotations, which can be time-consuming and costly. In this paper, we propose an annotation-efficient cell counting approach which injects cell counting networks into an active learning framework. By designing a multi-task learning in the cell counter network model, we leverage unlabeled data for feature representation learning and use deep clustering to group unlabeled data. Rather than labeling every cell in each training image, the deep active learning only suggests the most uncertain, diverse, representative and rare image regions for annotation. Evaluated on four widely used cell counting datasets, our cell counter trained by a small subset of training data suggested by the deep active learning, achieves superior performance compared to state-of-the-arts with full training or other suggestive annotations. Our code is available at https://github.com/cvbmi-research/AnnotationEfficient-CellCounting.

Keywords: Cell counting · Suggestive annotation · Active learning

1 Introduction

Cell counting aims to estimate the cell numbers within microscopy images. Cell numbers play an important role in biomedical discoveries and disease diagnosis. For example, the number of proliferative neural progenitor cells is closely linked to autism spectrum disorders [1]. Deep learning-based cell counting algorithms have demonstrated their effectiveness on this task [3,6,15]. The success of deep learning-based cell counting relies on the large number of annotated training data. However, it is laborious and expensive to label microscopy images for cell counting due to the following reasons: (1) a single microscopy image may contain hundreds of cells, and it is time-consuming to label them one-by-one over a large number of images; (2) a microscopy image may exhibit different levels of difficulties to label cells. Some regions may have high cell densities with irregular cell shapes and overlapping cell clusters; and (3) due to the microscopy image variations according to different biological experiments, deep learning models need specific sets of training data rather than a generic model able to count all types of cells. The above challenges inspire some **research questions** to think: *do we really need to annotate every individual cell in every training image to train a cell counting model? Can we just label some important cell regions in some training images to achieve the annotation-efficient cell counting?*

© Springer Nature Switzerland AG 2021
M. de Bruijne et al. (Eds.): MICCAI 2021, LNCS 12908, pp. 405–414, 2021.
https://doi.org/10.1007/978-3-030-87237-3_39

1.1   Related Work

Active learning [12] can be utilized to select the most effective samples for annotation during model training. In the medical image segmentation domain, several active learning-based suggestive annotation methods have been proposed to alleviate manual annotation efforts to achieve good results [4,5,9,14]. In [5], the most informative samples among unlabeled samples are identified for annotation, but the representativeness of the selected samples is overlooked. The representativeness of samples is considered in [17], but this method is a one-time pool-based suggestive annotation, rather than progressively selecting training samples based on the performance of the model being previously trained. An active-learning framework with progressive-training is proposed to select effective samples iteratively [16]. However, it only focuses on the uncertainty and representativeness of samples in each iteration independently. These existing methods do not consider epoch-wise uncertainty during model training. An efficient suggestive annotation framework is still open to be investigated. After surveying the state-of-the-arts, we have a few **observations**:

- In a cell image, some image regions may be more informative than the rest, so it is intuitive to suggest image regions in an image for partial labelling, instead of labeling the whole image;
- Image regions may contain redundancies, so similar image regions should be clustered together. Then, the suggestive samples can be selected from different clusters to preserve the sample diversity;
- The unlabeled data are overlooked when training the cell counting models. Semi-supervised learning that uses both labeled and unlabelled data can aid the suggestive annotation by learning the effective visual representation to select samples from the unlabeled dataset for annotation.

1.2   Our Proposal and Contributions

Motivated by the above research questions and observations, we propose an annotation-efficient cell counting by deep active learning, with the following contributions:

- A new active learning algorithm is designed based on a comprehensive set of metrics: for each unlabeled sample, we consider both the uncertainty on ensembled models and uncertainty among training epochs; unlabeled samples' diversity is preserved by the cluster information; the representativeness of unlabeled samples and the rarity compared with the previously labeled data are computed by encoded feature similarities.
- In our suggestive annotation procedure, only the important image regions (defined as image patches in this paper) are recommended for annotation. The partial labeling alleviates annotation workloads.
- Both the labeled samples and unlabeled samples are used in a semi-supervised way to train the cell counting model. For unlabeled samples, the augmentation consistency on unlabeled data is to help the representation learning on the entire dataset. The feature representation is used to generate cell density maps and suggest samples for annotation.

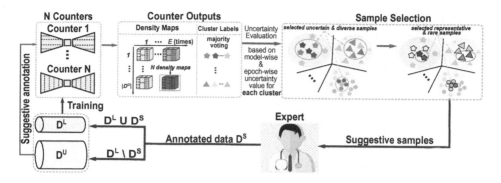

Fig. 1. The workflow of the proposed deep active learning framework.

- The proposed cell counting model is designed with multi-task learning, which counts the overall cell number in an image and predict the input image's cluster information.

2 Methodology

As shown in Fig. 1, the overall workflow of the proposed deep active learning framework contains the following steps: (1) each unlabeled sample is sent into N trained cell counters to generate $E \cdot N$ density maps over E epochs, and its cluster labels; (2) the grouped unlabeled data by deep clustering guarantees the diversity, and then the most uncertain, representative, and rare samples are recommended for annotation; and (3) the suggested samples are annotated, and the N cell counters are fine-tuned based on the updated unlabeled dataset D^U and labeled dataset D^L. This procedure is iterated until counter performance converges or label budget is exhausted.

2.1 Cell Counter

Our cell counter is based on multi-task deep learning networks and it is trained in a semi-supervised way, as illustrated in Fig. 2.

Multi-task Deep Learning. The cell counter model contains two tasks: a encoder-decoder branch to generate cell density map to estimate the cell number in an image patch; and a classification module to assign the cluster label to the input image patch based on the features extracted by the encoder. In the initial annotation round, the cluster labels are assigned by K-means. For the rest annotation rounds, we treat cluster predictions from the previous epoch as ground truth for the next clustering model training.

We use the first ten convolutional layers of the pre-trained VGG16 [13] model as the feature encoder. Each convolutional layer uses a 3×3 kernel. The max-pooling operation is followed by every two or three convolutional layers. There are three max-pooling layers inside the encoder. Then, the feature maps are passed through a feature enhancement module that contains a spatial attention mechanism, a channel-wise attention mechanism, and three dilated convolutional layers. The spatial attention mechanism is designed to pay attention to the important feature parts spatially. It consists of two convolutional layers, and a sigmoid function is applied after the second convolutional layer. The channel-wise attention mechanism assigns different weights to the feature maps for our tasks. It takes the input feature maps into a global average pooling layer. Then, the outputs are fed into two fully-connected layers, followed by a sigmoid function. Finally, the feature maps after the attention mechanisms are sent to three dilated convolutional layers [10] to extract features at different scales.

The enhanced features will be sent to two task branches. First, they are input to a decoder, which contains three convolutional layers followed by up-sampling layers to generate the final maps. The cell number is counted by summing all density values in a density map. Second, the enhanced features are input to a classification module that contains two convolutional layers followed by max-pooling layers and two fully-connected layers. The final output layer of the classification module contains a one-hot vector over the C clusters.

Semi-supervised Learning. When training the cell counter model, unlabeled samples can help the model learn the latent representation of the entire dataset, i.e., the encoder will be trained to generate effective feature representation to suggest unlabeled data for annotation. We employ the consistency learning into the semi-supervised learning (Fig. 2(b)): each unlabeled sample and its random augmented versions are expected to generate consistent outputs by the cell counter model.

Note, for a labeled patch, we zero-pad it with the same size as the original image during training. For unlabeled images, we crop it into some non-overlapped small patches and zero-pad them to the original image size. Both the unlabeled patch images and unlabeled full-size images are used in the consistency learning.

Function to Train the Cell Counter. For labeled samples, we employ the L_2 loss (MSE, Mean Squared Error) to compare the generated density map with the ground truth and a cluster label consistency loss between epochs (the first two terms in Eq. 1). For unlabeled samples, we propose a scalar count loss and a cross-entropy loss for comparing the consistency between an unlabeled sample and its random augmentation (the last two terms in Eq. 1). The total loss function to train our cell counter is:

$$Loss = \frac{1}{|D^L|} \sum_{j=1}^{|D^L|} \left\| \hat{\mathbf{Y}}_j - \mathbf{Y}_j \right\|_2^2 + \frac{\lambda_1}{|D^L|} \sum_{j=1}^{|D^L|} \left\| \hat{y}_{j,e} - \hat{y}_{j,e-1} \right\|_1$$

$$+ \frac{\lambda_2}{|D^U|} \sum_{i=1}^{|D^U|} \left\| \hat{ct}_i - \tilde{ct}_i \right\|_1 - \frac{\lambda_3}{|D^U|} \sum_{i=1}^{|D^U|} \sum_{c=1}^{C} \hat{y}_i^c \log\left(\tilde{y}_i^c\right), \tag{1}$$

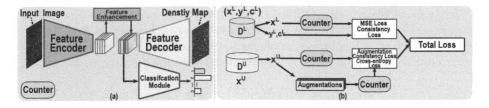

Fig. 2. The architecture of the proposed cell counter (a) and Training loss design (b).

where $\hat{\mathbf{Y}}_j$ is the predicted density map of the j-th labeled sample, $\mathbf{Y}_j$ is the corresponding ground truth density map. $|D^L|$ and $|D^U|$ denote the total number of labeled and unlabeled samples, respectively. $\hat{y}_{j,e}$ is the predicted cluster label of the j-th sample at epoch e. In the last two terms, $\hat{ct}_i = \sum_p \sum_q \hat{\mathbf{Y}}_i(p,q)$ is the estimated cell number of the i-th unlabeled image by summing over all pixel locations (p,q), and $\tilde{ct}_i = \sum_p \sum_q \tilde{\mathbf{Y}}_i(p,q)$ is the estimated cell number of the random augmented version of the i-th image. $\hat{y}_i$ and $\tilde{y}_i$ are the one-hot cluster label generated by the cell counter, for the i-th unlabeled sample and its augmentation, respectively. Besides, λ_1, λ_2, and λ_3 are weights for each loss components. In the experiment, they are set to 0.1, 0.1, and 0.01 based on cross validations.

2.2 Sample Suggestion

The trained cell counter estimates the density map and cluster label of an input image along with its encoded features, based on which we present the metrics and procedure to suggest unlabeled samples for annotation.

Uncertainty. We consider two uncertainties of an unlabeled sample: model-wise uncertainty and epoch-wise uncertainty. The model-wise uncertainty of an unlabeled sample relies on the bootstrapping strategy that trains N cell counters, each of which only randomly selects a subset of the suggested samples for training in each suggestive annotation round. The model-wise uncertainty is computed as the disagreement among the N models. Specifically, for each unlabeled image $I_i \in D^U$, we first use the N trained cell counters to generate N density maps $\{\hat{\mathbf{Y}}_i^{(n)}\}_{n=1...N}$ and corresponding counts $\{\hat{ct}_i^{(n)}\}_{n=1...N}$. Then, we compute the model-wise uncertainty score $u_M(I_i)$ as follows:

$$u_M(I_i) = \frac{1}{w \times h} \sum_{p=1}^{w} \sum_{q=1}^{h} \text{VAR}\left(\hat{\mathbf{Y}}_i^{(n)}(p,q)\right) + \text{VAR}\left(\hat{ct}_i^{(n)}\right), \quad n = 1, \cdots, N, \quad (2)$$

where the first term is the averaged pixel-wise uncertainty score over N models, and $\text{VAR}()$ evaluates the variance (disagreement) among N models. w and h denote the resolution of the density map. The second term is the count uncertainty score over N models.

In each suggestive annotation round, each cell counter is trained with R epochs, and we save the trained model every r epochs, leading to $E = \lfloor (R/r) \rfloor$ variants for every cell counter in one suggestive round. Thus, we can calculate an epoch-wise uncertainty score over the model-wise uncertainty, as follows:

$$u_{EP}(I_i) = \text{VAR}\left(u_M^{(e)}(I_i)\right), \quad e = 1, \cdots, E. \tag{3}$$

We use $u_{EP}(I_i)$ to denote the uncertainty score for unlabeled image I_i.

Diversity. In a single suggestive annotation round, an unlabeled sample is fed into N trained counters. Then, we can obtain N cluster labels for this sample and its corresponding encoded features. We use the majority-voting on the N cluster predictions to decide the cluster label for this unlabeled sample. If a tie appears during the majority voting, we assign this unlabeled to its nearest cluster. Besides, we follow [2] to prevent empty clusters.

Within each cluster c, unlabeled samples are sorted based on their uncertainty scores u_{EP}. Then, we select the top K uncertainty samples as the candidates, yielding the full candidate sets for all C clusters, $\{\text{Cand}^{(c)}\}_{c=1...C}$. These candidate samples preserve the diversity and uncertainty information simultaneously.

Representativeness and Rarity. For each cluster c, we have a candidate set, $\text{Cand}^{(c)}$, within which we aim to search for a subset $S^{(c)}$ ($S^{(c)} \subset \text{Cand}^{(c)}$) that contains s samples as the suggestive samples (i.e., $s = |S^{(c)}|$). The final suggestive samples are expected to have two properties: (1) Representativeness. They should represent unlabeled samples D^U well, so the newly selected samples improve the model generalization ability to unlabeled samples; and (2) Rarity. They should have the least similarity with the existing labeled samples D^L to avoid labeling redundancy. To capture these two properties, for cluster c, any suggestive sample $t \in S^{(c)}$ should maximize the following ratio score:

$$ratio_t = \frac{\sum_{i=1}^{|D^U|-s} \text{SIM}\left(f_t, f_i\right)}{\sum_{j=1}^{|D^L|+s} \text{SIM}\left(f_t, f_j\right)}, \tag{4}$$

where $\text{SIM}()$ represents the cosine similarity between features, f_t is the encoded feature of target sample t, f_i and f_j are the encoded features of i-th unlabeled sample, and j-th labeled sample, respectively. We choose s samples in $\text{Cand}^{(c)}$ with the top s ratio scores as the final suggested samples for cluster c. Finally, we obtain $C \times s$ samples as the suggested set D^S (i.e., $|D^S| = C \times s$) for annotation. The whole procedure of our sample suggestion is summarized in Algorithm 1.

3   Experiments

Datasets. Four public benchmark datasets are used to evaluate the proposed active learning framework. For fair comparisons, we follow [3,6,15] to randomly

Algorithm 1: The Sample Suggestion Algorithm

Input: $Ctr = \{Ctr^e | e = 1, \cdots, E\}$, $Ctr^e = \{Ctr_n^e | n = 1, \cdots, N\}$,
$Ctr_n^e = \{En_n^e, De_n^e | m = 1, \cdots, M\}$, $Cls = \{Cls_c | c = 1, \cdots, C\}$,
$D^U = \{I_i | i = 1, \cdots, |D^U|\}$, $D^L = \{I_j | j = 1, \cdots, |D^L|\}$, K, s, h, w;

Output: $D^S = \{I_d | d = 1, \cdots, C \times s\}$;

for $i \in [1, |D^U|]$ do
  for $e \in [1, E]$ do
    for $n \in [1, N]$ do
      $\hat{\mathbf{Y}}_n^{(e)}, \text{Cls}_n^{(e)} = Ctr_n^{(e)}(I_i)$
    $u_M^{(e)}(I_i) = \frac{1}{w \times h} \sum_{p=1}^{w} \sum_{q=1}^{h} \text{VAR}\left(\hat{\mathbf{Y}}_i^{(n)}(p, q)\right) + \text{VAR}\left(\hat{ct}_i^{(n)}\right), n = [1, N]$
  $u_{EP}(I_i) = \text{VAR}\left(u_M^{(e)}(I_i)\right), \text{Cls}(I_i)_i = \text{MAJORITY-VOTING}(\text{Cls}_n^{(E)}, n = [1, N])$

for $Cls_c \in Cls$ do
  for $i \in [1, |Cls_c|]$ do
    $f_i^{(c)} = \text{mean}(En_n^{(E)}(I_i), n = [1, N])$
  $\text{Cand}^{(c)} = \text{TOP K SELECT}\left(\text{SORT-DEC}(f_i^{(c)}, c = [1, |Cls_k|]), K\right)$
  Search: $\{S^{(c)}\}$ can maximize the following ratio. $(\{S^{(c)}\} \subset \{\text{Cand}^{(c)}\})$
  for $t \in S^{(c)}$ do
    $\text{ratio}_t = \frac{\sum_{i=1}^{|D^U|-s} \text{SIM}(f_t, f_i)}{\sum_{j=1}^{|D^L|+s} \text{SIM}(f_t, f_j)}$
  $D^S = D^S + t$
return D^S

split each dataset as follows: (1) VGG Cell [8]: a synthetic cell dataset with 50 training images and 100 testing images; (2) MBM [7]: a bone marrow dataset with 15 training images and 14 testing images; (3) ADI [3]: a dataset of human adipocyte cells with 50 training images and 100 testing images; and (4) DCC [11]: the Dublin cell counting dataset with 100 training images and 76 testing images. During the suggestive annotation for cell counter training, each training image is cropped into four non-overlapped patches and padded to the original size. To avoid overfitting, each patch is applied with horizontal flipping, vertical flipping, clockwise 90° rotation, and counterclockwise 90° rotation. Finally, the numbers of training samples for the four datasets are 1000, 300, 1000, and 2000, respectively. For model evaluation, mean absolute error (MAE) is used as the evaluation metric.

Implementation Details. In our project, we train 3 cell Counters ($N = 3$). For each annotation round, we divide unlabeled data into 5 clusters ($C = 5$), then we select the top 10 ($K = 10$) uncertain samples for each cluster, and our final suggested samples are 10% ($|D^S|$) of total training samples for each round. At the start of each round, all cell Counters are fine-tuned with all labeled samples and unlabeled samples. These numbers are set to achieve the balance of model performance and time cost.

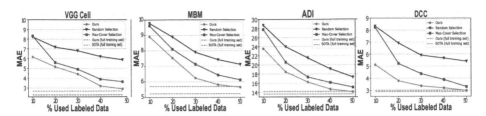

Fig. 3. Comparison on four public datasets. The green dash lines are the current state-of-the-art results using full training set. The red dash lines are the results of our proposed cell counter using full training set. The three solid curves are: ours (red), Max-Cover Selection [16] (blue), and random annotation (black). (Color figure online)

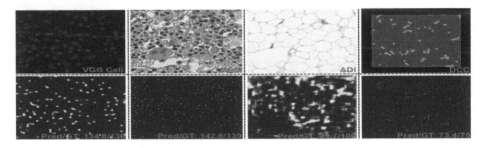

Fig. 4. Examples of cell images of the four public datasets and the corresponding generated density maps.

Experiment Result Analysis. First, we compared our cell counter with several state-of-the-art models [3,6] using full training sets. As shown in Fig. 3, our proposed cell counter achieves competitive counting performance (best in three of the four datasets). Though the four datasets exhibit various cell appearances, shapes, and densities, our model is suitable for cell counting with different imaging modalities. Second, we evaluate the proposed deep active learning framework on selecting effective samples for model training. For fair comparisons, we set the annotation cost budget from 10% to 50% of the overall training sets. Our framework is compared with (1) Random Selection: randomly select samples for annotation; and (2) Max-Cover Selection [16]: a SOTA active learning algorithm. As shown in Fig. 3, our proposed method outperforms the stat-of-the-art frameworks persistently. It demonstrates that our proposed suggestive annotation algorithm is effective for the cell counting task with limited training samples. Some qualitative samples of generated density maps by the proposed active learning framework with 50% training data are shown in Fig. 4, which illustrates the effectiveness of our framework on different cell counting scenarios. Additionally, we conducted an ablation study on the four datasets, and the results are summarized in Table 1. In the results, we see that the proposed epoch-wise uncertainty, active learning algorithm, and semi-supervised learning enable the model to produce accurate counting results.

Table 1. Ablation study on the four datasets, with MAE as the evaluation metric. **AL** stands for Active Learning, and **SSL** denotes semi-supervised learning.

Dataset.	Ours-w/o-EpochUncertainty	Ours-w/o-AL	Ours-w/o-SSL	Ours
VGG Cell [8]	3.5	5.9	3.4	2.9
MBM [7]	6.1	7.1	6.0	5.7
ADI [3]	14.5	17.3	14.4	14.1
DCC [11]	3.6	5.4	3.3	3.0

4 Conclusion

In this paper, we presented a deep active learning framework to alleviate the heavy burden of manual annotation for the microscopy cell counting task. The proposed framework provides several contributions: (1) the proposed new cell counter achieves state-of-the-art cell counting performances when using the full training data; (2) unlabeled samples are used to train the cell counter to learn effective feature representation; (3) a multi-task learning with counting and deep cluster facilitates the suggestive annotation based on a comprehensive set sample selection criteria. Our cell counter trained within the deep active learning framework achieves state-of-the-art cell counting performance by only using a portion of the annotated training data on four public datasets.

Acknowledgement. This project was supported by Stony Brook University - Brookhaven National Laboratory (SBU-BNL) seed grant on annotation-efficient deep learning.

References

1. Bernier, R., et al.: Disruptive CHD8 mutations define a subtype of autism early in development. Cell **158**(2), 263–276 (2014)
2. Caron, M., Bojanowski, P., Joulin, A., Douze, M.: Deep clustering for unsupervised learning of visual features. In: Ferrari, V., Hebert, M., Sminchisescu, C., Weiss, Y. (eds.) Computer Vision – ECCV 2018. LNCS, vol. 11218, pp. 139–156. Springer, Cham (2018). https://doi.org/10.1007/978-3-030-01264-9_9
3. Cohen, J.P., Boucher, G., Glastonbury, C.A., Lo, H.Z., Bengio, Y.: Count-ception: counting by fully convolutional redundant counting. In: 2017 IEEE International Conference on Computer Vision Workshops, ICCV Workshops 2017, Venice, Italy, 22–29 October 2017, pp. 18–26 (2017)
4. Dai, C., et al.: Suggestive annotation of brain tumour images with gradient-guided sampling. In: Martel, A.L., et al. (eds.) MICCAI 2020. LNCS, vol. 12264, pp. 156–165. Springer, Cham (2020). https://doi.org/10.1007/978-3-030-59719-1_16
5. Deng, Y., et al.: A new framework to reduce doctor's workload for medical image annotation. IEEE Access **7**, 107097–107104 (2019)

6. Guo, Y., Stein, J.L., Wu, G., Krishnamurthy, A.K.: SAU-Net: a universal deep network for cell counting. In: Proceedings of the 10th ACM International Conference on Bioinformatics, Computational Biology and Health Informatics, BCB 2019, Niagara Falls, NY, USA, 7–10 September 2019, pp. 299–306. ACM (2019)
7. Kainz, P., Urschler, M., Schulter, S., Wohlhart, P., Lepetit, V.: You should use regression to detect cells. In: Navab, N., Hornegger, J., Wells, W.M., Frangi, A.F. (eds.) MICCAI 2015. LNCS, vol. 9351, pp. 276–283. Springer, Cham (2015). https://doi.org/10.1007/978-3-319-24574-4_33
8. Lempitsky, V.S., Zisserman, A.: Learning to count objects in images. In: Lafferty, J.D., Williams, C.K.I., Shawe-Taylor, J., Zemel, R.S., Culotta, A. (eds.) Advances in Neural Information Processing Systems 23: 24th Annual Conference on Neural Information Processing Systems 2010. Proceedings of a meeting held 6–9 December 2010, Vancouver, British Columbia, Canada, pp. 1324–1332 (2010)
9. Li, H., Yin, Z.: Attention, suggestion and annotation: a deep active learning framework for biomedical image segmentation. In: Martel, A.L., et al. (eds.) MICCAI 2020. LNCS, vol. 12261, pp. 3–13. Springer, Cham (2020). https://doi.org/10.1007/978-3-030-59710-8_1
10. Li, Y., Zhang, X., Chen, D.: CSRNet: dilated convolutional neural networks for understanding the highly congested scenes. In: Proceedings of the IEEE Conference on Computer Vision and Pattern Recognition, pp. 1091–1100 (2018)
11. Marsden, M., McGuinness, K., Little, S., Keogh, C.E., O'Connor, N.E.: People, penguins and petri dishes: adapting object counting models to new visual domains and object types without forgetting. In: 2018 IEEE Conference on Computer Vision and Pattern Recognition, CVPR 2018, Salt Lake City, UT, USA, 18–22 June 2018, pp. 8070–8079. IEEE Computer Society (2018)
12. Ren, P., et al.: A survey of deep active learning. CoRR abs/2009.00236 (2020)
13. Simonyan, K., Zisserman, A.: Very deep convolutional networks for large-scale image recognition. In: Bengio, Y., LeCun, Y. (eds.) 3rd International Conference on Learning Representations, ICLR 2015, San Diego, CA, USA, 7–9 May 2015. Conference Track Proceedings (2015)
14. Xie, S., Feng, Z., Chen, Y., Sun, S., Ma, C., Song, M.: Deal: difficulty-aware active learning for semantic segmentation. In: Proceedings of the Asian Conference on Computer Vision (2020)
15. Xie, W., Noble, J.A., Zisserman, A.: Microscopy cell counting and detection with fully convolutional regression networks. CMBBE Imaging Visual. 6(3), 283–292 (2018)
16. Yang, L., Zhang, Y., Chen, J., Zhang, S., Chen, D.Z.: Suggestive annotation: a deep active learning framework for biomedical image segmentation. In: Descoteaux, M., Maier-Hein, L., Franz, A., Jannin, P., Collins, D.L., Duchesne, S. (eds.) MICCAI 2017. LNCS, vol. 10435, pp. 399–407. Springer, Cham (2017). https://doi.org/10.1007/978-3-319-66179-7_46
17. Zheng, H., et al.: Biomedical image segmentation via representative annotation. In: Proceedings of the AAAI Conference on Artificial Intelligence, pp. 5901–5908 (2019)

A Deep Learning Bidirectional Temporal Tracking Algorithm for Automated Blood Cell Counting from Non-invasive Capillaroscopy Videos

Luojie Huang, Gregory N. McKay, and Nicholas J. Durr[✉]

Department of Biomedical Engineering,
Johns Hopkins University, Baltimore, MD, USA
ndurr@jhu.edu

Abstract. Oblique back-illumination capillaroscopy has recently been introduced as an efficient method for non-invasive blood cell imaging in human capillaries. To apply this technique to clinical blood cell counting, solutions for automatic processing of acquired videos are needed. Here, we take the first step towards this goal, by introducing a novel deep learning multi-cell tracking model, named CycleTrack, which achieves accurate blood cell counting from capillaroscopic videos. CycleTrack combines two simple online tracking models, SORT and CenterTrack, and is tailored to features of capillary blood cell flow. Blood cells are tracked by displacement vectors in two opposing temporal directions between consecutive frames. This approach yields accurate tracking despite rapidly moving and deforming blood cells. The proposed model outperforms other baseline trackers, achieving 66.3% MOTA and 75.1% ID F1 score on test videos. CycleTrack achieves an average cell counting error of 3.42% among 8 1000-frame test videos, compared to 6.55% and 22.98% from original CenterTrack and SORT, with negligible time expense. It takes 800s to track and count approximately 8000 blood cells from 9,600 frames captured in a typical one-minute video. Moreover, the blood cell velocity measured by CycleTrack demonstrates a consistent, pulsatile pattern within the physiological range of heart rate. The project code is accessible online at: https://github.com/DurrLab/CycleTrack.

Keywords: Blood cell count · Multiple Object Tracking · Oblique back-illumination capillaroscopy

1 Introduction

The complete blood count (CBC) is the most common clinical test with approximately 34.5 million tests performed annually in the United States [1]. The CBC

This research was supported in part with a gift from Fifth Generation, Inc.

Electronic supplementary material The online version of this chapter (https://doi.org/10.1007/978-3-030-87237-3_40) contains supplementary material, which is available to authorized users.

© Springer Nature Switzerland AG 2021
M. de Bruijne et al. (Eds.): MICCAI 2021, LNCS 12908, pp. 415–424, 2021.
https://doi.org/10.1007/978-3-030-87237-3_40

measures the concentration of cells in patients' blood, including white blood cells (WBCs), red blood cells (RBCs), and platelets (PLTs). The CBC is useful in managing a wide range of conditions and diseases, such as infection, inflammation, as well as for prognostic monitoring of chemotherapy and radiation therapy [2]. The current clinical CBC is administered invasively through venipuncture in adults and heelstick in newborns. The drawn blood is then processed via a hematologic analyzer, typically analyzing scattering signal of each cell in a flow cytometer [3]. While the CBC is a ubiquitous clinical test, some vulnerable patients, such as immunocompromised cancer patients and neonates who are susceptible to infection and phlebotomy-induced anemia, would benefit from a non-invasive technique [4, 5].

In recent years, there are emerging advances towards minimal- and non-invasive point-of-care blood cell analysis. Hemocue (Ängelholm, Sweden) is a portable hemoglobinometer that can provide efficient hemoglobin concentration results with only 10 μL blood from finger prick [6]. Leuko Labs is translating a technology called the PointCheck, aiming at non-invasive screening for severe neutropenia in chemotherapy patients [7]. Recently, McKay et al. introduced oblique back-illumination capillaroscopy (OBC), an affordable technique that acquires high-quality images of blood cells flowing in tongue capillaries in vivo [8]. To enable OBC to complete non-invasive blood counting and analysis, we present a deep multi-object tracking framework named CycleTrack that accurately tracks and counts blood cells flowing through human capillaries. To our knowledge, this is the first work on deep learning algorithm for automated in-vivo blood cell tracking and counting.

2   Related Work

2.1   Oblique Back-Illumination Capillaroscopy

OBC is a non-invasive, label-free method for high-speed in-vivo blood cell imaging. OBC works regardless of skin tone and can be implemented with a simple camera, microscope objective, and LED. Blood cells in ventral tongue capillaries, normally 70–80 μm below the surface, can be clearly visualized using phase contrast generated by an illumination-detection offset, and hemoglobin absorption contrast from green LED illumination. The system simplicity and imaging efficiency makes it a promising non-invasive technology for blood cell counting and analysis. Therefore, there is a need for video analysis algorithms to efficiently process OBC data and achieve an accurate cell count.

2.2   Multiple Object Tracking (MOT)

For object counting task, counting-by-detection is the most intuitive method. Besides counting results, such method can also extract individual object information for extended studies. State-of-the-art MOT algorithms utilize Deep Learning based object detectors such as Fast-RCNN [9], MaskRCNN [10], and Center-Net [11]. Following the tracking-by-detection pipeline, these models first identify

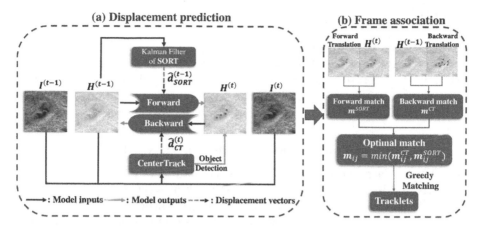

Fig. 1. Workflow of CycleTrack Framework. $H^{(t)} \in \mathbb{R}^{W \times H \times 1}$ represents the center heatmap of detected cells at time t.

objects in each frame with masks, bounding boxes or center points, and then associate detections across frames. Among these frameworks, appearance feature based association is particularly popular thanks to powerful convolutional feature extractors [12,13].

2.3 Our Motivation and Proposal

The task of OBC cell tracking is unique and challenging. Cells of a given class have similar appearances, with similar sizes, shapes, and granularity. Moreover, the shapes of individual cells tend to change from rotation and collision as they flow through crowded capillaries. Therefore, it is difficult to distinguish and track individual cells using appearance-based MOT models. To solve the above challenges, we use another kind of tracker that achieves object association based on position and movement information. For example, SORT [14], a predictive tracking model, tracks in a forward manner, assuming that objects move in a predictable and continuous pattern over time and space; CenterTrack [15], a tracking-by-detection model, works in a retrospective way by globally matching a constellation of current object centers backward to the previous frame. In OBC videos, blood cells move in fixed directions along capillaries, which approximately meets the SORT assumption. Blood cell tracking is also an appropriate use case for CenterTrack as relative positions among nearby cells in crowded capillaries tend to remain consistent throughout flow. Another benefit of combining SORT and CenterTrack is that SORT maintains a long-term memory of flow velocity by continuously recording the flow history, whereas CenterTrack allows for short-term changes in velocity while enforcing similar relative positions of detected cells. Following these intuitions, we introduce a novel architecture, called CycleTrack, by combining SORT and CenterTrack into a robust tracker that tracks objects in both temporal directions. Moreover, such position-based trackers are able to perform higher-speed blood cell analysis which is significant for point-of-care application.

3   Methods

The CycleTrack framework[1] is shown in Fig. 1. CycleTrack combines Center-Track and SORT to achieve backward and forward tracking between two consecutive frames. In this section, the description of CycleTrack is organized around its three key components of CenterTrack, SORT, and association of new cell detections with previously existing cell tracks, termed as tracklets.

3.1   Cell Detection and Backward Tracking via CenterTrack

CenterTrack is a single deep network that solves object detection and tracking jointly and is trained end-to-end. CenterTrack uses a CenterNet [11] detector, which takes a single image as the input and outputs object detections. Each detection $y = (p, s, c, id)$ is represented by its center location $(p \in \mathbb{R}^2)$, size of the bounding box $(s \in \mathbb{R}^2)$, a confidence score $(c \in [0, 1])$ and a detection id $(id \in \mathbb{Z}^+)$. The architecture of CenterTrack is nearly identical to CenterNet, simply expanding the input and output channels to achieve multiple tasks. Center-Track takes two consecutive frames: $I^{(t)} \in \mathbb{R}^{W \times H \times 1}$ and $I^{(t-1)} \in \mathbb{R}^{W \times H \times 1}$, and the prior tracked objects $O^{(t-1)} = \{y_0^{(t-1)}, y_1^{(t-1)}, ...\}$ as inputs, and outputs current object detections with an additional 2D displacement map $\hat{D}^{(t)} \in \mathbb{R}^{W \times H \times 2}$, where W and H represent the width and height of input frames. A displacement vector $\hat{d}^{(t)}$ for each object could then be extracted from $\hat{D}^{(t)}$.

To restrict displacement estimations to adhere to the assumption that all blood cells in the same frame should move in similar directions, we introduce a base vector $\hat{d}_{base}^{(t-1)}$, which is the average displacement vector of all cells from frame $(t-1)$. This base vector is used to refine displacement vector predictions from CenterTrack, $\hat{d}_{CT_i}^{(t)}$:

$$\hat{d}_{CT_i}^{(t)} = w_i \hat{d}_i^{(t)} + |1 - w_i| \hat{d}_{base}^{(t-1)} \tag{1}$$

where $w_i = \frac{\hat{d}_{base}^{(t-1)} \cdot \hat{d}_i^{(t)}}{|\hat{d}_{base}^{(t-1)}||\hat{d}_i^{(t)}|}$. This equation provides a weighted, corrective action on the conventional displacement vector prediction from CenterTrack. The more $\hat{d}^{(t)}$ deviates from $\hat{d}_{base}^{(t-1)}$, the more the refined vector $\hat{d}_{CT}^{(t)}$ would rely on $\hat{d}_{base}^{(t-1)}$.

3.2   Forward Tracking via SORT

SORT is an unsupervised tracking model, approximating each object's displacement from $(t-1)$ to (t) with a linear constant velocity model. This is accomplished with a Kalman filter, which is commonly used for state transition prediction in linear dynamic systems [16, 17]. A Kalman filter is created for each tracklet, and updated by the input state of each tracked object, modeled as $O_{sort} = (p_{sort}, s_{sort})$ with the center location $(p_{sort} \in \mathbb{R}^2)$ and the bounding box size $(s_{sort} \in \mathbb{R}^2)$. Finally, the displacement vector from $(t-1)$ to (t) is outputted for tracking:

---

[1] Supplementary material 1, Table 1 outlines a step-by-step detailed tracking workflow.

$$\hat{d}_{sort}^{(t-1)} = p_{sort}^{(t)} - p_{sort}^{(t-1)} \tag{2}$$

3.3   Association Between Consecutive Frames

CenterTrack outputs object displacement vectors from (t) to $(t-1)$. Using these displacements, we simply translate new detection centers backwards to the previous frame. The matching cost matrix $m^{CT} \in \mathbb{R}^{(N \times M)}$ is then computed as the Euclidean distances between the centers of N tracked objects and M translated detections. For the ith tracked object and the jth translated detection:

$$m_{ij}^{CT} = |p_i^{(t-1)} - (p_j^{(t)} + \hat{d}_{CT_j}^{(t)})| \tag{3}$$

From SORT, we get another forward matching cost matrix $m^{sort} \in \mathbb{R}^{(N \times M)}$ between N predicted locations of $(t-1)$ objects frame and M new detections at (t):

$$m_{ij}^{sort} = |(p_i^{(t-1)} + \hat{d}_{sort_j}^{(t-1)}) - p_j^{(t)}| \tag{4}$$

All the cell detections used in CycleTrack are outputted by the CenterNet backbone of CenterTrack. To combine the matching estimates from CenterTrack and SORT, we first generate the optimal matching cost matrix for CycleTrack by selecting the smaller distance for each element in these two matching cost matrices $m_{ij}^{Cycle} = min(m_{ij}^{CT}, m_{ij}^{sort})$. Then, a greedy matching algorithm is applied to match detections to the tracked objects with the closest mutual distances based on m_{ij}^{Cycle}. Moreover, as an additional restriction, if all the distances of a detection in the matrix are out of a reasonable range, which is defined as two times of the average diameters of cells in the current frame, it will be regarded as unmatched and a new tracklet will be created for it. The threshold is set adaptively to be the average distance between adjacent cells in the same frame.

4   Experiments

We trained and evaluated the proposed model on videos of human ventral tongue capillaries acquired by the OBC system with approval by the Johns Hopkins University Institutional Review Board (IRB00204985). The OBC system is fully described in [8] and uses a Green LED as the light source with an illumination-detection offset of around 200 μm Using a 40×1.15NA water immersion microscope objective, videos with a frame size of 1280×812 pixels were acquired at 160 Hz and 0.5 ms exposure time, with a 416×264 μm^2 field of view[2].

4.1   Data Preparation

We acquired videos from 4 different ventral tongue capillaries. During model hyperparameter tuning, we applied 4-fold cross validation by splitting the dataset based on capillaries to prevent capillary feature leakage. And with the optimal hyperparameters, the final model is trained on videos from 3 capillaries while

---

[2] Supplementary material 1, Fig. 1 shows the setup of OBC system.

Table 1. MOT metrics on comparative models.

Model	Detection		ID match			Trajectory				Overall	Speed (Hz)
	Prcn↑	Rcll↑	IDP↑	IDR↑	IDF1↑	MT↑	ML↓	IDSw↓	Frag↓	MOTA↑	
Tracktor++	88.3	83.8	63.6	57.3	61.1	31.1	24.8	**26.7**	**15.7**	46.4	1.5
MaskTrack	90.3	**85.8**	67.2	64.5	65.9	41.2	22.9	38.1	24.5	53.2	2.6
CN+SORT	**92.6**	82.7	68.5	64.0	66.1	51.7	18.5	69.1	43.4	57.4	**16.8**
CenterTrack	**92.6**	82.7	75.5	74.3	71.6	65.8	15.6	59.8	30.6	62.4	12.0
CycleTrack	**92.6**	82.7	**78.2**	**72.1**	**75.1**	**72.7**	**14.3**	34.5	21.8	**66.3**	12.0

*CN+SORT: CenterNet-based SORT; Prcn: precision; Rcll: recall; IDP/IDR: ID precision/recall; MT/ML (%): most tracked/lost trajectory; IDSw (%): an ID switches to a different tracklet; Frag (%): fragment tracklets from miss detection.

another capillary's videos were left for test. The training dataset contains 942 fully annotated frames from 9 different sequences with a total of 4570 masks for 607 cells. Manual annotations were created by a trained expert, each of which consists of a labeled mask and a tracking ID. All tracking IDs are consistent across frames for the same cell in a sequence. The testing dataset contained a sequence with 300 annotated frames, with 901 masks for 197 cells. For further validation of cell count accuracy, we applied CycleTrack to eight additional videos with 1000 frames each. These videos had manually determined cell counts as ground truth but no mask annotations.

4.2 Implementation Details

CycleTrack builds upon the CenterNet-based CenterTrack and SORT in Pytorch, with a modified DLA model [18] as a backbone. The training inputs were made up of frame pairs after standard normalization. To enhance the model generalization on the limited dataset, data augmentation, including rotation uniformly varying within 15°, vertical/horizontal flips, and temporal flips with a probability of 0.5, were applied to simulate various blood cell flows. To simulate variation of up to 3× flow velocity, frame pairs were randomly generated within the frame range of $[-3,3]$. During training, we used the focal loss in the original CenterNet work [11] for object detection and offset loss L_{off} [15] for displacement vector regression, optimized with Adam with a learning rate of 10^{-4} and batch size of 16 for 300 epochs. The learning rate was reduced by half every 60 epochs. We tested CycleTrack runtime on an Intel Xeon E5-2620 v4 CPU with a Titan V GPU. We only track detections with a confidence $\omega \geq 0.6$. We also used test-time detection errors simulation [15] to better tolerate the imperfect object detection by setting random false positive and false negative ratios as $\lambda_{fp} = 0.1$ and $\lambda_{fn} = 0.4$. For model evaluations, we compared our CycleTrack with several benchmark online MOT models including CenterNet-based SORT, CenterTrack, and appearance-based trackers such as Tracktor++ [21] and MaskTrack [22].

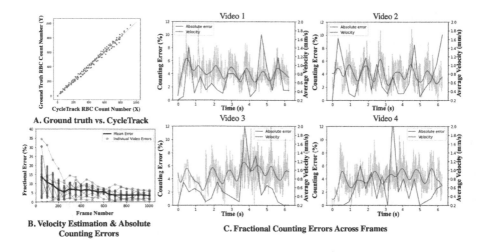

Fig. 2. A. Correlation between ground truth blood cell count and results from CycleTrack. B. Fractional Counting Errors Across Frames. Blue curve: individual absolute percentage counting errors; black curve is the mean, and grey bars are the standard deviations of errors over 8 test videos. **C. Velocity Estimation and Absolute Counting Errors Over 4 Different Test Videos.** The faded blue lines: average velocity of all objects; the solid blue lines: a lowpass filtered average velocity; the green lines: the absolute cell counting errors over the nearby 50 frames. (Color figure online)

5   Results and Discussions

5.1   MOT Evaluation

A quantitative analysis of performance is presented in Table 1, where we list the MOT metrics [19,20] of comparative models tested on an unseen 300-frame video with full annotations. With similar detection accuracy, we first observe that position-based trackers have better tracking performance over appearance-based trackers in our videos. It is also important to note that CycleTrack outperforms all other trackers in the tracking metrics, especially in terms of multiple object tracking accuracy (MOTA), which provides general evaluation of both object detection and tracking, and ID F1 score (IDFI). We also notice that, compared with local trackers without re-identification (Re-ID) models [21], like SORT and CenterTrack, the major improvement of our framework is in the significant reduction of ID switches. ID switches have widely shown to be a good metric that reflects stable long, consistent tracks [23,24]. For local trackers only focusing on two consecutive frames, a missed detection or biased displacement vector would cause an irreparable break of tracklets that leads to high ID switches and fragments. The reduction of ID switches demonstrates that local association refinement using back-and-forth tracking paths effectively compensate for tracking errors from unidirectional trackers, thus achieving stable long-term tracking.

5.2   Counting Results

We also evaluate the cell counting accuracy on 8 1000-frame videos with manually counted ground truth (without masks). The agreement between CycleTrack count and ground truth is shown Fig. 2. A. The correlation coefficient (γ) calculated from these experiments is 0.9960 which indicated a very strong positive relation between CycleTrack count and ground truth. Figure 2. B shows the percentage of absolute counting error change across time on these 8 videos. As frame number increases, we observe a descending trend in both average and variance of counting errors, which decrease quickly at first 300 frames and then become more stable as the base vector from CenterTrack gradually stabilizes to the right direction of capillary flow. When the frame number exceeds 600 when model typically has counted more than 400 cells, the average error stabilizes below 5%. This indicates that, to get a reliable counting in clinical scenarios, OBC videos are suggested to have at least 600 frames (3.75 s). By 1000 frames (6.25 s), the CycleTrack method reaches a state-of-the-art average counting accuracy of 96.58±2.43%, compared to 93.45% and 77.02% accuracy of original CenterTrack and SORT respectively. This demonstrates that, with the same object detector, stabler long-time tracking contributes to a great improvement to final counting accuracy. A verification study by Vis et al. [25] reported that the state-of-the-art analytical blood cell count accuracy of routine hematology is above 96.8%. And the average coefficient of variation of fingerprick blood cell counts from point-of-care instruments was higher by at least 3 times [26]. CycleTrack achieves a promising average accuracy of 96.58% on 1000-frame OBC videos compared with manual counting ground truths, which is close to the acceptable clinical accuracy as a point-of-care technique.

5.3   Runtime

The runtime mainly depends on the input image resolution and the number of objects detected and tracked. With 16-bit image inputs, CycleTrack ran at around 12 frames per second. The runtime of comparative models is shown in the last column in Table 1. Thanks to the efficiency of CenterNet, CycleTrack has a great advantage over other trackers in terms of speed while maintaining a good detection accuracy. Moreover, as SORT is a fast, unsupervised online tracking model capable of real-time tracking incorporating this model in CycleTrack adds no significant computational costs over the original CenterTrack.

5.4   Additional Physiological Information: Heart Rate

Fig. 2. C shows four examples of the estimated average velocity across frames from predicted displacement vectors with the absolute errors of the past 50 frames. From these data, we observe a clear sinusoidal signal at a frequency of 1 Hz. This falls within the expected normal physiological heartbeat of around 60 beats per minute. Therefore, we believe it may be possible to assess other significant physiological information beyond blood counts with this technology, such as blood flow metrics and vital signs. Moreover, these data show that the absolute error peaks tend to align with the peak blood flow velocity, which indicates a correlation between counting errors and flow velocity.

6 Conclusion

We presented a deep tracking model, called CycleTrack, that automatically counts blood cells from OBC videos. CycleTrack combines two online tracking models, SORT and CenterTrack, and predicts back-and-forth cell displacement vectors to achieve optimal matching between newly detected cells and previously tracked cells in two consecutive frames with minimal increase in runtime. We make two simple assumptions about blood flow that enhance the accuracy of our model: (1) cells in the same capillary tend to flow in similar directions in a single frame, and (2) individual cells move with a roughly linear constant velocity across frames. CycleTrack results outperform four existing multi-object tracking models and demonstrates robust cell counting with an average accuracy of 96.58% that is close to clinical acceptance accuracy. In addition, CycleTrack is a promising model to explore other valuable clinical biomarkers from OBC videos, like blood velocity and heartrate.

One limitation of capillary-based blood counting is the relatively few number of cells that we observe compared to the conventional invasive CBC. However, some studies have proven that capillary blood cell analysis can provide indications for various related diseases. For example, a clinical study on the superficial capillaroscopy video has shown a promising result on severe neutropenia detection by counting WBCs in 2–3 one-minute imaging sessions for each patient [27]. As a result, the OBC system is still in an exploratory research stage and further clinical study is needed to verify the robustness of OBC for clinical blood cell counting and assisting diagnosis of other diseases.

References

1. Agrawal, D., Sarode, R.: Complete blood count or complete blood count with differential: what's the difference? Am J Med. **130**(8), 915–916 (2017)
2. Carruthers, R., et al.: Systemic inflammatory response is a predictor of outcome in patients undergoing preoperative chemoradiation for locally advanced rectal cancer. Colorectal Dis. Off. J. Assoc. Coloproctol. Great Br. Irel. **14**(10), e701–7 (2012)
3. Barnes, P.W., et al.: The international consensus group for hematology review: suggested criteria for action following automated CBC and WBC differential analysis. Lab. Hematol. Off. Publ. Int. Soc. Lab. Hematol. **11**(2), 83–90 (2005)
4. Crawford, J., Dale, D.C., Lyman, G.H.: Chemotherapy-induced neutropenia. risks, consequences, and new directions for its management. Cancer **100**(2), 228–237 (2004)
5. Widness, J.A.: Pathophysiology of anaemia during the neonatal period. Including anaemia of prematurity. Neoreviews **9**(11), e520–e525 (2008)

6. Sanchis-Gomar, F., Cortell-Ballester, J., Pareja-Galeano, H., Banfi, G., Lippi, G.: Hemoglobin point-of-care testing: the HemoCue system. J. Lab. Autom. **18**, 198–205 (2013)

7. Bourquard, A., et al.: Non-invasive detection of severe neutropenia in chemotherapy patients by optical imaging of nailfold microcirculation. Sci. Rep. **8**, 5301 (2018)

8. McKay, G.N., et al.: Imaging human blood cells in vivo with oblique back-illumination capillaroscopy. Biomed. Opt. Exp. **11**(5), 2373–2382 (2020)

9. Girshick, R.: Fast R-CNN. In: ICCV, pp. 1440–1448 (2015)

10. He, K., Gkioxari, G., Dollár, P., Girshick, R.: Mask R-CNN. In: ICCV, pp. 2980–2988 (2017)

11. Duan, K., Bai, S., Xie, L., Qi, H., Huang, Q., Tian, Q.: CenterNet: keypoint triplets for object detection. In: ICCV, pp. 6568–6577 (2019)

12. Krizhevsky, A., Sutskever, I., Hinton, G.: ImageNet classification with deep convolutional neural networks. In: NIPS (2012)

13. He, K., Zhang, X., Ren, S., Sun, J.: Deep residual learning for image recognition. In: CVPR, pp. 770–778 (2016)

14. Bewley,A., Ge, Z., Ott, L., Ramos, F., Upcroft, B.: Simple online and realtime tracking. In: ICIP, pp. 3464–3468 (2016)

15. Zhou, X., Koltun, V., Krähenbühl, P.: Tracking objects as points. arXiv preprint. arXiv: 2004.01177 (2020)

16. Kalman, R.: A new approach to linear filtering and prediction problems. J. Basic Eng. **82**(Series D), 35–45 (1960)

17. Mehra, R.: On-line identification of linear dynamic systems with applications to Kalman filtering. IEEE Trans. Autom. Control **16**(1), 12–21 (1971)

18. Yu, F., Wang, D., Shelhamer, E., Darrell, T.: Deep layer aggregation. In: CVPR, pp. 2403–2412 (2018)

19. Milan, A., Leal-Taixé, L., Reid, I., Roth, S., Schindler, K.: Mot16: a benchmark for multi-object tracking. arXiv preprint. arXiv: 1603.00831 (2016)

20. Dendorfer, P., et al.: MOT20: a benchmark for multi object tracking in crowded scenes. arXiv preprint. arXiv:2003.09003 (2020)

21. Bergmann, P., Meinhardt, T., Leal-Taixé, L.: Tracking without bells and whistles. In: ICCV, pp. 941–951 (2019)

22. Yang, L., Fan, Y., Xu, N.: Video instance segmentation. In: ICCV, pp. 5188–5197 (2019)

23. Maksai, A., Fua, P.: Eliminating exposure bias and metric mismatch in multiple object tracking. In: CVPR, pp. 4639–4648 (2019)

24. Ciaparrone, G., et al.: Deep learning in video multi-object tracking: a survey. Neurocomputing **318**, 61–88 (2020)

25. Vis, J.Y., Huisman, A.: Verification and quality control of routine hematology analyzers. Int. J. Lab. Hematol. **38**(Suppl 1), 100–9 (2016)

26. Bond, M., Richards-Kortum, R.: Drop-to-drop variation in the cellular components of fingerprick blood: implications for point-of-care diagnostic development. Am. J. Clin. Pathol. **144**(6), 885–894 (2015)

27. Pablo-Trinidad, A., et al.: Automated detection of neutropenia using noninvasive video microscopy of superficial capillaries. Am. J. Hematol. **94**, E219–E222 (2019)

Cell Detection from Imperfect Annotation by Pseudo Label Selection Using P-classification

Kazuma Fujii[1(✉)], Daiki Suehiro[1,2], Kazuya Nishimura[1], and Ryoma Bise[1]

[1] Kyushu University, Fukuoka, Japan
fujii.kazuma@humna.ait.kyushu-u.ac.jp, bise@ait.kyushu-u.ac.jp
[2] RIKEN, AIP, Tokyo, Japan

Abstract. Cell detection is an essential task in cell image analysis. Recent deep learning-based detection methods have achieved very promising results. In general, these methods require exhaustively annotating the cells in an entire image. If some of the cells are not annotated (imperfect annotation), the detection performance significantly degrades due to noisy labels. This often occurs in real collaborations with biologists and even in public data-sets. Our proposed method takes a pseudo labeling approach for cell detection from imperfect annotated data. A detection convolutional neural network (CNN) trained using such missing labeled data often produces over-detection. We treat partially labeled cells as positive samples and the detected positions except for the labeled cell as unlabeled samples. Then we select reliable pseudo labels from unlabeled data using recent machine learning techniques; positive-and-unlabeled (PU) learning and P-classification. Experiments using microscopy images for five different conditions demonstrate the effectiveness of the proposed method. Our code is available at https://github.com/FujiiKazuma/CDFIAPLSUP.git.

Keywords: Cell detection · Imperfect annotation

1 Introduction

Cell detection is an essential task in cell image analysis, which has been widely used for cell counting and cell tracking. Many image processing based methods have been proposed for automatically detecting cells *e.g.*, using a thresholding [3,13,24], region growing [25] and graph cuts [1]. These methods are usually designed on the basis of image characteristics, so they may only work under certain conditions.

Recently, deep learning-based detection methods have shown to be effective for various types of cells if they are trained on enough training data for specific conditions [6,10,12,22]. Moreover, deep learning-based methods usually require fully annotating all the cells in an entire image for the network to learn both the foreground (cell) and the background area. If some of the cells are not annotated (*i.e.*, imperfect annotation), the non-annotated cell regions are mistakenly

© Springer Nature Switzerland AG 2021
M. de Bruijne et al. (Eds.): MICCAI 2021, LNCS 12908, pp. 425–434, 2021.
https://doi.org/10.1007/978-3-030-87237-3_41

treated as background regions in training. The detection performance significantly degrades due to such noisy labels. However, it is very costly to annotate all the cells in an image since there are as many as hundreds or thousands of cells in an image. Therefore, some of the current public data-sets only provide partially annotated cells (imperfect annotation).

The aim of our study is to make cell detection feasible from imperfect annotated data by using pseudo labeling. This would enable the use of imperfect datasets, which have already been made public, and reduce the annotation cost for biologists in real applications. In the proposed method, we first create a mask that covers only the annotated cells, in which the loss is ignored outside the mask. The masked loss facilitates the reduction of false negatives but produces many false positives since it learns part of the foreground (cell) region but not the background. When the detector is applied to the dataset that contains partially labeled cells (positive data), the detected positions excluding the labeled cell can be considered unlabeled data, which may contain both positive (cell) and negative (background) positions. To address the over-detection problem, we propose a semi-supervised method that selects reliable background as pseudo negative labels and additional foreground regions as pseudo positive labels from the unlabeled data and adds these to the training data in the next step. We applied positive and unlabeled (PU) learning [9] to extract the optimal image features that separate the feature distribution of positive (cell) and negative label (background). In order to minimize the risk of selecting incorrect labels as the pseudo labels, we performed ranking learning using P-classification [5] which aims to learn a ranking (scoring) function so that reliable positive samples are ranked higher. These processes are iteratively performed. This improves the performance of the detector network by adding reliable labels for both negative and positive positions. The experiments using microscopy images for five different conditions demonstrate the effectiveness of the proposed method.

2   Related Work

Object detection from imperfect annotation is more challenging than supervised object detection. Some methods have been proposed for this task in general object detection. Xu et al. [20] investigated the effects of imperfect annotation by changing the annotation rate using PASCAL VOC2007. They found that the performance of the current methods such as YOLO [15] and Faster-RCNN [16], drastically degraded as the rate lowered (e.g., from 0.7 to 0.45 when the rate was 0.2). Pseudo labeling has been often used for object detection in semi-supervised learning [2,8,10], and it could be used for learning from imperfect annotation. Misra et al. [11] proposed semi-supervised learning for object detection from imperfect annotation. In their study, the target object was cars in a video. This method selects the reliable positive objects (cars) by tracking candidate objects in the inputted video. However, they used random images from the internet as negative labels, which cannot be used for cell detection tasks. Recently, Yang et al. [21] proposed a PU-learning [9] based method for

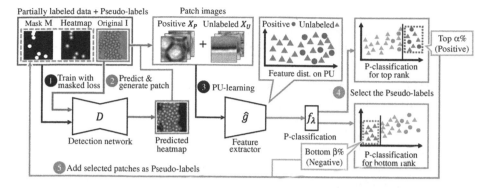

Fig. 1. Overview of the proposed method. Given the partially labeled data, to improve the detection network D, the proposed method iteratively adds the pseudo labels for both positives and negatives by iteratively performing the five steps; 1) training D with the masked loss using partially labeled data; 2) predicting the position heatmaps and generates patch images from detected points; 3) training the feature extractor $\hat{g}$ using PU learning; 4) training the ranking function f_λ and selecting pseudo labels for positive and negative samples based on the ranking score; 5) adding the selected patches as pseudo labels to be used for the next iteration.

general object detection from imperfect annotation. In this method, the positive objects are directly selected using PU learning without re-training the detector. PU learning requires the prior (the proportion of positive samples in the data), and the method assumes a small number of the same class objects in an image. However, in our target, there are many cells in an image, so it is difficult to estimate the prior, in our preliminary work, PU learning was not effective.

Unlike the previous methods, our method incrementally improves the detector by selecting reliable pseudo positive and negative labels using recent machine learning techniques.

3   Cell Detection from Imperfect Annotation

Figure 1 shows an overview of the proposed method. Given the original images I with the imperfect annotation of the cell position C, the method iteratively trains the detection network D that estimates the position heatmap [12] by pseudo labeling. In the estimated heatmap, a cell centroid becomes a peak with a Gaussian distribution as shown in the estimated image in Fig. 1. The method consists of the following five steps: 1) training the detection network D using the imperfect annotation for cell centroid positions C; 2) generating patch images based on the detection results; 3) training the feature extractors using PU-learning [9] with positive and unlabeled patch images; 4) training the ranking function that estimates the score that a sample belongs to positive or negative using P-classification [5]; 5) selecting reliable pseudo-labels using the estimated scores, and adding the center positions of the selected patches as the pseudo-labels C_P

to be used for training in the next iteration. These steps are iteratively performed and these improve the detection performance of D using the reliable pseudo labels for both positive (cell) and negative (background) positions.

Cell Detection with Masked Loss and Patch Generation: We use a cell position heatmap that has shown a good performance [12]. The detection network D is trained using the set of the annotated cell centroid positions to predict a heatmap so that a cell centroid becomes a peak with a Gaussian distribution. We use the U-net architecture for D. The method requires all cells in an image to be annotated as training data since the network is trained to produce zero values on the background area (non-annotated area). If we train the network using the imperfect training data, it affects the detection performance. Therefore, we use the masked loss function which gives the loss only around the given ground-truth of the cell centroids. A mask M_k is generated for the k-th image so that a circular area within radius r from an annotated position becomes the foreground (loss is calculated) and otherwise background. The radius of the mask should be large enough to cover a Gaussian distribution in the heat-map. Examples of the heatmap and mask are shown in the training data in Fig. 1.

Next, the trained model predicts the heatmap for all the original images I. Local maximum points that are larger than a threshold th in the heatmap are detected as cell positions. The masked loss facilitates the reduction of the false negatives but produces many false positives. We have to select the reliable detection results from the noisy prediction to effectively perform pseudo labeling. The patch images are first generated by cropping the cell image based on the detected points. The patch image with the annotated positions C can be considered positive labeled samples $X_P = \{x_i^p\}_{i=1,\dots,N_p}$, and the patch images except X_P can be considered the unlabeled samples $X_U = \{x_i^u\}_{i=1,\dots,N_u}$.

Feature Extraction Using PU-leaning: The aim of the 3rd step is to extract optimal image features that separate the feature distribution of positive (cell) and negative label (background), which is useful to select reliable labels. To achieve this, we use PU learning [9] which uses positive labeled samples and unlabeled samples as training data, so the unlabeled samples can be classified as positive or negative.

Let g be the classifier CNN that classifies an input patch image x_i into positive ($+1$: cell) or negative (-1: background), where training is performed using positive and unlabeled data. In PU-learning, the following non-negative risk function [9] is used as the CNN loss:

$$R_{pu}(g) = \pi_p R_p^+(g) + \max\{0, R_u^-(g) - \pi_p R_p^-(g)\}, \tag{1}$$

where π_p represents *prior* probability of the positive samples (*i.e.*, the proportion of the positive samples in the data), $R_p^+(g) = (1/N_p)\sum_{i=1}^{N_p} l(g(x_i^p), +1)$, $R_p^-(g) = (1/N_p)\sum_{i=1}^{N_p} l(g(x_i^p), -1)$ and $R_u^-(g) = (1/N_u)\sum_{i=1}^{N_u} l(g(x_i^u), -1)$. l is by default the *zero-one* loss, namely $l_{01}(t, y) = (1 - \text{sign}(ty))/2$.

After training, we obtain the feature extraction layers $\hat{g}$ by removing the FC classifier layer from g. We use the image features $\hat{g}(x_i)$ in the next step.

Pseudo-label Selection Using P-classification: Although PU learning aims to extract optimal features for distinguishing positive and negative samples, the proportion is unknown in real application and the distribution of the features depends on the dataset. Therefore, it is difficult to directly determine the discriminant plane in the feature space, and it may contain many incorrect labels. Instead, we take the pseudo labeling approach to select reliable samples from the unlabeled data X_U based on the extracted features.

To minimize the risk of selecting incorrect labels as pseudo labels, we use P-classification [5] which is a technique for learning to rank. The advantage of using P-classification is that we can emphasize the classification performance at the top of the ranked list. More precisely, P-classification aims to learn a ranking (scoring) function which gives large scores to (possibly a limited number of) reliable positive samples rather than gives large scores for all positive samples. This indicates that we can reduce the risk that the high rank scored samples contain negative (incorrect) samples, (*i.e.*, the precision on the higher-ranked samples becomes high).

Given the positive $\{x_i^p\}_{i=1}^{N_p}$ and negative samples $\{x_k^n\}_{k=1}^{N_n}$, P-classification optimizes the parameters of a scoring linear function $f_\lambda := \sum_j \lambda_j g_j$, in which g_j is the j-th feature of $\hat{g}(X_i)$, using the following loss:

$$\mathcal{R}^{PC}(\lambda) := \sum_{i=1}^{N_p} e^{-f_\lambda(x_i^p)} + \frac{1}{p} \sum_{k=1}^{N_n} e^{f_\lambda(x_k^n)}, \tag{2}$$

where $p\ (\geq 1)$ is a hyper-parameter which controls the degree of concentration at the top of the list. Roughly speaking, when we set $p = 1$, the method maximizes AUC (Area Under the receiver operating characteristic Curve), which is a standard scoring/ranking performance measure. When we set a larger p, the method maximizes the leftmost portion of the curve (*i.e.*, performance at the top of the ranked list). This method only trains the discriminant layer, and thus we used $\hat{g}$ as the feature extractor network.

In this study, the negative samples are unknown and the objective is to reduce the risk of selecting incorrect labels as the pseudo-labels. Therefore, we use the unlabeled data X_U as $\{x_k^n\}_{k=1,\ldots,N_n}$, instead. Then we select the top α of the ranked unlabeled data is selected as the positive pseudo-labels. In addition, we also have to select the negative samples (background) from X_U to reduce the false positives. To select bottom-negatives, we use P-classification by opposing the labels. Then, the bottom β of the ranked unlabeled data is selected as the negative pseudo-labels.

From the selected pseudo-labels, we re-generate the pseudo ground-truth of the position heatmap and the mask that will be used in the next iteration. The center positions of the selected positive pseudo patches are additionally registered as pseudo labels C_P. It is used for both generating pseudo position

| Control | FGF2 | BMP2 | FGF2 + BMP2 | BF-C2DL-HSC |

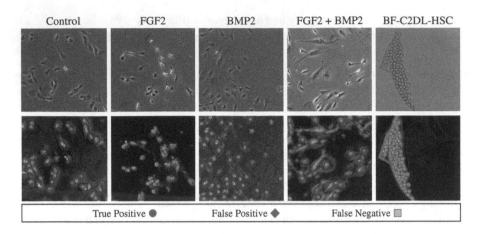

True Positive ●   False Positive ◆   False Negative ■

Fig. 2. Examples of enlarged images of detection results in each condition.

heatmap and the mask for the training loss. The center positions of the selected negative pseudo patches are used for generating the mask, where a position in the pseudo heatmap has a value of 0 in the background. These steps are iteratively performed and improve the detection performance of D using the reliable pseudo labels for both positive (cell) and negative (background) positions.

4   Experiment

Dataset and Performance Metric: In the experiments, we used the five conditioned data from two datasets, BF-C2DL-HSC (HSC) from the Cell Tracking Challenge at ISBI [14,18] and C2C12 [7]. HSC has a resolution of 1010 × 1010 pixels. Since we assume that a large number of cells exist in a single image and only some of them can be annotated, we used frames with a large number of cells for our experiments. We used 264 images containing over 80 cells. Thirteen images with partially labeled cells were used for training, in which the total number of annotated cells is 125. The other unlabeled cells in the partially labeled images were used for unlabeled data. We used the other 251 images for test. In this data, noises appeared on the well, and many false positives were detected in the initial estimation. In C2C12 [7], myoblast cells were captured by phase contrast microscopy at a resolution of 1040 × 1392 pixels and cultured on four different conditions: Control (no growth factor), where 10 images with partially labeled cells and 90 images are used as training and test data, respectively; FGF2 (fibroblast growth factor), with 38 images for training and 342 images for testing; BMP2 (bone morphogenetic protein), with 10 images for training and 90 images for test, 2–4) FGF2+BMP2, with 10 images for training and 90 images for test. These cells have more varied cell appearances compared with HSC. In detection, the heatmap was normalized from 0 to 255 and the threshold th was set to 128, and Mean squared error was used as loss function. The proportions

Table 1. Performance of the compared methods on each dataset.

Data	Condition	Nishimura [12]	With mask	Vicar [19]	Yang [21]	Ours	Fully supervised[12]
C2C12	Control	0.477	0.239	0.802	0.239	**0.834**	0.922
	FGF2	0.318	0.361	0.648	**0.768**	**0.768**	0.924
	BMP2	0.609	0.217	0.739	**0.809**	0.769	0.978
	FGF2 + BMP2	0.105	0.257	0.539	0.257	**0.578**	0.962
HSC		0.157	0.393	0.475	0.108	**0.952**	0.998
	Average	0.333	0.293	0.6406	0.436	**0.780**	0.971

of the labeled cells in a training image were 0.1 and the number of iterations was 2 in all experiments. The percentages of pseudo labels to be selected, α and β, were set to 5 % in all our experiments, in which we did not perform optimal parameter search for a fair comparison. These parameters work well as long as it is not set to an extremely large value. For p in P-classification, we used 4, which was used in the reference paper [5]. This p-value will work if it is not too small or too large.

We used F-score as the detection performance metric. To compute F-score, we first assigned the positions in detection and ground-truth by one-by-one matching with a certain distance threshold, defined by the cell radius. We used 15 pixels for all data. Then we defined a detection position successfully assigned to a ground-truth as true positives, un-associated detected positions as false positives, and un-associated ground-truths as false negatives.

Evaluation: We evaluated the performance of our method using five data with three methods as ablation study; 1) Nishimura [12] that was a supervised detection method, it was simply trained using missing labels; 2) With mask, in which the detector [12] was trained with the masked loss; 3) Vicar [19] that is an image processing-based method using Yin [23] and distance transform [17]; 4) Yang [21] that uses PU-learning to directly determine the labels without pseudo labeling, in which the class prior was estimated by [4]. The idea was simply applied to our model, Table 1 shows the F-scores of these methods. The performance of our method was significantly better than the baseline method (Nishimura). The baseline method treated a lot of cells as background and thus degraded its performance. Supervised detection with masked loss is also worse. The performance from Vicar that is not a learning method is better than the baseline, however, it depends on the image characteristic and thus the performance was not well in some conditions. Yang [21] improved the performance in some data-sets. However, the performances in some data were significantly worse. In our method, detection results using the detection CNN trained by sparse supervised data is unstable, and thus the prior of the positive and negative samples in the test data is also unstable. Even if we use the correct prior in training, the prior in the test may be different from that in training. In this case, the PU-learning could not

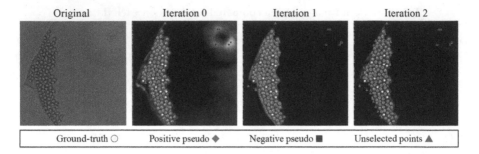

Fig. 3. Examples of selected pseudo labels in each iteration. (Color figure online)

Table 2. Improvements in training.

ittr.	precision	recall	F-score
0	0.337	0.999	0.504
1	0.732	0.997	0.844
2	0.963	0.998	0.980
3	0.956	0.997	0.976
4	0.946	0.995	0.970
5	0.952	0.996	0.973

Table 3. Improvements in test.

ittr.	Precision	Recall	F-score
0	0.245	0.999	0.394
1	0.622	0.999	0.767
2	0.910	0.999	0.952
3	0.896	0.998	0.944
4	0.918	0.997	0.956
5	0.888	0.998	0.940

work well as the discriminator. For HSC, results of our method achived accuracy close to that of the fully-supervised. Our method further improved the performance in most of the data. For FGF2+BMP2, the further iteration improved the performance (0.750 at iteration 5). Figure 2 shows the examples of our final detection results in each condition. In the results, there are several false positives (two peaks appear in a cell region) but few false negatives.

Improvement Process in Training: Figure 3 shows the improvement process in iterations using HSC. In this experiments, the yellow points are given as the initial partial labels (Ground-truth). The green points are predicted to be cells by the detection network but not selected as pseudo-labeled points via P-classification. The image at iteration 0 indicates the prediction results, where the background region also has high values, so there are false positives. In iteration 0, the positive (red) and negative (blue) positions were successfully selected as pseudo labels. In iteration 1, the estimation of the background was improved. After the first iteration, the unselected detection points (green) are also good. We can observe that the positive pseudo positions (red) increase with the iteration.

Tables 2 and 3 show the precision, recall, and F-score in each iteration under train and test data, respectively. 'ittr.' indicates the number of iteration for pseudo labeling. In the training phase, the recall of the initial estimation is very high but the precision is low. It supports our assumption that the results estimated using the masked loss have many false positives but few false negatives. We can observe that the precision was improved with keeping high recall by applying our method. Here, the improvements were saturated after the second iteration in both train and test data. This shows that our iterative pseudo learning approach improved the precision and F-score, and the few iterations worked enough. We consider that the small number of iteration does not affect the performance and improves the performance for many datasets, even though the additional iteration may improve the performance. It is our future work to find an optimal iteration using the relationship between the feature distribution and the selected pseudo labels.

5 Conclusion

We propose a cell detection method that can train the detection network from imperfect annotation, where only partial cells are annotated in an image. To archive this, our method selects reliable positive and negative samples from the over-detection results using the recent machine learning approaches: positive-and-unlabeled learning and P-classification. The experiments using microscopy images for five different conditions demonstrated the effectiveness of the proposed method, which can significantly improve the performance using very few labeled cells (only 10% of the total cells).

Acknowledgment. This work was supported by JSPS KAKENHI Grant Number JP19K22895 and JP20H04211.

References

1. Al-Kofahi, Y., Lassoued, W., Lee, W., Roysam, B.: Improved automatic detection and segmentation of cell nuclei in histopathology images. IEEE Trans. Biomed. Eng. **57**(4), 841–852 (2009)
2. Bertasius, G., Feichtenhofer, C., Tran, D., Shi, J., Torresani, L.: Learning temporal pose estimation from sparsely labeled videos. In: NeurIPS (2019)
3. Bise, R., Sato, Y.: Cell detection method from redundant candidates under the non-overlapping constraints. In: Proceedings of the IEEE Transaction on Medical Imaging, pp. 1417–1427 (2015)
4. Du Plessis, M.C., Niu, G., Sugiyama, M.: Class-prior estimation for learning from positive and unlabeled data. In: Proceedings of Asian Conference on Machine Learning, pp. 221–236 (2016)
5. Ertekin, S., Rudin, C.: On equivalence relationships between classification and ranking algorithms. J. Mach. Learn. Res. **12**, 2905–2929 (2011)
6. Fujita, S., Han, X.H.: Cell detection and segmentation in microscopy images with improved mask R-CNN. In: Proceedings of the Asian Conference on Computer Vision (2020)
7. Ker, D.F.E., et al.: Phase contrast time-lapse microscopy datasets with automated and manual cell tracking annotations. Sci. Data **5**(1), 1–12 (2018)

8. Kikkawa, R., Sekiguchi, H., Tsuge, I., Saito, S., Bise, R.: Semi-supervised learning with structured knowledge for body hair detection in photoacoustic image. In: ISBI, pp. 1411–1415 (2019)
9. Kiryo, R., Niu, G., Du Plessis, M.C., Sugiyama, M.: Positive-unlabeled learning with non-negative risk estimator. In: Proceedings of NeurIPS (2017)
10. Li, J., et al.: Signet ring cell detection with a semi-supervised learning framework. In: Chung, Albert C. S.., Gee, James C.., Yushkevich, Paul A.., Bao, Siqi (eds.) IPMI 2019. LNCS, vol. 11492, pp. 842–854. Springer, Cham (2019). https://doi.org/10.1007/978-3-030-20351-1_66
11. Misra, I., Shrivastava, A., Hebert, M.: Watch and learn: semi-supervised learning of object detectors from videos. In: Proceedings of the IEEE Conference on Computer Vision and Pattern Recognition (2015). https://doi.org/10.1109/CVPR.2015.7298982
12. Nishimura, Kazuya, Ker, Dai Fei Elmer., Bise, Ryoma: Weakly supervised cell instance segmentation by propagating from detection response. In: Shen, D., et al. (eds.) MICCAI 2019. LNCS, vol. 11764, pp. 649–657. Springer, Cham (2019). https://doi.org/10.1007/978-3-030-32239-7_72
13. Otsu, N.: A threshold selection method from gray-level histograms. IEEE Trans. Syst. Man Cybern. $9(1)$, 62–66 (1979)
14. Redmon, J., Divvala, S., Girshick, R., Farhadi, A.: You only look once: unified, real-time object detection. In: Proceedings of the IEEE Conference on Computer Vision and Pattern Recognition, pp. 779–788 (2016)
15. Redmon, J., Farhadi, A.: Yolov3: an incremental improvement. arXiv (2018)
16. Ren, S., He, K., Girshick, R., Sun, J.: Faster R-CNN: towards real-time object detection with region proposal networks. In: Proceedings of NeurIPS (2015)
17. Thirusittampalam, K., Hossain, M.J., Ghita, O., Whelan, P.F.: A novel framework for cellular tracking and mitosis detection in dense phase contrast microscopy images. IEEE J. Biomed. Health Inform. $17(3)$, 642–653 (2013)
18. Ulman, V., et al.: An objective comparison of cell-tracking algorithms. Nat. Methods $14(12)$, 1141–1152 (2017)
19. Vicar, T., et al.: Cell segmentation methods for label-free contrast microscopy: review and comprehensive comparison. BMC Bioinform. $20(1)$, 1–25 (2019)
20. Xu, M., Bai, Y., Ghanem, B.: Missing labels in object detection. In: Proceedings of the IEEE Conference on Computer Vision and Pattern Recognition Workshop, pp. 1–10 (2017)
21. Yang, Y., Liang, K.J., Carin, L.: Object detection as a positive-unlabeled problem. In: Proceedings of BMVC, pp. 1–14 (2020)
22. Yi, J., et al.: Multi-scale cell instance segmentation with keypoint graph based bounding boxes. In: Shen, D., et al. (eds.) MICCAI 2019. LNCS, vol. 11764, pp. 369–377. Springer, Cham (2019). https://doi.org/10.1007/978-3-030-32239-7_41
23. Yin, Z., Kanade, T., Chen, M.: Understanding the phase contrast optics to restore artifact-free microscopy images for segmentation. Med. Image Anal. $16(5)$, 1047–1062 (2012)
24. Yuan, Y., et al.: Quantitative image analysis of cellular heterogeneity in breast tumors complements genomic profiling. Sci. Trans. Med. $4(157)$, 157ra143–157ra143 (2012)
25. Zhou, Y., Starkey, J., Mansinha, L.: Segmentation of petrographic images by integrating edge detection and region growing. Comput. Geosci. $30(8)$, 817–831 (2004)

Learning Neuron Stitching
for Connectomics

Xiaoyu Liu[1], Yueyi Zhang[1,2]([✉]), Zhiwei Xiong[1,2], Chang Chen[1], Wei Huang[1],
Xuejin Chen[1,2], and Feng Wu[1,2,3]

[1] University of Science and Technology of China, Hefei, China
[2] Institute of Artificial Intelligence, Hefei Comprehensive National Science Center,
Hefei, China
[3] CAS Center for Excellence in Brain Science and Intelligence Technology,
Shanghai, China

Abstract. The pipeline of connectomics usually divides the large-scale
electron microscopy volumes into multiple 3D blocks and segments them
independently. The segmentation results in adjacent blocks demand subtle merging so that corresponding neurons can be correctly stitched. In
this paper, we propose the first deep learning based neuron stitching
method for connectomics. Specifically, we densely slide a 3D window
along the shared face of two adjacent blocks to generate the training and
testing input. A classifier based on a 3D convolutional neural network
is utilized to identify whether two instance objects from adjacent blocks
should be merged. The stitching label is obtained from the in-block segmentation of dedicated blocks. Experimental results on isotropic and
anisotropic datasets demonstrate that our stitching method outperforms
state-of-the-art methods.

Keywords: Neuron stitching · Convolutional neural network ·
Connectomics

1 Introduction

To reconstruct a connectome at the level of synapses, researchers need to manage large-scale electron microscope (EM) volumes of the brain with an unprece-
dented amount of data [6,10,23]. For example, a complete electron microscopy
volume of the brain of an adult drosophila melanogaster consists of more than
21 million images, occupying a storage of 106 terabytes [25]. Limited by computing resources, it is impossible to segment such big data directly. The typical
pipeline of connectomics, which is shown in Fig. 1(a), divides EM images into
multiple blocks and segments them independently (in-block segmentation). Then
the segmented adjacent blocks are merged so that the corresponding neurons are
stitched. The global segmentation is achieved after neuron stitching, which is of

Electronic supplementary material The online version of this chapter (https://
doi.org/10.1007/978-3-030-87237-3_42) contains supplementary material, which is
available to authorized users.

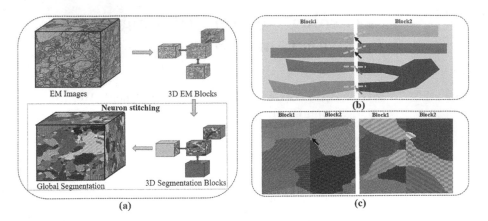

Fig. 1. (a) A typical pipeline for connectome reconstruction. (b, c) Illustration of cases which lead to stitching errors. Black arrows: Boundary Shift. Red arrows: Neuronal Branching. (Color figure online)

great benefit for connectome reconstruction. Although many methods have been proposed, neuron stitching is still challenging because of boundary shift and neuronal branching [19]. Figure 1(b, c) show several segmentation cases that may lead to stitching errors.

To figure out the neuron stitching problem for connectomics, a heuristic stitching algorithm that is based on the overlapping area between adjacent blocks was proposed in [9,19]. In this algorithm, two objects that have overlapping voxels above a given threshold, are judged as merge-pairs. Although the overlap-based method is simple and fast, uniform thresholds still fail to cover various edge cases. Matveev and Meirovitch [12,14] simplified the problem of identifying merge-pairs by treating it as a special case of agglomeration of over-segmentation. Agglomeration algorithms [5,15,17,18] originally target clustering the over-segmentation results generated by the watershed in the in-block segmentation. Their method analyzes a thin volume around the shared face of adjacent blocks by constructing a regional adjacency graph (RAG). A random forest classifier is trained to identify which adjacent vertices in RAG are merge-pairs across the adjacent blocks. However, constructing RAGs and extracting the regional features are time-consuming. Moreover, the stitching performance is sensitive to different extracted features. Subsequent remedies are needed to identify remaining merge-pairs. Recently, deep learning based methods which utilize deep neural network for feature generation, have been applied to the error-correction task [3,11,27] and provide beneficial inspirations for us to solve the neuron stitching problem.

In this paper, we propose a CNN-based framework for neuron stitching to extract the regional features for accurate merge-pair identification. Different from the graph-based method which has to construct complicated RAGs, we turn to analyze the region around the shared face of adjacent blocks to identify merge-pairs by sliding a window. A 3D ResNet-style network is adopted as a classifier to identify merge-pairs. The classifier takes the patches obtained by sliding a

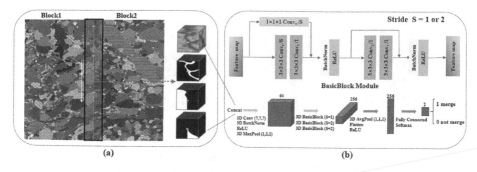

Fig. 2. Workflow of our proposed neuron stitching method. (a) The input patch of the network is a 4-channel volume which is obtained by densely sliding a window (red box) along the shared face of two adjacent blocks. (b) Illustration of the network architecture and the BasicBlock Module. (Color figure online)

3D window as input, and outputs the probability indicating whether the two segments are a merge-pair or not. Given there are no enough annotated labels for training our network, we devise a simple but effective method to synthesize the ground-truth by segmenting dedicated blocks which contains the shared face of adjacent blocks. We evaluate our stitching method on different EM datasets. Experimental results demonstrate improved numerical and perceptual results of our method over existing other solutions.

In summary, this paper makes the following contributions: 1) We convert the neuron stitching problem to a binary classification problem and first propose a deep learning based framework for merge-pair classification. 2) We utilize the in-block segmentation of a dedicated block to generate the stitching labels, which supervises the training of our network and avoids the usage of manual annotated data. 3) Our proposed method outperforms previous methods on both isotropic and anisotropic EM datasets.

2   Methodology

Overall Architecture. After dividing EM images into multiple 3D blocks and segmenting them independently, each instance object is assigned a unique ID. We need to stitch them to reconstruct complete neurons across multiple adjacent blocks. Our proposed stitching method simplifies the problem of identifying merge-pairs to a binary classification of segmentation masks of two objects from different blocks. Figure 2 shows the workflow of our proposed CNN-based stitching method.

Classification Network. The input patch of our network is a combination of four channels, which are the original EM grayscale volume, the boundary probability volume and two mask volumes. All the four volumes share the same size and are cropped from the same position identified by a 3D window densely slid along the shared face of two adjacent blocks. The boundary probability 3D

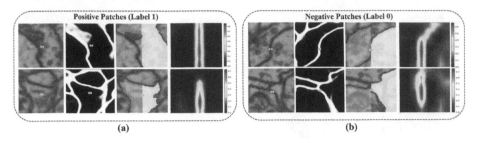

Fig. 3. (a) Two positive patches. The four columns present the EM grayscale patches, the probability maps for segmentation, the mask images for the two objects and the class activation maps [26] for the predicted class. (b) Two negative patches.

patch is generated from the segmentation stage. Within the sliding window, we pick the central two voxels which are from both sides of the shared face as two anchors. For each anchor, we generate a mask volume for the object containing the anchor. Then we get two mask volumes for both anchors. Figure 2(a) illustrates the sliding window and the procedures to get the input patch.

Our CNN network, which is inspired by the classic ResNet [4], is deployed to identify whether there is a merge-pair in the sliding window. It consists of four 3D convolution layers, one flatten layer and one fully connected layer. The first convolution layer is a 3D convolution followed by 3D batch normalization, ReLU activation and MaxPooling. The subsequent three convolution layers are three BasicBlock modules. The architecture of the basic block module, which is shown in Fig. 2(b), is quite similar to the ResBlock module [4]. The difference is that our BasicBlock module is adjustable in choosing stride number. The flatten layer transforms the fed feature map to a 256-dimension vector. The fully connected layer produces the final 2D vector indicating whether there is a merge-pair.

Training and Inference. For the neuron stitching task, we expect after-stitching segmentation results of the two divided EM blocks should be consistent with the segmentation results based on undivided EM blocks. This inspires us that we can use the segmentation results of the EM block which contains the shared face as the ground-truth. Thus by generating the label ourselves, our method avoids the usage of manually annotated data. In practice, for each pair of two adjacent blocks, a dedicated EM block, consisting of the shared face of the two adjacent blocks, is constructed and segmented. Then we adopt a method, which is similar to the method proposed in [15], to find correspondences between the objects from two adjacent blocks and the dedicated block. After that, we acquire the information that whether two objects in the two adjacent blocks should be merged, which will be utilized as labels to guide the training of our network. Figure 3 shows some representative patches belonging to different merge cases. The positive patch means that the two objects identified by the central anchor voxels within the patch need merging. The negative patch means the opposite.

For training, we adopt binary cross entropy as the loss function for our classification network. After densely sliding the 3D window along the shared face, we get a large amount of patches. However, the number of positive patches is far more than that of negative patches. We randomly pick the positive patches so that the numbers of positive and negative patches are the same. Then we generate the labels in the one-hot form for each patch with the aforementioned method. For testing, we slide a window as densely as possible to cover more unique object-pairs. This operation generates many redundant patches with the same object-pair. To speedup the processing, we do not feed the patches with identified merge-pair to the network.

3   Experiments

Datasets. We evaluate our neuron stitching method on three popular EM datasets: FAFB [25], CREMI [1] and FIB-25 [24]. FAFB is an anisotropic large-scale dataset, which is imaged from a complete adult drosophila brain at $4 \times 4 \times 40$ nm resolution with the ssTEM technique [22]. It consists of 7062 sections and the resolution for each section is $286,720 \times 155,648$. To validate the effectiveness of our stitching method, we only utilize a portion of the FAFB dataset. The resolution of the portion is $7780 \times 7780 \times 861$. We divide it into blocks with overlap and apply the segmentation algorithm to the blocks. After segmentation, each block has a resolution of $2660 \times 2660 \times 56$. The CREMI dataset is originally produced for the segmentation task with annotated labels. Essentially it is a subset of the FAFB dataset, so it is also anisotropic. The image resolution of the CREMI dataset is $1250 \times 1250 \times 125$. After segmentation, we obtain the blocks with resolution $544 \times 988 \times 61$. FIB-25 is an isotropic EM dataset, imaged at $8 \times 8 \times 8$ nm resolution from a drosophila brain obtained with the FIB-SEM technique [8]. The whole dataset consists of 8090 sections with a resolution of 6426×6423. FIB-25 provides segmentation groundtruth for a small portion of the dataset, which has the resolution $520 \times 520 \times 520$. The size of segmented blocks is $200 \times 308 \times 492$.

Implementation Details. All stitching experiments are based on the block-wise results from a state-of-the-art neuron segmentation method [2]. The size of the overlap is set as 100 voxels in the lateral (X/Y) direction and 30 voxels in the axial (Z) direction for all the datasets. The overlap of adjacent blocks is only utilized for overlap-based stitching method. For our CNN-based and the graph-based methods, half of the overlapping area is removed to form a shared face for training and testing.

On the anisotropic datasets, we train two models on FAFB for the lateral and axial directions respectively. For the lateral direction, we select 30 block-pairs and generate corresponding ground-truth, of which 20 pairs are used to generate training and validation samples and the remaining 10 pairs are used for testing. The size of the 3D sliding window is $100 \times 100 \times 23$, which is appropriate to cover most objects without efficiency dropping. After patch re-sampling, we generate 240,244 patches for training and 15,015 patches for validation. A similar evaluation scheme is adopted for FAFB in the axial direction. In addition, we test our trained models on the labeled CREMI dataset as well.

Table 1. Quantitative stitching results of different methods on the FAFB, CREMI and FIB-25 EM datasets.

Dataset	Method	VOI	ARAND	Time (s)
FAFB-X	No stitching	1.5098	0.3908	–
	Overlap-based	0.7662	0.1379	1.61
	Graph-based (33f)	0.8029	0.1264	58.91
	Graph-based (61f)	0.7825	0.1163	595.24
	CNN-Ours	**0.7379**	**0.0765**	10.46
FAFB-Z	No stitching	1.6576	0.3694	–
	Overlap-based	1.1541	0.1736	10.24
	Graph-based (33f)	1.1550	0.1591	406.95
	Graph-based (61f)	1.1358	**0.1506**	31669.49
	CNN-Ours	**1.1313**	0.1558	63.93
CREMI-X	No stitching	1.6415	0.3288	–
	Overlap-based	0.9621	0.1167	0.36
	Graph-based (33f)	1.0581	0.1228	29.58
	Graph-based (61f)	0.9887	0.0928	221.37
	CNN-Ours	**0.9293**	**0.0873**	2.01
CREMI-Z	No stitching	1.7887	0.3692	–
	Overlap-based	1.0028	0.1136	0.83
	Graph-based (33f)	1.1832	0.1577	68.59
	Graph-based (61f)	1.1125	0.1310	393.34
	CNN-Ours	**0.9833**	**0.0937**	4.03
FIB-25	No stitching	1.7999	0.3077	–
	Overlap-based	1.1607	0.0839	1.40
	Graph-based (33f)	1.1832	0.0751	130.57
	Graph-based (61f)	1.1747	0.0742	1169.15
	CNN-Ours	**1.1480**	**0.0721**	9.35

On the isotropic FIB-25 dataset, we train one model for all directions. We use 10 pairs of unlabeled adjacent blocks to generate patches of size $50 \times 50 \times 50$. In total, there are 53,120 patches for training and 8,739 patches for validation. Then we test on the labeled adjacent blocks using the trained model.

We implement the proposed method with the PyTorch framework. Our models are trained and tested on one NVIDIA TitanXP GPU. The batch size is set 32. Adam optimizer [7] is adopted during the training with $\beta_1 = 0.9$ and $\beta_2 = 0.99$. The initial learning rate is 10^{-4}, which is decayed by a half when the accuracy stops improving in 10 epochs. The train epochs on FAFB are 61 for the lateral direction and 48 for the axial direction. For FIB-25, the epoch number is 74.

To evaluate the performance of our proposed CNN-based stitching method, we compare it with the overlap-based method and the graph-based method in both quantitative and qualitative ways. For the overlap-based method, we utilize the release implementation [21]. The overlap-based method [9] is sensitive to

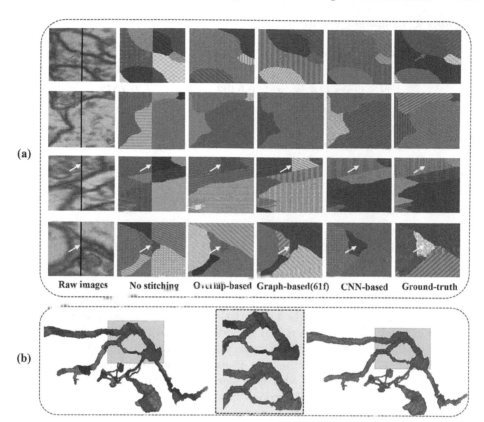

Fig. 4. (a) Qualitative comparison of stitching results of different methods. The red and yellow arrows highlight a wrong merge-pair and a missed merge-pair identified by other methods. (b) The 3D visualization of two objects across multiple adjacent blocks before and after applying our stitching method. (Color figure online)

thresholds. For a fair comparison, we choose the thresholds empirically. As for the graph-based method, we implement the algorithm ourselves with the help of Gala library [16]. we deploy two versions: One extracts 33 features for each object and the other extracts 61 features.

Experimental Results. We utilize two metrics for the quantitative comparison: Variation of Information (VOI) [13] and Adapted Rand Error (ARAND) [20]. The computational scope of the metrics are the areas which are traversed by the sliding windows.

The quantitative comparison results are shown in Table 1. The method 'No stitching' means we do not merge adjacent blocks, the result of which can be regarded as over-segmentation. In the dataset column, there are two suffixes '-X' and '-Z', which mean we evaluate the performance on the lateral direction and axial direction respectively. It can be seen that our CNN-based stitching method outperforms other methods in most cases. Especially, our proposed method

Table 2. Comparison of stitching results from networks with different depths

Architecture	Validation Accuracy	VOI
Variant-8 (8 layers)	0.9379	0.7420
CNN-Ours (14 layers)	**0.9403**	**0.7379**
Variant-28 (28 layers)	0.9283	0.7518

Table 3. Comparison of stitching results from networks with different input channels

Input Channel	Validation Accuracy	VOI
Mask	0.9152	0.7560
Mask+Boundary	0.9192	0.7537
Mask+Raw	0.9231	0.7474
mask+Boundary.+Raw.	**0.9403**	**0.7379**

achieves 3.7% improvement for VOI and 34.2% improvement for ARAND compared with the second best method on FAFB-X. We also list the running time of stitching methods. It can be seen that although our method runs slightly slower than the overlap-based method, it is much faster than the graph-based method.

For the qualitative comparison, we visualize some representative stitching results in Fig. 4(a). It can be seen that our CNN-based method can identify merge-pairs more accurately and reduce wrong or missing merge-pairs. In addition, we perform an experiment to test our method on a larger EM volume. The EM volume, which is also cropped from the FAFB dataset, is divided to 288 blocks. All the blocks are segmented independently and stitched with our pre-trained models. We select two complete objects across multiple blocks and show 3D visualization of the two objects before and after stitching in Fig. 4(b). As can be observed, after stitching, the two objects are recovered accurately.

Ablation. To investigate the contributing area of our CNN network, we visualize Class Activation Map (CAM) [26] for the patches demonstrated in Fig. 3. We can see that the CAM images highlight the regions close to the shared face of two adjacent blocks, which is reasonable because these regions provide most information relevant to the predicted class.

We perform experiments on the FAFB-X dataset to analyze the impact of network depth on the stitching performance. Based on our network that has 14 layers, we decrease and increase the usage of convolution operation, constructing two variants Variant-8 and Variant-28. The two variants have 8 layers and 28 layers respectively. Table 2 shows the quantitative comparison of validation accuracy and VOI score for these two variants and the original method. The validation accuracy is the accuracy of classification for the patches in the validation set. It can be seen that the network with 14 layers, which is the configuration of the original network, achieves the best performance for the neuron stitching task.

We further perform an ablation experiment to investigate the impact of different input channels. The results are shown in Table 3. It can be seen that the raw image and boundary map provide useful texture and structure information respectively for classification decision, and the input combination composed of binary mask, raw image and boundary image has the best performance.

4   Conclusion

In this paper, we propose a deep learning based method to solve the neuron stitching problem for connectomics. The proposed method is based on a 3D ResNet-style neural network. The input patches are obtained by sliding a 3D window along the shared face of two adjacent blocks. The stitching labels are generated by the in-block segmentation of dedicated blocks, which solves the problem of lack of ground-truth. Experimental results on isotropic and anisotropic datasets demonstrate that our proposed method outperforms existing leading neuron stitching methods.

Acknowledgement. This work was supported in part by Key Area R&D Program of Guangdong Province with grant No. 2018B030338001, Anhui Provincial Natural Science Foundation under grant No. 1908085QF256, National Natural Science Foundation of China under grant No. 61901435, 62076230 and University Synergy Innovation Program of Anhui Province No. GXXT-2019-025.

References

1. CREMI: MICCAI challenge on circuit reconstruction from electron microscopy images (2016). https://cremi.org/
2. Funke, J., et al.: Large scale image segmentation with structured loss based deep learning for connectome reconstruction. IEEE Trans. Pattern Anal. Mach. Intell. **41**(7), 1669–1680 (2018)
3. Haehn, D., Kaynig, V., Tompkin, J., Lichtman, J.W., Pfister, H.: Guided proofreading of automatic segmentations for connectomics. In: Proceedings of the IEEE Conference on Computer Vision and Pattern Recognition, pp. 9319–9328 (2018)
4. He, K., Zhang, X., Ren, S., Sun, J.: Deep residual learning for image recognition. In: Proceedings of the IEEE Conference on Computer Vision and Pattern Recognition, pp. 770–778 (2016)
5. Januszewski, M., et al.: High-precision automated reconstruction of neurons with flood-filling networks. Nat. Methods **15**(8), 605–610 (2018)
6. Kasthuri, N., et al.: Saturated reconstruction of a volume of neocortex. Cell **162**(3), 648–661 (2015)
7. Kingma, D.P., Ba, J.: Adam: a method for stochastic optimization. arXiv preprint arXiv:1412.6980 (2014)
8. Kizilyaprak, C., Daraspe, J., Humbel, B.: Focused ion beam scanning electron microscopy in biology. J. Microsc. **254**(3), 109–114 (2014)
9. Knowles-Barley, S., et al.: RhoanaNet pipeline: dense automatic neural annotation. arXiv preprint arXiv:1611.06973 (2016)

10. Lichtman, J.W., Pfister, H., Shavit, N.: The big data challenges of connectomics. Nat. Neurosci. **17**(11), 1448–1454 (2014)
11. Matejek, B., Haehn, D., Zhu, H., Wei, D., Parag, T., Pfister, H.: Biologically-constrained graphs for global connectomics reconstruction. In: 2019 IEEE/CVF Conference on Computer Vision and Pattern Recognition (CVPR), pp. 2084–2093. IEEE (2019)
12. Matveev, A., et al.: A multicore path to connectomics-on-demand. In: Proceedings of the 22nd ACM SIGPLAN Symposium on Principles and Practice of Parallel Programming, pp. 267–281 (2017)
13. Meilă, M.: Comparing clusterings by the variation of information. In: Schölkopf, B., Warmuth, M.K. (eds.) COLT-Kernel 2003. LNCS (LNAI), vol. 2777, pp. 173–187. Springer, Heidelberg (2003). https://doi.org/10.1007/978-3-540-45167-9_14
14. Meirovitch, Y., et al.: A multi-pass approach to large-scale connectomics. arXiv preprint arXiv:1612.02120 (2016)
15. Nunez-Iglesias, J., Kennedy, R., Parag, T., Shi, J., Chklovskii, D.B.: Machine learning of hierarchical clustering to segment 2D and 3D images. PloS One **8**(8), e71715 (2013)
16. Nunez-Iglesias, J., Kennedy, R., Plaza, S.M., Chakraborty, A., Katz, W.T.: Graph-based active learning of agglomeration (GALA): a python library to segment 2D and 3D neuroimages. Front. Neuroinform. **8**, 34 (2014)
17. Parag, T., Chakraborty, A., Plaza, S., Scheffer, L.: A context-aware delayed agglomeration framework for electron microscopy segmentation. PloS one **10**(5), e0125825 (2015)
18. Plaza, S.M.: Focused proofreading to reconstruct neural connectomes from EM images at scale. In: Carneiro, G., et al. (eds.) LABELS/DLMIA -2016. LNCS, vol. 10008, pp. 249–258. Springer, Cham (2016). https://doi.org/10.1007/978-3-319-46976-8_26
19. Plaza, S.M., Berg, S.E.: Large-scale electron microscopy image segmentation in spark. arXiv preprint arXiv:1604.00385 (2016)
20. Rand, W.M.: Objective criteria for the evaluation of clustering methods. J. Am. Stat. Assoc. **66**(336), 846–850 (1971)
21. RhoANA: dense automatic neural annotation (2016). https://github.com/Rhoana/rhoana/
22. Stevens, J.K., Davis, T.L., Friedman, N., Sterling, P.: A systematic approach to reconstructing microcircuitry by electron microscopy of serial sections. Brain Res. Rev. **2**(1–3), 265–293 (1980)
23. Takemura, S.y., et al.: A visual motion detection circuit suggested by drosophila connectomics. Nature **500**(7461), 175–181 (2013)
24. Takemura, S.Y., et al.: Synaptic circuits and their variations within different columns in the visual system of drosophila. Proc. Nat. Acad. Sci. **112**(44), 13711–13716 (2015)
25. Zheng, Z., et al.: A complete electron microscopy volume of the brain of adult drosophila melanogaster. Cell **174**(3), 730–743 (2018)
26. Zhou, B., Khosla, A., Lapedriza, A., Oliva, A., Torralba, A.: Learning deep features for discriminative localization. In: Proceedings of the IEEE Conference on Computer Vision and Pattern Recognition, pp. 2921–2929 (2016)
27. Zung, J., Tartavull, I., Lee, K., Seung, H.S.: An error detection and correction framework for connectomics. In: Proceedings of the 31st International Conference on Neural Information Processing Systems, pp. 6821–6832 (2017)

CA$^{2.5}$-Net Nuclei Segmentation Framework with a Microscopy Cell Benchmark Collection

Jinghan Huang[1], Yiqing Shen[2] , Dinggang Shen[3,4], and Jing Ke[5,6,7( )]

[1] School of Physics and Astronomy, Shanghai Jiao Tong University, Shanghai, China
teddyhuang@sjtu.edu.cn
[2] School of Mathematical Sciences, Shanghai Jiao Tong University, Shanghai, China
shenyq@sjtu.edu.cn
[3] School of Biomedical Engineering, ShanghaiTech University, Shanghai, China
dgshen@shanghaitech.edu.cn
[4] Shanghai United Imaging Intelligence Co., Ltd., Shanghai, China
[5] Department of Computer Science and Engineering, Shanghai Jiao Tong University, Shanghai, China
kejing@sjtu.edu.cn
[6] School of Computer Science and Engineering, University of New South Wales, Sydney, Australia
[7] BirenTech Research, Shanghai, China

Abstract. Nuclei segmentation is an indispensable prerequisite for microscope image analyses. However, a successful instance segmentation result is still challenging attributable to the ubiquitous presence of clustered nuclei, as well as the morphological variation among dissimilar phenotype of cells. In this paper, a novel contour-aware 2.5-path decoder network (CA$^{2.5}$-Net) is proposed for nuclei segmentation in microscope images. In contrast to the regular two-path decoders in many previous contour-aware networks, a shared decoder path is employed when the clustered-edge problem is severe. The range of recognizability difficulty generated by the extra half path also serves as a natural proxy to construct a curriculum-learning model, where training samples are sequenced for a better segmentation performance. Last, in this paper, we publicize two well-annotated privately-owned datasets covering a wide range of difficulty in the nuclei segmentation task, comprising 500 confocal microscopy image patches of deep-sea archaea and drosophila embryos obtained from 2013 to 2020. In the benchmark test of these two own datasets and one open-source set, our model outperforms the state-of-the-art nuclei segmentation approaches by a large margin, evaluated by the metrics of Average Jaccard Index and Dice score. Empirically, the proposed structure triples the training convergence speed in comparison with the competing CIA-net and BRP-net structures in nuclei segmentation.

Keywords: Clustered nuclei segmentation · Fluorescence microscopy dataset · Curriculum learning

© Springer Nature Switzerland AG 2021
M. de Bruijne et al. (Eds.): MICCAI 2021, LNCS 12908, pp. 445–454, 2021.
https://doi.org/10.1007/978-3-030-87237-3_43

1 Introduction

Instance nuclei segmentation is an essential prerequisite for medical and biology research. For example, an instance-level mask has often been a necessity in the single-cell analysis to explore the signal correlation between different channels. As the manual labeling work is considered time-consuming and tedious, it has been a growing interest in computer-aided methods development. However, given the complexity of clustered nuclei, which might also be challenging for human experts, there is no easy cure for non-machine learning algorithms with deterministic parameters. To give an example, conventional algorithms such as gradient algorithms [8] or watershed [9] are capable to locate boundaries well when the brightness contrast between two touching nuclei is sharp, or the adjacent edge is short. However, they are prone to fail in more complicated scenarios, when two clustered nuclei share a similar brightness or more nuclei are tightly clustered.

The recent years have witnessed many successful applications of image segmentation with the advent of deep learning. One of the most revolutionary architectures for instance segmentation is Mask RCNN [3], which has been almost dominant in natural image analysis and also employed in some of the microscopy analysis tasks [4]. However, in the microscope discipline, the defect has arisen at the contour identification task in the appearance-homogeneous scenarios, and this is also the case with BRP-Net [2] and other two-stage learning frameworks [5]. On the basis of the two-step learning framework [3], a deep contour-aware neural network (DCANs) [1] adds an extra decoder path to the definitive UNet architecture [10] to predict the contour. More recently, a CIA-net [12] incorporates additional information aggregation modules to the decoder path, aiming at a leverage of the feature maps between the two task-specific decoders. However, the literature works still have the limitation in the complicated cases when nuclei are severely clustered.

To address the problem discussed above, we propose a novel one-stage DCAN architecture in this paper. The major contributions of our work are summarized as follows:

1. We proposed a novel architecture for nuclei segmentation without human interpretation, namely $CA^{2.5}$-Net. It is the decomposition of a tough instance segmentation task into sequenced subtasks, in which the clustered-edge segmentation task promisingly tackle the severely clustered-nuclei problem.
2. Instead of the routine random shuffling, it is the first attempt at the fine-granularity quantification of nuclei-segmentation difficulty by curriculum learning, and the outcome of sequenced training directly leads to a large margin in performance improvement.
3. A well-annotated collection of microscope images is publicized. It consists a number of 500 512 × 512 confocal microscopy images, curated from a large private dataset of 10,000 fluorescence images. Instance-level masks were annotated by three biologists. It is valuable in a comprehensive evaluation of future

segmentation models. The benchmark set is freely available at https://www.kaggle.com/hjh415/ca25net.

2   Methodology

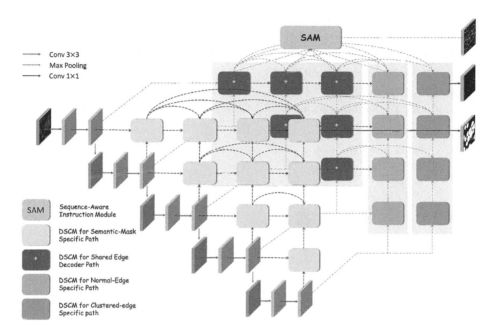

Fig. 1. The overall architecture for the proposed Contour-Aware network with 2.5-decoder paths (CA$^{2.5}$-Net). One path targets at semantic mask output, denoted in aqua. The other 1.5 path work for clustered-edge mask and normal-edge mask, with a proportion of Deep Skip-Connection Module (DSCM) shared and marked by the olive color. (Color figure online)

A novel deep contour-aware network (DCAN) with an extra output channel for clustered edge is introduced in this section. It consists of three differential output channels for semantic segmentation, regular contour segmentation, and clustered edge segmentation respectively. The proposed Contour-Aware architecture with 2.5-Decoder Paths Networks (CA$^{2.5}$-Net) is depicted in Fig. 1.

2.1   Ground Truth Preparation

The manually annotated images, namely the instance-level masks, are not well-suited to train a clustered-edge aware structure [1]. Subsequently, we incorporate a couple of intermediate stages to derive semantic mask, normal-edge mask and clustered-edge mask, which will be taken as salient input masks associated a raw image in the succeeding segmentation architecture, as shown in (Fig. 3). We write the conventional dataset storage format, which is ubiquitous for most instance segmentation tasks, as $\mathcal{D}_{\text{raw}} = \{(\mathbf{x}_i, \mathbf{y}_i)\}_{i=1}^{N}$, where N denotes the number of data instances. The ith grey microscopy image patch $\mathbf{x}_i \in \mathbb{R}^{l \times w}$ is sized at $l \times w$ pixels, $\mathbf{y}_i \in \mathbb{N}^{l \times w}$ standing for its associated pixel-level instance mask (Fig. 3). Consequently, the value of each patch $\mathbf{x}_i$ is linearly normalized into the range of $[0, 1]$. For each mask $\mathbf{y}_i \in N^{l \times w}$, $\mathbf{y}_i(m, n) = k \in \mathbb{N}$ represents the pixel value in the kth nucleus area, where the associated one-single nuclei mask $\Omega_i^{(k)}$ at coordinate (m, n) is defined as 1 if $\mathbf{y}_i(m, n) = k$, else $\Omega_i^{(k)} = 0$.

Given one-nuclei-one-mask ground truth pair $(\mathbf{x}_i, \mathbf{y}_i)$ and $\Omega_i^{(k)}$, we can obtain three binary-valued ground truth masks, namely the semantic mask $\{\mathbf{y}_i^{(sem)}\}_{i=1}^{N}$, the normal-edge mask $\{\mathbf{y}_i^{(nor)}\}_{i=1}^{N}$, and the clustered-edge mask $\{\mathbf{y}_i^{(clu)}\}_{i=1}^{N}$. They are taken as training groundtruth for a robust segmentation structure.

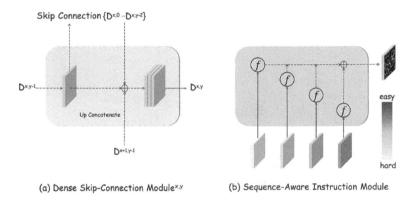

(a) Dense Skip-Connection Module^{x,y} (b) Sequence-Aware Instruction Module

Fig. 2. The detailed decoder module in the proposed architecture in Fig. 1. (a) The Dense Skip-Connection Module (DSCM), (b) Sequence-Aware Instruction Module (SAM).

A semantic mask $\{\mathbf{y}_i^{(sem)}\}_{i=1}^{N}$ is defined as the composition of a sign function (sgn) and an instance mask $\mathbf{y}_i$, where the value 0 stands for the background and 1 for the nuclei area, $\mathbf{y}_i^{(sem)}(m, n) = \text{sgn}(\mathbf{y}_i(m, n))$, where $\forall(m, n) \in \mathbb{N}^2$. A normal-edge mask is a subtraction of erosion from dilation of nuclear area $\Omega_i^{(k)}$ in the ith patch, with the same kernel K e.g. $(1)_{3 \times 3}$, to minimize the manual labeling deviation on the edges i.e.,

$$\mathbf{y}_i^{(nor)} = \text{sgn}\Big\{ \sum_{k \in \mathbb{N}} \big(\Omega_i^{(k)} \oplus K - \Omega_i^{(k)} \ominus K\big) \Big\}. \tag{1}$$

The clustered-edge mask outlines the clustered edge area in the microscopy as follows:

$$\mathbf{y}_i^{(clu)} = \mathbb{I}_{>1}\Big\{ \sum_{k \in \mathbb{N}} \big(\Omega_i^{(k)} \oplus K - \Omega_i^{(k)} \ominus K \big) \Big\}. \tag{2}$$

The indicator function $\mathbb{I}_{>1}(x)$ is assigned with the value 1 if and only if $x > 1$ holds, otherwise it is valued 0. Representative examples of three masks are illustrated in Fig. 3.

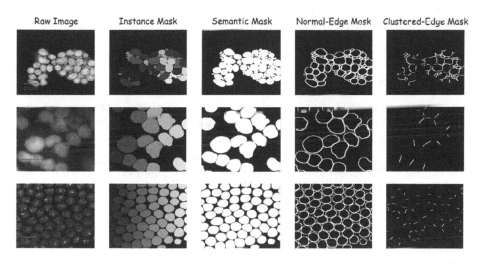

Fig. 3. A few examples of images and their masks. From the left column to the right one presents raw images, instance masks with original manual label, semantic masks, normal-edge masks and the clustered-edge masks, where the latter three column are constructed by the proposed algorithms. The input images are selected from an open-source set [6] and two private sets respectively.

2.2 The Contour-Aware Architecture with 2.5 Decoder Paths (CA$^{2.5}$)

The novel 2.5 decoder output paths are designed for semantic segmentation, normal-edge segmentation, and clustered-edge segmentation respectively, where the latter two share a proportion of convolutional operations and upsampling results on the morphological feature interpretation, marked by the olive color. A notable difference is the extra half path for the clustered-edge segmentation (DSCMs marked by grass green in Fig. 1) together with the sequence-aware instruction module, which distinguishes the CA$^{2.5}$-Net from any conventional contour-aware network.

Different from a direct skip connection between the corresponding encoder block and decoder block in a U-Net based architecture, we apply a couple of dense skip-connection modules targeting fusing semantically similar features. In each dense skip-connection module, a concatenation layer merges the output from its previous convolution layer in the same dense block, together with the relevant upsampling result from the lower dense block. After the fusion of latent features, the concatenated feature maps resume being processed by two 3×3 convolutional layers as shown in Fig. 2a. As we take the clustered edge as a special case of the normal contour, we add the extra interpretation of the former after a general prediction of contour in our method. In this scenario, in the first dense block, a sequence-aware instruction (SAM) module is integrated to learn the priority to handle the multiple cases of edges. The output of the shared-edge decoder and normal-edge decoder are applied with a 1×1 convolutional operation respectively, and followed by a weighted aggregation, as depicted in Fig. 2b.

2.3   Curriculum Learning for CA$^{2.5}$-Net

The accurate contour of clustered-edge is difficult to obtain from a nuclei segmentation network. In other medical image analyses e.g., histology [11], curriculum learning has been proposed to tackle this issue. However, in training a contour-aware network, a satisfying curriculum score is always challenging to find. Innovatively, we propose a curriculum learning model to determine the training sequence by a training difficulty score denoted as $S(\mathbf{x}_i, \mathbf{y}_i^c)$, mainly up to the brightness variation between adjacent nuclei. The sequenced image progressively and efficiently trains the CA$^{2.5}$-Net towards a robust network at the clustered-edge segmentation. The formulation of the $S(\mathbf{x}_i, \mathbf{y}_i^c)$ is constructed as follows.

To quantify the segmentation difficulty coming from the variation of brightness, we first define the averaged brightness as $b : \mathbb{R}^{l \times w} \times \mathbb{N}^{l \times w} \mapsto \mathbb{R}$ of a nuclear area as follows $b(\mathbf{x}_i, \Omega_i^k) = \frac{|\Omega_i^k \cdot \mathbf{x}_i|}{|\Omega_i^k|}$, where $|\cdot|$ is the L^1-norm for matrix. Consequently, our patch-level score function S is computed as follows:

$$S(\mathbf{x}_i, \mathbf{y}_i) = \frac{\sum\limits_{k_1 < k_2} f(\mathbf{x}_i, \Omega_i^{k_1}, \Omega_i^{k_2}) \cdot |\Omega_i^{k_1} \bigwedge \Omega_i^{k_2}|}{\sum\limits_{k_1 < k_2} |\Omega_i^{k_1} \bigwedge \Omega_i^{k_2}|}, \tag{3}$$

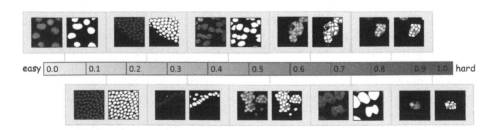

Fig. 4. An example of the sequence result of segmentation difficulty degree level by curriculum learning, with the image and ground truth pair presented from easy to hard.

where matrix $\Omega_i^{k_1} \bigwedge \Omega_i^{k_2} = \left(\min\{a_{i,j}, b_{i,j}\}\right)_{l \times w}$ for $\Omega_i^{k_1} = (a_{i,j})_{l \times m}$ and $\Omega_i^{k_2} = (b_{i,j})_{l \times w}$. And the score function f for one paired clustered-nuclei is defined as

$$f(\mathbf{x}_i, \Omega_i^{k_1}, \Omega_i^{k_2}) = \left(1 - \frac{|b(\mathbf{x}_i, \Omega_i^{k_1}) - b(\mathbf{x}_i, \Omega_i^{k_2})|}{b(\mathbf{x}_i, \Omega_i^{k_1}) + b(\mathbf{x}_i, \Omega_i^{k_2})}\right) \cdot \left(\frac{2b(\mathbf{x}_i, \Omega_i^{k_1} \bigwedge \Omega_i^{k_2})}{b(\mathbf{x}_i, \Omega_i^{k_1}) + b(\mathbf{x}_i, \Omega_i^{k_2})}\right). \quad (4)$$

Particularly, when two clustered nuclei share exactly the same brightness, the first term of f reaches the value of 1.0, associated with a harder training instance. The second term measures the signal decay at the clustered edge, which drastically reduce the difficulty of instance segmentation. In this way, we have all the images in sequence along with their paired masks with their difficulty score in a ascending pattern (Fig. 4).

3   The Privately-Collected Dataset

The experimental dataset consists of 524 fluorescence images sized at 512×512 from an open-source dataset [6] and two privately collected datasets. Our privately collected dataset is comprised of 152 well-annotated images with immunofluorescence staining, dyed with DAPI or fits, favored by biologists for gene regulation analysis. The images were scanned under the Zeiss confocal microscope (LSM880) by the 63× objectives magnifications. The Nuclei in IF images were first annotated automatically with existing non-machine learning methods and then manually annotated by five trained biologists. This dataset distinguishes itself for its severity in nuclei clustering and variety in segmentation difficulty. The collected drosophila nuclei are highly variated in brightness, challenging for semantic segmentation while the deep-sea archaea images are exceptionally complex in clustering. Additionally, its variety is applicable to test a curriculum learning mode.

4   Experimental Results

4.1   Implementations

We implement our network using Pytorch version 1.3.1 in a Python environment version 3.7. The learning rate was set to 10^{-4} at the beginning and with a 0.02 decay rate for every 2 epochs. The batch size is 8. We adopt only IoU loss for semantic masks and both the Smooth Truncated Loss [12], and IoU loss for normal-edge and clustered-edge masks. The overall loss of epoch ep is a weighted composition of 30% semantic mask loss ($\mathcal{L}_{sem}$), 35% normal-edge loss ($\mathcal{L}_{nor}$), and 35% clustered-edge loss ($\mathcal{L}_{clu}$), denotede as:

$$\mathcal{L}^{ep} = 0.3\mathcal{L}_{sem} + 0.35\mathcal{L}_{nor} + 0.35\mathcal{L}_{clu}. \quad (5)$$

The normal-edge mask and clustered-edge mask are merged straightforwardly to obtain the raw segmentation result. Afterwards, the edges are sharpened to achieve a precise boundary. Finally, a subtraction of the precisely-located-edge mask from the semantic mask is performed.

| Raw Image | Ground Truth | CIA-Net | BRP-Net | CA²·⁵-Net (Ours) |

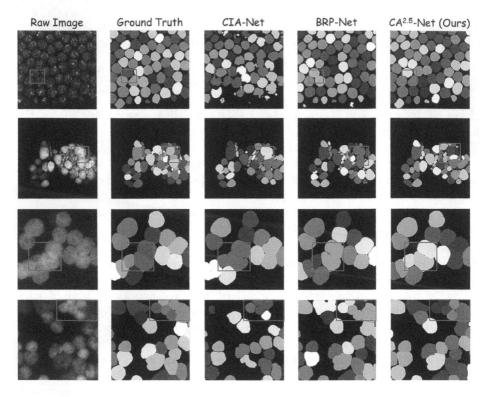

Fig. 5. The segmentation results of our method in comparison with the current competing approaches. The red-color rectangles highlight our advantages over the others on the most challenging scenarios of severely clustered nuclei. A successfully contoured nucleus is marked out by a differential pixel value, whereas the same color across two nuclei is a failed segmentation result. (Color figure online)

4.2   Evaluations

We evaluate our model by comparison on semantic segmentation with DCAN, Unet++, CIA-net, and BRP-net, regarding their prevalence and outstanding performance in the medical image and natural-scene images (Fig. 5). The ablation study is carried out in the benchmark test to verify the effectiveness of our proposal. The results outperform the state-of-the-art networks at the metrics of the Dice score, the Average Jaccard Index (AJI) [7], and the IoU (Table 1). Specifically, the advantages in the AJI evaluation are noticeable, which has been a widely accepted method to quantify the instance-level segmentation performance. The above comparisons demonstrate the effectiveness of $CA^{2.5}$-Net on clustered nuclei segmentation.

Table 1. The experimental results. A comparison of the state-of-the-art approaches is listed in the first 4 rows. CA$^{2.0}$-Net, CANS$^{2.5}$-Net and CArs$^{2.5}$-Net denotes CA$^{2.5}$-Net without clustered-edge specific path, CA$^{2.5}$-Net without sequence-aware instruction module and CA$^{2.5}$-Net with random shuffling respectively. CA$^{2.0}$-Net and CANS$^{2.5}$-Net are the ablation study of clustered-edge path and SAM module, while the row of CArs$^{2.5}$-Net validates the performance of our curriculum learning model. The proposed CA$^{2.5}$-Net demonstrates an observable performance improvement.

	Dice (semantic)	AJI (instance)	IoU (semantic)
DCAN [1]	0.848	0.460	0.751
Unet++ [13]	0.897	0.458	0.821
CIA-Net [12]	0.886	0.622	0.808
BRP-Net [2]	0.918	0.710	0.826
CA$^{2.0}$-Net	0.864	0.643	0.728
CANS$^{2.5}$-Net	0.923	0.759	0.863
CArs$^{2.5}$-Net	0.923	0.753	0.862
CA$^{2.5}$-Net (Ours)	**0.945**	**0.801**	**0.898**

5 Conclusion

In this research, we propose a novel CA$^{2.5}$-Net for nuclei instance segmentation on microscopy images, which has a noticeable performance at tackling clustered-edge nuclei. We also share two privately-collected and well-labeled datasets for further researches in nuclei instance segmentation. All in all, the proposed framework can outperform other competing methods on both the public dataset and the private images, particularly in the most challenging cases where the clustered nuclei are extensive in the image.

References

1. Chen, H., Qi, X., Yu, L., Heng, P.A.: DCAN: deep contour-aware networks for accurate gland segmentation. In: Proceedings of the IEEE conference on Computer Vision and Pattern Recognition, pp. 2487–2496 (2016)
2. Chen, S., Ding, C., Tao, D.: Boundary-assisted region proposal networks for nucleus segmentation. In: Martel, A.L., et al. (eds.) MICCAI 2020. LNCS, vol. 12265, pp. 279–288. Springer, Cham (2020). https://doi.org/10.1007/978-3-030-59722-1_27
3. He, K., Gkioxari, G., Dollár, P., Girshick, R.: Mask R-CNN. In: Proceedings of the IEEE International Conference on Computer Vision, pp. 2961–2969 (2017)
4. Johnson, J.W.: Adapting Mask-RCNN for automatic nucleus segmentation. arXiv preprint arXiv:1805.00500 (2018)
5. Kang, Q., Lao, Q., Fevens, T.: Nuclei segmentation in histopathological images using two-stage learning. In: Shen, D., et al. (eds.) MICCAI 2019. LNCS, vol. 11764, pp. 703–711. Springer, Cham (2019). https://doi.org/10.1007/978-3-030-32239-7_78

6. Kromp, F., et al.: An annotated fluorescence image dataset for training nuclear segmentation methods. Sci. Data **7**(1), 1–8 (2020)
7. Kumar, N., Verma, R., Sharma, S., Bhargava, S., Vahadane, A., Sethi, A.: A dataset and a technique for generalized nuclear segmentation for computational pathology. IEEE Trans. Med. Imaging **36**(7), 1550–1560 (2017)
8. Lin, C.H., Chan, Y.K., Chen, C.C.: Detection and segmentation of cervical cell cytoplast and nucleus. Int. J. Imaging Syst. Technol. **19**(3), 260–270 (2009)
9. Malpica, N., et al.: Applying watershed algorithms to the segmentation of clustered nuclei. Cytometry J. Int. Soc. Anal. Cytol. **28**(4), 289–297 (1997)
10. Ronneberger, O., Fischer, P., Brox, T.: U-net: convolutional networks for biomedical image segmentation. In: Navab, N., Hornegger, J., Wells, W.M., Frangi, A.F. (eds.) MICCAI 2015. LNCS, vol. 9351, pp. 234–241. Springer, Cham (2015). https://doi.org/10.1007/978-3-319-24574-4_28
11. Wei, J., et al.: Learn like a pathologist: curriculum learning by annotator agreement for histopathology image classification. In: Proceedings of the IEEE/CVF Winter Conference on Applications of Computer Vision, pp. 2473–2483 (2021)
12. Zhou, Y., Onder, O.F., Dou, Q., Tsougenis, E., Chen, H., Heng, P.-A.: CIA-net: robust nuclei instance segmentation with contour-aware information aggregation. In: Chung, A.C.S., Gee, J.C., Yushkevich, P.A., Bao, S. (eds.) IPMI 2019. LNCS, vol. 11492, pp. 682–693. Springer, Cham (2019). https://doi.org/10.1007/978-3-030-20351-1_53
13. Zhou, Z., Siddiquee, M.M.R., Tajbakhsh, N., Liang, J.: Unet++: redesigning skip connections to exploit multiscale features in image segmentation. IEEE Trans. Med. Imaging **39**(6), 1856–1867 (2019)

Automated Malaria Cells Detection from Blood Smears Under Severe Class Imbalance via Importance-Aware Balanced Group Softmax

Canfeng Lin[1], Huisi Wu[1(✉)], Zhenkun Wen[1], and Jing Qin[2]

[1] College of Computer Science and Software Engineering, Shenzhen University,
Shenzhen, China
hswu@szu.edu.cn
[2] Centre for Smart Health, School of Nursing,
The Hong Kong Polytechnic University, Hung Hom, Hong Kong

Abstract. Malaria is one of the main threats to global health. Manual examination of thick and thin blood smears is the current gold standard for diagnosing malaria. However, it is of extremely low throughput and susceptible to human bias, and hence, automated detection tools are highly demanded in practice. Developing an automated detection algorithm is a quite challenging due to (1) the wide range of variations in bright field microscopy images, and (2) more importantly, the severe class imbalance problem in this task. While recently proposed balanced group softmax is somehow able to alleviate the problem of class imbalance, the crucial prerequisite for its success is that the samples can be *correctly* categorized into different classes. We present a novel importance-aware BGS (*IaBGS*) to address the class imbalance problem and thereby improve the detection performance. Our main idea is to introduce a *relation module (RM)* before the group softmax module in the network to learn the *relationships* between different cells. We then figure out the feature of a cell by considering the relationships between this cell and other cells in the input image with different cells having different learned weights. In the RM module, we leverage both the appearance features and locations to calculate the feature of each cell to take full advantage of the relationships to obtain more discriminative features for BGS. We conducted extensive experiments on a famous dataset to evaluate the proposed *IaBGS*. Experimental results demonstrate the effectiveness of the proposed approach, consistently outperforming state-of-the-art methods. Codes will be released upon publication.

Keywords: Malaria · Class imbalance · Relationship · Cells detection

1 Introduction

Malaria is a disease caused by the plasmodium parasite. It is one of the main threats to global health; more than 200 million people are infected each year and

© Springer Nature Switzerland AG 2021
M. de Bruijne et al. (Eds.): MICCAI 2021, LNCS 12908, pp. 455–465, 2021.
https://doi.org/10.1007/978-3-030-87237-3_44

more than 400,000 die from the disease [17]. For malaria and other microbial infections, due to the low cost and high flexibility of reagents and instruments, manual examination of thick and thin blood smears by trained microscopists is still the gold standard for parasite detection and stage determination [5]. The concentration of infected cells in the blood of patients at different stages of malaria is different, and hence prescribing the right medicine for patients at different stages is a key part of the treatment of malaria [2,23,24]. In this regard, in order to calculate the concentration, we need to detect and count all types of cells in the field of view during manual examination. However, manual detection and count are of extremely low throughput and susceptible to human bias. Therefore, automatic detection and count tools are highly demanded in practice, as such tools make the diagnosis of malaria much faster, more accurate, and more cost-effective, obtaining the results without consuming huge time and manpower.

Developing such an automatic and reliable detection and count algorithm is, however, a challenging task due to (1) the wide range of variations in bright field microscopy images, and (2) more importantly, the severe class imbalance problem. In the BBBC041 dataset [12], which is also the dataset we use, there are 77523 uninfected cells, accounting for 96.77% of all cells, and infected cells 2590, accounting for 3.23%, which shows the severity of the class imbalance problem in this task.

Under most circumstances, normal red blood cells account for the vast majority in a field of view, which makes red blood cells dominate in the microscopy images. In such a case, a detector tends to categorize all cells into red blood cells, as this will not obviously reduce the entire accuracy of the detector, but, simultaneously and unfortunately, the accuracy of infections is usually very low, which will greatly harm the reliability of the computer-assisted detection system.

Some methods have been proposed for automatically detecting cells in blood smears to assist malaria diagnosis. Early investigations employed hand-crafted features to capture the characteristics of different cells for automated detection [1,13,14,20]. However, these methods are incapable of tackling the wide range of variations in bright field microscopy images and hence cannot reach the clinical use level [18]. Later, some researchers proposed to harness deep learning models to address this challenging task [6,13,15,16,25]. These models still cannot solve the problem of class imbalance well, resulting in their performance is still not satisfactory.

On the other hand, a lot of effort has been dedicated to addressing the problem of class imbalance. These methods can be roughly divided into two categories. The first category is re-sampling, which achieves the goal of balancing the training data by oversampling of low-shot classes or down-sampling of many-shot classes [7,21]. However, re-sampling based methods may lead to the risk of over-fitting to low-shot classes. The other line of research is based on re-weighting, which aims at set different weights for different class to alleviate the class imbalance problem [3,4,8,22]. But these re-weighting based methods are very sensitive to hyper-parameters. Recently, some researchers reported that the standard softmax function may amplify the adverse effects of class imbalance [10]. To tackle this, they proposed an approach, called balanced group softmax (BGS), to putting classes with similar number of samples in a group for softmax and loss calculation. However, while BGS is somehow able to alleviate the problem of class imbalance, the crucial prerequisite for its success is that the samples can be *correctly* categorized into different classes. Otherwise, it will not only make the class imbalance unsolved but also hurt the detection accuracy. Due to severe class imbalance, the features of samples in infrequent class (infected class) are easily diluted or ignored. Our idea is to allow each cell to take into account the difference in appearance characteristics and location information with other cells, so as to make up for the impact of insufficient training examples.

In this paper, we present a novel importance-aware balanced group softmax (*IaBGS*) to address severe class imbalance problem in this challenging task. Our main idea is to introduce a *relation module (RM)* before the group softmax module in the network to learn the *relationships* between different cells. In this case, we figure out the feature of a cell by considering the relationships between this cell and other cells in the input image with different cells having different weights. In the RM module, we leverage both the appearance features and locations to calculate the feature of each cell to take full advantage of the relationships to obtain more discriminative features for BGS. By this way, the proposed *IaBGS* is able to more effectively and accurately solve the class imbalance problem, and thereby achieve better detection performance. We conducted extensive experiments on a famous dataset (BBBC041) [12] to evaluate the proposed *IaBGS*. Experimental results demonstrate the effectiveness of the proposed approach, consistently outperforming state-of-the-art methods.

2   Methodology

We use Faster-rcnn [19] as our baseline model. The overall framework of our method is shown in Fig. 1. The process of multi-scale feature extraction and proposal extraction is consistent with the baseline model. The resulting feature maps consist of multiple scales, each scale performs *IaBGS* respectively. In the figure, we select one of the scale feature map to illustrate.

2.1   Balanced Group Softmax

Our task contains two foreground categories (infected and uninfected), so we set up three groups: $g0$ for background group, $g1$ for infected group, and $g2$ for uninfected group. Nevertheless, since each group conducts its own softmax, each group will have a highest confidence, which makes the final prediction results have multiple categories and adds a lot of false positives. Therefore, we add an *others* category to each group. This category represents other categories that do not belong to the categories in the current group. Apart from this, because of the calculation way of the softmax function, the original category labels need to be converted into the group label. The index of the group label start from

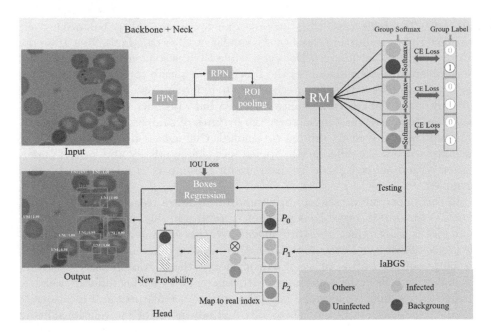

Fig. 1. The overall architecture of our method. CE denotes cross entropy. After the input image is extracted by backbone and neck to extract the ROI under multiple scales, it is input to *RM* and *BGS*. When training, only need to calculate the loss function to update the weight. When testing, it needs to go through the *Head* and finally output. I and UNI denote infected category and uninfected category.

0, which means the *others* category, and 1 means other categories in the group. During training and testing, the process of BGS is different, we will elaborate on it below.

Training. For the feature map of each scale, we use the fully connected layer to connect it with the elements in each group. Each group performs softmax respectively, and calculate the cross-entropy loss after obtaining the in-group probability of each category. In the training process, the probability of i category obtained by group softmax is expressed as:

$$P_n^i = \frac{e^{x_n^i}}{e^{x_n^0} + e^{x_n^1}}, \tag{1}$$

where n denotes the group g_n, 0 and 1 represent the two elements in the group, x refers to the output values of fully connected layers. The three groups of probabilities P_0, P_1, P_2 obtained in this way are calculated for cross-entropy loss with the group labels. The loss function is:

$$\mathcal{L} = -\sum_{n=0}^{2} \sum_{i=0}^{1} y_n^i \log(P_n^i), \tag{2}$$

where y_n denotes the group label of group g_n. For boxes regression branch, we use the simple IOU loss.

Testing. Because there is a difference between the group label and original label, it is necessary to map the group label back to the real label index when testing. As shown in Fig. 1, after the probabilities of each group P_n obtained by group softmax, take the probabilities of the two foreground groups, ignore the *others* category among them, concatenate the remaining probabilities, and multiply them with the *others* category of the background group. Because in the background group, the *others* category represents the sum of the probabilities of all foreground category, we need to multiply it with all foreground category for a calibration. After the calibrated foreground category probability is obtained, it is concatenate with the background class probability in the background group to obtain the final new probability. The category with the highest value in the new probability is the final classification given by the model. Note that the sum of the new probabilities is not equal to 1.

2.2 Relation Module

The premise for better classification is to have more discriminative features map. However, in imbalanced categories problem, the features of the few-shot classes are often diluted or ignored due to insufficient training. Therefore, our idea is to let each cell consider the appearance features differences and locations information with other cells to obtain the relationship. The importance of this relationship are reflected by the set weight.

Under this task, we can think of a cell amount to an object. Assuming that there are n objects in the feature map input to RM, we define it as a set $O = \{f_1, f_2, ..., f_n\}$. We divide the feature map into locations and appearance features, which are defined as f^L and f^A. Locations refer to the information of bounding boxes, which contains the positional relationship between objects. On the other hand, appearance features includes the texture, color, and shape of the objects, which are obtained by feature maps through the fully connected layer. Note that appearance features also need bounding boxes information as input. In order for the model to learn which feature relationships between objects are more important for detection, we introduce location weight ω^L and appearance features weight ω^A. The location weight of the objects i to the object j is calculated as:

$$\omega_{ij}^L = max\{0, W_G \cdot D(f_i^L, f_j^L)\} \tag{3}$$

$$D(f_i^L, f_j^L) = (\log(\frac{|x_i - x_j|}{w_j}), \log(\frac{|y_i - y_j|}{h_j}), \log(\frac{w_i}{w_j})^{\mathrm{T}}, \log(\frac{h_i}{h_j})), \tag{4}$$

where (x, y, w, h) are bounding boxes information, W_G denotes fully connected layer parameters. As for appearance features weight of objects i to the object j, it is computed as:

$$\omega_{ij}^A = \frac{dot(W_Q f_i^A, W_K f_j^A)}{\sqrt{d_k}}, \tag{5}$$

where W_Q and W_K are also fully connected layer parameters, and d_k is a hyper-parameter which represents the key feature dimension, and we set it as 64 in this paper. dot is the dot product calculation.

We calculate these two feature relations separately to refine the calculation of the two relations, but in the end they will work together. Therefore, after obtaining the two weights separately, we need to consider them together. Thus, we define ω_{ij} to express the combined weights:

$$\omega_{ij} = \frac{\omega_{ij}^L \cdot \exp(\omega_{ij}^A)}{\sum_{k=1}^n \omega_{ik}^L \cdot \exp(\omega_{ik}^A)} \tag{6}$$

Here, the relation between object i and other n objects $f_R(i)$ is defined as:

$$f_R(i) = \sum_{j=1}^n \omega_{ij} \cdot (W_V \cdot f_j^A), \tag{7}$$

where W_v is a linear transformation operation, implemented by 1×1 convolution.

Finally, after all the relational features are concatenated, they are added to the original feature maps. The channel of each $f_R(i)$ is $1/n$ of f_i^A, and after concatenating their channel are the same:

$$f_i^A = f_i^A + Concat[f_R^1(i), ..., f_R^n(i)] \tag{8}$$

So far, we have obtained new feature maps which consider the locations and appearance features between each object.

The RM leverages both appearance features and location information to figure out the relation between cells and then generates a new feature map by integrating the relation into original feature map generated from RPN. The new feature map is fed into BSG to help tackle class imbalance. The shape and dimensions of the features remain unchanged after passing through the RM, which also makes the RM plug-and-play.

2.3   Implementation Details

Our experimental environment is pytorch, the GPU device is RTX 2080Ti, and our method is implemented under the framework of mmdetection. The backbone is pre-trained on ImageNet. The original image size is 1600×1200. In order to reduce the memory usage and training time, we resize the image to a size of 1333×800 before training, and then perform random flip as data augmentation. We use SGD with 0.9 momentum as the learning rate strategy, and the initial learning rate is 0.001 and the batch size is 4. Learning rate is reduced in the 9th and 11th epochs. After training for 20 epochs, the weights that perform best on the validation set are selected for testing. We performed five-fold cross-validation on all experiments to prove the effectiveness and robustness of our method.

Table 1. Statistical comparisons of ablation studies. The following numerical results represent (mean) ± (standard deviation)

Method	AP(UNI)	AP(I)	mAP
Baseline	0.951 ± 0.0017	0.657 ± 0.0016	0.804 ± 0.0020
Baseline+BGS	0.945 ± 0.0010	0.829 ± 0.0008	0.887 ± 0.0009
Baseline+RM	0.967 ± 0.0014	0.694 ± 0.0018	0.831 ± 0.0016
Ours (Baseline+BGS+RM)	$\mathbf{0.964 \pm 0.0016}$	$\mathbf{0.846 \pm 0.0016}$	$\mathbf{0.905 \pm 0.0016}$

3 Experiments and Result

3.1 Dataset and Evaluation Metrics

We use P. vivax (malaria) infected human blood smears (BBBC041) [12] as the dataset to validate our method. The dataset includes 1208 training images and 120 test images. We randomly divide 100 pictures from the training set as a validation set to guide the experiment. The cells in the dataset image are divided into 7 categories, but for the diagnosis and cell counting of malaria, currently only need to distinguish whether the cells are infected or normal can meet the requirements. Therefore, we combined RBCs and leukocytes into uninfected categories, and combined other categories into infected categories. For the metrics, Average Precision (AP) and mean Average Precision (mAP) are commonly used metrics in the field of object detection, In this paper, all AP and mAP refer to AP:50 and mAP:50.

3.2 Ablation Studies

We choose Faster-rcnn with the Resnet-50 backbone as the baseline model for ablation experiments. The experimental results and visualization results are shown in Table 1 and Fig. 2, respectively. In the baseline method, due to the imbalance in the number of training instances, the model is not clear about the classification of infected cells, so it predicts two bounding boxes with low confidence. To make matters worse, in some difficult to distinguish cases, the model directly considers the infected cells to be normal cells and gives high confidence. After adding the BGS, the model weakens the suppression effect of many-shot on the few-shot, which greatly improves the AP of the infected categories. After introducing the relation module, the model has improved its ability to detect occluded cells and irregularly shaped cells. In addition, RM also has a calibration effect on object confidence. It can be proved that the appearance features and locations information between the objects extracted by RM improves the detecting ability of model.

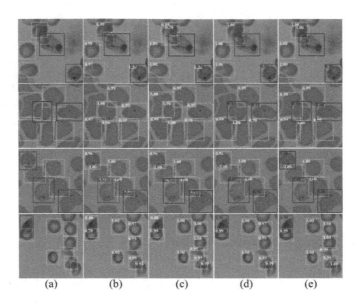

| | | | | |
| (a) | (b) | (c) | (d) | (e) |

Fig. 2. Visual comparison for ablation studies. (a), (b), (c), (d) and (e) represent ground truth, baseline, baseline with RM, baseline with BGS and baseline with RM and BGS, respectively. The green box represents the uninfected category while the red box represents the infected category. The green box represents the uninfected category while the red represents the infected category. (Color figure online)

3.3   Comparison with State-of-the-Art Methods

In order to prove the superiority of our method, we implemented multiple state-of-the-art methods under the detection framework of Faster-rcnn [19] and conducted experiments on the BBBC041 dataset [12], including the weakly supervised method multiple objects feature fusion (MOFF) [15], re-sample method repeat factor sampling (RFS) [7], transfer learning method Open long-tailed Recognition (OLTR) [11], re-weight method class-balanced softmax (CB Softmax) [4], decoupling method τ normalization [9]. For a fair comparison, we conducted experiments in the experimental environment of Sect. 3.2 and adjusted the hyper-parameters of all methods. The experimental statistical results are shown in Table 2, and the visualization results are shown in Fig. 3. We observed the results and found that MOFF only uses image-level labels for detection and did not solve the problem of data imbalance, so the performance is not ideal. RFS, τ normalization and OLTR prove that the methods of re-sample, re-weight and transfer learning are helpful for the problem of data imbalance, but there are still limitations. They do not perform well under the detection of some heavily occluded cells, and the confidence in infected category is not too high. But our method do well in solving these problems, and achieves the best performance in the infected and uninfected class.

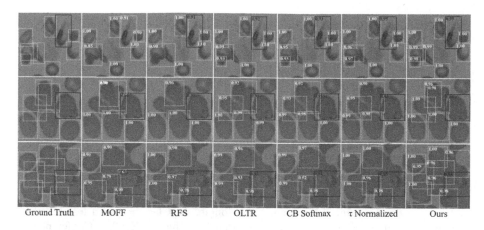

Fig. 3. Visual comparison with state-of-the-art methods. The green box represents the uninfected category while the red represents the infected category. (Color figure online)

Table 2. Statistical comparisons of state-of-the-art methods. The following numerical results represent (mean) ± (standard deviation)

Method	Year	Category	AP(UNI)	AP(I)	mAP
MOFF [15]	2020	Weakly Supervised	0.954 ± 0.0016	0.673 ± 0.0014	0.814 ± 0.0015
RFS [7]	2019	Re-sample	0.950 ± 0.0012	0.742 ± 0.0008	0.846 ± 0.0010
OLTR [11]	2019	Transfer Learning	0.955 ± 0.0008	0.810 ± 0.0006	0.883 ± 0.0007
CB Softmax [4]	2019	Re-weight	0.950 ± 0.0022	0.812 ± 0.0018	0.881 ± 0.0020
τ Normalization [9]	2020	Decoupling	0.957 ± 0.0006	0.821 ± 0.0005	0.889 ± 0.0005
Ours	2021	IaBGS	**0.964 ± 0.0016**	**0.846 ± 0.0016**	**0.905 ± 0.0016**

4   Conclusions

We propose an novel automatic method for malaria blood smear cells detection based on the importance-aware balanced group softmax, which is realized by introducing the RM before the balanced group softmax module. RM take advantage of appearance features and locations of each cell to model relationships, so that model can learn the importance of relationships. Thus, RM can provide more discriminative feature maps for BGS to make up for the shortcomings of BGS. Experiments show that our method improves the ability of the model to detect occluded cells while solving the imbalance of data categories. We compare our method with the state-of-the-art methods, and the result proves that our method defeated all rivals and achieved the optimal performance.

Acknowledgement. This work was supported in part by grants from the National Natural Science Foundation of China (No. 61973221), the Natural Science Foundation of Guangdong Province, China (Nos. 2018A030313381 and 2019A1515011165), the COVID-19 Prevention Project of Guangdong Province, China (No. 2020KZDZX1174), and the Hong Kong Research Grants Council (Project No. PolyU 152035/17E and 15205919).

References

1. Arco, J.E., Górriz, J.M., Ramírez, J., Álvarez, I., Puntonet, C.G.: Digital image analysis for automatic enumeration of malaria parasites using morphological operations. Expert Syst. Appl. **42**(6), 3041–3047 (2015)
2. Ashley, E.A., et al.: Spread of artemisinin resistance in plasmodium falciparum malaria. N. Engl. J. Med. **371**(5), 411–423 (2014)
3. Cao, K., Wei, C., Gaidon, A., Arechiga, N., Ma, T.: Learning imbalanced datasets with label-distribution-aware margin loss. arXiv preprint arXiv:1906.07413 (2019)
4. Cui, Y., Jia, M., Lin, T.Y., Song, Y., Belongie, S.: Class-balanced loss based on effective number of samples. In: Proceedings of the IEEE/CVF Conference on Computer Vision and Pattern Recognition, pp. 9268–9277 (2019)
5. Das, D.K., Mukherjee, R., Chakraborty, C.: Computational microscopic imaging for malaria parasite detection: a systematic review. J. Microsc. **260**(1), 1–19 (2015)
6. Doering, E., Pukropski, A., Krumnack, U., Schaffand, A.: Automatic detection and counting of malaria parasite-infected blood cells. In: Su, R., Liu, H. (eds.) MICAD 2020. LNEE, vol. 633, pp. 145–157. Springer, Singapore (2020). https://doi.org/10.1007/978-981-15-5199-4_15
7. Gupta, A., Dollar, P., Girshick, R.: LVIS: a dataset for large vocabulary instance segmentation. In: Proceedings of the IEEE/CVF Conference on Computer Vision and Pattern Recognition, pp. 5356–5364 (2019)
8. Huang, C., Li, Y., Loy, C.C., Tang, X.: Deep imbalanced learning for face recognition and attribute prediction. IEEE Trans. Pattern Anal. Mach. Intell. **42**(11), 2781–2794 (2019)
9. Kang, B., et al.: Decoupling representation and classifier for long-tailed recognition. arXiv preprint arXiv:1910.09217 (2019)
10. Li, Y., et al.: Overcoming classifier imbalance for long-tail object detection with balanced group softmax. In: Proceedings of the IEEE/CVF Conference on Computer Vision and Pattern Recognition, pp. 10991–11000 (2020)
11. Liu, Z., Miao, Z., Zhan, X., Wang, J., Gong, B., Yu, S.X.: Large-scale long-tailed recognition in an open world. In: Proceedings of the IEEE/CVF Conference on Computer Vision and Pattern Recognition, pp. 2537–2546 (2019)
12. Ljosa, V., Sokolnicki, K.L., Carpenter, A.E.: Annotated high-throughput microscopy image sets for validation. Nat. Methods **9**(7), 637 (2012)
13. Loddo, A., Di Ruberto, C., Kocher, M.: Recent advances of malaria parasites detection systems based on mathematical morphology. Sensors **18**(2), 513 (2018)
14. Loddo, A., Di Ruberto, C., Kocher, M., Prod'Hom, G.: MP-IDB: the malaria parasite image database for image processing and analysis. In: Lepore, N., Brieva, J., Romero, E., Racoceanu, D., Joskowicz, L. (eds.) SaMBa 2018. LNCS, vol. 11379, pp. 57–65. Springer, Cham (2019). https://doi.org/10.1007/978-3-030-13835-6_7
15. Manescu, P., Bendkowski, C., Claveau, R., Elmi, M., Brown, B.J., Pawar, V., Shaw, M.J., Fernandez-Reyes, D.: A weakly supervised deep learning approach for detecting malaria and sickle cells in blood films. In: International Conference on Medical Image Computing and Computer-Assisted Intervention. pp. 226–235. Springer (2020)

16. Mehanian, C., et al.: Computer-automated malaria diagnosis and quantitation using convolutional neural networks. In: Proceedings of the IEEE International Conference on Computer Vision Workshops, pp. 116–125 (2017)

17. World Health Organization et al.: World malaria report 2020: 20 years of global progress and challenges (2020)

18. Poostchi, M., Silamut, K., Maude, R.J., Jaeger, S., Thoma, G.: Image analysis and machine learning for detecting malaria. Transl. Res. **194**, 36–55 (2018)

19. Ren, S., He, K., Girshick, R., Sun, J.: Faster R-CNN: towards real-time object detection with region proposal networks. arXiv preprint arXiv:1506.01497 (2015)

20. Rosado, L., Da Costa, J.M.C., Elias, D., Cardoso, J.S.: Automated detection of malaria parasites on thick blood smears via mobile devices. Procedia Comput. Sci. **90**, 138–144 (2016)

21. Shen, L., Lin, Z., Huang, Q.: Relay backpropagation for effective learning of deep convolutional neural networks. In: Leibe, B., Matas, J., Sebe, N., Welling, M. (eds.) ECCV 2016. LNCS, vol. 9911, pp. 467–482. Springer, Cham (2016). https://doi.org/10.1007/978-3-319-46478-7_29

22. Shu, J., et al.: Meta-weight-net: learning an explicit mapping for sample weighting. arXiv preprint arXiv:1902.07379 (2019)

23. Slater, H.C., et al.: The temporal dynamics and infectiousness of subpatent plasmodium falciparum infections in relation to parasite density. Nat. Commun. **10**(1), 1–16 (2019)

24. White, N.: The parasite clearance curve. Malaria J. **10**(1), 1–8 (2011)

25. Zhao, O.S., et al.: Convolutional neural networks to automate the screening of malaria in low-resource countries. PeerJ **8**, e9674 (2020)

Non-parametric Vignetting Correction for Sparse Spatial Transcriptomics Images

Bovey Y. Rao[1,2], Alexis M. Peterson[2], Elena K. Kandror[2],
Stephanie Herrlinger[1,2], Attila Losonczy[1,2,3], Liam Paninski[2,4,5,6],
Abbas H. Rizvi[2(✉)], and Erdem Varol[2,4,5,6(✉)]

[1] Department of Neuroscience, Columbia University, New York, NY, USA
[2] Zuckerman Mind Brain Behavior Institute, Columbia University,
New York, NY, USA
abbas.rizvi@columbia.edu
[3] Kavli Institute for Brain Sciences, Columbia University, New York, NY, USA
[4] Department of Statistics, Columbia University, New York, NY, USA
[5] Grossman Center for the Statistics of the Mind, Columbia University,
New York, NY, USA
[6] Center for Theoretical Neuroscience, Columbia University, New York, NY, USA
ev2430@columbia.edu

Abstract. Spatial transcriptomics techniques such as STARmap [15] enable the subcellular detection of RNA transcripts within complex tissue sections. The data from these techniques are impacted by optical microscopy limitations, such as shading or vignetting effects from uneven illumination during image capture. Downstream analysis of these sparse spatially resolved transcripts is dependent upon the correction of these artefacts. This paper introduces a novel non-parametric vignetting correction tool for spatial transcriptomic images, which estimates the illumination field and background using an efficient iterative sliced histogram normalization routine. We show that our method outperforms the state-of-the-art shading correction techniques both in terms of illumination and background field estimation and requires fewer input images to perform the estimation adequately. We further demonstrate an important downstream application of our technique, showing that spatial transcriptomic volumes corrected by our method yield a higher and more uniform gene expression spot-calling in the rodent hippocampus. Python code and a demo file to reproduce our results are provided in the supplementary material and at this github page: https://github.com/BoveyRao/Non-parametric-vc-for-sparse-st.

B. Y. Rao and A. M. Peterson—These authors contributed equally.

Electronic supplementary material The online version of this chapter (https://doi.org/10.1007/978-3-030-87237-3_45) contains supplementary material, which is available to authorized users.

© Springer Nature Switzerland AG 2021
M. de Bruijne et al. (Eds.): MICCAI 2021, LNCS 12908, pp. 466–475, 2021.
https://doi.org/10.1007/978-3-030-87237-3_45

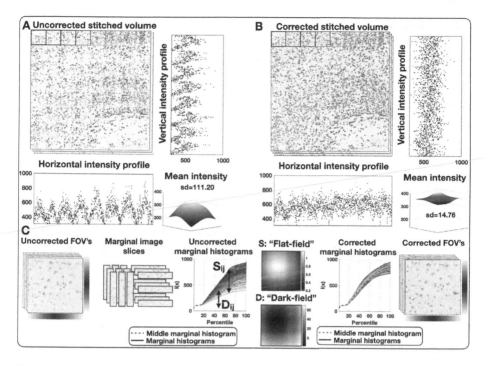

Fig. 1. Overview of the proposed method. A: Vignetting in individual FOVs results in discontinuities in pixel intensities in stitched volumes. B: After applying our proposed technique, the pixel intensities are made uniform across the entire FOV, yielding seamless intensity profiles in stitched volumes. C: Our method estimates the "flat-field" and "dark-field" pixel transformation matrices by iteratively scaling and shifting the histograms of vertical and horizontal strips of all FOVs to match the histograms of "central" strips of the FOVs. The iteratively estimated parameters are then used to derive "flat-field" and "dark-field" matrices. These matrices are then applied to each FOV to ensure that all marginal histograms match closely with the histogram of central regions, ensuring uniformity of pixel intensities throughout all FOVs, countering the effects of vignetting.

1   Introduction

Complex neural representations necessitate experimental and analytical schemes to assess genetically defined cellular populations with spatial resolution. *in situ* sequencing [6,7] affords the ability to interrogate neural circuits within a histological context but is subject to optical limitations. Uneven illumination fields, optical vignetting, chromatic aberration, and detection noise are inherent to imaging platforms and are a significant obstacle to accurately determine the precise number and location of gene expression *in situ*.

In addition to a wealth of literature on vignetting correction in natural images [3,17], several techniques have been introduced in recent years for microscopy applications [9–12]. These techniques address non-uniformity in illumination but underperform when applied to spatial transcriptomic images, given the inherent sparsity. Furthermore, they often require tedious parameter settings to reflect the sparsity of the cell population under view.

In this paper, we posit that if there was no vignetting, aggregated marginal regions of images in a large sample would follow roughly similar intensity distributions due to spatial randomization of objects in view. This property exists regardless of the sparsity of cells in the field of view (FOV), but rather as a consequence of the uniform distribution of objects in arbitrarily imaged tissue sections. Thus, the objective of vignetting correction can be cast as a marginal histogram matching problem [4] aiming to minimize differences in the intensity profiles across different regions of images. To accomplish this, we propose an algorithm that first generates histograms corresponding to horizontal and vertical strips from each FOV. Then, these histograms are iteratively normalized to a reference histogram. The scaling and offsets used to normalize histograms are then used to estimate global transformation terms that reflect the level of spatial amplification needed to uniformize the pixel intensities throughout the slice samples within each FOV.

We extensively evaluate our method in a real rodent spatial transcriptomics dataset and show that it significantly outperforms the state-of-the-art microscopy vignetting correction tools, BASIC [9,10] and CIDRE [12]. Furthermore, we demonstrate an important downstream application of our method by using it to assist in STARmap [15] *in situ* sequencing imaging-based detection of transcripts within the CA1 region of the mouse hippocampus, demonstrating significantly enhanced detection of transcript specific barcodes [1].

2   Method

We first introduce notation. Let $I \in \mathbf{R}^{N,M}$ denote a $(N \times M)$ observed spatial transcriptomics FOV such that $I_{i,j}$ denotes the pixel intensity at the (i, j)th pixel (row/column). We model the observed pixel value as having been transformed from the "true" pixel value, $I_{i,j}^0$, through a transformation by a multiplicative "flat-field" matrix, $S \in \mathbf{R}^{N,M}$ and an additive "dark-field" matrix, $D \in \mathbf{R}^{N,M}$:

$$I_{i,j} = I_{i,j}^0 S_{i,j} + D_{i,j} + \epsilon \tag{1}$$

The "flat-field" and "dark-field" matrices model the shading inhomogeneities of foreground and background of the images, respectively [9].

Next, we make an observation that the pixel intensity profiles captured at different rows and columns of many random images would be indicative of potential vignetting artefacts. For example, in a large set of images, if the objects in the bottom right of the image always tend to be darker than the objects in the center of the image, regardless of the objects in view, we can posit that the pixels in the bottom right of the image is subject to lower values of flat-field transformations.

We can quantify pixel intensities using marginal histograms sampled at different rows and columns of images. To estimate the transformation matrices S

and $\boldsymbol{D}$, we propose to normalize histograms obtained from horizontal and vertical strips of the FOV slices to match the histograms of a "central" reference strip (the robustness is addressed in the Supplementary Materials). We then use the histogram normalization parameters to decode a full spatial estimate of the "flat-field" ($\boldsymbol{S}$) and "dark-field" ($\boldsymbol{D}$) matrices. The key idea behind this procedure is that a properly corrected set of images should have indistinguishable histograms in different regions of the image space. See Fig. 1 for an illustration.

In detail, let $F_{I_{i,:}}^{-1}(q)$ denote the inverse cumulative distribution function (iCDF), evaluating the qth quantile ($0 \leq q \leq 1$) of the ith row of the **all** FOVs and $F_{I_{:,j}}^{-1}(q)$ denote the same thing for the jth column. Furthermore, let $F_{I_0}^{-1}(q)$ denote the iCDF of a reference strip of the FOV. Note that discretely sampling iCDF is equivalent to generating histograms. Thus, the objective of linearly normalizing the marginally sliced histograms to the reference histogram can be formulated as a linearly parametrized sliced Wasserstein distance [4] minimization problem:

$$\min_{s,d} \int_0^1 ||F_{I_0}^{-1}(q) - F_{I_{i,:}}^{-1}(q)s - d||_2^2 dq \longrightarrow [s \ d]^T = [F_{I_{i,:}}^{-1} \ \mathbf{1}]^\dagger F_{I_0}^{-1} \quad (2)$$

Here the scalars s and d account for the scaling and additive offsetting of the ith horizontal marginal histogram to match the reference histogram. These terms can be derived by sampling the iCDFs at a discrete number of bins and solving a linear regression problem with the closed form solution: $[s \ d]^T = [F_{I_{i,:}}^{-1} \ \mathbf{1}]^\dagger F_{I_0}^{-1}$, with $\dagger$ denoting the Moore–Penrose pseudoinverse. If this operation is repeated for all horizontal slices, we get the vectors $\boldsymbol{S}^{\text{horiz}}, \boldsymbol{D}^{\text{horiz}} \in \mathbf{R}^N$. Next, this procedure can be repeated for all vertical slices to yield $\boldsymbol{S}^{\text{vert}}, \boldsymbol{D}^{\text{vert}} \in \mathbf{R}^M$. If we repeat this procedure, estimating the iterates of $\boldsymbol{S}^{t,\text{horiz}}, \boldsymbol{D}^{t,\text{horiz}}, \boldsymbol{S}^{t,\text{vert}}, \boldsymbol{D}^{t,\text{vert}}$ at the tth round whilst simultaneously normalizing the corresponding sliced histograms, we arrive at the following formula to derive an estimate of the "flat-field" and "dark-field" terms:

$$\boldsymbol{S} = \mathbf{1}\mathbf{1}^T \oslash \boldsymbol{S}', \quad \boldsymbol{D} = -\boldsymbol{D}' \oslash \boldsymbol{S}' \quad (3)$$

where $\oslash$ denotes elementwise division and $\boldsymbol{S}'$ and $\boldsymbol{D}'$ are given by:

$$\boldsymbol{S}' = \left(\prod_t \text{diag}(\boldsymbol{S}^{t,\text{horiz}}) \mathbf{1}\mathbf{1}^T \prod_t \text{diag}(\boldsymbol{S}^{t,\text{vert}}) \right) \quad (4)$$

$$\boldsymbol{D}' = \sum_t \boldsymbol{D}^{t,\text{horiz}} \odot \left(\prod_{T-t} \text{diag}(\boldsymbol{S}^{t,\text{horiz}}) \mathbf{1}\mathbf{1}^T \prod_{T-t} \text{diag}(\boldsymbol{S}^{t,\text{vert}}) \right) +$$
$$\left(\prod_{T-t} \text{diag}(\boldsymbol{S}^{t,\text{horiz}}) \mathbf{1}\mathbf{1}^T \prod_{T-t} \text{diag}(\boldsymbol{S}^{t,\text{vert}}) \right) \odot \boldsymbol{D}^{t,\text{vert}}.$$

Here $\odot$ denotes row-wise or column-wise multiplication and $\text{diag}(\cdot)$ denotes diagonal matrix. The pseudocode for the routine is provided in Algorithm 1.

Parameter Setting and Histogram Slicing: Note that the procedure to derive sliced iterates of S and D is convergent since each minimization round monotonically reduces the Wasserstein distance to the reference histogram. Importantly, unlike in BASIC [10] where the user has to specify the sparsity penalty, our routine only requires the setting of the level of histogram discretization by a number of bins. Higher number of bins provides more emphasis to middle quantiles of pixel intensities and lower number bins emphasizes the extremes, such as min and max and may provide higher contrast levels in corrected images.

Also, the slicing of marginal histograms does not need to be at a single pixel resolution, and "strips" consisting of multiple contiguous sets of image rows/columns can be utilized and share the same scaling and additive terms. Alternatively, images can be downsampled and sliced along single pixel row/columns to estimate the transformation terms which then can be upsampled to correct full resolution images.

Rank-One Assumption of the Vignetting Field: The estimated "flat-field" and "dark field" are presumed to be rank one by construction. In practice such an assumption is sufficient to capture the convex shaped vignetting field observed in most imaging setups and is due to how we structure the histograms (by rows/columns). Hypothetically, we can normalize arbitrary shapes of histograms, it is possible to sample "checkerboard" patterns of histograms and model any arbitrary rank/shape of vignetting fields.

Algorithm 1. Iterative sliced histogram normalization

Input: Observed set of n FOV's: $I = \{I^{u(1),v(1)}, \ldots, I^{u(n),v(n)}\} \in \mathbf{R}^{N,M}$

1: **for** $t = 1, \ldots$ number of iterations **do**
2:     **Horizontal normalization:** Estimate linear regression terms to match ith horizontal histogram to the reference histogram
3:     **for** $i = 1, \ldots, N$ **do**
4:         $[S_i^{(t,\mathrm{horiz})} \; D_i^{(t,\mathrm{horiz})}]^T = \min_{s,d} \int_0^1 ||F_{I_0}^{-1}(q) - F_{I_{i,:}}^{-1}(q)s - d||_2^2 dq$
5:     **end for**
6:     $I \longleftarrow S^{(t,\mathrm{horiz})} \mathbf{1}_M^T \odot I + D^{(t,\mathrm{horiz})} \mathbf{1}_M^T$ for all FOV's
7:     **Vertical normalization:** Estimate linear regression terms to match jth vertical histogram to the reference histogram
8:     **for** $j = 1, \ldots, M$ **do**
9:         $[S_j^{(t,\mathrm{vert})} \; D_i^{(t,\mathrm{vert})}]^T = \min_{s,d} \int_0^1 ||F_{I_0}^{-1}(q) - F_{I_{:,j}}^{-1}(q)s - d||_2^2 dq$
10:     **end for**
11:     $I \longleftarrow \mathbf{1}_N S^{(t,\mathrm{vert})T} \odot I + \mathbf{1}_N D^{(t,\mathrm{vert})T}$ for all FOV's
12: **end for**
13: **return** Corrected set of FOV's: $\{I^{u(1),v(1)}, \ldots, I^{u(n),v(n)}\} \in \mathbf{R}^{N,M}$
    "flat-field" S and "dark-field" D estimates, using Eq. (3).

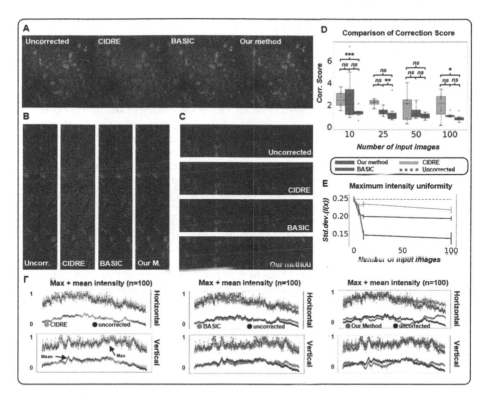

Fig. 2. Vignetting correction evaluation. A: Maximum projection comparison using 3 methods with 100 input images. B: Representative left-right overlap. C: Representative top-bottom overlap. D: Correction scores from 4 left-right and 4 top-bottom overlapping sections. E: Uniformity metric of bootstrapped 0.1% samples of Gaussian filtered maximum projections. F: Vertical and horizontal intensity profiles for max and mean projections compared to that of the raw image. Our method produces flatter images for maximum projections, while having a lower uniformity metric and equal or lower correction scores (*p < 0.05, **p < 0.01, and $* * *$p < 0.001 for paired t-test). *See Supplementary Materials for additional panels.* (Color figure online)

3   Results

Data and Imaging System Description: STARmap based *in situ* sequencing was performed as previously described [15], utilizing five rounds (of 4 color channels each) of sequencing by ligation to detect 44 transcripts in 20 micron sections of the murine hippocampus. Samples were imaged using an Andor Dragonfly spinning disk confocal microscope [8] utilizing Borealis conditioning for each excitation wavelength and sCMOS based detection of fluorescent output to yield 2048×2048 pixel FOV's that cover $200\,\mu\text{m} \times 200\,\mu\text{m}$ area at $60\times$ magnification. The depth slices are acquired at increments of $0.22\,\mu\text{m}$. Imaged sequencing rounds were rigidly registered using fast-Fourier-transform-based phase correlation [2]. Our vignetting correction was applied to this field of view with a downsample factor of 50 and bin size 40, over 5 iterations. After registration, BarDensr [1] was used for spot detection using a detection threshold of 0.95, blur level 2 pixels, tile size of 250×250 pixels, and $5\times$ downsample level.

Evaluation Approaches: For real microscopy images where the ground truth is not available, a thorough evaluation of vignetting correction methods is not trivial. One approach is to compare the estimated flat-field term, $\hat{S}$, with a reference flat-field, S_{ref}, obtained from a calibration experiment [14]. The key challenge of such a validation is to acquire a reliable reference. As we did not have that option, for one metric, we measured the uniformity of illumination in corrected FOV's by taking the std of pixel intensities in aggregated mean or maximum projected images. This evaluation metric can be formulated as:

$$\textbf{Uniformity metric: } u(I,\sigma) = \sqrt{(1/NM)\sum_{i,j}\left(f(I,\sigma)_{i,j} - (1/NM)\sum_{i,j}f(I,\sigma)_{i,j}\right)^2} \quad (5)$$

where $f(I,\sigma)_{i,j}$ denotes i,jth pixel of the max or mean image that has been Gaussian filtered with a kernel width of σ pixels. We evaluate this metric on z-scored pixel intensities (evaluated across the entire FOV) to keep the scale of this metric normalized and enable comparison across different methods.

In addition to the Uniformity metric we described, we also implemented the correction score (I^{corr}) based strategy of measured differences in overlapping regions [9]. This value is formulated as:

$$\textbf{Correction score [9]: } \Gamma'(I^{corr}) = \frac{\sum_x |I_a^{corr}(x) - I_b^{corr}(x)|}{\sum_x |I_a^{meas}(x) - I_b^{meas}(x)|} \quad (6)$$

This correction score generates a metric where 0 is a perfect correction, <1 is an improvement from the uncorrected images, 1 is the same as the uncorrected images, and >1 is worse than the uncorrected images.

Vignetting Correction Comparisons with the State-of-the-Art: We compared our method with CIDRE [12] and BASIC [9,10]. CIDRE was the first method to estimate both light and dark fields for image correction [12]. BASIC is another image correction method that estimates the light and dark field and uses sparse and low-rank decomposition to correct vignetting [9,10]. For BASIC and CIDRE, we utilized the respective ImageJ plugins with their default parameters, while using the parameters mentioned above for our method in Python. Our test image stack was from the murine spatial transcriptomic experiment with dimensions of $2048 \times 2048 \times 191$. We selected random subsets of 5, 10, 25, 50, and 100 image slices to build correction models for all three methods.

All three methods showed some level of vignetting correction from the uncorrected images (Fig. 2A). We applied the correction score methodology on 8 sets of overlapping regions (4 top-bottom, 4 left-right) (Fig. 2B-C). Our correction score results across all numbers of input images were equal or lower than both

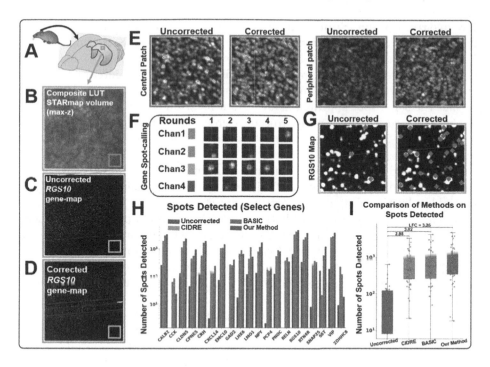

Fig. 3. Vignetting correction improves spot calling and gene detection. A: STARmap based detection of 44 transcripts within CA1. B: Data was rigidly registered and projected across the depth axis. C: Detection of the RGS10 transcript in uncorrected image yields uneven spot calling and uneven localization. D: Vignetting correction enhances spot detection of RGS10. E: Magnified fields of view from central (red) and peripheral (blue) regions. F: RGS10 spot detected using BarDensr following vignetting correction G: RGS10 has a higher rate of detection post vignetting correction (green). H: Absolute gene count for uncorrected (blue) versus vignetting corrected images using CIDRE (orange), BASIC (green), and our method (red). I: Gene spots detected in uncorrected and corrected images with average log fold change (LFC). Our method improves spot detection as compared to CIDRE and BASIC correction methods. (Color figure online)

CIDRE and BASIC (Fig. 2D). We also bootstrapped 0.1% samples of Gaussian filtered pixels and computed the Uniformity metric, where our method had the lowest value (Fig. 2E). We also observed the maximum and mean intensities along the horizontal and vertical axes to provide another qualitative metric for the corrected stack's flatness (Fig. 2F and in the Supplementary Materials). Our vignetting correction method works more effectively on maximum intensities than BASIC and CIDRE with roughly equivalent results for mean intensities.

Gene spot calling techniques like BarDensr [1] utilize thresholding of high-intensity pixels across multiple rounds of barcode imaging, so our technique, which corrects higher quantiles such as the maximum projection, is functionally more relevant for such types of downstream analysis.

Downstream Gene Spot Calling Analysis: We examined the utility of our method towards spot detection, a process critical to *in situ* sequencing. We performed STARmap multiplexed *in situ* sequencing of the mouse CA1 hippocampal region over five rounds, probing 44 distinct transcripts of interest (Fig. 3A). Sample drift was accounted for by rigidly registering [2] spots round-by-round so that the same spot appeared in a constant location across all rounds. Following registration, the data were projected across the depth axis (Z) to create a $5 \times 4 \times 2048 \times 2048$ (rounds × channels × image area in pixels) matrix as input into BarDensr (Fig. 3B).

We focused on RGS10, an enriched gene in the hippocampus [5]. In the uncorrected image, detection of RGS10 was sparse and nonuniform, with poor spatial localization (Fig. 3C). Vignetting correction using our approach increased spot calls and their spatial distribution (Fig. 3D). It also improved homogeneity and spot visualization when comparing uncorrected and corrected spots in the central region (red) and periphery (blue) (Fig. 3E). An example of an RGS10 spot fitting these criteria is shown in Fig. 3F. The detection rate of RGS10 improved overall after vignetting correction, and is highlighted specifically in the central region (Fig. 3G).

Absolute gene count was quantified in the uncorrected data and data corrected using CIDRE, BASIC, and our method. As compared to uncorrected data, overall transcript detection increased by an order of magnitude. Previously undetected transcripts, such as GAD2, a marker for interneurons [16], were observed. Many markers were enhanced using our method as compared to CIDRE and BASIC (Fig. 3H and Fig. S15). We compared the average log fold change of spots detected using each vignetting corrected method with the uncorrected data, and our method provided the most consistent increase in spot detection (Fig. 3I). Correction of uneven illumination field using our method offers enhanced analysis of transcriptional activation and localization in tissue.

Conclusion: The approach we describe offers a generalized method to contend with uneven illumination fields, resulting in heightened quantification of multiplexed *in situ* data. Our approach may offer value to time resolved photobleaching, enabling enhanced discrimination of metabolic flux in tissue and address depth based intensity dropoff effects that result from scattering occurring during deep tissue imaging. Although we highlight the application of this algorithm in murine hippocampal tissue, we anticipate it will offer value towards translational applications including spatially resolved transcriptomic studies of cancer and neurodegenerative diseases as well as other imaging modalities such as 2-photon calcium imaging [13].

Acknowledgements. BYR, SH, and AL are supported by NIMH 1R01MH124047 and 1R01MH124867; and NINDS 1U19NS104590 and 1U01NS115530. SH also is supported by NIMH 5K00MH121382. AMP, EKK, and AHR are funded from CZF2019-002460 and 1R01MH124047-01. LP, EV are supported by Simons Foundation 543023, NSF 1912194, NSF NeuroNex Award 1707398 and The Gatsby Charitable Foundation GAT3708.

References

1. Chen, S., Loper, J., Chen, X., Zador, T., Paninski, L.: Barcode demixing through non-negative spatial regression (BarDensr). bioRxiv (2020)
2. Guizar-Sicairos, M., Thurman, S.T., Fienup, J.R.: Efficient subpixel image registration algorithms. Opt. Lett. **33**(2), 156–158 (2008)
3. Kim, S.J., Pollefeys, M.: Robust radiometric calibration and vignetting correction. IEEE Trans. Pattern Anal. Mach. Intell. **30**(4), 562–576 (2008)
4. Kolouri, S., Zou, Y., Rohde, G.K.: Sliced Wasserstein kernels for probability distributions. In: Proceedings of the IEEE Conference on Computer Vision and Pattern Recognition, pp. 5258–5267 (2016)
5. Lee, J.K., Chung, J., Druey, K.M., Tansey, M.G.: Rgs10 exerts a neuroprotective role through the PKA/C-AMP response-element (CREB) pathway in dopaminergic neuron-like cells. J. Neurochem. **122**(2), 333–343 (2012)
6. Lee, J.H., et al.: Highly multiplexed subcellular RNA sequencing in situ. Science **343**(6177), 1360–1363 (2014)
7. Mitra, R.D., Shendure, J., Olejnik, J., Church, G.M., et al.: Fluorescent in situ sequencing on polymerase colonies. Anal. Biochem. **320**(1), 55–65 (2003)
8. Oreopoulos, J., Berman, R., Browne, M.: Spinning-disk confocal microscopy: present technology and future trends. Methods Cell Biol. **123**, 153–175 (2014)
9. Peng, T., et al.: A basic tool for background and shading correction of optical microscopy images. Nat. Commun. **8**(1), 1–7 (2017)
10. Peng, T., Wang, L., Bayer, C., Conjeti, S., Baust, M., Navab, N.: Shading correction for whole slide image using low rank and sparse decomposition. In: Golland, P., Hata, N., Barillot, C., Hornegger, J., Howe, R. (eds.) MICCAI 2014. LNCS, vol. 8673, pp. 33–40. Springer, Cham (2014). https://doi.org/10.1007/978-3-319-10404-1_5
11. Piccinini, F., Bevilacqua, A., Smith, K., Horvath, P.: Vignetting and photo-bleaching correction in automated fluorescence microscopy from an array of overlapping images. In: 2013 IEEE 10th International Symposium on Biomedical Imaging, pp. 464–467. IEEE (2013)
12. Smith, K., et al.: CIDRE: an illumination-correction method for optical microscopy. Nat. Methods **12**(5), 404–406 (2015)
13. Stosiek, C., Garaschuk, O., Holthoff, K., Konnerth, A.: In vivo two-photon calcium imaging of neuronal networks. Proc. Natl. Acad. Sci. **100**(12), 7319–7324 (2003)
14. Tomaževič, D., Likar, B., Pernuš, F.: Comparative evaluation of retrospective shading correction methods. J. Microsc. **208**(3), 212–223 (2002)
15. Wang, X., et al.: Three-dimensional intact-tissue sequencing of single-cell transcriptional states. Science **361**(6400) (2018)
16. Zeisel, A., et al.: Cell types in the mouse cortex and hippocampus revealed by single-cell RNA-Seq. Science **347**(6226), 1138–1142 (2015)
17. Zheng, Y., Lin, S., Kambhamettu, C., Yu, J., Kang, S.B.: Single-image vignetting correction. IEEE Trans. Pattern Anal. Mach. Intell. **31**(12), 2243–2256 (2008)

Multi-StyleGAN: Towards Image-Based Simulation of Time-Lapse Live-Cell Microscopy

Christoph Reich, Tim Prangemeier, Christian Wildner, and Heinz Koeppl[✉]

Centre for Synthetic Biology, Department of Electrical Engineering
and Information Technology, Department of Biology,
Technische Universität Darmstadt, Darmstadt, Germany
heinz.koeppl@bcs.tu-darmstadt.de

Abstract. Time-lapse fluorescent microscopy (TLFM) combined with predictive mathematical modelling is a powerful tool to study the inherently dynamic processes of life on the single-cell level. Such experiments are costly, complex and labour intensive. A complimentary approach and a step towards *in silico* experimentation, is to synthesise the imagery itself. Here, we propose Multi-StyleGAN as a descriptive approach to simulate time-lapse fluorescence microscopy imagery of living cells, based on a past experiment. This novel generative adversarial network synthesises a multi-domain sequence of consecutive timesteps. We showcase Multi-StyleGAN on imagery of multiple live yeast cells in microstructured environments and train on a dataset recorded in our laboratory. The simulation captures underlying biophysical factors and time dependencies, such as cell morphology, growth, physical interactions, as well as the intensity of a fluorescent reporter protein. An immediate application is to generate additional training and validation data for feature extraction algorithms or to aid and expedite development of advanced experimental techniques such as online monitoring or control of cells.

Code and dataset is available at https://git.rwth-aachen.de/bcs/projects/tp/multi-stylegan.

Keywords: Generative adversarial networks · Deep learning · Time-lapse fluorescence microscopy · Systems biology · Synthetic biology

1 Introduction

Time-lapse fluorescent microscope (TLFM) is a powerful tool to study the inherently dynamic processes of life on the single-cell level [6,23,24,27,29]. TLFM

C. Reich and T. Prangemeier—Both authors contributed equally.

Electronic supplementary material The online version of this chapter (https://doi.org/10.1007/978-3-030-87237-3_46) contains supplementary material, which is available to authorized users.

M. de Bruijne et al. (Eds.): MICCAI 2021, LNCS 12908, pp. 476–486, 2021.
https://doi.org/10.1007/978-3-030-87237-3_46

yields vast amounts of multi-domain imagery from which pertinent quantitative measures can be extracted. These domains are typically a brightfield (BF) channel that captures the spatial structure and organisation of cells (Fig. 1 top), and one or more fluorescent channels (Fig. 1 bottom) upon which the abundance of biomolecular species can be quantified from fluorescence intensities [23,24,28–30]. These quantitative measures promise to constitute the backbone for understanding and *de novo* design of biomolecular functionality with explanatory and predictive mathematical models in systems and synthetic biology [13,27,29,38]. Ideally, computer-aided engineering of biological systems will become as routine and reliable as it is today for mechanical or electrical systems, for example.

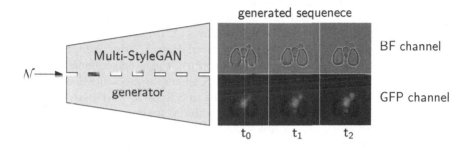

Fig. 1. Multi-StyleGAN simulation of yeast TLFM imagery consisting of three consecutive multi-domain timesteps; brightfield top row, fluorescent channel bottom row.

TLFM experiments yield valuable high-throughput time-lapse fluorescence data on the single-cell level, however, they are costly, labour intensive, and complex [23,24,29]. A complimentary approach to predictive modelling of the pertinent features extracted from these experiments, and a further step towards *in silico* experimentation, is to simulate experiments by synthesising the imagery itself. While this approach is primarily descriptive in nature, it may be able to capture the broader context of cell morphology and the spatio-temporal structure of multiple cells, or other biophysical features which are not routinely extracted from the imagery. In the future, interfacing quantitatively predictive modelling of biomolecular circuitry and the spatio-temporal description of multi-cell behaviour is expected to advance our ability to engineer more complex biological microsystems and biomaterials [10,36]. More immediate applications for synthetic microscope imagery are as a means to generate additional data for training and validating of feature extraction algorithms, or to aid and expedite development of advanced experimental techniques such as online monitoring or control of cells [3,28,30,31,36].

Generative adversarial networks (GANs) are a recent approach to synthesise images [9]. They implicitly learn a high-dimensional dataset distribution through unsupervised adversarial training where a *generator* and a *discriminator* play a minimax game [9]. While the generator synthesises images, the discriminator distinguishes between synthetic *fake* images and *real* images from a training set. GANs have been employed to synthesise a wide range of imagery, such as handwriting, paintings, medical imagery, natural images and faces [9,17]. StyleGAN2 is the current state-of-the-art for high-resolution images [19].

The generation of synthetic cell imagery dates back to the late 1990s [36]. Recently GANs have been employed, for example, to synthesise fluorescent microscope images of isolated *Schizosaccharomyces pombe* or human cells in the centre of the frame [8,16,26]. Synthetic images of multiple blood cells were generated for data augmentation with conditional GANs [2]. GANs have also been employed to infer one microscope modality, such as fluorescence or enhanced contrast imagery from another modality [12,21,22,40] or to increase image spatial resolution [41]. The spatial organisation of tissue on electron microscopy imagery has been simulated with supervised GANs [11]. The interpolation of video frames between recorded TLFM timesteps has also recently been demonstrated [7]. To date, we are not aware of any GAN simulations of brightfield imagery of multiple yeast cells, nor of any simulations that capture the growth and spatio-temporal development of cells in future timestep sequences.

In this study, we propose Multi-StyleGAN to synthesise sequences of multi-domain TLFM imagery of multiple yeast cells in microstructured environments. We introduce a novel dual-styled-convolutional block with separate convolutional paths for each domain. This enables the Multi-StyleGAN generator to learn multi-domain microscope images. We present the corresponding TLFM dataset recorded in our laboratory. Both the brightfield and a fluorescent channel are simulated at three consecutive timesteps. Dynamic behaviour such as changes in morphology, cell growth, their movement, their mechanical interactions with each other and the environment are captured. To the best of our knowledge, this is the first GAN to synthesise brightfield and fluorescence yeast microscopy, the first to simulate multiple yeast cells, as well as the first multi-domain simulation over multiple timesteps.

2   Dataset

Optical access to living cells is generally enabled by confining these to a monolayer within the focal plane of a microscope (Fig. 2). The monolayer is achieved by loading cells into a gap approximately the size of a cell diameter between a cover slip and microstructured polydimethylsiloxane [23,29]. In the microfluidic configuration we consider here, the microchip is perfused with a constant flow of yeast growth media and maintained at temperatures conducive to yeast growth. The cells are hydrodynamically trapped in the microstructures, constraining these horizontally [23,29]. The flow enables long term imaging of up to several days, by removing daughter cells and preventing chip crowding. Examples of the routine employ of this configuration include Fig. 2 and [15,23,28–30].

The training dataset was recorded from one yeast TLFM experiment in our laboratory. The dataset is structured in sequences of at least nine timesteps and includes slight variations in focal plane. Images were selected to each contain less than twelve cells, the majority of which remain inside the frame throughout

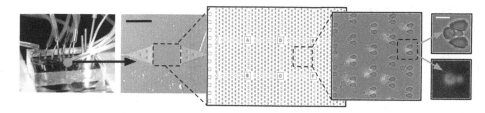

Fig. 2. TLFM setup. Microfluidic chip on microscope table (left). The imaging chamber (green rectangle) contains an array of approximately 1000 traps. Overlay of brightfield and fluorescent channel showing fluorescent cells in traps. A brightfield sample with a pair of trap microstructures and two yeast cell, as well as the corresponding fluorescent channel sample (right). Black scale bar 1 mm, white scale bar 10 μm. (Color figure online)

the sequence. The dataset includes 9696 images of both brightfield and green fluorescent protein (GFP) channels at a resolution of 256×256 (Fig. 2 (right) and Fig. 5 (left)). 8148 sequences are available to train Multi-StyleGAN when utilising overlapping sequences of three images.

3   Methodology

We propose Multi-StyleGAN (Fig. 3) for high-resolution (256^2) multi-domain image sequence generation. The architecture is influenced by the recent Style-GAN2 [17] and star-shaped GAN [26]. The latter utilises a generator with two convolutional paths to synthesise a low-resolution (48×80) two-domain image. We applied this idea to the StyleGAN2 architecture to develop Multi-StyleGAN.

Initially, we naively adapted StyleGAN2 for sequences of multi-domain imagery, which became the basis of the baselines in this study. Both domains and the time dimension were modeled in the channel dimension. We also employed a StyleGAN2 with 3D convolutions. StyleGAN2 3D models the time dimension in the third convolution dimension. The GFP and BF domains were modeled in the channel dimension. However, even with the use of a U-Net discriminator [33] and adaptive discriminator augmentation (ADA) [17], these only converged to equilibria with poor generative performance. Samples for the StyleGANs with the best convergence are depicted in Fig. S2 (supplement). We modified the architecture resulting in Multi-StyleGAN, as the StyleGAN2 and StyleGAN2 3D samples are qualitatively unrealistic and not biophysically sensible, in particular for the fluorescent domain which bears a strong resemblance to the BF.

The Multi-StyleGAN generator utilises a mapping network f and two separate 2D convolutional paths, conditioned on the latent vector w, to generate a matching BF and GFP image sequence (Fig. 3). The time dimension is modeled within the feature dimension. A U-Net [33] serves as the Multi-StyleGAN discriminator network, returning both a scalar and pixel-wise real/fake prediction. This reinforces local and global coherence in the synthesised imagery [33].

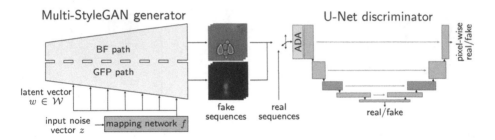

Fig. 3. Architecture of Multi-StyleGAN. The style mapping network f (purple) transforms the input noise vector $z \sim \mathcal{N}_{512}(0, 1)$ into a latent vector $w \in \mathcal{W}$, which in turn is passed to each stage of the generator (yellow) by three dual-styled-convolutional blocks (Fig. 4). The generator predicts a sequence of three consecutive images for both the BF and GFP channels. The U-Net discriminator with ADA distinguishes between real and a fake sequences by making both a scalar and a pixel-wise real/fake prediction. Residual discriminator blocks in gray and non-local blocks [39] in blue. (Color figure online)

The dual-styled-convolutional (DSC) block is the main component of the Multi-StyleGAN generator. It uses two separate convolutional paths (Fig. 4 BF/GFP path) to generate the BF and GFP domains separately. A single style vector modulates [19] the convolutional weights of both paths, enforcing consistency between the domains. Multi-StyleGAN utilises three DSC blocks in each of the seven resolution stages. Similarly to the StyleGAN2 output skip architecture [19], two blocks build the main path, and one serves as the output mapping.

Multi-StyleGAN trains unsupervised on the top-k [34] non-saturating GAN loss [9] for both the scalar and pixel-wise prediction of the U-Net discriminator [33]. Similarly to the original StyleGAN2 training process, path length [19] and R_1 [25] regularization are employed in a lazy fashion [19]. Additionally, CutMix augmentation and consistency regularization [33] is applied to the U-Net discriminator. To enforce learning of time dependencies, real disordered sequences are fed to the discriminator as fake samples. We emloyed ADA [17] to prevent the discriminator from overfitting. Due to the used dataset characteristics, only pixel blitting and geometric transformations are applied as augmentations.

We employ the Inception Score [32] (IS), Fréchet Inception Distance [14] (FID) and Fréchet Video Distance [37] (FVD) as quantitative metrics to analyse Multi-StyleGANs performance and to facilitate future comparisons. These widespread metrics measure image quality and diversity relative to the training dataset. Technically, the FID measures the similarity between the generated distribution and the dataset distribution in the Inception-Net latent space [14]. FVD is the related measure for sequences [37]. One frame was sampled uniformly from the predicted sequence to compute both the IS and the FID. A trained Inception-Net V3 [35] provided by Torchvision[1] predicted the statistics

---

[1] https://github.com/pytorch/vision.

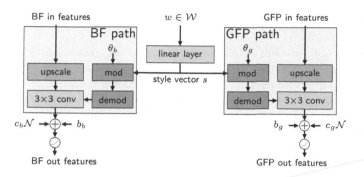

Fig. 4. Dual-styled-convolutional block of Multi-StyleGAN. The incoming latent vector w is transformed into the style vector s by a linear layer. This style vector modulates (mod) [19] the convolutional weights θ_b and θ_g, which are optionally demodulated (demod) [19] before convolving the (optionally bilinearly upsampled) incoming features of the previous block. Learnable biasses (b_b and b_g) and channel-wise Gaussian noise ($\mathcal{N}$) scaled by a learnable constant (c_b and c_g), are added to the features. The final output features are obtained by applying a leaky ReLU activation.

for the FID and the IS. We utilised a trained I3D network[2] [5] to compute the FVD [37]. All validation metrics were computed over the whole dataset length (8148 sequences). While these are the most widespread and suitable metrics available, they have some limitations for the scenario studied here [4,17]. The FID tends to be dominated by an inherent bias given limited real samples [17]. Both the Inception-Net and the I3D network are trained on natural images or videos, respectively [14,32,37]. These may not fully capture the domain-specific features of the trapped yeast cell dataset, in particular for the fluorescent channel.

We implemented Multi-StyleGAN using PyTorch[3], and ADA with Kornia[4]. Each of the seven generator stages employs 512 features. The mapping network f is an eight-layered fully connected neural network. The input to f is a 512-dimensional input noise vector. The U-Net discriminator encoder consists of five blocks with 128, 256, 384, 768, and 1024 features. The decoder employs 768, 384, 256, and 128 features in each respective block. We trained Multi-StyleGAN for 100 epochs with Adam optimizer [20] and the hyperparameters $\beta_1 = 0$, $\beta_2 = 0.99$. The generator and discriminator learning rates were $2 \cdot 10^{-4}$ and $6 \cdot 10^{-4}$. Exponential-moving-average of the generator weights were used. The learning rate for the mapping network was $2 \cdot 10^{-6}$. Training took approximately one day on four Nvidia Tesla V100 (32 GB) with a batch size of 24. An overview of all hyperparameters is given in the supplement (Table S1).

---

[2] https://github.com/piergiaj/pytorch-i3d.
[3] https://pytorch.org/.
[4] https://kornia.github.io/.

4   Results

We demonstrate Multi-StyleGAN's performance at synthesising sequences of consecutive multi-domain TLFM time-points by simulating yeast cells in microstructured environments. Sample sequences are depicted in Fig. 5 (right) and Fig. S2 (supplement). In the brightfield domain, the network successfully captures the microstructures at the correct positions as well as multiple cells at various stages of growth and cell cycle. Cell growth is most evident in the newly budded daughter cells, and as expected biophysically, growth slows for larger cells. Cell fluorescence, and changes thereof, is exhibited on the corresponding channel. Both the BF and GFP domains are aligned.

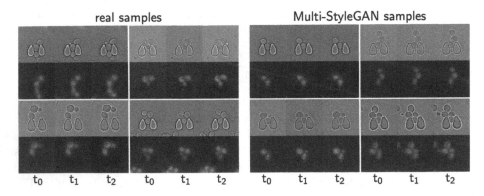

Fig. 5. Real BF & GFP sequences, three timesteps (left). Multi-StyleGAN generated BF & GFP sequences (right). BF channel in grayscale and GFP channel in green.

In addition to capturing the biophysical features and time dependencies, Multi-StyleGAN synthesises image sequences with a high degree of variation in cell and trap configurations. The fine texture of the cells is captured. The generated samples include slight variations in microscope focus between sequences, leading to light or dark outer *halos* around the cell contours (Fig. 5). The GAN samples show a similar distribution of these *halos* or focus variations.

We consider quantitative metrics to analyse Multi-StyleGAN's performance and to facilitate future comparisons (Table 1). Multi-StyleGAN yields better scores than StyleGAN2 and StyleGAN 3D, in both FID and FVD, on both domains. This is in agreement with visual assessment of the achieved results (supplement Fig. S2). The BF domain achieves significantly better scores than the GFP domain for all methods, in all but one case. This may be caused by a mismatch between the domain-specific features of the GFP channel and the networks used to evaluate the metrics that are trained on natural imagery or videos. Multi-StyleGAN achieved an IS of 1.864 and 2.437 for the BF and GFP channel, respectively. Both scores are close to the dataset IS of 2.021 for the BF channel and 2.479 for the GFP channel. This supports the qualitative observation that the imagery generated by Multi-StyleGAN are sharp and diverse in comparison to the dataset.

Table 1. Evaluation metrics for Multi-StyleGAN and baselines.

Method	FID [14] ↓		FVD [37] ↓	
	BF	GFP	BF	GFP
Multi-StyleGAN (ours)	**33.3687**	**207.8409**	**4.4632**	**30.1650**
StyleGAN2 + ADA + U-Net dis.	200.5408	224.7860	45.6296	35.2169
StyleGAN2 3D + ADA + U-Net dis.	76.0344	298.7545	14.7509	31.4771

Multi-StyleGAN utilises two separate convolutional paths in the generator. This decouples the convolutional weights, which are subsequently learnt for the individual domains. The transitions between images are smooth when interpolating through the latent space (see supplementary video), indicating the network does not merely memorise the training data. Multi-StyleGAN preserves the style mixing property of StyleGAN [18], allowing images to be manipulated in the latent space [1]. This is demonstrated in Fig. S1 (supplement) where the latent vectors of two samples are mixed at different stages of the generator.

5 Discussion

The proposed Multi-StyleGAN successfully synthesises a multi-domain microscope imagery sequence of live cells at three consecutive timesteps. Both the brightfield and fluorescent channels capture underlying biophysical factors realistically (Fig. 5). While some cells bud within the simulated sequence, longer time series over 9 timesteps, corresponding to the doubling time of yeast or more are needed to fully capture and simulate the complete cell cycle including the budding process. In the future, this limitation could be counteracted by adapting Multi-StyleGAN for training on longer sequences.

The trained Multi-StyleGAN we present can be applied to a range of scenarios. A typical application for synthesised microscope imagery is as a data augmentation technique to train feature extraction algorithms [6,36] such as cell segmentation tools [24,28–30]. The simulations of consecutive TLFM timesteps themselves can be employed as *in silico* experiments, for example to develop advanced experimental techniques such as online monitoring of cells or optimal experimental design techniques with cell segmentation in the loop [3,6,31,36].

Currently, Multi-StyleGAN learns an implicit high-dimensional representation of a single experiment. A promising direction for future research is to extend our approach to a whole campaign of experiments. This would allow generating image sequences conditioned on given experimental parameters such as organism type or temperature. In a further step towards *in silico* TLFM experimentation, the descriptive simulations Multi-StyleGAN offers may be interfaced with explanatory and predictive models of specific biomolecular circuitry.

6   Conclusion

In summary, we propose Mult-StyleGAN to synthesise multi-domain image sequences and showcase it by simulating TLFM imagery *in silico*. To the best of our knowledge, this is the first network to simulate temporal sequences of yeast brightfield imagery, in particular with multiple cells in a microstructured environment. Trained on the presented dataset, the simulations capture the spatio-temporal organisation of multiple yeast cells. Biophysical factors and time-dependencies, such as cell morphology and growth, are realistically simulated concurrently to the cell fluorescence. Immediate applications for Multi-StyleGAN are to generate additional training data for segmentation algorithms or to expedite the development of advanced experimental techniques such as optimal experimental design. While the Multi-StyleGAN simulations are descriptive in nature, they are a step towards more complete *in silico* experimentation, especially if interfaced with predictive mathematical models in the future.

Acknowledgements. We thank Markus Baier for aid with the computational setup, Klaus-Dieter Voss for aid with the microfluidics fabrication, and Tim Kircher, Tizian Dege, and Florian Schwald for aid with the data preparation.

This work was supported by the Landesoffensive für wissenschaftliche Exzellenz as part of the LOEWE Schwerpunkt CompuGene. H.K. acknowledges support from the European Research Council (ERC) with the consolidator grant CONSYN (nr. 773196).

References

1. Abdal, R., Qin, Y., Wonka, P.: Image2StyleGAN++: how to edit the embedded images? In: CVPR, pp. 8296–8305 (2020)
2. Bailo, O., Ham, D., Shin, Y.M.: Red blood cell image generation for data augmentation using conditional generative adversarial networks. In: CVPRW (2019)
3. Bandiera, L., Hou, Z., Kothamachu, V.B., Balsa-Canto, E., Swain, P.S., Menolascina, F.: On-line optimal input design increases the efficiency and accuracy of the modelling of an inducible synthetic promoter. Processes **6**(9) (2018)
4. Barratt, S., Sharma, R.: A note on the inception score. In: ICML Workshop (2018)
5. Carreira, J., Zisserman, A.: Quo vadis, action recognition? A new model and the kinetics dataset. In: CVPR, pp. 6299–6308 (2017)
6. Chessel, A., Carazo Salas, R.E.: From observing to predicting single-cell structure and function with high-throughput/high-content microscopy. Essays Biochem. **63**(2), 197–208 (2019)
7. Comes, M.C., et al.: Multi-scale generative adversarial network for improved evaluation of cell-cell interactions observed in organ-on-chip experiments. Neural. Comput. Appl. **33**, 3671–3689 (2020)

8. Goldsborough, P., Pawlowski, N., Caicedo, J.C., Singh, S., Carpenter, A.E.: Cyto-GAN: generative modeling of cell images. BioRxiv, p. 227645 (2017)
9. Goodfellow, I., et al.: Generative adversarial nets. In: NeurIPS, vol. 27, pp. 2672–2680 (2014)
10. Hall, M.S., Decker, J.T., Shea, L.D.: Towards systems tissue engineering: elucidating the dynamics, spatial coordination, and individual cells driving emergent behaviors. Biomaterials **255**, 120189 (2020)
11. Han, L., Murphy, R.F., Ramanan, D.: Learning generative models of tissue organization with supervised GANs. In: WACV, pp. 682–690 (2018)
12. Han, L., Yin, Z.: Transferring microscopy image modalities with conditional generative adversarial networks. In: CVPRW, pp. 851–859 (2017)
13. Henningsen, J., Schwarz-Schilling, M., Leibl, A., Gutiérrez, J., Sagredo, S., Simmel, F.C.: Single cell characterization of a synthetic bacterial clock with a hybrid feedback loop containing dCas9-sgRNA. ACS Synth. Biol. **9**(12), 3377–3387 (2020)
14. Heusel, M., Ramsauer, H., Unterthiner, T., Nessler, B., Hochreiter, S.: GANs trained by a two time-scale update rule converge to a local nash equilibrium. In: NeurIPS, vol. 30, pp. 6626–6637 (2017)
15. Hofmann, A., et al.: A tightly regulated and adjustable CRISPR-dCas9 based AND gate in yeast. Nucleic Acids Res. **47**(1), 509–520 (2019)
16. Johnson, G.R., Donovan-Maiye, R.M., Maleckar, M.M.: Generative modeling with conditional autoencoders: building an integrated cell. arXiv:1705.00092 (2017)
17. Karras, T., Aittala, M., Hellsten, J., Laine, S., Lehtinen, J., Aila, T.: Training generative adversarial networks with limited data. In: NeurIPS, vol. 33, pp. 12104–12114 (2020)
18. Karras, T., Laine, S., Aila, T.: A style-based generator architecture for generative adversarial networks. In: CVPR, pp. 4401–4410 (2019)
19. Karras, T., Laine, S., Aittala, M., Hellsten, J., Lehtinen, J., Aila, T.: Analyzing and improving the image quality of StyleGAN. In: CVPR, pp. 8110–8119 (2020)
20. Kingma, D.P., Ba, J.: Adam: a method for stochastic optimization. In: ICLR (2015)
21. Lee, G., Oh, J.W., Her, N.G., Jeong, W.K.: DeepHCS++: bright-field to fluorescence microscopy image conversion using multi-task learning with adversarial losses for label-free high-content screening. Med. Image Anal. **70**, 101995 (2021)
22. Lee, G., Oh, J.-W., Kang, M.-S., Her, N.-G., Kim, M.-H., Jeong, W.-K.: DeepHCS: bright-field to fluorescence microscopy image conversion using deep learning for label-free high-content screening. In: Frangi, A.F., Schnabel, J.A., Davatzikos, C., Alberola-López, C., Fichtinger, G. (eds.) MICCAI 2018. LNCS, vol. 11071, pp. 335–343. Springer, Cham (2018). https://doi.org/10.1007/978-3-030-00934-2_38
23. Leygeber, M., et al.: Analyzing microbial population heterogeneity - expanding the toolbox of microfluidic single-cell cultivations. J. Mol. Biol. **431**, 4569–4588 (2019)
24. Lugagne, J., Lin, H., Dunlop, M.: DeLTA: automated cell segmentation, tracking, and lineage reconstruction using deep learning. PLOS Comput. Biol. **16**(4) (2020)
25. Mescheder, L., Geiger, A., Nowozin, S.: Which training methods for GANs do actually converge? In: ICML, pp. 3481–3490 (2018)
26. Osokin, A., Chessel, A., Carazo Salas, R.E., Vaggi, F.: GANs for biological image synthesis. In: ICCV (2017)
27. Pepperkok, R., Ellenberg, J.: High-throughput fluorescence microscopy for systems biology. Nat. Rev. Mol. Cell Biol. **7**(9), 690–696 (2006)
28. Prangemeier, T., Wildner, C., Françani, A.O., Reich, C., Koeppl, H.: Multiclass yeast segmentation in microstructured environments with deep learning. In: IEEE CIBCB, pp. 1–8 (2020)

29. Prangemeier, T., Lehr, F.X., Schoeman, R.M., Koeppl, H.: Microfluidic platforms for the dynamic characterisation of synthetic circuitry. Curr. Opin. Biotechnol. **63**, 167–176 (2020)
30. Prangemeier, T., Reich, C., Koeppl, H.: Attention-based transformers for instance segmentation of cells in microstructures. In: IEEE BIBM, pp. 700–707 (2020)
31. Prangemeier, T., Wildner, C., Hanst, M., Koeppl, H.: Maximizing information gain for the characterization of biomolecular circuits. In: Proceedings of the 5th ACM/IEEE NanoCom, pp. 1–6 (2018)
32. Salimans, T., et al.: Improved techniques for training GANs. In: NeurIPS, vol. 29, pp. 2234–2242 (2016)
33. Schonfeld, E., Schiele, B., Khoreva, A.: A U-Net based discriminator for generative adversarial networks. In: CVPR, pp. 8207–8216 (2020)
34. Sinha, S., Zhao, Z., Goyal, A., Raffel, C.A., Odena, A.: Top-k training of GANs: improving GAN performance by throwing away bad samples. In: NeurIPS, vol. 33, pp. 14638–14649 (2020)
35. Szegedy, C., Vanhoucke, V., Ioffe, S., Shlens, J., Wojna, Z.: Rethinking the inception architecture for computer vision. In: CVPR, pp. 2818–2826 (2016)
36. Ulman, V., Svoboda, D., Nykter, M., Kozubek, M., Ruusuvuori, P.: Virtual cell imaging: a review on simulation methods employed in image cytometry. Cytometry A **89**(12), 1057–1072 (2016)
37. Unterthiner, T., van Steenkiste, S., Kurach, K., Marinier, R., Michalski, M., Gelly, S.: FVD: a new metric for video generation. In: ICLR Workshop (2019)
38. Wang, N.B., Beitz, A.M., Galloway, K.: Engineering cell fate: applying synthetic biology to cellular reprogramming. Curr. Opin. Syst. Biol. **24**, 18–31 (2020)
39. Wang, X., Girshick, R., Gupta, A., He, K.: Non-local neural networks. In: CVPR, pp. 7794–7803 (2018)
40. Wieslander, H., Gupta, A., Bergman, E., Hallström, E., Harrison, P.J.: Learning to see colours: generating biologically relevant fluorescent labels from bright-field images. bioRxiv (2021)
41. Zhang, H., et al.: High-throughput, high-resolution deep learning microscopy based on registration-free generative adversarial network. Biomed. Opt. Express **10**(3), 1044–1063 (2019)

Deep Reinforcement Exemplar Learning for Annotation Refinement

Yuexiang Li[1(✉)], Nanjun He[1], Sixiang Peng[2], Kai Ma[1], and Yefeng Zheng[1]

[1] Tencent Jarvis Lab, Shenzhen, China
vicyxli@tencent.com
[2] Tencent Health, Shenzhen, China

Abstract. Due to the inter-observer variation, the ground truth of lesion areas in pathological images is generated by majority-voting of annotations provided by different pathologists. Such a process is extremely laborious, since each pathologist needs to spend hours or even days for pixel-wise annotations. In this paper, we propose a reinforcement learning framework to automatically refine the set of annotations provided by a single pathologist based on several exemplars of ground truth. Particularly, we treat each pixel as an agent with a shared pixel-level action space. The multi-agent model observes several paired single-pathologist annotations and ground truth, and tries to customize the strategy to narrow down the gap between them with episodes of exploring. Furthermore, we integrate a discriminator to the multi-agent framework to evaluate the quality of annotation refinement. A quality reward is yielded by the discriminator to update the policy of agents. Experimental results on the publicly available Gleason 2019 dataset demonstrate the effectiveness of our reinforcement learning framework—the segmentation network trained with our refined single-pathologist annotations achieves a comparable accuracy to the one using majority-voting-based ground truth.

Keywords: Exemplar learning · Deep reinforcement learning · Annotation refinement

1 Introduction

Deep learning has achieved a great success on medical image segmentation tasks such as organ segmentation [5,6,17] and lesion segmentation [7,8,10]. Nevertheless, existing methods heavily rely on a large amount of pixel-wise labeled data, which is laborious to acquire. Such a problem becomes more intractable while dealing with extremely high-resolution pathological images. Furthermore, due to the inter-observer variation, the ground truth of pathological images is generated by majority-voting of annotations provided by different pathologists, as shown in Fig. 1, which rapidly increases the overall annotation workload.

Exemplar learning is a potential solution to reduce the workload, which has not been extensively explored. Historically, the theory of example-based learning

© Springer Nature Switzerland AG 2021
M. de Bruijne et al. (Eds.): MICCAI 2021, LNCS 12908, pp. 487–496, 2021.
https://doi.org/10.1007/978-3-030-87237-3_47

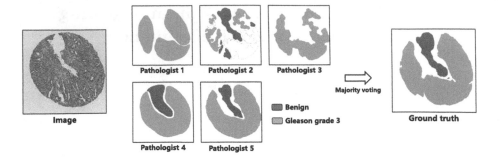

Fig. 1. The ground truth for pathological images is often generated by majority-voting. Such a process is extremely expensive and laborious.

was first uncovered by Sweller *et al.* [16]. One of the core findings is the worked example effect—it is better for initial cognitive skill acquisition to study examples than to learn by problem solving. The idea has been introduced to the area of machine learning in recent years. The conventional setup of example-based machine learning is only having a single positive exemplar for the model to learn. For example, the exemplar support vector machine (Exemplar-SVM) [12] has been one of the driving methods for exemplar based learning. Each Exemplar-SVM classifier is defined by a single positive instance (worked example) and a large set of negatives. Since the deep learning models require more training data to converge, researchers [1,18,19] loose the requirement to multiple positive samples in recent studies. However, most of existing studies focus on image classification [1,12,15] and image translation [18,19].

In this paper, we explore the potential of applying exemplar learning to address a practically relevant yet previously untouched problem, *i.e.*, annotation refinement. Concretely, we train a model and expect it to act as an annotation quality inspector, who acquires the skill of correcting the annotation mistakes made by the single pathologist via observing the worked exemplars, *i.e.*, several pathological images with pair-wise single-pathologist annotations and majority-voting-based ground truth.[1] In this regard, we adopt the technique of deep reinforcement learning [2,11,13], which encourages machines to imitate humans' behaviors, to address the problem. Particularly, we treat each pixel as an agent with a shared pixel-level action space. During the episodes of exploring, the multi-agent model is encouraged to customize the strategy to revise the annotation mistakes produced by the single pathologist, by exhaustively observing the worked examples. We further integrate a discriminator to the multi-agent framework to evaluate the quality of annotation refinement. A quality reward is yielded by the discriminator to update the policy of agents. Experimental results on the publicly available Gleason 2019 dataset demonstrate the effectiveness of our reinforcement-learning-based framework—the segmentation network trained

---

[1] The pathologists are required to annotate only the worked examples, instead of the full set of images, which significantly reduces the overall workload of annotation.

with our refined single-pathologist annotations achieves a comparable accuracy to the one using majority-voting-based ground truth (Fig. 2).

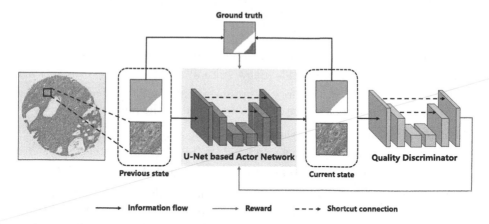

Fig. 2. The pipeline of our reinforcement learning framework, which consists of an actor network and a quality discriminator. The actor network is jointly supervised by two reward functions.

2   Method

In this section, we introduce the proposed reinforcement exemplar learning framework in details. Since the actions of reinforcement learning framework is highly related to the target task, we briefly introduce the dataset and the annotations used in this study—the Gleason 2019 dataset[2] [8] released for the development of automated prostate cancer Gleason grading system. The dataset consists of 244 high-resolution tissue microarrays (TMAs), which were annotated by six pathologists, *i.e.*, assigning a label (0–normal and 1 to 5–Gleason grades) to each pixel. Clinically, the pathologist diagnoses the severity of prostate tumors based on the Gleason grades, *i.e.*, the higher grade means the severer.

2.1   Overview

The pipeline of our deep reinforcement exemplar learning framework, consisting of an actor network (G) and a quality discriminator (D), is presented in Fig. 1. Let $x = (x_1, \cdots, x_N)$ be one tile cropped from an exemplar, where N is the number of pixels, and x_i is the ith pixel of x. Each x_i is treated as an agent with a pre-defined policy $\pi_i(a_i^{(t)}|s_i^{(t)})$, where $s_i^{(t)}$ and $a_i^{(t)}$ are the state (*i.e.*, image and annotation information) and action for x_i at the step t. For each episode, a set of

---

[2] https://gleason2019.grand-challenge.org/.

Table 1. The action pool defined for annotation refinement.

Action	± 0	± 1	± 2	± 3	± 4	± 5	Erosion	Dilation	Open	Close
Kernel	–	–	–	–	–	–	(5×5)	(5×5)	(5×5)	(5×5)

actions $\boldsymbol{a}^{(t)} = (a_1^{(t)}, \cdots, a_N^{(t)})$ is taken to the corresponding pixels for annotation refinement, and accordingly yields a new state $\boldsymbol{s}^{(t+1)} = (s_1^{(t+1)}, \cdots, s_N^{(t+1)})$ and a reward $\boldsymbol{r}(t) = (r_1^{(t)}, \cdots, r_N^{(t)})$ for the optimization of actor network. The state, action and reward of a single agent x_i are detailed in the following.

State. As illustrated in Fig. 1, the state for agent x_i at step t is a concatenation of its pixel value v_i and the label l_i, i.e., $s_i^{(t)} = [v_i, l_i^{(t)}]$. The initial state $s_i^{(0)}$ is obtained by assigning the labels generated by the single-pathologist to $\boldsymbol{l}^{(0)}$.

Action. Since the single-pathologist annotations mainly suffer from the inaccurate Gleason grade and shape of annotated areas, compared to the ground truth, we thereby define a pool of actions to simultaneously refine the annotations in terms of the two aspects, as listed in Table 1.[3] For each time step t, the agent x_i selects one action from the pool to revise its label $l_i^{(t)}$.

2.2 Reward Functions

Our framework consists of two reward functions for the optimization of actor network—a conventional relative improvement reward and a novel refinement quality reward. The former term is similar to the ones defined by existing approaches:

$$\tilde{r}_i^{(t)} = \mathcal{X}_i^{(t-1)} - \mathcal{X}_i^{(t)} \tag{1}$$

where $\mathcal{X}_i^{(t)} = |l_i^{(t)} - l_i^{(gt)}|$, and $l_i^{(gt)}$ is the ground truth via majority voting; $|.|$ calculates the absolute value.

Refinement Quality Reward. To further improve the performance of annotation refinement, we propose a novel reward function, namely quality reward, generated by a quality discriminator. The underlying principle of quality discriminator is similar to the one used in adversarial generative network (GAN) [3], i.e., distinguishing the 'fake' pixels (refined by the actor network) from the 'real' ones (ground truth). To this end, we randomly sample the tiles $\tilde{x}$ from exemplars with ground truth to train the discriminator, together with $\boldsymbol{s}^{(t)}$. The quality reward can be formulated as:

$$\hat{r}_i^{(t)} = \hat{\mathcal{X}}_i^{(t)} - \hat{\mathcal{X}}_i^{(t-1)}, \tag{2}$$

$$\hat{\mathcal{X}}_i^{(t)} = \mathbb{E}_{s \sim p_{\tilde{x}}} \|(D(s_i^{(gt)}) - 1)^2\| + \mathbb{E}_{s \sim p_x} \|(D(G(s_i^{(t)})))^2\| \tag{3}$$

---

[3] The implementation of morphological-kernel-based actions (erosion, dilation, open and close) is similar to [2].

where $s_i^{(gt)}$ is the state formed by the pixel value v_i and ground truth $l_i^{(gt)}$.

Overall Reward. With the previously defined reward functions, the accumulated reward of an exploration for an agent can be written as:

$$R_i = \sum_{t=1}^{T} \gamma^{t-1}(\tilde{r}_i^{(t)} + \mathcal{T}\hat{r}_i^{(t)}) \tag{4}$$

where T is the number of episode steps, and γ is the discount factor with a value in $(0, 1]$; $\mathcal{T}$ is a temperature factor controlling the contribution made by our quality reward, which is defined as:

$$\mathcal{T} = \frac{e}{e_{max}} \tag{5}$$

where e and e_{max} are the current epoch and the number of total training epochs, respectively. The underlying principle for the setting of $\mathcal{T}$ is that since the under-trained quality discriminator may lead to an incorrect evaluation of actions, the $\mathcal{T}$ is set to a lower value at the beginning of training. After several epochs of training, the quality discriminator can provide promising evaluation; therefore, $\mathcal{T}$ accordingly increases. It is worthwhile to mention that, similar to GAN, our actor network is trained to fool the quality discriminator, *i.e.*, a smaller distance between our refined annotation and the ground truth in the latent space. Hence, a larger loss yielded by the quality discriminator at step t, compared to $t - 1$, results in a more positive reward to the corresponding actions (refer to Eq. (2)).

2.3   Technical Details

Network Architecture. To fit the asynchronous advantage actor-critic (A3C) algorithm [13], the actor network G has a similar architecture to [2,11], *i.e.*, a policy head and a value head are connected to the end of the backbone network (*i.e.*, U-Net [14]). The two heads generate gradients to optimize actor network based on the accumulated reward. The detailed process of gradient calculation and model optimization can be found in [2,11]. The quality discriminator D yields pixel-wise penalty for the actor network. To achieve that, we adopt the fully convolutional network (*i.e.*, U-Net) as its backbone.

Optimization Process. Similar to the training process of GAN, the actor network and quality discriminator are iteratively optimized. Specifically, we first train the actor network G with a fixed quality discriminator D, and then fix G to train D using an adversarial loss [3].

Implementation. The proposed deep reinforcement exemplar learning framework is implemented using Chainer. The mini-batch size for training is set to 16. The initial learning rates for actor network and quality discriminator are set to 0.0001 and 0.001, respectively. The Adam solver [9] is used for network optimization. Parameter setting is as follows: $T = 5$ and $\gamma = 0.95$.

3   Experiments

In this section, we introduce the Gleason 2019 dataset in details, and present the experimental results. As aforementioned, the Gleason 2019 dataset [8] used in this study consists of 244 tissue microarrays (TMAs), which are annotated by six pathologists. However, the numbers of annotations provided by the pathologists are different—the six pathologists annotate 244, 141, 242, 244, 244 and 65 TMAs, respectively. In this regard, we select 136 TMAs with the annotations yielded by the same five pathologists from the dataset for network training and evaluation. Since the pathologists annotating Gleason 2019 dataset are with different years of experiences (ranging from one year to 27 years), the sets of annotations generated by the middle-level (15 years) pathologist are employed for refinement.[4] The resolution of each TMA is around $5,000 \times 5,000$ pixels. To process such a high-resolution image, we crop 512×512 tiles from the TMAs, which are then resized to 256×256 pixels and fed into our framework.

Exemplar Selection. The selection of exemplars, containing the rich information for Gleason grading, is a crucial step for our deep reinforcement exemplar learning framework. To this end, we invite an experienced pathologist to perform the exemplar selection. Finally, six TMAs are chosen as the exemplars for our framework to observe and learn—the single-pathologist annotations and ground truth of these six exemplars are used to train the proposed deep reinforcement exemplar learning framework.

Testing Protocol. Apart from the selected exemplars, we randomly separate the rest TMAs into training, validation and test sets according to the ratio of 70:10:20. Our reinforcement-learning-based framework trained with selected exemplars is adopted to refine the single-pathologist annotations of training and validation sets, which are then used to train a segmentation network (ResU-Net [4,14]) to perform Gleason grading area segmentation. The performance of the well-trained ResU-Net is evaluated on the test set within majority-voting-based ground truth. To assess the performance of our reinforcement-learning-based framework on annotation refinement, we also train ResU-Nets using training and validation sets with original single-pathologist annotations and ground truth, respectively. The segmentation accuracy on the ground-truth-based test set of these ResU-Nets serves as the lower and upper bound for our refinement framework. Consistent to [8], we group the Gleason grades into three categories, *i.e.,* benign (grade 1 and 2), low-grade (grade 3) and high-grade (grade 4 and 5), for segmentation performance evaluation. In this study, the mean Dice coefficient (DSC), obtained by averaging the DSCs [11] of different Gleason grades, is adopted as the metric for segmentation performance evaluation.

---

[4] The middle-level pathological annotations are easier to acquire and more cost-friendly than the high-level ones, while much more accurate than the low-level pathologists with less than five years experiences—the extremely low-quality annotations often lead to a model collapse during our reinforcement learning.

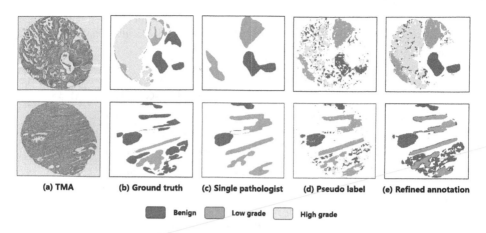

(a) TMA   (b) Ground truth   (c) Single pathologist   (d) Pseudo label   (e) Refined annotation

Benign   Low grade   High grade

Fig. 3. Examples of annotations generated by different approaches and the corresponding TMA and ground truth. Although the single pathologist provides incomplete annotations, the proposed method still works well.

Table 2. Mean absolute error (MAE) between annotations and the ground truth. The MAE is the smaller the better. (S.-P.–single-pathologist)

	Original S.-P.	Pseudo label	Refined S.-P. (ours)
Benign	0.5759	0.9924	**0.5167**
Low-grade	0.9125	0.9510	**0.8240**
High-grade	0.8743	1.1707	**0.6455**
Mean	0.7876	1.0380	**0.6621**

3.1 Quality Analysis of Refined Annotation

To validate the effectiveness of our reinforcement exemplar learning framework, we conduct experiments to analyze the quality of refined annotations. For visual comparison, we present the examples of ground truth and different annotations in Fig. 3. Note that the pseudo label generated by exemplar-trained segmentation network is also adopted as the baseline for comparison—we trained a ResU-Net using only exemplars and adopted the predictions on the training and validation sets as pseudo labels. It can be observed that our reinforcement-learning-based approach significantly refines the single-pathologist annotations by adding high-grade areas and revising the benign pixels to low grade, as shown in the first and second rows of Fig. 3, respectively. In contrast, the exemplar-trained segmentation network is observed to generate incomplete Gleason grading areas and assign incorrect grade to pixels, which demonstrate the additional single-pathologist annotations employed by our reinforcement-learning-based framework can provide useful guidelines for annotation refinement. To quantitatively evaluate the performance of annotation refinement, we calculate the average absolute error (MAE) between annotations and ground truth for different Gleason grades. The

Table 3. Segmentation accuracy on the test set yielded by U-Nets trained with different annotations and the corresponding annotation workload. (S.-P.–single-pathologist; G.–grade)

	Workload*	Dice coefficient (%)			
		Benign	Low-G.	High-G.	Mean
Exemplar only	5 × 6	35.83	53.48	38.84	42.72
Pseudo label	5 × 6	54.89	51.45	54.32	53.33
Original S.-P.	1 × 130	58.89	60.34	63.14	60.79
Refined S.-P. w/o D	5 × 6 + 1 × 130	61.17	63.32	69.31	64.60
Refined S.-P. (ours)	5 × 6 + 1 × 130	**63.33**	**64.56**	**71.31**	**66.40**
Ground truth	5 × 130	63.77	66.03	71.96	67.25

* Calculated by *the number of pathologists* × *the number of TMAs*.

evaluation results in Table 2 show that our refined single-pathologist annotations are much closer to the ground truth, compared to the original one, *i.e.*, smaller MAEs are achieved.

3.2   Performance on Gleason Grading Area Segmentation

To further evaluate the performance of our reinforcement-learning-based annotation refinement framework, we use the refined annotations to train the segmentation network (ResU-Net) and compared with the ones trained under different strategies on the same ground-truth-based test set. The segmentation accuracy of different Gleason grading areas is presented in Table 3.

As shown in Table 3, the ResU-Net trained with our refined single-pathologist annotations achieves a comparable mean DSC, *i.e.*, 66.40%, to the one using ground truth (67.25%), which is significantly higher than the original one (60.79%). The network trained with exemplars only achieves the lowest mean DSC, due to the lack of sufficient training data. The pseudo labels generated by such an exemplar-only network are not reliable, which result in a mean DSC of 53.33%, *i.e.*, −7.46% lower than the one using original single-pathologist annotations. Table 3 also lists the annotation workload for different training strategies. Compared to training with ground truth, our reinforcement-learning-based approach remarkably reduces the overall workload (160 *vs.* 650 *cf.* Table 3).

Ablation Study. To validate the effectiveness of our refinement quality reward, we conduct an ablation study and present the result in Table 3. The entry of 'Refined S.-P. w/o D' lists the segmentation accuracy achieved by the ResU-Net trained with the annotations refined by our reinforcement learning framework without quality discriminator (D). The experimental result demonstrates the benefits yielded by our refinement quality reward to the annotation refinement— a degradation of −1.8% to the mean DSC is observed caused by the removal of quality discriminator.

4 Conclusion

In this paper, we proposed a reinforcement learning framework to automatically refine the set of annotations provided by a single pathologist based on several exemplars of ground truth. We trained a multi-agent model and expected it to act as an annotation quality inspector, who acquired the skill of correcting the annotation mistakes made by the single pathologist via observing the worked exemplars. Experimental results on the publicly available Gleason 2019 dataset demonstrated the effectiveness of our multi-agent framework.

Acknowledgements. This work was funded by Key-Area Research and Development Program of Guangdong Province, China (No. 2018B010111001), and the Scientific and Technical Innovation 2030–"New Generation Artificial Intelligence" Project (No. 2020AAA0104100).

References

1. Bautista, M.A., Sanakoyeu, A., Sutter, E., Ommer, B.: CliqueCNN: deep unsupervised exemplar learning. In: Advances in Neural Information Processing Systems, pp. 3853–3861 (2016)
2. Furuta, R., Inoue, N., Yamasaki, T.: Fully convolutional network with multi-step reinforcement learning for image processing. In: AAAI Conference on Artificial Intelligence, pp. 3598–3605 (2019)
3. Goodfellow, I., et al.: Generative adversarial nets. In: Advances in Neural Information Processing Systems, pp. 2672–2680 (2014)
4. He, K., Zhang, X., Ren, S., Sun, J.: Deep residual learning for image recognition. In: IEEE Conference on Computer Vision and Pattern Recognition, pp. 770–778 (2016)
5. Huang, R., Zheng, Y., Hu, Z., Zhang, S., Li, H.: Multi-organ segmentation via co-training weight-averaged models from few-organ datasets. In: Martel, A.L., et al. (eds.) MICCAI 2020. LNCS, vol. 12264, pp. 146–155. Springer, Cham (2020). https://doi.org/10.1007/978-3-030-59719-1_15
6. Jiang, X.: Multi-phase and multi-level selective feature fusion for automated pancreas segmentation from CT images. In: Martel, A.L., et al. (eds.) MICCAI 2020. LNCS, vol. 12264, pp. 460–469. Springer, Cham (2020). https://doi.org/10.1007/978-3-030-59719-1_45
7. Kalapahar, A., Silva-Rodríguez, J., Colomer, A., López-Mir, F., Naranjo, V.: Gleason grading of histology prostate images through semantic segmentation via residual U-Net. In: IEEE International Conference on Image Processing, pp. 2501–2505 (2020)
8. Karimi, D., Nir, G., Fazli, L., Black, P.C., Goldenberg, L., Salcudean, S.E.: Deep learning-based Gleason grading of prostate cancer from histopathology images-role of multiscale decision aggregation and data augmentation. IEEE J. Biomed. Health Inform. **24**(5), 1413–1426 (2020)
9. Kingma, D.P., Ba, J.: Adam: a method for stochastic optimization. arXiv preprint arXiv:1412.6980 (2014)
10. Li, Z., Pan, J., Wu, H., Wen, Z., Qin, J.: Memory-efficient automatic kidney and tumor segmentation based on non-local context guided 3D U-Net. In: Martel, A.L., et al. (eds.) MICCAI 2020. LNCS, vol. 12264, pp. 197–206. Springer, Cham (2020). https://doi.org/10.1007/978-3-030-59719-1_20

11. Liao, X., et al.: Iteratively-refined interactive 3D medical image segmentation with multi-agent reinforcement learning. In: IEEE Conference on Computer Vision and Pattern Recognition, pp. 9394–9402 (2020)
12. Malisiewicz, T., Gupta, A., Efros, A.A.: Ensemble of exemplar-SVMs for object detection and beyond. In: International Conference on Computer Vision, pp. 89–96 (2011)
13. Mnih, V., et al.: Asynchronous methods for deep reinforcement learning. In: International Conference on Machine Learning, pp. 1928–1937 (2016)
14. Ronneberger, O., Fischer, P., Brox, T.: U-Net: convolutional networks for biomedical image segmentation. In: Navab, N., Hornegger, J., Wells, W.M., Frangi, A.F. (eds.) MICCAI 2015. LNCS, vol. 9351, pp. 234–241. Springer, Cham (2015). https://doi.org/10.1007/978-3-319-24574-4_28
15. Shapovalova, N., Mori, G.: Clustered exemplar-SVM: discovering sub-categories for visual recognition. In: IEEE International Conference on Image Processing, pp. 93–97 (2015)
16. Sweller, J., Cooper, G.A.: The use of worked examples as a substitute for problem solving in learning algebra. Cogn. Instr. **2**(1), 59–89 (1985)
17. Wang, G., Aertsen, M., Deprest, J., Ourselin, S., Vercauteren, T., Zhang, S.: Uncertainty-guided efficient interactive refinement of fetal brain segmentation from stacks of MRI slices. In: Martel, A.L., et al. (eds.) MICCAI 2020. LNCS, vol. 12264, pp. 279–288. Springer, Cham (2020). https://doi.org/10.1007/978-3-030-59719-1_28
18. Wang, M., et al.: Example-guided style-consistent image synthesis from semantic labeling. In: IEEE Conference on Computer Vision and Pattern Recognition, pp. 1495–1504 (2019)
19. Zhang, P., Zhang, B., Chen, D., Yuan, L., Wen, F.: Cross-domain correspondence learning for exemplar-based image translation. In: IEEE Conference on Computer Vision and Pattern Recognition, pp. 5143–5153 (2020)

Modalities - Histopathology

Instance-Aware Feature Alignment for Cross-Domain Cell Nuclei Detection in Histopathology Images

Zhi Wang[1], Xiaoya Zhu[2], Lei Su[1], Gang Meng[2], Junsheng Zhang[2], Ao Li[1], and Minghui Wang[1(✉)]

[1] School of Information Science and Technology, University of Science and Technology of China, Hefei 230026, China
mhwang@ustc.edu.cn
[2] School of Basic Medicine, Anhui Medical University, Hefei 230026, China

Abstract. Robust nuclei detection is crucial prerequisite for histologic characteristics of nuclei that can assist various clinical tasks such as disease diagnosis and cancer grading. Despite of their success, most existing nuclei detection methods ignore the case where the testing (target) domain has different data distribution with the training (source) domain, which is known as the problem of domain shift. In fact, the domain shift problem is prevalent in histopathology images due to various reasons such as different staining procedures and organ specific nuclear morphology. Thus, the performance of a nuclei detection model in the source domain will be hurt if it is directly applied to the target domain. To address this problem, we propose a novel instance-aware domain adaption framework for nuclei detection in histopathology images, which includes both image-level alignment (IMA) and instance-level alignment (INA) components to minimize the domain shift. Especially, INA component extracts instance-level features by using nuclei locations as the guidance and effectively aligns the instance-level features via adversarial training. Furthermore, to facilitate instance-level feature alignment, a Temporal Ensembling based Nuclei Localization (TENL) module is introduced in INA component to automatically generate candidate nuclei locations in the target domain. We evaluate the proposed method on different benchmark settings and obtain remarkable improvements compared to existing methods on the challenging problem of cross-domain cell nuclei detection.

Keywords: Nuclei detection · Digital pathology · Domain adaptation

1 Introduction

The histologic characteristics of nuclei play a key role in disease diagnosis, prognosis and analysis. Therefore, robust nuclei detection is crucial prerequisite for cellular morphology processing and identification of tissue structures, which can assist various clinical tasks including diagnosis of several medical conditions and automated grading of cancer tissue specimens [1].

© Springer Nature Switzerland AG 2021
M. de Bruijne et al. (Eds.): MICCAI 2021, LNCS 12908, pp. 499–508, 2021.
https://doi.org/10.1007/978-3-030-87237-3_48

Despite the success of deep learning based methods for nuclei detection [2–4], they all require that training and testing data have the same distribution [5]. However, if a detection model is trained in the source (training) domain and directly applied to the target (testing) domain that has different data distribution with the source domain, the detection performance will be severely hurt, which is known as the problem of domain shift [6, 7]. As shown in Fig. 1, since the domain shift problem is prevalent in histopathology images due to various reasons such as different staining procedures [5, 8] and organ specific nuclear morphology, a nuclei detection model with excellent performance in the source domain may instead be ineffective in the target domain. Furthermore, due to the time cost and expertise required for manual annotation of cell nuclei, training data available for nuclei detection still remains very limited for the development of deep learning based methods in real-world applications. Therefore, there is urgent need for transferring knowledge from the source domain to the target domain for accurate cross-domain nuclei detection.

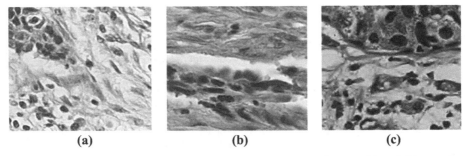

(a)   **(b)**   **(c)**

Fig. 1. Examples of the domain shift problem in histopathology images. (a) and (b) are colon cancer histopathology images with different staining procedures. (c) is a histopathology image of breast cancer that shows different nuclear morphology with colon cancer histopathology images.

In recent years, domain adaptation technique has been developed to deal with the problem of domain shift, which includes pixel-wise adaptation [12–14] and feature-wise adaptation [6, 7, 15]. Concretely, to reduce the domain shift pixel-wise methods first translate images of source domain to the target domain, and then train task models with generated source images with label. Nevertheless, it is very difficult to guarantee the quality of generated images, which in consequence may reduce the adapted performance [16]. Alternatively, feature-wise adaptation based methods align the features for alleviating the problem of domain shift. Such methods can be applied conveniently and perform well, making them becoming a main branch in domain adaptation [16]. In this category, there are several methods applying feature alignment to histopathology image classification [8, 17, 18]. Although excellent results have been achieved, these classification methods only align images as a whole, which may lead to limited improvement in nuclei detection that, by nature, focuses on local nuclei regions [3].

In this paper, we propose a novel end-to-end instance-aware (here instance stands for nucleus) domain adaption framework for cross-domain cell nuclei detection in histopathology images (see Fig. 2). To successfully mitigate the domain shift problem on both image (e.g., image magnification, staining, etc.) and instance (e.g., nuclei size, appearance, etc.) levels, we introduce two feature alignment components, namely image-level alignment (IMA) and instance-level alignment (INA), to work together with a nuclei detection model, and minimize the domain shift on both levels by training domain discriminators with adversarial learning strategy. Importantly, INA component leverages nuclei locations to extract instance-level features obtained from local nuclei regions, and then effectively aligns the instance-level features by a domain discriminator. Moreover, as nuclei locations are not available for the target domain, INA component also includes a Temporal Ensembling based Nuclei Localization (TENL) module that is designed to automatically generate candidate nuclei locations to facilitate instance-level feature alignment. To validate our proposed method, extensive experiments are conducted on two benchmark settings for cross-domain nuclei detection, including CoNSeP [19] to CRCHisto [3], and CoNSeP to an in-house dataset BCNuP (Breast Cancer Nuclear Phenotypes). The experimental results show that our method outperforms existing domain adaptation methods by large margin.

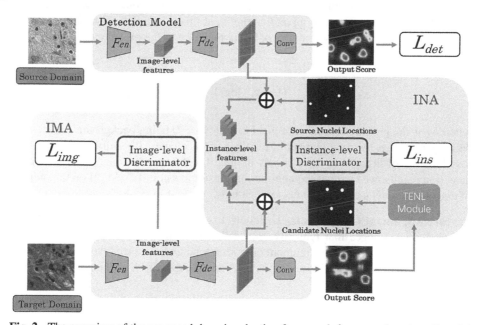

Fig. 2. The overview of the proposed domain adaption framework for cross-domain cell nuclei detection.

2 Method

2.1 Problem Formulation

In the task of cross-domain nuclei detection, we are given an annotated source domain $D_s = \left\{ \left(x_i^s, y_i^s \right) \right\}_{i=1}^{N_s}$, where x_i^s and $y_i^s = \left\{ \left(m_{i,j}^s, n_{i,j}^s \right) \right\}_{i=1}^{N_i^s}$ indicate the i-th image and its corresponding annotations, i.e., the coordinates of nuclei centroids. N_s and N_i^s denote the number of source images and the number of annotations in x_i^s respectively. Additionally, we have an unannotated target domain $D_t = \{x_i^t\}_{i=1}^{N_t}$, where N_t denotes the number of target images. We try to utilize the knowledge from D_s to improve the detection performance in D_t.

2.2 Framework Overview

As shown in Fig. 2, we introduce an instance-aware domain adaption framework for cross-domain cell nuclei detection in histopathology images, which contains a detection model and two feature alignment components.

Detection Model. The goal of detection model is to obtain a mapping translation between a histopathology image and its nuclei positions. Similar to [20], we adopt an encoder-decoder architecture that consists of three encoding blocks and three decoding blocks, and a 1×1 convolutional layer followed by a softmax nonlinearity as our detection model. Formally, for every pixel k in the input image, the detection model outputs the score p_k indicating its probability of being nuclei, and the model can be trained by minimizing:

$$L_{\text{det}} = -\frac{1}{N} \sum_{k=1}^{N} ((1 - y_k) \log(1 - p_k) + y_k \log p_k), \tag{1}$$

where y_k is the ground truth label of pixel k, with $y_k = 0$ being background and $y_k = 1$ being nuclei. N is the total number of pixels in input images. It's worth noting that the loss function of detection model is only applied for the source domain. To obtain the detection results, we conduct the non-maximum suppression (NMS) [2] on the outputs of detection model to obtain the nuclei locations.

Feature Alignment Components. Different from most of the existing studies of histopathology images that typically reduce the domain shift by aligning images as a whole, we conduct feature alignment on both image and instance levels. In summary, we design two powerful components, i.e., IMA and INA, to fulfill instance-aware feature alignment.

2.3 Image-Level Alignment

IMA component aims to align global features obtained from the whole image to alleviate the problem of domain shift, for which a domain discriminator D_{img} with the same architecture as [21] is trained via adversarial alignment [22]. Concretely, given image-level features extracted from encoder of detection model F_{en}, D_{img} aims to identify whether the image-level features come from the source or the target domain, while F_{en} is trained to fool D_{img}. Accordingly, D_{img} and F_{en} can be optimized by an image-level adaptation loss, which can be written as:

$$L_{img} = -\frac{1}{N_s} \sum_{i=1}^{N_s} (1 - z_i) \log(1 - D_{img}(F_{en}(x_i^s))) - \frac{1}{N_t} \sum_{i=1}^{N_t} z_i \log(D_{img}(F_{en}(x_i^t))). \tag{2}$$

F_{en} parameters are updated to minimax the image-level adaptation loss, whereas the discriminator D_{img} is updated to maximin the loss.

2.4 Instance-Level Alignment

In this study, a powerful INA component is developed that allows us to focus on extracting and aligning instance-level features. To this end, we train a domain discriminator for effectively aligning instance-level features obtained from local nuclei regions. Also, a TENL module is employed in INA component to automatically generate candidate nuclei locations in the target domain with high efficiency.

Perform Alignment. We use nuclei locations, i.e., the coordinates of nuclei centroids, as the guidance to our INA component. Given the centroid coordinates $\left(m_{i,j}, n_{i,j}\right)$ of the j-th nuclei in input image x_i, we first create a local rectangular region that is defined by a four-tuple $\left(m_{i,j} - (w-1)/2, n_{i,j} - (h-1)/2, m_{i,j} + (w-1)/2, n_{i,j} + (h-1)/2\right)$, with h and w being the height and width of the local region. After that, by applying these local rectangular regions to high-resolution feature map generated by decoder F_{de}, we extract a series of instance-level features from these local nuclei regions, and feed them into a domain discriminator D_{ins} with five 3×3 convolutional layers, a 1×1 convolutional layer and a FC layer to perform instance-level feature alignment. Let $r_{i,j}$ denotes the instance-level features of the j-th nuclei region in x_i. The instance-level adaptation loss is defined as:

$$L_{ins} = -\frac{1}{N_s}\sum_{i=1}^{N_s}(1-z_i)\log(1-\frac{1}{N_i^s}\sum_{j=1}^{N_i^s}D_{ins}(r_{i,j}^s)) - \frac{1}{N_t}\sum_{i=1}^{N_t}z_i\log\frac{1}{N_i^t}\sum_{j=1}^{N_i^t}D_{ins}(r_{i,j}^t),$$

(3)

where N_i^t denotes the number of local nuclei regions in $x_i^t \cdot \frac{1}{N_i}\sum_{j=1}^{N_i}D_{ins}\left(r_{i,j}\right)$ represents average output of D_{ins} for the local nuclei regions in x_i. z_i represents domain label and is set as 0 and 1 for the source and target domain, respectively.

Generate Candidate Nuclei Locations. We desire to utilize nuclei locations to perform instance-level feature alignment, but nuclei locations are unavailable in the target domain. A natural idea is that during the t-th training epoch we can use the pixel-wise output $p_k^{(t-1)}$ of the detection model in the previous training epoch to generate candidate nuclei locations in the target domain. Nevertheless, we are still facing one challenge that the output from the detection model at the most recent training epoch is often noisy, which in consequence hampers the localization of candidate nuclei in the target domain and instance-level feature alignment. To alleviate this problem, inspired by temporal ensembling technique [23] we incorporate an efficient TENL module into INA component. Specifically, TENL module tries to aggregate the predictions of multiple previous outputs of the detection model into an ensemble output $P_k^{(t-1)}$, which can be formulated as:

$$P_k^{(t-1)} = \alpha P_k^{(t-2)} + (1-\alpha)p_k^{(t-1)},$$

(4)

where α is a momentum term controlling how far the ensemble reaches into training history [23]. After that, TENL module determines the positions of the candidate nuclei centers by finding local maxima in $P_k^{(t-1)}$ exceeding a certain threshold β via NMS.

2.5 Network Optimization

The training procedure of our proposed end-to-end domain adaptation framework is as follow: 1) The supervised detection loss L_{det} is only used in the annotated source domain; 2) We align image-level features by optimizing L_{img}; 3) At first, candidate nuclei locations are generated in the target domain. Then we update instance-level features adaptively. Finally, instance-level feature alignment is achieved by optimizing L_{ins}.

With the terms aforementioned, the overall loss is:

$$L_{total} = L_{det} + \lambda L_{img} + \eta L_{ins}, \tag{5}$$

Where λ and η weight the importance of IMA and INA components, respectively.

3 Experiments and Results

3.1 Datasets

We evaluate our method on two benchmark settings for domain adaptation: 1) train on CoNSeP [19] and test on CRCHisto [3] dataset; 2) train on CoNSeP and test on in-house dataset BCNuP. The CoNSeP dataset contains 41 hematoxylin and eosin (H&E) stained images of colorectal adenocarcinoma. We use the dataset as our source domain on two benchmark settings and all images and annotations in CoNSeP are used for training [6, 22]. As the dataset just provides the coordinates of nuclei centroids, by following [4] we employ a 5×5 rectangular mask centered at each centroid as the ground truth when training the detection model. The CRCHisto dataset includes 100 H&E stained histology images of colorectal adenocarcinoma. We randomly split the dataset into two subsets of 50 images each, one for training and one for testing [14], and then randomly split 20% images out of training subset for validation. We follow [6] to use the training subset of CRCHisto as the target domain (without annotations), and report the results on the test subset of CRCHisto, including the metrics for evaluating the performances of various methods, i.e., precision, recall and F1 score [3].

In this study, a new dataset is introduced, which we term as the Breast Cancer Nuclear Phenotypes (BCNuP) dataset to evaluate our method. The dataset involves 100 H&E stained breast cancer histology images. All images have a size of 512×512 pixels at 20 $\times$ objective magnification, and are cropped without overlapping from areas of WSIs obtained using an KFBIO KF-PRO-005 scanner (http://www.kfbio.cn/). Manual annotation of nuclei is conducted by three experienced pathologists and for detection purposes a total number of 18000 nuclei are marked at the center. This dataset is split and evaluated in the same way as CRCHisto.

3.2 Implementation Details

In our experiments, we adopt data augmentation such as rotation and horizontal/vertical flipping when training model [2]. Domain discriminators are trained by the Adam optimizer [24] with the learning rate of 10^{-3}. The nuclei detection model is trained by the Adam optimizer for 30 epochs with the learning rate of 10^{-3}, and we reduce it to 10^{-4} for another 70 epochs. To prevent the instance-level alignment suffering from less-accurate candidate nuclei locations in the early training epoch, we perform instance-level alignment after 20 training epochs. We set the parameter values as: $\alpha = 0.3$ in Eq. (4) and $\lambda = 0.1$, $\eta = 0.02$ in Eq. (5). We set h and w to 9 when extracting instance-level features and use $\beta = 0.5$ when generating candidate nuclei locations in TENL module.

3.3 Results

Comparison with Existing Methods. We implement several existing domain adaptation methods for comparison, including a color normalization method (SPCN) [10], a classical pixel-wise adaptation method (CycleGAN) [12] and feature-wise adaptation methods (ADDA [15] and DA Faster R-CNN [6]). It is noteworthy that we choose to compare domain adaptation components in [6] that take instance-level features extracted by our method as input, since region proposals used in [6] is not applicable to our datasets. In addition, we also conduct the "Oracle" results to know how much domain shift our method reduces, in which the detection model is trained in a supervised manner on the target domain [7, 16]. As shown in Table 1, for the adaptation of CoNSeP-to-CRCHisto, our final model (IMA + INA + TENL) achieves a higher performance over these domain adaptation methods. In particular, on F1 score our final model outperforms SPCN [10], CycleGAN [12], ADDA [15] and DA Faster R-CNN [6] by 6.7%, 4.8%, 5.4% and 3.1%, respectively. Additionally, our final model helps to reduce the performance gap between

Table 1. Results of different methods for the adaptation of CoNSeP-to-CRCHisto and CoNSeP-to-BCNuP. "P", "R" and "F1" represent precision, recall, and F1 score.

	CoNSeP-to-CRCHisto			CoNSeP-to-BCNuP		
	P	R	F1	P	R	F1
SPCN [10]	0.693	0.774	0.732	0.709	0.764	0.735
CycleGAN [12]	0.692	0.797	0.741	0.716	0.777	0.745
ADDA [15]	0.688	0.789	0.735	0.677	0.776	0.723
DA Faster R-CNN [6]	0.712	0.811	0.758	0.685	0.796	0.736
Baseline	0.662	0.809	0.728	0.658	0.766	0.708
Ours (IMA)	0.678	0.826	0.745	0.695	0.785	0.737
Ours (IMA + INA)	0.691	0.887	0.777	0.723	0.791	0.756
Ours (IMA + INA + TENL)	0.721	0.872	0.789	0.730	0.812	0.769
Oracle	0.811	0.861	0.836	0.772	0.858	0.813

domain adaptation model and the oracle model to about 5% on F1 score. Not surprisingly, in Table 1 we also find that our final model obtains the best results among all the counterparts for the adaptation of CoNSeP-to-BCNuP.

Furthermore, we compare our final model with fully supervised deep learning methods including POI [4], U-Net [9] and FCN [11], which are trained with both images and annotations in the target domain. As shown in Table 2, we see that our final model is comparable to or even better than these methods on both two datasets. Taken together, these results demonstrate the strength of our method for cross-domain nuclei detection in histopathology images.

Table 2. Comparison with fully supervised methods in the target domain. For our method that does not use any annotations in the target domain, we report the performances for the adaptation of CoNSeP-to-CRCHisto and CoNSeP-to-BCNuP.

	CoNSeP-to-CRCHisto			CoNSeP-to-BCNuP		
	P	R	F1	P	R	F1
FCN [11]	0.668	0.874	0.757	0.675	0.843	0.750
U-Net [9]	0.691	0.819	0.750	0.777	0.749	0.763
POI [4]	0.802	0.872	0.836	0.757	0.850	0.801
Ours (IMA + INA + TENL)	0.721	0.872	0.789	0.730	0.712	0.769

Ablation Analysis. We study the contribution of each key component in our framework. The reference baseline is the detection model that is trained in the source domain and applied to the target domain directly. In addition, two variants of our method are evaluated: 1) IMA, which is the detection model with IMA component only; 2) IMA + INA, which is the detection model with IMA component and INA component that feeds only pixel-wise output $p_k^{(t-1)}$ in the previous training epoch into NMS to generate candidate nuclei locations in the target domain. As shown in Table 1, for both CoNSeP-to-CRCHisto and CoNSeP-to-BCNuP, IMA performs better than the baseline by aligning image-level features, and IMA + INA further improves the performance via extracting and aligning instance-level features. Notably, for the adaptation of CoNSeP-to-CRCHisto, our final model outperforms the baseline by 6.1% on F1 score, 6.3% on recall and 5.9% on precision, demonstrating the capability of our feature alignment components to deal with the domain shift problem.

To further assess the influence of height and width of local region for extracting in-stance-level features, we conduct an ablation study on CRCHisto dataset. The experimental comparisons under different height and width settings are shown in Table 3. The best overall performance can be achieved when the height and width are both set to 9. Smaller height and width may lead to insufficient discriminative information for instance-level alignment, and therefore the performance is not satisfactory in target domain. Using height and width larger than 9 shows no substantial benefit and a too large region results in decreased performance probably due to the background noises.

Table 3. The ablation study on height and width of the local region for extracting instance-level features.

Height × Width	Precision	Recall	F1 score
5 × 5	0.708	0.859	0.777
6 × 6	0.721	0.872	0.789
7 × 7	0.721	0.867	0.787
8 × 8	0.720	0.863	0.785
9 × 9	0.704	0.863	0.775

4 Conclusion

We present a novel instance-aware adversarial domain adaptation framework for cell nuclei detection in histopathology images. Specifically, IMA and IINA components effectively align the features on both image and instance levels by domain discriminators via adversarial training. Additionally, to facilitate instance-level feature alignment, TENL module is introduced to automatically generate candidate nuclei locations in the target domain. Extensive experiments confirm the effectiveness of our method on cross-domain nuclei detection.

Acknowledgement. This work was partly supported by the National Natural Science Foundation of China (61871361, 61971393, 61471331, 61571414).

References

1. Hou, L., et al.: Sparse autoencoder for unsupervised nucleus detection and representation in histopathology images. Pattern Recogn. **86**, 188–200 (2019)
2. Zhou, Y., Dou, Q., Chen, H., Qin, J., Heng, P.A.: SFCN-OPI: detection and fine-grained classification of nuclei using sibling FCN with objectness prior interaction. In: AAAI, pp. 2374–3468 (2018)
3. Sirinukunwattana, K., Raza, S.E.A., Tsang, Y.W., Snead, D.R., Cree, I.A., Rajpoot, N.M.: Locality sensitive deep learning for detection and classification of nuclei in routine colon cancer histology images. IEEE Trans. Med. Imaging **35**(5), 1196–1206 (2016)
4. Li, X., Wei, L., Ran, T.: Staged detection–identification framework for cell nuclei in histopathology images. IEEE Trans. Instrum. Meas. **69**(1), 183–193 (2020)
5. Alirezazadeh, P., Hejrati, B., Monsef-Esfahani, A., Fathi, A.: Representation learning-based unsupervised domain adaptation for classification of breast cancer histopathology images. Biocybernet. Biomed. Eng. **38**(3), 671–683 (2018)
6. Chen, Y., Li, W., Sakaridis, C., Dai, D., Van Gool, L.: Domain adaptive faster r-cnn for object detection in the wild. In: CVPR, pp. 3339–3348 (2018)
7. Hsu, C.-C., Tsai, Y.-H., Lin, Y.-Y., Yang, M.-H.: Every pixel matters: center-aware feature alignment for domain adaptive object detector. In: Vedaldi, A., Bischof, H., Brox, T., Frahm, J.-M. (eds.) Computer Vision – ECCV 2020: 16th European Conference, Glasgow, UK, August 23–28, 2020, Proceedings, Part IX, pp. 733–748. Springer International Publishing, Cham (2020). https://doi.org/10.1007/978-3-030-58545-7_42

8. Ren, J., Hacihaliloglu, I., Singer, E.A., Foran, D.J., Qi, X.: Adversarial domain adaptation for classification of prostate histopathology whole-slide images. In: Frangi, A.F., Schnabel, J.A., Davatzikos, C., Alberola-López, C., Fichtinger, G. (eds.) MICCAI 2018. LNCS, vol. 11071, pp. 201–209. Springer, Cham (2018). https://doi.org/10.1007/978-3-030-00934-2_23

9. Ronneberger, O., Fischer, P., Brox, T.: U-Net: convolutional networks for biomedical image segmentation. In: Navab, N., Hornegger, J., Wells, W.M., Frangi, A.F. (eds.) MICCAI 2015. LNCS, vol. 9351, pp. 234–241. Springer, Cham (2015). https://doi.org/10.1007/978-3-319-24574-4_28

10. Vahadane, A., et al.: Structure-preserving color normalization and sparse stain separation for histological images. IEEE Trans. Med. Imaging **35**(8), 1962–1971 (2016)

11. Long, J., Shelhamer, E., Darrell, T.: Fully convolutional networks for semantic segmentation. In: CVPR, pp. 3431–3440 (2015)

12. Zhu, J.Y., Park, T., Isola, P., Efros, A.: Unpaired image-to-image translation using cycle-consistent adversarial networks. In: ICCV, pp. 2223–2232 (2017)

13. Hoffman, J., et al.: CyCADA: cycle-consistent adversarial domain adaptation. In: ICML, pp. 1989–1998 (2018)

14. Xing, F., Bennett, T., Ghosh, D.: Adversarial domain adaptation and pseudo-labeling for cross-modality microscopy image quantification. In: Shen, D., et al. (eds.) MICCAI 2019. LNCS, vol. 11764, pp. 740–749. Springer, Cham (2019). https://doi.org/10.1007/978-3-030-32239-7_82

15. Tzeng, E., Hoffman, J., Saenko, K., Darrell, T.: Adversarial discriminative domain adaptation. In: CVPR, pp. 2962–2971 (2017)

16. Zheng, Y., Huang, D., Liu, S., Wang, Y.: Cross-domain object detection through coarse-to-fine feature adaptation. In: CVPR, pp. 13766–13775 (2020)

17. Zhang, Y., et al.: From whole slide imaging to microscopy: deep microscopy adaptation network for histopathology cancer image classification. In: Shen, D., et al. (eds.) MICCAI 2019. LNCS, vol. 11764, pp. 360–368. Springer, Cham (2019). https://doi.org/10.1007/978-3-030-32239-7_40

18. Lafarge, M.W., Pluim, J.P.W., Eppenhof, K.A.J., Moeskops, P., Veta, M.: Domain-adversarial neural networks to address the appearance variability of histopathology images. In: Cardoso, M.J., et al. (eds.) DLMIA/ML-CDS -2017. LNCS, vol. 10553, pp. 83–91. Springer, Cham (2017). https://doi.org/10.1007/978-3-319-67558-9_10

19. Graham, S., et al.: Hover-net: simultaneous segmentation and classification of nuclei in multi-tissue histology images. Med. Image Anal. **58**, 101563 (2019)

20. Xie, Y., Xing, F., Shi, X., Kong, X., Su, H., Yang, L.: Efficient and robust cell detection: a structured regression approach. Med. Image Anal. **44**, 245–254 (2018)

21. Pan, F., Shin, I., Rameau, F., Lee, S., Kweon, I.S.: Unsupervised intra-domain adaptation for semantic segmentation through self-supervision. In: CVPR, pp. 3764–3773 (2020)

22. Zhu, X., Pang, J., Yang, C., Shi, J., Lin, D.: Adapting object detectors via selective cross-domain alignment. In: CVPR, pp. 687–696 (2019)

23. Laine, S., Aila, T.: Temporal ensembling for semi-supervised learning. In: ICLR, pp. 1–13 (2016)

24. Kingma, D.P., Ba, J.: Adam: a method for stochastic optimization. In: ICLR, pp. 1–15 (2015)

Positive-Unlabeled Learning for Cell Detection in Histopathology Images with Incomplete Annotations

Zipei Zhao[1], Fengqian Pang[2], Zhiwen Liu[1(✉)], and Chuyang Ye[1(✉)]

[1] School of Information and Electronics, Beijing Institute of Technology,
Beijing, China
{zwliu,chuyang.ye}@bit.edu.cn
[2] School of Information Science and Technology, North China University
of Technology, Beijing, China

Abstract. Cell detection in histopathology images is of great value in clinical practice. *Convolutional neural networks* (CNNs) have been applied to cell detection to improve the detection accuracy, where cell annotations are required for network training. However, due to the variety and large number of cells, complete annotations that include every cell of interest in the training images can be challenging. Usually, incomplete annotations can be achieved, where positive labeling results are carefully examined to ensure their reliability but there can be other positive instances, i.e., cells of interest, that are not included in the annotations. This annotation strategy leads to a lack of knowledge about true negative samples. Most existing methods simply treat instances that are not labeled as positive as truly negative during network training, which can adversely affect the network performance. In this work, to address the problem of incomplete annotations, we formulate the training of detection networks as a positive-unlabeled learning problem. Specifically, the classification loss in network training is revised to take into account incomplete annotations, where the terms corresponding to negative samples are approximated with the true positive samples and the other samples of which the labels are unknown. To evaluate the proposed method, experiments were performed on a publicly available dataset for mitosis detection in breast cancer cells, and the experimental results show that our method improves the performance of cell detection given incomplete annotations for training.

Keywords: Cell detection · Positive-unlabeled learning · Incomplete annotation

1 Introduction

Clinical medicine relies largely on cell detection and counting in histopathology images to assess the degree of tissue damage. However, conventional detection

---

Z. Zhao and F. Pang—Equal contribution.

© Springer Nature Switzerland AG 2021
M. de Bruijne et al. (Eds.): MICCAI 2021, LNCS 12908, pp. 509–518, 2021.
https://doi.org/10.1007/978-3-030-87237-3_49

methods [18] are complicated and inefficient, and they cannot cope with the large amount of image data. In recent years, the application of *convolutional neural networks* (CNNs) to object detection has shown unparalleled advantages, and CNN-based algorithms are increasingly used in the cell detection task with remarkable results [2,14,17,19].

For training CNN-based detectors, high-quality annotations (bounding boxes in most cases) of the cells of interest are needed. Ideally, every cell of interest in the training images should be annotated by experts. However, due to the large number and diverse morphology of cells in histopathology images, completely annotating all instances becomes very challenging. In practice, experts can prefer to only ensure that all instances labeled as positive are correct [10], and the annotation may even be sparse in the image if a large number of images are to be annotated [9]. In this case, the rest of the instances may not be all true negatives, and there still exist unannotated positive instances with high probability. In other words, the annotations are incomplete and only include a subset of the cells of interest. Most existing methods simply treat unannotated areas as negative instances during network training [16]. Although this training strategy may still achieve promising results given a relatively large number of annotated positive instances, it neglects the existence of false negative training data due to incomplete annotations and is thus suboptimal.

Very recently, the problem of incomplete annotations for training CNN-based cell detectors draws attention [9]. In [9], motivated by the significant density difference between the regression boxes of positive and negative instances, *Boxes Density Energy* (BDE) is proposed to calibrate the training loss. The assumption of BDE is that negative samples are inclined to possess a lower density of regression boxes. Therefore, among the instances that are not annotated as positive, the regions with a higher density of regression boxes are less likely to be truly negative, and their losses as negative samples are calibrated to be smaller. Compared with methods that neglect the problem of incomplete annotations, the detection performance is improved with BDE. To the best of our knowledge, this is the only existing work that addresses the problem of incomplete annotations for cell detection[1], and the development of cell detection methods with incomplete annotations is still an open problem.

In this work, we continue to explore the problem of incomplete annotations for CNN-based cell detection in histopathology images. Since the regions without annotated instances may include both positive and negative samples, we treat the instances in these regions as unlabeled data and propose to reformulate the classification part of the detection problem as a *positive-unlabeled* (PU) learning problem [1,4]. In particular, the classification loss for network training is revised, where the terms about negative samples are approximated with the annotated positive instances and unlabeled instances. The revised classification loss is then integrated with the localization loss to train the detection network. To evaluate the proposed method, we performed experiments on a publicly available dataset

---

[1] The work in [10] requires the annotated mask of each instance in addition to the bounding box, and thus it addresses a different problem.

for mitosis detection in breast cancer histopathology images. For demonstration, Faster R-CNN [13] was used as our backbone detection network, which has been previously applied to various cell detection tasks [16,21]. Experimental results show that our method leads to improved cell detection performance given incomplete annotations for training.

2   Methods

2.1   Background: Cell Detection with Complete Annotations for Training

In typical deep learning based methods of object detection, e.g., Faster R-CNN [13], the network generates a bounding box to indicate the position of each instance and the corresponding class probability, i.e., the likelihood of the instance belonging to a certain category. In this work, we are interested in cell detection, which usually aims at the detection of a certain type of cells, e.g., cells related to cancer [2,15,19]. Thus, we assume that the classification is binary, i.e., the ground truth label z of the bounding box x is binary: $z \in \{0,1\}$. Note that x is generally initially produced by a region proposal module, such as a region proposal network [13]. The localization of the bounding box x given by the network is denoted by $v = \{X, Y, W, H\}$, where X, Y, W, and H represent the x-coordinate, y-coordinate, width, and height of the bounding box, respectively. The probability of a bounding box being positive—i.e., $z = 1$—predicted by the network is denoted by $c \in [0,1]$.

Conventionally, to train a detection network, all positive instances should be annotated for the training images, and the loss comprising both localization and classification error is minimized. The localization loss $\mathcal{L}_{\mathrm{loc}}$ is computed from the predicted location v and the ground truth location $b = \{X_b, Y_b, W_b, H_b\}$ of the positive instances. For example, a typical choice of $\mathcal{L}_{\mathrm{loc}}$ is the smooth L_1 loss function [9], where

$$\mathcal{L}_{\mathrm{loc}} = \frac{1}{N_{\mathrm{p}}} \sum_{i=1}^{N_{\mathrm{p}}} \sum_{\substack{(v^i, b^i) \in \{(X^i, X_b^i), (Y^i, Y_b^i), \\ (W^i, W_b^i), (H^i, H_b^i)\}}} \mathrm{smooth}_{L_1}(v^i - b^i) \tag{1}$$

$$\text{with} \quad \mathrm{smooth}_{L_1}(a) = \begin{cases} a^2/2, & \text{if } |a| \leq 1 \\ |a| - 0.5, & \text{otherwise} \end{cases}. \tag{2}$$

Here, i and N_{p} are the index and the total number of positive training samples, respectively. The classification loss $\mathcal{L}_{\mathrm{cls}}$ is computed from the predicted classification probability and the corresponding ground truth label as follows

$$\mathcal{L}_{\mathrm{cls}} = \frac{1}{N_{\mathrm{n}} + N_{\mathrm{p}}} \left(\sum_{j=1}^{N_{\mathrm{n}}} H(c_{\mathrm{n}}^j, 0) + \sum_{i=1}^{N_{\mathrm{p}}} H(c_{\mathrm{p}}^i, 1) \right). \tag{3}$$

Here, j and N_n are the index and the total number of negative training samples (samples that have no overlap or do not have a sufficiently large overlap with the labeled positive instances), respectively; c_p^i and c_n^j represent the predicted probability of the positive sample x_p^i and the negative sample x_n^j being positive, respectively; and most commonly $H(\cdot, \cdot)$ is a cross-entropy loss function that measures the difference between the prediction and ground truth [12]. With the complete annotations where every positive instance in the training images is labeled, the sum of the two losses $\mathcal{L}_{loc}$ and $\mathcal{L}_{cls}$ is minimized to learn the weights of the detection network.

2.2   PU Learning for Cell Detection with Incomplete Annotations

For cell annotations on histopathology images, because there are usually a huge number of cells with various appearances, it is challenging to annotate every positive instance. Experts may only ensure that the annotated cells are truly positive, and the annotated cells may even appear sparse in the image to reduce the annotation load [9]. In this case, the training set only contains a subset of the positive instances and misses other positive instances. In other words, in this incompletely annotated dataset, the regions with no instances labeled as positive are not necessarily all truly negative. Therefore, given incomplete annotations, training the detection network with the classification loss described in Eq. (3) is no longer accurate and could cause performance degradation.

Since the regions that are not labeled as positive may comprise both positive and negative samples, the instances in these regions can be considered unlabeled. This means that the incompletely annotated training dataset contains both positively labeled and unlabeled training samples (x_p and x_u, respectively). Thus, to address the problem of incomplete annotations for cell detection, we propose to exploit PU learning, so that the classification loss that is originally computed with complete annotations can be approximated with incomplete annotations.

To derive the approximation of the classification loss, we notice that $\mathcal{L}_{cls}$ is an approximation (empirical mean) of the expectation $\mathbb{E}_{(x,z)}[H(c,z)]$ that measures the difference between the predicted probability c of x being a positive sample and the ground truth label z. The computation of $\mathbb{E}_{(x,z)}[H(c,z)]$ can be reformulated as

$$\mathbb{E}_{(x,z)}[H(c,z)]$$
$$= \Pr(z=0) \int p(x|z=0)H(c,0)\mathrm{d}x + \Pr(z=1) \int p(x|z=1)H(c,1)\mathrm{d}x \quad (4)$$
$$= (1-\pi)\mathbb{E}_{x|z=0}[H(c,0)] + \pi\mathbb{E}_{x|z=1}[H(c,1)]. \quad (5)$$

Here, $p(\cdot)$ represents a probability density function, and $\pi = \Pr(z=1)$ is the positive class prior.

Since positive training samples are available yet negative training samples are unavailable, we can directly compute the second term in Eq. (5) with the training samples but not the first term. However, it is possible to approximate the first term with both positive and unlabeled training samples [8]. Because $p(x) = \Pr(z = 0)p(x|z = 0) + \Pr(z = 1)p(x|z = 1)$, we have

$$\Pr(z = 0)p(x|z = 0) = p(x) - \Pr(z = 1)p(x|z = 1), \qquad (6)$$

and the first term $(1 - \pi)\mathbb{E}_{x|z=0}[H(c, 0)]$ in Eq. (5) becomes

$$\Pr(z = 0) \int p(x|z = 0)H(c, 0)\mathrm{d}x$$

$$= \int p(x)H(c, 0)\mathrm{d}x - \Pr(z = 1) \int p(x|z = 1)H(c, 0)\mathrm{d}x \qquad (7)$$

$$= \mathbb{E}_x[H(c, 0)] - \pi\mathbb{E}_{x|z=1}[H(c, 0)]. \qquad (8)$$

Then, based on Eq. (5), $\mathbb{E}_{(x,z)}[H(c, z)]$ becomes

$$\mathbb{E}_{(x,z)}[H(c, z)] = \mathbb{E}_x[H(c, 0)] - \pi\mathbb{E}_{x|z=1}[H(c, 0)] + \pi\mathbb{E}_{x|z=1}[H(c, 1)]. \qquad (9)$$

Now, the second and third terms on the right hand side of Eq. (9) can be computed with positive samples, and the first term $\mathbb{E}_x[H(c, 0)]$ still needs to be determined.

In PU learning for classification problems, it is assumed that the distribution of the unlabeled data x_u is the same as the distribution of x, so that $\mathbb{E}_x[H(c, 0)]$ can be approximated by $\mathbb{E}_{x_u}[H(c, 0)]$. Previous work has directly applied such approximation to an object detection problem [20]. However, simply applying the PU learning strategy developed for classification to the detection problem can be problematic, because in detection problems the unlabeled samples and positively labeled samples originate from the same images. Some positive samples are excluded from the distribution of x_u, and thus the approximation is biased. Instead, if we combine the positively labeled and unlabeled samples in the same images, they provide samples drawn from the distribution of x, and $\mathbb{E}_x[H(c, 0)]$ can be approximated using the combination of these samples:

$$\mathbb{E}_x[H(c, 0)] \approx \frac{1}{N_u + N_p} \left(\sum_{k=1}^{N_u} H(c_u^k, 0) + \sum_{i=1}^{N_p} H(c_p^i, 0) \right), \qquad (10)$$

where k and N_u are the index and the total number of unlabeled training samples, respectively, and c_u^k represents the predicted probability of the unlabeled sample x_u^k. In this way, all terms on the right hand side of Eq. (9) can be approximated with the training samples. Note that in practice an expressive CNN may overfit the data and produce negative values for the approximation of $(1 - \pi)\mathbb{E}_{x|z=0}[H(c, 0)]$ in Eq. (8). Thus, we follow [8] and use a nonnegative approximation of $(1 - \pi)\mathbb{E}_{x|z=0}[H(c, 0)]$, which leads to

$$\mathbb{E}_x[H(c, 0)] - \pi\mathbb{E}_{x|z=1}[H(c, 0)]$$

$$\approx \max\left\{ 0, \frac{1}{N_u + N_p} \left(\sum_{k=1}^{N_u} H(c_u^k, 0) + \sum_{i=1}^{N_p} H(c_p^i, 0) \right) - \frac{\pi}{N_p} \sum_{i=1}^{N_p} H(c_p^i, 0) \right\}.$$

$$(11)$$

Then, we have the revised classification loss that approximates $\mathbb{E}_{(x,z)}[H(c,z)]$ with the PU learning framework:

$$\mathcal{L}_{\text{cls}}^{\text{pu}} = \max \left\{ 0, \frac{1}{N_{\text{u}} + N_{\text{p}}} \left(\sum_{k=1}^{N_{\text{u}}} H(c_{\text{u}}^k, 0) + \sum_{i=1}^{N_{\text{p}}} H(c_{\text{p}}^i, 0) \right) - \frac{\pi}{N_{\text{p}}} \sum_{i=1}^{N_{\text{p}}} H(c_{\text{p}}^i, 0) \right\}$$

$$+ \frac{\pi}{N_{\text{p}}} \sum_{i=1}^{N_{\text{p}}} H(c_{\text{p}}^i, 1). \tag{12}$$

Note that the class prior π in $\mathcal{L}_{\text{cls}}^{\text{pu}}$ is assumed to be known. Since it is difficult to directly estimate π using incompletely annotated training samples, π can be considered a hyperparameter and determined with a validation set (see Sect. 3.2).

With the revised classification loss, the complete loss function for training the detection network with incomplete annotations is

$$\mathcal{L} = \mathcal{L}_{\text{loc}} + \mathcal{L}_{\text{cls}}^{\text{pu}}. \tag{13}$$

This loss function can be integrated with different state-of-the-art backbone detection networks that are based on the combination of localization and classification losses, e.g., Faster R-CNN [13] that is widely applied to object detection problems including cell detection.

3   Results

3.1   Dataset Description and Experimental Settings

To evaluate the proposed method, we performed experiments on the publicly available MITOS-ATYPIA-14 dataset[2], which aims to detect mitosis in breast cancer cells. The dataset comprises 393 images, and the image size is 1600×1600. In this dataset, experienced pathologists have annotated each mitosis with a key point, and like [9] for each key point we generated a 32×32 bounding box centered around it.

The images were split into a training, validation, and test set with a ratio of about 4:1:1, and we performed 5-fold cross-validation for evaluation, where the validation set was fixed and the training and test sets were regrouped in each fold. Since the size of the original image is large, we cropped the images into 500 × 500 patches with an overlap of 100 pixels horizontally and vertically between adjacent patches. In addition, to simulate the scenario where incomplete annotations are performed, like [9] for each image in the training or validation set, we randomly deleted the annotations until there was only one annotation per image patch. The annotations in the test set were intact.

For demonstration, we used Faster R-CNN [13] as the baseline network to detect the mitosis, as it has been previously used for similar detection tasks [16,21]. The Faster R-CNN had been pretrained on ImageNet [3] for a

---

[2] https://mitos-atypia-14.grand-challenge.org/.

better initialization of network weights.[3] For each patch, at most 100 prediction boxes were generated according to the confidence score (greater than 0.5) in descending order [13]. For test images, the detection result on each patch was merged to produce the final prediction. Specifically, we generated prediction boxes for each 500×500 patch, mapped the coordinates of these boxes back into the image, and performed non-maximum suppression [11] to merge duplicate bounding boxes.

The Adam optimizer [7] was used for minimizing the loss function, where the initial learning rate was set to 10^{-3}. To ensure training convergence, the detection network was trained with 20 epochs, and the training procedure took about 4 h on an NVIDIA GeForce GTX 1080 Ti GPU.

3.2 Detection Accuracy

As described in Sect. 2.2, the class prior π was determined based on the validation set. The candidate values of π ranged from 0.02 to 0.06 with an increment of 0.01. Because there were only incompletely annotated images in the validation set, precision could not be used to evaluate the performance on the validation set [16]. Thus, we selected π according to the best average recall computed from the validation set. Note that π was selected for each fold independently, and the selected value was consistent (0.04 or 0.05) across the folds.

We compared the proposed method with two competing methods, which, for fair comparison, used the same backbone Faster R-CNN detection network. In the first competing method, the Faster R-CNN model (initialized with the pretraining on ImageNet) was trained using the incomplete annotations, where the unlabeled regions were simply considered negative. This Faster R-CNN is referred to as the baseline method. In the second competing method, we integrated the BDE method [9] with the baseline Faster R-CNN, so that weights were added to the unlabeled samples to calibrate the classification loss according to the density of regression boxes. Note that in the BDE method, the samples in the unlabeled areas are still considered negative, but their weights are adjusted based on how likely they are to be really negative, whereas in our method the samples in the unlabeled areas are considered to have unknown classes, and they are used together with positively labeled samples to approximate the classification loss in a principled framework.

We first qualitatively evaluated the proposed method. Examples of the detection results of each method on test patches are shown in Fig. 1, together with the full annotations. The numbers of *true positive* (TP) and *false positive* (FP) detection results are also indicated in the figure for each case. In these cases, our method compares favorably with the competing methods by either producing more TP boxes than the competing methods without increasing the number of FP boxes or reducing the number of FP boxes with preserved TP boxes.

Next, we quantitatively compared the proposed method with the competing methods. We computed the average recall and average precision of the detection

---

[3] The VGG16 [6] backbone was selected here, but similar results (not reported) were achieved with the ResNet50 and ResNet101 [5] backbones.

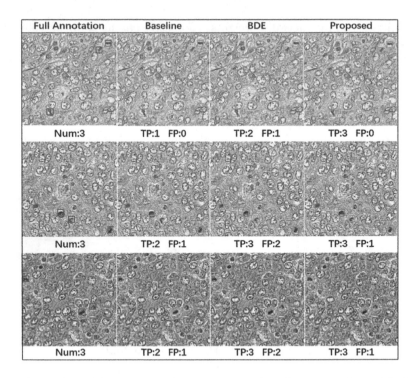

Full Annotation	Baseline	BDE	Proposed
Num:3	TP:1 FP:0	TP:2 FP:1	TP:3 FP:0
Num:3	TP:2 FP:1	TP:3 FP:2	TP:3 FP:1
Num:3	TP:2 FP:1	TP:3 FP:2	TP:3 FP:1

Fig. 1. Examples of detection results on test patches shown together with the full annotations. The numbers of TP and FP detection results and the number of mitoses in the annotation are also indicated for each case.

results on the test set for each fold, and they are shown in Table 1. Compared with the competing methods, the proposed method has higher recall and precision values, which indicate the better detection accuracy of the proposed method.

We also computed the means and standard deviations of the average recall and average precision of the five folds, and compared the proposed method with the competing methods using paired Student's t-tests. These results are shown in Table 2. Consistent with Table 1, the proposed method has higher recall and precision. In addition, the improvement of our method is statistically significant.

Finally, to confirm the benefit of the approximation developed in Eq. (10) for detection problems, we performed experiments with the original PU learning strategy for classification problems as in [20] for comparison. The means of the average recall and average precision of the five folds were computed, which are 0.770 and 0.503, respectively. Although the recall is comparable to the result (0.771) of the proposed method, the mean precision is much worse than the result (0.530) of the proposed method (see Table 2). The mean precision is even worse than the BDE result (0.516) and close to the baseline result (0.501) reported in Table 2. These comparisons confirm that directly applying the PU learning strategy developed for classification problems may not be suitable for cell detection in histopathology images.

Table 1. The average recall and average precision on the test set for each fold. The results of the proposed method are highlighted in bold.

Method	Fold 1		Fold 2		Fold 3		Fold 4		Fold 5	
	Recall	Precision	Recall	Precision	Recall	Precision	Recall	Precision	Recall	Precision
Baseline	0.778	0.533	0.733	0.506	0.753	0.543	0.710	0.510	0.649	0.412
BDE	0.821	0.552	0.792	0.529	0.789	0.557	0.725	0.528	0.670	0.415
Proposed	**0.842**	**0.567**	**0.802**	**0.547**	**0.801**	**0.559**	**0.738**	**0.541**	**0.670**	**0.435**

Table 2. The means and *standard deviations* (stds) of the average recall and average precision of the five folds. The results of the proposed method are highlighted in bold. Asterisks indicate that the difference between the proposed method and the competing method is significant using a paired Student's t-test. ($^*p < 0.05$, $^{**}p < 0.01$)

	Recall			Precision		
	Baseline	BDE	Proposed	Baseline	BDE	Proposed
Mean	0.725	0.750	**0.771**	0.501	0.516	**0.530**
Std	0.044	0.055	**0.060**	0.047	0.052	**0.048**
p	**	*	–	**	*	–

4   Conclusion

In this work, we seek to address the problem of network training with incomplete annotations for cell detection in histopathology images. We propose to apply PU learning to cell detection, so that the classification loss is more appropriately computed from the incompletely annotated data during network training. The experimental results on a publicly available dataset show that our method can improve the performance of cell detection given incomplete annotations.

Acknowledgements. This work is supported by National Natural Science Foundation of China (62001009).

References

1. Charles, E., Keith, N.: Learning classifiers from only positive and unlabeled data. In: International Conference on Knowledge Discovery and Data Mining, pp. 213–220 (2008)
2. Cireşan, D.C., Giusti, A., Gambardella, L.M., Schmidhuber, J.: Mitosis detection in breast cancer histology images with deep neural networks. In: Mori, K., Sakuma, I., Sato, Y., Barillot, C., Navab, N. (eds.) MICCAI 2013. LNCS, vol. 8150, pp. 411–418. Springer, Heidelberg (2013). https://doi.org/10.1007/978-3-642-40763-5_51
3. Deng, J., Dong, W., Socher, R., Li, L.J., Li, K., Fei-Fei, L.: ImageNet: a large-scale hierarchical image database. In: IEEE Conference on Computer Vision and Pattern Recognition, pp. 248–255 (2009)
4. Fabien, L., Francois, D., Remi, G.: Learning from positive and unlabeled examples. In: Algorithmic Learning Theory, pp. 71–85 (2000)

5. He, K., Zhang, X., Ren, S., Sun, J.: Deep residual learning for image recognition. In: IEEE Conference on Computer Vision and Pattern Recognition, pp. 770–778 (2016)
6. Karen, S., Andrew, Z.: Very deep convolutional networks for large-scale image recognition. arXiv preprint arXiv:1409.1556 (2015)
7. Kingma, D.P., Ba, J.: Adam: a method for stochastic optimization. arXiv preprint arXiv:1412.6980 (2014)
8. Kiryo, R., Niu, G., Marthinus, P., Masashi, S.: Positive-unlabeled learning with non-negative risk estimator. In: Advances In Neural Information Processing Systems, pp. 1674–1684 (2017)
9. Li, H., et al.: A novel loss calibration strategy for object detection networks training on sparsely annotated pathological datasets. In: Martel, A.L., et al. (eds.) MICCAI 2020. LNCS, vol. 12265, pp. 320–329. Springer, Cham (2020). https://doi.org/10.1007/978-3-030-59722-1_31
10. Li, J., et al.: Signet ring cell detection with a semi-supervised learning framework. In: Chung, A.C.S., Gee, J.C., Yushkevich, P.A., Bao, S. (eds.) IPMI 2019. LNCS, vol. 11492, pp. 842–854. Springer, Cham (2019). https://doi.org/10.1007/978-3-030-20351-1_66
11. Neubeck, A., Van Gool, L.J.: Efficient non-maximum suppression. In: International Conference on Pattern Recognition, pp. 850–855 (2006)
12. Phan, T.H., Yamamoto, K.: Resolving class imbalance in object detection with weighted cross entropy losses. arXiv preprint arXiv:2006.01413 (2020)
13. Ren, S., He, K., Girshick, R., Sun, J.: Faster R-CNN: towards real-time object detection with region proposal networks. In: Advances in Neural Information Processing Systems, pp. 91–99 (2015)
14. Schmidt, U., Weigert, M., Broaddus, C., Myers, G.: Cell detection with star-convex polygons. In: Frangi, A.F., Schnabel, J.A., Davatzikos, C., Alberola-López, C., Fichtinger, G. (eds.) MICCAI 2018. LNCS, vol. 11071, pp. 265–273. Springer, Cham (2018). https://doi.org/10.1007/978-3-030-00934-2_30
15. Sirinukunwattana, K., Raza, S.E.A., Tsang, Y.W., Snead, D.R., Cree, I.A., Rajpoot, N.M.: Locality sensitive deep learning for detection and classification of nuclei in routine colon cancer histology images. IEEE Trans. Med. Imaging 35(5), 1196–1206 (2016)
16. Sun, Y., Huang, X., Molina, E.G.L., Dong, L., Zhang, Q.: Signet ring cells detection in histology images with similarity learning. In: International Symposium on Biomedical Imaging, pp. 37–48 (2020)
17. Tzu-Hsi, S., Victor, S., Hesham, E.: Simultaneous cell detection and classification in bone marrow histology images. IEEE J. Biomed. Health Inform. 23(4), 1469–1476 (2018)
18. Veta, M., Pluim, J.P., Van Diest, P.J., Viergever, M.A.: Breast cancer histopathology image analysis: a review. IEEE Trans. Biomed. Eng. 61(5), 1400–1411 (2014)
19. Xu, J., Lei, X., Liu, Q., Hannah, G., Wu, J.: Stacked sparse autoencoder (SSAE) for nuclei detection on breast cancer histopathology images. IEEE Trans. Med. Imaging 35(1), 119–130 (2015)
20. Yang, Y., Liang, K.J., Carin, L.: Object detection as a positive-unlabeled problem. In: British Machine Vision Conference (2020)
21. Zhang, J., Hu, H., Chen, S.: Cancer cells detection in phasecontrast microscopy images based on faster R-CNN. In: International Symposium on Computational Intelligence and Design, pp. 363–367 (2016)

GloFlow: Whole Slide Image Stitching from Video Using Optical Flow and Global Image Alignment

Viswesh Krishna[(✉)], Anirudh Joshi[(✉)], Damir Vrabac, Philip Bulterys,
Eric Yang, Sebastian Fernandez-Pol, Andrew Y. Ng, and Pranav Rajpurkar

Stanford University, Stanford, CA 94305, USA
{viswesh,anirudhjoshi}@cs.stanford.edu

Abstract. The application of deep learning to pathology assumes the existence of digital whole slide images of pathology slides. However, slide digitization is bottlenecked by the high cost of precise motor stages in slide scanners that are needed for position information used for slide stitching. We propose GloFlow, a two-stage method for creating a whole slide image using optical flow-based image registration with global alignment using a computationally tractable graph-pruning approach. In the first stage, we train an optical flow predictor to predict pairwise translations between successive video frames to approximate a stitch. In the second stage, this approximate stitch is used to create a neighborhood graph to produce a corrected stitch. On datasets of simulated video scans of pathology slides, we find that our method outperforms known approaches to slide-stitching, and stitches images resembling those produced by slide scanners. Our method allows for creation of whole slide images using widely-available low cost microscopes.

1 Introduction

Although the application of deep learning to pathology requires digital whole slide images (WSIs), the majority of pathology slides across the world are not digitized [10]. Conventional slide scanning technology uses precise sub-micron motor stages to capture image tiles at a magnification and stitch them together, and can cost upwards of $70,000 [6,8,13]. An alternative is to use cheaper hardware with less precise position information and more sophisticated computer vision methods to stitch the slide together [1,18,26].

The creation of a whole slide image from a video scan can be cast as an image stitching problem. Sequential pairwise registration has been a well studied way to solve this problem. Sequential pairwise methods include optical flow methods like Lucas Kanade and FlowNet [5,7,12,16] and homography based methods like RANSAC [9]. However, purely sequential pairwise image registration can accumulate errors in the creation of the overall image stitch [3]. These errors can be corrected using global image alignment algorithms that optimize which pairwise

Electronic supplementary material The online version of this chapter (https://doi.org/10.1007/978-3-030-87237-3_50) contains supplementary material, which is available to authorized users.

© Springer Nature Switzerland AG 2021
M. de Bruijne et al. (Eds.): MICCAI 2021, LNCS 12908, pp. 519–528, 2021.
https://doi.org/10.1007/978-3-030-87237-3_50

registrations are more likely than others [19, 25]. However these algorithms are computationally intractable as they attempt to produce pairwise translations between all possible images.

To tackle the slide-stitching problem, we propose GloFlow, a two-stage method for creating a whole slide image using optical flow-based image registration with global alignment using a computationally tractable graph-pruning approach. In the first stage, we train an optical flow predictor to predict pairwise translations between successive video frames to approximate a stitch. In the second stage, this approximate stitch is used to create a neighborhood graph to produce a corrected stitch. We also extend our method to incorporate information from a low resolution map to piece together multiple tissue sections that may be present on a slide.

The key contributions of our work include:

- We introduce a position-free method (GloFlow) for slide stitching from video that is 36× more accurate than pairwise sequential registration methods and 10× as computationally efficient as global alignment methods (Fig. 1).
- We develop an evaluation metric called Re-EPE that captures the stitching error while being translationally invariant to the location of the stitched regions in the global stitch.
- We develop an extension to GloFlow that incorporates information from a low resolution thumbnail to align multiple tissue sections that may be present in a slide.

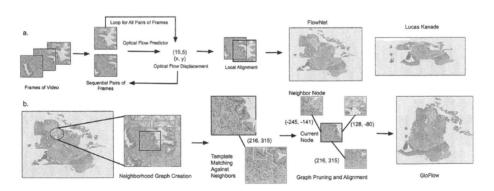

Fig. 1. Overview of GloFlow (a) Optical flow is computed using pairwise sequential frames of video. Each pair of frames is aligned to produce an approximate stitch. (b) Using the approximate WSI, we create a neighborhood graph that uses template matching for refining the stitch.

2   Related Work

Image Stitching in Microscopy. Image stitching in microscopy requires alignment of multiple images to create a single whole slide digital image. Techniques for image stitching in modern scanners have relied on position information of images captured to align images across rows [2, 6, 8, 17, 23, 25, 26]. Closely related to our work, Pellikka et al. demonstrated producing digital slides without any prior position information of the images [19]. However their method relies on good initialization of image positions for the least squares optimization to converge to a reasonable outcome. They compute translations between all possible pairs of images to compensate for not having position information which makes the method extremely computationally expensive.

Pairwise Image Registration. Approaches to image stitching have relied on sequential pairwise registration [3, 5]. Linear transformations provided by optical flow [16] have been used in image registration problems to compute displacements between images. Certain images captured in microscopy have rotations based on the camera angle and work in homographies capture warping, rotations and translations between pairs of images [22]. Features computed with Shi-Tomasi [21], Harris corners [11] and SIFT [15] have been used to compute correspondences used to determine the homography or linear transformation for use in panoramas and mosaics [3, 4]. Recently work in deep learning has demonstrated that neural networks can be used for pairwise image registration [7, 12, 24] by learning to infer optical flow between the pairs. As opposed to iterative approaches to image registration like RANSAC, neural network based flow predictors estimate optical flow in a single forward pass and can learn features specific to the training distribution that are needed for correspondences.

3   Methods

Task. The creation of WSIs from a video scan can be cast as an image stitching problem. The input of the task is a video over the slide where each frame of the video is a small section of the slide. The output for the task is a stitched WSI.

Data. We develop a procedure to simulate video capture of slides under a microscope using digitized WSIs. This provides a simple testbed for the comparison of approaches and ground truth for the whole-slide image stitch. We extract 512×512 patches of a digital WSI at constant magnification with small translational displacements. In order to simulate the general movement of a slide under a microscope, we extract patches in a boustrophedonic manner - i.e. alternating left to right horizontal passes over the vertical length of the image beginning at the top-left corner. After each horizontal pass, we extract successive patches with vertical displacements until we cross a specified height after which we begin the next horizontal pass in the opposite direction. These images, when considered sequentially simulate a video capture of a slide moved under a microscope without associated local or global location data. Methods are developed and validated on 40 videos (200,000 frames) generated from 5 hematoxylin and eosin

(H&E) stained cervical tissue slides collected from surgical pathology in a large academic medical center.

3.1 GloFlow

We propose GloFlow, a two-stage method for creating a whole slide image using optical flow-based sequential pairwise image registration and global alignment through a computationally tractable graph pruning. In the first stage, we train an optical flow predictor to predict pairwise translations between successive video frames to approximate a stitch. In the second stage, this approximate stitch is used to initialize a neighborhood graph which is then pruned to produce a corrected stitch.

Stage 1: Creating Approximate Stitch Using Sequential Pairwise Registration. The task in the stage 1 is to create an approximate WSI from a video capture. On extracting a sequence of images from video, we compute pairwise translations for each sequential pair. These predicted pairwise translations can then be used to stitch an approximate WSI. We implement two optical flow methods to compute translations between image pairs. The first method is Lucas-Kanade (LK) optical flow [16] that uses Shi-Tomasi feature points [5].

FlowNetMod. The second method is our modification of FlowNet, a deep learning-based flow predictor [7]. FlowNet trains a neural network to output a dense pixel-wise (x, y) translation map between two input images. In this method called *FlowNetMod* (FNM) we train a neural network to output the translation in the x and y coordinates between two frames as opposed to the dense pixel-wise output from FlowNet. We leverage just the encoder from FlowNet in our setting since we can enforce the constraint that every pixel has the same displacement. The input to the network for each forward pass is two sequential frames from the video concatenated channelwise. The $L1$ loss is computed using the predicted and ground truth flows.

Stage 2: Correcting Approximate Stitch Using Neighborhood Graph. In the second stage, the approximate stitch produced in the first stage is used to create and prune a neighborhood graph that produces a corrected stitch. A neighborhood graph is created as follows. All frames within a radius of twice the frame width from the upper left coordinate of a chosen frame in the approximate stitch are considered to be neighbors of that frame. These neighbors are added as connected nodes to the original frame and this process is repeated for each frame in the approximate WSI to create a neighborhood graph.

Using this neighborhood graph, we recompute image registrations to produce a corrected stitch. For each frame, Shi-Tomasi feature point neighborhoods are aggregated via dilation to form templates which are matched with neighbors to create a set of possible translations from the frame for each neighbor. A weighted directed multigraph is created with each frame as a vertex. Each translation between the source vertex and its neighbors is added as a directed edge to this multigraph. The weight is assigned to each edge corresponds to the maximum correlation coefficient computed during template matching. The multigraph is then pruned to form a directed graph by first aggregating similar translations and then removing edges with low weights.

In order to ensure that the translation between a pair of nodes is consistent, each pair of translations in the directed graph between a given pair of nodes are checked to be equal in magnitude and opposite in direction which guarantees that they correspond to the same translation. This enables us to convert the directed graph is converted to an undirected graph. Global coordinates are computed for every frame using the neighborhood translations to create final stitch. In order to reduce computational costs but still ensure a high quality stitch, we sample every 20th frame from the original video.

The full algorithm is also described formally in the Supplement.

Evaluation Metrics. We generate global coordinates for each frame from the stage 1 optical flow and the stage 2 graph alignment translations which are used for error computation. We use four evaluation metrics - End-Point-Error (EPE), Intersection over Union (IOU), Structural Similarity Index Measure (SSIM), and our new metric *Re-centered End-Point Error* (Re-EPE) which extends EPE by being invariant to global offsets between stitched regions while measuring the accuracy of local location predictions. Re-EPE is calculated by averaging the EPEs computed between the predicted and ground truth location vectors which are recentered over each node (patch) in a single connected component (tissue section).

$$L_{\text{EPE}}(P, T) = \sum_{i=1}^{N} \sqrt{(P[i] - T[i])^2}$$

$$L_{\text{RE-EPE}} = \frac{1}{N} \sum_{i=1}^{N} L_{\text{EPE}} \left(P - (P[i] \cdot \mathbf{1}), T - (T[i] \cdot \mathbf{1}) \right) \tag{1}$$

where P is the predicted location vector, T is the ground truth location vector, N is the number of nodes in the connected component and L_{EPE} is End Point Error.

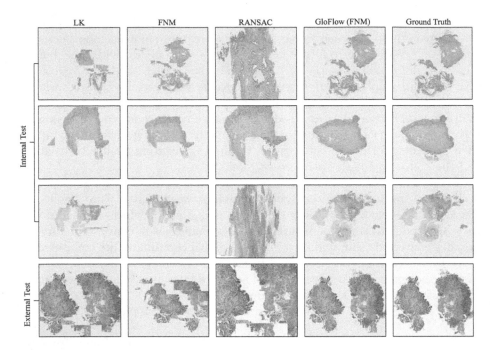

Fig. 2. Stage 1 Comparisons Whole slide image stitches produced from sequential pairwise methods compared to GloFlow (with FNM initialization) and the ground truth. The top three rows are from the cervical cancer dataset (Internal) while the bottom row is from the external dataset of intestinal cancer.

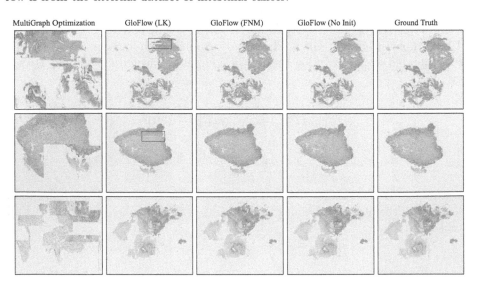

Fig. 3. Stage 2 Comparisons Whole slide image stitches produced with MultiGraph Optimization, different initializations of GloFlow, and the ground truth. Blue rectangles highlight small, but perceptible errors, seen with GloFlow (LK) that are not seen with GloFlow (FNM/No Init). (Color figure online)

Table 1. Comparison of sequential pairwise registration methods and global alignment methods to GloFlow.

Method	EPE	Re-EPE	SSIM	IOU	Time (s)
Sequential Pairwise					
LK	12.52	1386.08	0.73	0.07	382
FN	**6.27**	1118.99	**0.76**	0.15	172
FNM	7.10	**705.17**	0.75	**0.16**	**163**
RANSAC	120.95	2361.63	0.72	0.03	275
Global Alignment					
MultiGraph Optimization	214.80	863.56	0.70	0.21	>9999
GloFlow (No Init) (ours)	**184.37**	**426.79**	**0.76**	**0.81**	**7078**
GloFlow					
LK Init (ours)	27.15	48.98	0.78	0.88	2177
FN Init (ours)	**16.00**	**01.73**	**0.82**	**0.89**	1379
FNM Init (ours)	16.75	37.64	0.78	0.87	**929**

4   Experiments

We first compare GloFlow, a two-stage methodology, to sequential pairwise registration methods (stage 1 of GloFlow), and to global alignment (stage 2 of GloFlow). We then compare the performance of GloFlow with different initialization strategies. Finally, we develop and evaluate an extension of our method to align multiple separated tissue sections to form a single image stitch utilizing a low resolution image of the slide.

4.1   Comparisons for Stage 1 - Sequential Pairwise Registration

We compare GloFlow to four sequential pairwise registration methods. The first three methods are optical flow methods: Lucas-Kanade (LK) with Shi-Tomasi features, a pre-trained FlowNet (FN) and FlowNetMod (FNM), all described previously in 3.1. The fourth method we implement is RANSAC using ORB feature detectors [20] to compute the homography between successive pairs of images and produce a stitched image using the translations [14].

Results. We find that GloFlow significantly outperforms all sequential pairwise methods (LK, FN, FNM, RANSAC), as seen in Table 1. On IOU and Re-EPE, GloFlow outperforms pure pairwise methods by 8.4× and 36.8× respectively. On IOU, the best GloFlow method (using FN initialization) achieves a score of 0.89 while LK, FN, FNM, and RANSAC achieve a score of 0.07, 0.15, 0.16, and 0.03 respectively. On Re-EPE, the best GloFlow method (using FN initialization) achieves an error of 37.64 while LK, FN, FNM, and RANSAC achieve errors of 1386.08, 1118.99, 705.17, and 2361.63 respectively. SSIM and EPE values can be found in Table 1.

Qualitative Evaluation. We find that GloFlow produces locally and globally accurate stitches that capture the local structural integrity and global positional information of individual tissue sections in the ground truth. Sequential pairwise methods while locally accurate on individual rows, produce unusable global stitches that do not resemble the ground truth. These methods suffer from accumulation of errors between pairwise predictions and cannot accurately determine positioning of rows as seen in Fig. 2. GloFlow with the FNM initialization produces stitches that closely resemble the ground truth.

4.2   Comparison for Stage 2 - Global Alignment

We compare GloFlow to a global alignment method for slide-stitching [19] described in detail in the supplemental materials (Fig. 3).

Results. GloFlow outperforms MultiGraph Optimization on all metrics, as seen in Table 1. On IOU, GloFlow with FN initialization achieves a score of 0.89 and is 4.2× better than MultiGraph Optimization which achieves a score of 0.21. On Re-EPE, GloFlow with FN initialization incurs an error of 31.73 and is 27.2× better than MultiGraph Optimization which incurs an error of 863.56. Moreover, we find that GloFlow with no initialization - only global alignment in stage 2 against all pairs - also outperforms Multigraph Optimization on all metrics, as seen in Table 1.

For one dataset MultiGraph Optimization does not converge on the first optimization problem. In experiments for which MultiGraph Optimization does converge, it takes 3+ hours which is infeasible for deployment purposes. Furthermore, results are still significantly lower than those from GloFlow, both qualitatively and quantitatively. This may be due to the method converging to a local optima in the first non-convex optimization problem.

4.3   Comparing GloFlow Initializations

We compare the performance of GloFlow with different initialization strategies.

We find that GloFlow with FN, FNM and No Init achieves nearly identical Re-EPE (FN = 31.73, FNM = 37.64, No Init = 33.00), IOU (FN = 0.89, FNM = 0.87, No Init = 0.81) and SSIM (FN = 0.82, FNM = 0.78, No Init = 0.76). On Re-EPE, GloFlow with LK initialization incurs an error of 48.98. With all initializations, GloFlow still performs 10× better than do sequential pairwise methods (LK, FN, FNM, RANSAC) on Re-EPE and IOU metrics.

Qualitatively, GloFlow with FN, FNM, and No Init produces accurate stitches that match the ground truth. GloFlow with LK produces an accurate stitch with the exception of small missing sections. As observed in quantitative metrics, GloFlow with FN, FNM and no initialization produce similarly accurate stiches, while GloFlow with LK initialization performs comparatively worse.

Time. While GloFlow produces stitches of comparable quality across different initializations, we find large differences in time efficiency. GloFlow with FN takes 684s on average for producing a WSI stitch, over 10x faster than the GloFlow without a stage 1 initialization 7512 s). While global graph alignment without optical flow neighborhoods needs $O(n^2)$ pairwise comparisons to compute translations against all possible pairs, GloFlow only needs $O(n)$ with a constant k neighbors.

5   Conclusion

The purpose of this work was to develop a method to create an accurate whole slide image stitch from a video scan in a computationally tractable manner. We introduce GloFlow, a method that combines optical flow with graph alignment, and demonstrate superior performance to optical flow and graph based methods on a dataset of simulated pathology slide video scans. GloFlow significantly improves on quality of slide stitching as well as computational efficiency. Moreover, we develop an extension to GloFlow which incorporates a low resolution thumbnail for alignment of connected components in a higher resolution stitch. Our work can be extended to more challenging datasets of video scans collected using a variety of lab microscopes and sample types. We hope that this work will lower the barrier to digitization in pathology enabling access to digital pathology in low resource settings.

References

1. Beckstead, J.A., et al.: High-throughput high-resolution microscopic slide digitization for pathology. In: Advanced Biomedical and Clinical Diagnostic Systems, vol. 4958, pp. 149–159. International Society for Optics and Photonics (2003)
2. Botan, R., Coco, K.F., Komati, K.S.: Implementation of an image stitching algorithm to a low-cost digital microscope, pp. 285–291 (2017)
3. Brown, M., Lowe, D.G.: Automatic panoramic image stitching using invariant features. Int. J. Comput. Vision **74**(1), 59–73 (2007). https://doi.org/10.1007/s11263-006-0002-3
4. Brown, M., Szeliski, R., Winder, S.: Multi-image matching using multi-scale oriented patches. In: 2005 IEEE Computer Society Conference on Computer Vision and Pattern Recognition (CVPR'05), vol. 1, pp. 510–517. IEEE (2005)
5. Carozza, L., Bevilacqua, A., Piccinini, F.: An incremental method for mosaicing of optical microscope imagery. In: 2011 IEEE Symposium on Computational Intelligence in Bioinformatics and Computational Biology (CIBCB), pp. 1–6. IEEE (2011)
6. Chalfoun, J., et al.: Mist: accurate and scalable microscopy image stitching tool with stage modeling and error minimization. Sci. Rep. **7**(1), 1–10 (2017)
7. Dosovitskiy, A., et al.: FlowNet: learning optical flow with convolutional networks. In: Proceedings of the IEEE International Conference on Computer Vision, pp. 2758–2766 (2015)

8. Farahani, N., Parwani, A.V., Pantanowitz, L.: Whole slide imaging in pathology: advantages, limitations, and emerging perspectives. Pathol. Lab. Med. Int. **7**(23–33), 4321 (2015)
9. Fischler, M.A., Bolles, R.C.: Random sample consensus: a paradigm for model fitting with applications to image analysis and automated cartography. Commun. ACM **24**(6), 381–395 (1981)
10. Hanna, M.G., et al.: Whole slide imaging equivalency and efficiency study: experience at a large academic center. Mod. Pathol. **32**, 1 (2019)
11. Harris, C.G., Stephens, M., et al.: A combined corner and edge detector. In: Alvey Vision Conference, vol. 15, pp. 10–5244. Citeseer (1988)
12. Ilg, E., Mayer, N., Saikia, T., Keuper, M., Dosovitskiy, A., Brox, T.: FlowNet 2.0: evolution of optical flow estimation with deep networks. In: Proceedings of the IEEE conference on Computer Vision and Pattern Recognition, pp. 2462–2470 (2017)
13. Isse, K., Lesniak, A., Grama, K., Roysam, B., Minervini, M.I., Demetris, A.J.: Digital transplantation pathology: combining whole slide imaging, multiplex staining and automated image analysis. Am. J. Transplant. **12**(1), 27–37 (2012)
14. Jeon, H.K., Jeong, J.M., Lee, K.Y.: An implementation of the real-time panoramic image stitching using ORB and PROSAC. In: 2015 International SoC Design Conference (ISOCC), pp. 91–92. IEEE (2015)
15. Lowe, D.G.: Distinctive image features from scale-invariant keypoints. Int. J. Comput. Vision **60**(2), 91–110 (2004). https://doi.org/10.1023/B:VISI.0000029664.99615.94
16. Lucas, B.D., Kanade, T., et al.: An iterative image registration technique with an application to stereo vision (1981)
17. Ma, B.: Use of autostitch for automatic stitching of microscope images. Micron **38**(5), 492–499 (2007)
18. Montalto, M.C., McKay, R.R., Filkins, R.J.: Autofocus methods of whole slide imaging systems and the introduction of a second-generation independent dual sensor scanning method. J. Pathol. Inform. **2** (2011)
19. Pellikka, M., Lahtinen, V.: A robust method for image stitching. arXiv preprint arXiv:2004.03860 (2020)
20. Rublee, E., Rabaud, V., Konolige, K., Bradski, G.: Orb: an efficient alternative to sift or surf. In: 2011 International Conference on Computer Vision, pp. 2564–2571. IEEE (2011)
21. Shi, J., et al.: Good features to track. In: 1994 Proceedings of IEEE Conference on Computer Vision And Pattern Recognition, pp. 593–600. IEEE (1994)
22. Shum, H.Y., Szeliski, R.: Panoramic image mosaics (1997)
23. Steckhan, D., Bergen, T., Wittenberg, T., Rupp, S.: Efficient large scale image stitching for virtual microscopy. In: 2008 30th Annual International Conference of the IEEE Engineering in Medicine and Biology Society, pp. 4019–4023. IEEE (2008)
24. Sun, D., Yang, X., Liu, M.Y., Kautz, J.: PWC-Net: CNNs for optical flow using pyramid, warping, and cost volume. In: Proceedings of the IEEE Conference on Computer Vision and Pattern Recognition, pp. 8934–8943 (2018)
25. Yu, Y., Peng, H.: Automated high speed stitching of large 3D microscopic images. In: 2011 IEEE International Symposium on Biomedical Imaging: From Nano to Macro, pp. 238–241. IEEE (2011)
26. Zarella, M.D., et al.: A practical guide to whole slide imaging: a white paper from the digital pathology association. Arch. Pathol. Lab. Med. **143**(2), 222–234 (2019)

Multi-modal Multi-instance Learning Using Weakly Correlated Histopathological Images and Tabular Clinical Information

Hang Li[1,2], Fan Yang[2], Xiaohan Xing[2,3], Yu Zhao[2], Jun Zhang[2], Yueping Liu[4], Mengxue Han[4], Junzhou Huang[2], Liansheng Wang[1(✉)], and Jianhua Yao[2(✉)]

[1] School of Informatics, Xiamen University, Xiamen, China
lswang@xmu.edu.cn
[2] AI Lab, Tencent, Shenzhen, China
[3] The Department of Electronic Engineering, The Chinese University of Hong Kong, Hong Kong, China
[4] Department of Pathology, The Fourth Hospital of Hebei Medical University, Shijiazhuang, Hebei, China

Abstract. The fusion of heterogeneous medical data is essential in precision medicine to assist medical experts in treatment decision-making. However, there is often little explicit correlation between data from different modalities such as histopathological images and tabular clinical data. Besides, attention-based multi-instance learning (MIL) often lacks sufficient supervision to assign appropriate attention weights for informative image patches and thus generates a good global representation for the whole image. In this paper, we propose a novel multi-modal multi-instance joint learning method, which fuses different modalities and magnification scales as a cross-modal representation to capture the potential complementary information and recalibrate the features in each modality. Furthermore, we leverage the information from tabular clinical data to optimize the MIL bag representation in the imaging modality. The proposed method is evaluated on a challenging medical task, *i.e.*, lymph node metastasis (LNM) prediction of breast cancer, and achieves the state-of-the-art performance with AUC of 0.8844, outperforming the AUC of 0.7111 using histopathological images or the AUC of 0.8312 using tabular clinical data alone. An open-source implementation of our approach can be found at https://github.com/yfzon/Multi-modal-Multi-instance-Learning.

Keywords: Multi-modal multi-instance learning · Histopathological image analysis · Multi-scale

---

H. Li and F. Yang contributed equally to this work.

© Springer Nature Switzerland AG 2021
M. de Bruijne et al. (Eds.): MICCAI 2021, LNCS 12908, pp. 529–539, 2021.
https://doi.org/10.1007/978-3-030-87237-3_51

1 Introduction

Precision medicine refers to making full use of comprehensive information in all aspects (*i.e.*, medical images, genes, and medical reports) to tailor the disease prognosis or treatment plans for each patient, instead of one-size-fits-all treatments [6,11]. One of the typical applications is to combine the histopathological images and tabular clinical data (*i.e.* age, gender, genes, tumor location, *etc.*) to perform preoperative prediction of breast lymph node metastasis (LNM) so that individualized axillary treatment may be planned to avoid unnecessary lymphadenectomy surgeries.

In the real clinical scenario, doctors usually use the microscope to observe the biopsy slides at different scales and refer to medical reports to make the final diagnosis. To mimic this real clinical scenario, we integrate the information of heterogeneous healthcare data from different modalities by employing multi-modal learning (MML). MML has been successfully applied in multi-modal action recognition in videos, audio-visual speech enhancement, and hand gesture recognition scenarios [3,10,12]. There is also a survey on recent advances in the MML area and presents them in a common taxonomy [2]. However, there are specific issues in the medical field that challenge the existing MML methods.

First, there are also successful intermediate fusion methods for the multi-modal multi-instance tasks, like multi-modal CNN for multi-instance multi-label image classification (MMCNN-MIML) [19]. However, the existing multi-modal multi-instance methods could not fully solve the specific multi-modal multi-instance medical task in this study. The medical data from imaging modality and tabular modality cannot be aligned and merged as cross-modal instances like those in MMCNN-MIML. Nevertheless, these two modalities potentially have complementary information since they reflect the same patient from different perspectives and may influence each other (*i.e.*, the gene alternation may induce the cell morphologic changes in tumor regions) [21]. Therefore, a method that can tackle the misaligned information from image and tabular modalities and make full use of the potential complementary to improve the learning in each modality is in need.

Second, the histopathological images have gigantic image sizes (which is around 130000×50000 pixels in this study) and are often *tiled into patches* for processing [16,20,29]. Multi-instance learning (MIL) such as attention-based MIL is conventionally employed to extract latent features from those patches and then fuse patch-level features to generate a *WSI-level representation* for downstream tasks, including classification [17,24], metastasis prediction [28], genome mutation detection [4,23], and survival analysis [16,27]. However, attention-based MIL, as a weakly supervised learning approach, still cannot effectively reduce the weights of the unrelated patches and strengthen the weights of the discriminative patches. At present, MIL is mainly based on the guidance of the knowledge from the imaging modality alone and overlooks useful supplementary knowledge from real scenarios to guide the instance-level attention. It's worth exploring how to borrow useful knowledge from another modality (*i.e.*, tabular modality) to guide the MIL in imaging modality to optimally distribute the instance-level attention weights in terms of network performance.

Third, histopathological images are generally analyzed at multiple scales to capture different levels of information [18,26]. For instance, histopathological images at 5× power magnification reveal tissue-level structure, while histopathological images at 20× magnification reflect the cell-level information. How to utilize multi-scale information in MML is also a problem to be solved.

To tackle the above challenges, we proposed a unified joint MMMI learning model for breast LNM prediction tasks. Our contributions in this work can be summarized as follow:

- We propose a novel MMMI joint learning model with a Multi-modal Multi-instance Fusion (M3IF) module that can generate a cross-modal representation of different modalities to recalibrate the features in each modality and capture the relation, alleviating the bad effect of the data misalignment between modalities.
- We leverage the cross-modal representation to guide the attention-based MIL to strengthen the attention on informative instances in the imaging modality.
- Multi scale images provide a more comprehensive representation of the imaging modality.

2   Methodology

The overall architecture of our method is shown in Fig. 1. For the imaging modality, a pre-trained CNN is adopted to extract high-level image features from the patches at different magnification scales simultaneously. For the clinical data, a tabular model is used to extract embedding representations. Then our proposed multi-modal multi-instance fusion module (M3IF) module learns cross-modal representation, which guides the instance aggregation procedure in the imaging modality, and recalibrate features in the tabular modality.

2.1   MIL Problem Formulation

We formulate the learning process of imaging modality as a MIL problem, which is a typical weakly supervised learning problem, where only bag-level (WSI in this paper) labels are available. Therefore, it's important to embed instance-level features of patches from each WSI into a compact bag-level representation and then map this representation to the bag label. In our problem, each sample is represented by a WSI x_n, clinical information t_n, and the corresponding class label y_n. The dataset is denoted as $\{(x_n, t_n, y_n)\}_{n=1}^{N}$, where N is the number of cases. For each WSI, we crop 512×512 patches at different scales. Let $s \in [S]$ denote the level of magnification scales. The collection of tiled patches (bag) of n_{th} WSI at s_{th} magnification scales is denoted by $\mathfrak{B}_n^s$ and each patch (instance) in the bag is denoted as $\mathfrak{I}_b^s$ (for simplicity, the subscripts of bag index n can be safely omitted here without confusion) for $b \in \mathfrak{B}_n$ and $s \in [S]$. Then the WSI x_n can be represented as $\{\mathfrak{I}_b^s | \text{for } b \in \mathfrak{B}_n \text{ and } s \in [S]\}$, i.e. a bag of instance features at different scales.

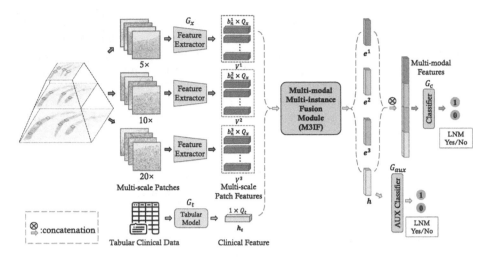

Fig. 1. The schematic illustration of our proposed multi-modal multi-instance network (MMMI). Our model takes imaging modality data and tabular data as inputs, the M3IF module learns a cross-modality representation.

EfficientNet-B0 [22] is adopted as the patch-level feature extractor G_x. For the n_{th} patient, G_x maps patches into a batch of Q dimension features $V^s \in \mathbb{R}^{b_n^s \times Q}$, here b_n^s is the number of patches in n_{th} WSI at magnification scale s, we denote it as: $V^s = G_x(\{\mathfrak{I}_j^s\}_{j=1}^{b_n^s}; \theta_x)$, where θ_x is the parameter of G_x. To integrate the instance-level feature into bag representation, an attention mechanism is usually adopted, which will be explained in detail in the next few sections.

2.2 Tabular Modality Feature Extractor

Clinical information is extracted from a patient's report via a text pattern matching algorithm. By that, our algorithm generates structured data for each patient, such as age, genes, menopausal status, tumor location in the breast, etc., a total of eighteen attributes are extracted. We adopt an advanced tabular network [1] as the tabular modality feature extractor G_t encoding tabular clinical data into compact representations to be integrated tightly with our framework for end-to-end learning. For the n_{th} patient, G_t maps the tabular record t_n into a vector $h_n \in \mathbb{R}^{Q_t}$: $h_n = G_t(t_n; \theta_t)$, where θ_t is the parameters of G_t. The tabular feature h_t will join the MML in the next stage.

2.3 Multi-modal Multi-instance Fusion

Figure 2 overviews our proposed M3IF module, which integrates image features V^s and tabular features h in our MML framework.

Multi-modal Joint Instance Aggregate Learning. Most existing MIL methods do not take other modal information into account when generating the

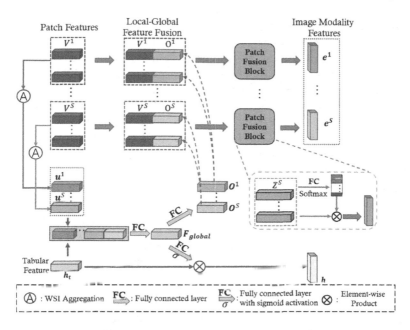

Fig. 2. The schematic illustration of the proposed multi-modal multi-instance fusion (M3IF) module. This module learns a cross-modal representation from different modalities and guides the instance aggregation procedure.

representation of a bag. However, in our scenario, only relying on the pathology modality is insufficient to assign instance attention correctly, and complementary information from other modalities may help to improve the aggregation procedure. In this regard, we propose to utilize the tabular modality information to guide the patch feature aggregation procedure. Through explicitly leveraging the multi-modality fusion information in a cross-modal manner, the global feature can be complemented for better instance-wise attention.

As shown in Fig. 2, the M3IF module takes features from all modalities as inputs and then compresses them into a global cross-modal representation. Let V^s represents the features from s_{th} imaging modality data, since b_n^s varies from different patients and different scales, which makes it difficult to merge V^s from different magnification scales, we compress it into a global representation vector $u^s \in \mathbb{R}^{1 \times Q_x}$ via mean pooling across different instances. After that, h from the medical report and features u^s from WSI (s at different magnification scales of $20\times$, $10\times$, and $5\times$) are concatenated together and a nonlinear transformation is applied to generate the cross-modal global representation F_{global}. Then a recalibrated clinical feature representation h' is generated by $h' = h_n \cdot \sigma(W_r F_{global})$, here W_r is the parameters of a fully connected layer and σ is sigmoid activation function. For imaging modality, a scale-specified feature O^k is produced by a linear transform $O^k = W_k F_{global}$, here W_k is the weight of parameter matrix, and O^k is used to guide the instance-level attention in the next section.

Global-Aware Instance Aggregation. We devise a global-aware instance aggregation block to generate the embedding feature with the guidance of global WSI information and the message from the tabular modality, thus each output of the M3IF module carries the information from other modalities. We treat this cross-modality representation O^k as global-feature and the corresponding patches feature V^s as local-feature, the local-global fused features are obtained by concatenating them together. Then, we obtain the joint representation $Z^s \in \mathbb{R}^{b_n^s \times Q}$ by transforming the fused features: $Z^s = W[V^s, REPT(O_k)] + b$. Here, $[\cdot, \cdot]$ represents the concatenation operation, $REPT$ represents the repeat operation at the instance dimension, $W \in \mathbb{R}^{2Q_x \times Q_x}$ are the weights and $b \in \mathbb{R}^{Q_x}$ are the biases of the fully connected layers. Let z_k^s to be the k_{th} instance of Z^s, then we apply the attention-based weighed aggregation to the embedding feature: $e^s = \sum_{k=1}^{b_n^s} a_k z_k^s$, where:

$$a_k = \frac{\exp\left\{ \boldsymbol{w}^T \left(\tanh(\boldsymbol{M} \boldsymbol{z}_k^s) \odot \sigma(\boldsymbol{U} \boldsymbol{z}_k^s) \right) \right\}}{\sum_{j \in \mathcal{I}_b^s} \exp\left\{ \boldsymbol{w}^T (\tanh(\boldsymbol{M} \boldsymbol{z}_j^s) \odot \sigma(\boldsymbol{U} \boldsymbol{z}_j^s)) \right\}}, k \in \mathcal{I}_b^s. \tag{1}$$

Here, $(\boldsymbol{w}, \boldsymbol{M}, \boldsymbol{U})$ are network parameters, $\odot$ is element-wise multiplication and σ is the sigmoid operation. Therefore, the instance aggregation procedure is supervised by cross-modality representation. Supposing we use WSI at three magnification scales along with clinical information, the embedding bag features are then concatenated to form a joint representation: $p = [h, e^1, e^2, e^3]$. Then p is fed into a classifier G_c to output the probability of breast LNM.

Overall Loss Function. Since different numbers of instances are contained in different WSIs, the batch size of the instances is dynamic, which can vary from 20 to more than 1000. This causes some numerically unstable issues during model training. According to the convergence difficulty of different parts of the model, several learning rates are empirically selected. Besides, a multi-head classifier (*i.e.*, G_c, G_{aux}) is adopted to help the tabular model converge more quickly and stably [15]. The overall loss function (denoted as $\mathcal{L}$) for our network training is defined as follow:

$$\mathcal{L} = \sum_{\{x_n, t_n, y_n\} \in D} \left(\mathcal{L}_{fusion}(x_n, t_n, y_n) + \beta \mathcal{L}_{tab}(x_n, t_n, y_n) \right), \tag{2}$$

where $\mathcal{L}_{fusion}$ denotes the supervised loss for the n_{th} image-text-label pair $\{x_n, t_n, y_n\}$ at the fusion branch while $\mathcal{L}_{tab}$ is the loss for tabular clinical data from the same patient at the tabular model branch, and β is the hyper-parameter to balance the two losses.

3   Experiments and Results

Datasets and Experimental Setting. Our experimental dataset of breast LNM is composed of 3990 clinical cases. We collected WSIs along with their

Table 1. Quantitative results of our network and other baseline networks in the ablation study. A-MIL [13], Tabnet [1].

Method		Input modalities	AUC	F1-score	Precision	Recall
Tabular model	TabNet	Tab	.8312	.7465	.6969	.8037
A-MIL based model	A-MIL-5×	WSI 5×	.6786	.6659	.5675	.8055
	A-MIL-10×	WSI 10×	.6745	.6695	.5535	.8472
	A-MIL-20×	WSI 20×	.6636	.6507	.5487	.7994
	A-MIL-MS	WSI MS	.7111	.6688	.5424	**.8718**
Ours (w/o M3IF)	Our-w/o-MS	Tab, WSI MS	.8420	.7700	.7180	.8300
Ours (w M3IF)	Our-w-MS	Tab, WSI MS	**.8844**	**.7942**	**.7544**	.8344

associated medical reports from our collaborating hospital. The diagnostic conclusion was made by consensus of two expert pathologists. All WSIs of the H&E stained slides were scanned at 20× magnification (0.5 μm/pixel).

We utilized four metrics (Area Under the Curve of the receiver operating characteristic curve (AUC), F1 score (F1), Precision, and Recall) for quantitative evaluation. The confidence intervals (CIs) are computed with Delong's method [7].

Experimental Setup. We randomly split the dataset into 60%, 20%, and 20% for training, validation, and test sets respectively. EfficientNet-B0 [22] pretrained with ImageNet [8] was employed as the feature extractor $G_x(\cdot, ; \theta_x)$. All experiments were conducted on a standard PC with eight NVIDIA TESLA P40 GPUs. During training, we employed the Adam [14] algorithm with momentum 0.9, weight decay 5e-4, and batch size 8. The learning rate of the tabular model part, the classifier (G_x, G_{aux}), and the rest of the model parameters were set to $\{1 \times 10^{-2}, 1 \times 10^{-3}, 1 \times 10^{-4}\}$ respectively. The hyper-parameter β was set to 1. The best model was chosen according to the performance on the validation set.

Ablation Study. To evaluate the effectiveness of the components of our proposed model, we compared our method that was trained on tabular clinical data and WSI data at three magnification scales with M3IF module (denoted as "Ours-w-MS") against six baseline models constructed as follows: (I) The first baseline network (denoted as "TabNet") was constructed by only considering the tabular clinical data. (II, III, IV) The next three models (denoted as "A-MIL-5×", "A-MIL-10×", "A-MIL-20×") were trained with only WSI data at three magnification scales (5×, 10×, 20×), respectively. (V) The fifth baseline network (denoted as "A-MIL-MS") was trained with WSI data at three magnification scales jointly. (VI) the sixth baseline network was constructed by replacing our proposed M3IF module with a simple concatenation operation, denoted as "Ours-w/o-MS".

The results are shown in Table 1. "TabNet" model achieves the AUC of 0.8312, indicating that medical reports contain rich information for breast LNM prediction. The combination of multi-scales results in performance gain, indicat-

Table 2. Comparison with recent clinical research (ANN) and state-of-the-art methods. Tab: Medical reports. WSI MS: WSI with all three magnification scales.

Fusion method	Input modalities	AUC	F1-score	Precision	Recall
ANN [9]	Tab	.7752	.7039	.6674	.7446
Gating attention [5]	Tab, WSI MS	.8570	.7594	.7375	.7827
M3DN [25]	Tab, WSI MS	.8117	.7302	.7046	.7576
Ours	Tab, WSI MS	**.8844**	**.7942**	**.7544**	**.8344**

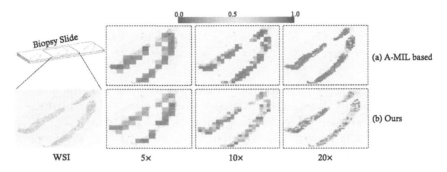

Fig. 3. Visual comparison of attention weights at different magnification scales produced by different methods.

ing that there exists complementary information from WSI at different scales. The multi-modal fusion method outperforms every single modality and achieves the AUC of 0.8844, proving the contribution of the complementary information between these two modalities. The comparison of the methods of "Ours-w/o-MS" and "Ours-w-MS" shows that the M3IF module generates more effective multi-modal multi-scale global representation than simply aggregating the features from each modality.

Comparison with Recently Clinical Research Results and State-of-the-Art Methods. We compared our method against a recent clinical research method [9] and two state-of-the-art methods. The recent clinical research method employed a shallow artificial neural network (denoted as "ANN"). The two SOTAs are both deep learning-based methods, *i.e.*, gating-based attention (denoted as "G-Attention") [5] to fuse the tabular modality features and the aggregated WSI features before the final classifier, and a bag-concept layer (denoted as "M3DN") [25] to concatenate the features from different modalities. We adopted their public implementations into our experimental pipeline for fair comparisons.

As shown in Table 2, our method (AUC: 0.8844, 95%CI: 0.8605–0.9083) greatly surpasses the recent clinical research that simple applies ANN (AUC: 0.7752, 95%CI: 0.7358–0.8004). Even the tabular modality baseline "TabNet" shows a remarkable performance boost (AUC: 0.8312, 95%CI: 0.8032–0.8592), proving that a well-designed TabNet method is more effective in dealing with structured medical reports. Our method shows superior performance than the SOTA multi-modal fusion method (Gating Attention, AUC: 0.8570, 95%CI: 0.8313–0.8828), mainly thanks to M3IF (AUC: 0.8844 vs 0.8420, P-value: 0.0002505, AUC and Delong's test on our method with and without M3IF). Furthermore, our method greatly surpasses the SOTA MMMI method M3DN (AUC: 0.8117, 95%CI: 0.785–0.8458). Our experiments have proved that intermediate fusion benefits the model, and the novelly designed M3IF module achieves better performance than a simple fusion of each modality.

Qualitative Evaluation. We qualitatively compare the attention map produced by A-MIL [13] and our method. Figure 3 shows heatmaps of a breast LNM positive example. In A-MIL, the attention weights of most instances are relatively equal, making the fusion approach of the attention-based MIL similar to average pooling. In contrast, our method can assign widely varying attention weights to instances at different regions compared to those in a single modality, which is prone to assigning more attention to discriminative instances and thus results in better performance.

4   Conclusions

In this work, we propose an MMMI learning solution to tackle the challenges of fusing histopathological images and tabular clinical data to predict whether LNM exists in breast cancer patients, which is critical in preoperative decision-making. The proposed method is designed for MIL and fully considers joint learning based on complementary information across modalities. Extensive experiments have demonstrated that our method surpasses the recent clinical research method in the breast cancer LNM task, providing a novel and efficient MMMI method for further application in precision medicine. Furthermore, our method outperforms the SOTA MMMI method in combining weakly correlated image and tabular modalities for the breast LNM prediction task.

Acknowledgements. This work was partially funded by National Key R&D Program of China (2018YFC2000702).

References

1. Arik, S.O., Pfister, T.: TabNet: attentive interpretable tabular learning. arXiv preprint arXiv:1908.07442 (2019)
2. Baltrušaitis, T., Ahuja, C., Morency, L.P.: Multimodal machine learning: a survey and taxonomy. IEEE Trans. Pattern Anal. Mach. Intell. **41**(2), 423–443 (2018)
3. Camgoz, N.C., Hadfield, S., Koller, O., Bowden, R.: Using convolutional 3D neural networks for user-independent continuous gesture recognition. In: 2016 23rd International Conference on Pattern Recognition (ICPR), pp. 49–54. IEEE (2016)
4. Cao, R., et al.: Development and interpretation of a pathomics-based model for the prediction of microsatellite instability in colorectal cancer. Theranostics **10**(24), 11080 (2020)

5. Chen, R.J., et al.: Pathomic fusion: an integrated framework for fusing histopathology and genomic features for cancer diagnosis and prognosis. IEEE Trans. Med. Imaging (2020)
6. Collins, F.S., Varmus, H.: A new initiative on precision medicine. N. Engl. J. Med. **372**(9), 793–795 (2015)
7. DeLong, E.R., DeLong, D.M., Clarke-Pearson, D.L.: Comparing the areas under two or more correlated receiver operating characteristic curves: a nonparametric approach. Biometrics **44**, 837–845 (1988)
8. Deng, J., Dong, W., Socher, R., Li, L.J., Li, K., Fei-Fei, L.: ImageNet: a large-scale hierarchical image database. In: 2009 IEEE Conference on Computer Vision and Pattern Recognition, pp. 248–255. IEEE (2009)
9. Dihge, L., Ohlsson, M., Edén, P., Bendahl, P.O., Rydén, L.: Artificial neural network models to predict nodal status in clinically node-negative breast cancer. BMC Cancer **19**(1), 610 (2019)
10. Egger, P., Borges, P.V., Catt, G., Pfrunder, A., Siegwart, R., Dubé, R.: Posemap: lifelong, multi-environment 3d lidar localization. In: 2018 IEEE/RSJ International Conference on Intelligent Robots and Systems (IROS), pp. 3430–3437. IEEE (2018)
11. Krieken, J.H.: Precision medicine. J. Hematop. **6**(1), 1 (2013). https://doi.org/10.1007/s12308-013-0176-x
12. Hou, J.C., Wang, S.S., Lai, Y.H., Tsao, Y., Chang, H.W., Wang, H.M.: Audio-visual speech enhancement using multimodal deep convolutional neural networks. IEEE Trans. Emerging Topics Comput. Intell. **2**(2), 117–128 (2018)
13. Ilse, M., Tomczak, J., Welling, M.: Attention-based deep multiple instance learning. In: International Conference on Machine Learning, pp. 2127–2136 (2018)
14. Kingma, D.P., Ba, J.: Adam: a method for stochastic optimization. In: International Conference on Learning Representations (ICLR) (2015)
15. Lee, C.Y., Xie, S., Gallagher, P., Zhang, Z., Tu, Z.: Deeply-supervised nets. In: Artificial Intelligence and Statistics, pp. 562–570 (2015)
16. Li, R., Yao, J., Zhu, X., Li, Y., Huang, J.: Graph CNN for survival analysis on whole slide pathological images. In: Frangi, A.F., Schnabel, J.A., Davatzikos, C., Alberola-López, C., Fichtinger, G. (eds.) MICCAI 2018. LNCS, vol. 11071, pp. 174–182. Springer, Cham (2018). https://doi.org/10.1007/978-3-030-00934-2_20
17. Nazeri, K., Aminpour, A., Ebrahimi, M.: Two-stage convolutional neural network for breast cancer histology image classification. In: Campilho, A., Karray, F., ter Haar Romeny, B. (eds.) ICIAR 2018. LNCS, vol. 10882, pp. 717–726. Springer, Cham (2018). https://doi.org/10.1007/978-3-319-93000-8_81
18. Schmitz, R., et al.: Multi-scale fully convolutional neural networks for histopathology image segmentation: from nuclear aberrations to the global tissue architecture. Med. Image Anal. **70**, 101996 (2021)
19. Song, L., et al.: A deep multi-modal CNN for multi-instance multi-label image classification. IEEE Trans. Image Process. **27**(12), 6025–6038 (2018)
20. Srinidhi, C.L., Ciga, O., Martel, A.L.: Deep neural network models for computational histopathology: a survey. Med. Image Anal. **67**, 101813 (2020)
21. Tai, W., Qin, B., Cheng, K.: Inhibition of breast cancer cell growth and invasiveness by dual silencing of HER-2 and VEGF. Mol. Pharm. **7**(2), 543–556 (2010)
22. Tan, M., Le, Q.: EfficientNet: rethinking model scaling for convolutional neural networks. In: International Conference on Machine Learning, pp. 6105–6114 (2019)
23. Wang, T., et al.: Microsatellite instability prediction of uterine corpus endometrial carcinoma based on H&E histology whole-slide imaging. In: 2020 IEEE 17th International Symposium on Biomedical Imaging (ISBI), pp. 1289–1292. IEEE (2020)

24. Wang, X., et al.: Weakly supervised deep learning for whole slide lung cancer image analysis. IEEE Trans. Cybern. **50**(9), 3950–3962 (2019)

25. Yang, Y., Fu, Z.Y., Zhan, D.C., Liu, Z.B., Jiang, Y.: Semi-supervised multi-modal multi-instance multi-label deep network with optimal transport. IEEE Trans. Knowl. Data Eng. **33**, 696–709 (2019)

26. Yang, Z., Ran, L., Zhang, S., Xia, Y., Zhang, Y.: EMS-Net: ensemble of multiscale convolutional neural networks for classification of breast cancer histology images. Neurocomputing **366**, 46–53 (2019)

27. Yao, J., Zhu, X., Huang, J.: Deep multi-instance learning for survival prediction from whole slide images. In: Shen, D., et al. (eds.) MICCAI 2019. LNCS, vol. 11764, pp. 496–504. Springer, Cham (2019). https://doi.org/10.1007/978-3-030-32239-7_55

28. Zhao, Y., et al.: Predicting lymph node metastasis using histopathological images based on multiple instance learning with deep graph convolution. In: Proceedings of the IEEE/CVF Conference on Computer Vision and Pattern Recognition, pp. 4837–4846 (2020)

29. Zhao, Z., Lin, H., Chen, H., Heng, P.-A.: PFA-ScanNet: pyramidal feature aggregation with synergistic learning for breast cancer metastasis analysis. In: Shen, D., et al. (eds.) MICCAI 2019. LNCS, vol. 11764, pp. 586–594. Springer, Cham (2019). https://doi.org/10.1007/978-3-030-32239-7_65

Ranking Loss: A Ranking-Based Deep Neural Network for Colorectal Cancer Grading in Pathology Images

Trinh Thi Le Vuong[1], Kyungeun Kim[2], Boram Song[2], and Jin Tae Kwak[1]([envelope])

[1] School of Electrical Engineering, Korea University, Seoul 02841, Korea
jkwak@korea.ac.kr
[2] Department of Pathology, Sungkyunkwan University of Medicine, Seoul 06355, Korea

Abstract. In digital pathology, cancer grading has been widely studied by utilizing hand-crafted features and advanced machine learning and deep learning methods. In most of such studies, cancer grading has been formulated as a multi-class categorical classification problem, likely overlooking the relationship among different cancer grades. Herein, we propose a ranking-based deep neural network for cancer grading in pathology images. Utilizing deep neural networks, pathology images are mapped into a latent space. Built based upon a triplet loss, a ranking loss is devised to maximize the inter-class distance among cancer grades in the latent space with respect to the aggressiveness of cancer, leading to the correct ordering or rank of pathology images. To evaluate the proposed method, a number of colorectal pathology images have been employed. The experimental results demonstrate that the proposed approach is capable of predicting cancer grades with high accuracy, outperforming the deep neural networks without the ranking loss.

Keywords: Colorectal cancer grading · Multi-class classification · Ranking loss · Triplet loss · Convolutional neural network

1 Introduction

Cancer is a primary disease worldwide [1]. Once diagnosed with cancer, a cancer grade is assigned upon the histologic assessment of tissue specimens by pathologists under a microscope, describing how abnormal cancer cells are in comparison to healthy (or normal) cells, i.e., the aggressiveness of the cancer. Although it is dependent on the types of cancer and grading system, cancer grading mainly adopts 1–3 (or –4) grading scale such as well, moderately, and poorly differentiated (or undifferentiated) cancer, in other words, the low, intermediate and high grade cancer. In clinics, the cancer grade is used as a primary determinant in treatment planning and patient care [2]; thus, accurate cancer grading not only leads to an improved patient outcome but also a substantial reduction in the cost and complexity of cancer treatment. However, there are several factors that limit the accuracy and efficiency of the current practice of cancer grading: 1) *low-throughput*: cancer grading is, by and large, manually conducted, i.e., time-consuming; 2) *subjective*:

© Springer Nature Switzerland AG 2021
M. de Bruijne et al. (Eds.): MICCAI 2021, LNCS 12908, pp. 540–549, 2021.
https://doi.org/10.1007/978-3-030-87237-3_52

cancer grading is mainly based upon qualitative measures, prone to inter- and intra-observer variability [3]; 3) *workload*: pathology services are under increasing pressure due to the upsurge of the volume and complexity of workloads per pathologist [4], leading to over-fatigue and burnout of pathologists as well as decrease in the quality of the service. Therefore, an alternative digital pathology tool that can permit automated, prompt, and objective decision-making for tissue specimens could aid in improving diagnostic yield and accuracy of cancer grading.

Many digital pathology tools have been developed to improve the accuracy, efficiency and robustness of cancer pathology [5]. Earlier works, in general, conducts cancer grading in two steps – feature extraction and classification. The feature extraction step includes a set of statistical, morphological and/or texture features, so called hand-crafted features. The classification step mainly utilizes supervised machine learning algorithms such as support vector machine (SVM) [6], decision tree [7], Bayes [8] and boosting [9]. This approach has been applied to cancer grading in prostate [7], brain [10], and colon [11]. Nowadays, deep convolutional neural networks (CNNs) are extensively utilized for digital pathology; for instance, tissue segmentation [12], nuclei detection [13] and segmentation [14], cancer detection [15], and pathology image synthesis [16]. Several efforts have been also made to develop CNN models for cancer grading in prostate [17], breast [18], and brain [19]. Such models have been built based upon the state-of-the-art network architectures, including inception module [20], residual layout [21], densely-connected layers [22], and depth-wise separable convolutions [23]. In most of the previous works, cancer grading has been studied as a multi-class categorical problem. These methods have been sought to either classify tissue specimens into multiple classes at once or classify tissue specimens in a cascaded manner. However, cancer grades are not independent to each other. The higher the grade is, the more aggressive the cancer is, i.e., it is an ordinal classification problem. Distinguishing high grade cancer from intermediate grade cancer is more difficult than from low grade cancer or healthy tissue. The hierarchy of cancer grades has not been fully utilized in developing digital pathology tools for cancer grading.

In this paper, we propose a ranking-based deep convolutional neural network (RankCNN) for colorectal cancer grading in pathology images. The proposed network is built based upon the following principles: 1) there exists a function f that maps tissues into data points (or embeddings) in an Euclidean latent (or embedding) space; 2) the similarity/dissimilarity between tissues (of the same or differing cancer grades) is measurable using distance metrics in the latent space; 3) the more (semantically) similar tissues are, the (metrically) closer the corresponding data points are; 4) the difference in the cancer grades of the tissues is directly related to the distance between the corresponding embeddings in the latent space. The mapping function f can be obtained via the-state-of-the-art deep convolutional neural networks. The distance between the embeddings can be measured using distance metrics, e.g., a Euclidean distance. To enforces the constraints of the distance between tissues in the latent space, we, in particular, introduce a ranking loss that could aid in obtaining the correct order of tissues. Built based upon the triplet loss [24], the ranking loss aims to maximize the relative distance between the tissues of differing grades in regard to the order of pathology grades.

2 Methodology

The overview of the proposed approach is illustrated in Fig. 1. It utilizes a deep convolutional neural network to conduct cancer grading. To exploit the nature ordering of cancer grades, we devise a loss function, so called ranking loss, and utilize to optimize the network. The ranking loss extends and generalizes triplet loss. We first introduce the triplet loss and then present the proposed ranking loss.

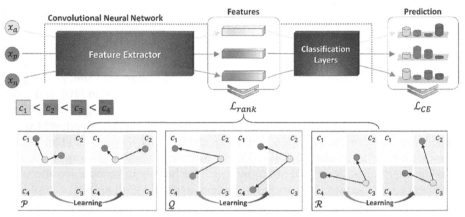

Fig. 1. The overview of the proposed method. x_a, x_p, and x_n denote an anchor, positive, and negative sample, respectively. c_1, c_2, c_3, and c_4 are the four classes that are ordered as $c_1 < c_2 < c_3 < c_4$. $\mathcal{P}$ denotes triples where x_a and x_p belong to the same class. $\mathcal{Q}$ and $\mathcal{R}$ include triplets from three different classes. In $\mathcal{Q}$, the class label of x_a is closer to the class label of x_p than that of x_n. In $\mathcal{R}$, the class label of x_a is equidistant from that of x_p and x_n, but x_p is ranked higher than x_a. $\mathcal{L}_{rank}$ and $\mathcal{L}_{CE}$ are ranking loss and cross entropy loss, respectively

2.1 Loss Functions

Two loss functions are employed to optimize the neural network as follows:

$$\mathcal{L} = \mathcal{L}_{CE} + \lambda \mathcal{L}_{rank} \tag{1}$$

where $\mathcal{L}_{CE}$ and $\mathcal{L}_{rank}$ denote cross entropy loss and ranking loss, respectively. λ is a weight factor that is associated with $\mathcal{L}_{rank}$ ($\lambda = 2$). $\mathcal{L}_{CE}$ has been widely accepted for the (categorical) classification task. $\mathcal{L}_{rank}$ is the loss function that is designed to capture the natural ordering of class labels, i.e., the ordinal classification task.

Let $\{(x_i, y_i)\}_{i=1}^{N}$ be a set of pathology images and ground truth labels where $x_i \in \mathbb{R}^{w \times h \times d}$ is the ith pathology image, $y_i \in C = \{c_1, c_2, \ldots, c_K\}$ is the ground truth label and N is the number of images. w, h and d denote the width, height and the number of channels, respectively. K is the cardinality of the class label. For the categorical classification, $\mathcal{L}_{CE}$ is used to measure the total entropy between the prediction and ground truth as follows:

$$\mathcal{L}_{CE} = -\sum_{i}^{N} \sum_{j}^{K} I_k(y_i) \log(o_{i,k}) \tag{2}$$

where $I_k(y)$ is a binary indicator where $I_k(y)$ is 1 if $k \in y$ and 0 otherwise. $o_{i,k}$ is the prediction for the image x_i and class label k.

$\mathcal{L}_{rank}$ utilizes the relative distance among the images with different class labels. It is defined on an embedding or feature representation of an image x_i, not the final prediction on the image. In the feature space $\mathbb{R}^D$, the relative distance among the images may be associated with the class labels. In other words, the distance between the images that belong to the same class or are closer to each other with respect to the class label becomes smaller than the distance between the images that are farther away from the perspective of the class labels. $\mathcal{L}_{rank}$ is built based upon the triplet loss. Thus, we first introduce the triplet loss and then provide the detailed description of the ranking loss.

Triplet Loss. The triplet loss is defined on a series of triplets $\{x_a, x_p, x_n\}, y_a = y_p \neq y_n$. For an (anchor) image x_a, the triplet loss is designed to have x_a is closer to all other (positive) images x_p of the same class than it is to any (negative) image x_n with a different class label from x_a. The triplet loss is formulated as:

$$\mathcal{L}_{tri} = \sum_{\substack{x_a, x_p, x_n \\ y_a = y_p \neq y_n}} \left[D(x_a, x_p) - D(x_a, x_n) + \alpha \right]_+ \tag{3}$$

where $[z]_+ = max(z, 0)$ and α is a margin. $D(x_i, x_j) = \|f(x_i) - f(x_j)\|_2^2$ where $f(x_i)$ is the feature representation of an image x_i. It should be noted that the number of all possible triplets grows exponentially. It is not necessary to consider all the triplets since most of the trivial triplets are easily and quickly separated in the feature space. Hence it is common to utilize only the *hard* (or *moderately hard*) triplets to compute $\mathcal{L}_{tri}$ [25]. For an anchor image x_a, the *hard* positive image is the one that is furthest away from x_a and *hard* negative image is the one that is closest to x_a. Thus, Eq. (3) can be rewritten as:

$$\mathcal{L}_{tri} = \sum_{(i,j,k) \in \mathcal{P}} \sum_a^{N_i} \mathcal{H}\left(x_a^{c_i}, x_p^{c_j}, x_n^{c_k}, \alpha\right), \tag{4}$$

$$\mathcal{H}\left(x_a^{c_i}, x_p^{c_j}, x_n^{c_k}, \alpha\right) = \left[\max_{p=1,\ldots,N_j} D\left(x_a^{c_i}, x_p^{c_j}\right) - \min_{n=1,\ldots,N_k} D\left(x_a^{c_i}, x_n^{c_k}\right) + \alpha \right]_+ \tag{5}$$

where $\mathcal{P} = \{(i, j, k) : c_i = c_j \neq c_k\}$, $x_a^{c_i}$ is an image with a class label c_i and N_i is the number of images in the class c_i.

Ranking Loss. In cancer pathology, there is a natural ordering of cancer grades $y \in \{c_1, c_2, \ldots, c_K\}$. Without loss of generality, let $c_1, c_2, \ldots, c_K$ be the values that are related on an ordinal scale; for example, $c_1 = 1, c_2 = 2, \ldots, c_K = K$. In the ordinal classification, the goal of a ranking function h is to learn the relative rank among the images, i.e., for any pair of images $\{x_i, x_k\}$ it holds that

$$h(x_i) > h(x_k), y_i > y_k. \tag{6}$$

This can be easily extended to any triplets $\{x_i, x_j, x_k\}$:

$$h(x_i, x_j) > h(x_i, x_k), y_i = y_j > y_k. \tag{7}$$

Replacing h with D, it is trivial to rewrite the formula as follows:

$$D(x_i, x_j) + \alpha > D(x_i, x_k), y_i = y_j > y_k. \tag{8}$$

This indicates that the rank between the images can be expressed with respect to the triplets, i.e., the triplet loss. However, the triplet loss can partially handle the rank among the images of multiple classes since the loss only considers a pair of class labels at a time. To extend the triplet loss and to fully exploit the ordering of the class labels, the ranking loss takes the triplets from three different classes into account. The ranking loss is formulated as:

$$\mathcal{L}_{rank} = \sum_{(i,j,k)\in\mathcal{P}} \sum_a^{N_i} \mathcal{H}\left(x_a^{c_i}, x_p^{c_j}, x_n^{c_k}, \alpha_\mathcal{P}\right) + \sum_{(i,j,k)\in\mathcal{Q}} \sum_a^{N_i} \mathcal{H}\left(x_a^{c_i}, x_p^{c_j}, x_n^{c_k}, \alpha_\mathcal{Q}\right)$$
$$+ \sum_{(i,j,k)\in\mathcal{R}} \sum_a^{N_i} \mathcal{H}\left(x_a^{c_i}, x_p^{c_j}, x_n^{c_k}, \alpha_\mathcal{R}\right)$$

$$\tag{9}$$

where $\mathcal{Q} = \{(i,j,k) : |c_i - c_j| < |c_i - c_k|, c_i \neq c_j \neq c_k\}$, $\mathcal{R} = \{(i,j,k) : |c_i - c_j| = |c_i - c_k|, c_i \neq c_j \neq c_k, c_j > c_k\}$, and $\alpha_\mathcal{P}$, $\alpha_\mathcal{Q}$, and $\alpha_\mathcal{R}$ are the margins ($\alpha_\mathcal{P} = 1.0$, $\alpha_\mathcal{Q} = 1.0$, and $\alpha_\mathcal{R} = -0.5$). The first term is the same as the triple loss. It focuses on minimizing the relative distance among the images in the same class with respect to the images of different classes. The second and third term include the triplets from three different classes. The second term is to consider the cases where the anchor images are closer to positive images than to negative images with respect to class labels. The third term is the constraint on the cases where positive and negative images are equidistant from anchor images with respect to the class labels, but positive images are ranked higher than negative images. These two terms aim to push negative images further away, forcing the minimum distance between anchor and negative images to be larger than the maximum distance between anchor and positive images, following the ordering of the class labels.

2.2 Network Architecture

We employed three different types of backbone CNNs, which are widely used and built based upon different principles, to evaluate the effectiveness of the proposed ranking loss. The three types include 1) DenseNet (DenseNet121): uses all the subsequent layers via concatenation and scales the network by its depth, [22], MoblieNet (MobileNetV2) [23]: is a light-weight network using depthwise separable convolutions, and 3) EfficientNet (EfficientNet-B0) [26]: adopts a compound scaling method that balances the width, depth, and image resolution. Given a pathology image x_i, all three types of architectures generate two distinct outputs: 1) the high dimensional features $f(x_i)$: the output of the last convolutional block and 2) the prediction result o_i: the output of the classification layers given $f(x_i)$. Due to the difference in the input size from the original implementation, the average-pooling layer (AvgPool) in the classification layers of the three architectures is replaced by the gobal AvgPool. The cross entropy loss is utilized to assess the prediction results and the ranking loss is adopted to evaluate the high dimensional features.

2.3 Evaluation Metrics

We quantitatively evaluate the performance of the proposed method using five evaluation metrics: 1) accuracy (ACC), 2) recall (REC), 3) Cohen's kappa (κ), 4) Matthews correlation coefficient (MCC) [27], and 5) macro-average F1-score ($F1_{mac}$).

3 Experiments and Results

3.1 Datasets

Colorectal tissue samples were stained with hematoxylin and eosin (H&E) and scanned at x20 optical magnification. The tissue samples were collected from six colorectal tissue microarrays (TMAs) and three whole slide images (WSIs). An experienced pathologist reviewed the tissue samples and identified and delineated distinct histological regions, including benign (BN) and well-differentiated (WD), moderately-differentiated (MD), and poorly-differentiated (PD) tumors. From the WSIs and TMAs, tissue patches of size 1024×1024 pixels were extracted and resized to 512×512. ~10,000 image patches, including 1600 BN, 2322 WD, 4105 MD, and 1830 PD patches, were generated and further divided into a training (898 BN, 1615 WD, 2623 MD, and 1245 PD), validation (444 BN, 374 WD, 810 MD, and 238 PD), and test (262 BN, 334 WD, 672 MD, and 347 PD) dataset. We note that the data partition was conducted at WSI- and TAM-level.

3.2 Implementation Details

All the networks are optimized using Adam optimizer with parameter values ($\beta_1 = 0.5$, $\beta_2 = 0.999$, $\varepsilon = 1e-8$). The learning rate is set to $1e-4$. After 30 epochs, it is decayed by 10. λ is set to 2 after cross-validation experiments within the training set only. We train the networks for 60 epochs. The best model on the validation dataset is chosen for the evaluation on the test dataset. During training, the following data augmentation techniques are applied: 1) a random rotation in a range of [0, 60] degree, 2) a random scaling in a range of [0.8, 1.2], 3) a random translation in a range of [0.02, 0.02] with respect to the width and height of the input image, and 4) a random change in the brightness, contrast, saturation, and hue with a factor in a range of [0.95, 1.05]. For the loss calculation, We set the weighting factor for the ranking loss (λ) to 2.0 and the margins α_P, α_Q, and α_R to 1.0, 1.0, and -0.5, respectively. Setting $\alpha_R = -0.5$, we relax the constraint for the equidistant cases.

3.3 Results and Discussions

The experimental results of colorectal cancer grading are available in Table 1. Equipped with the proposed $\mathcal{L}_{rank}$, RankCNNs with different backbone networks, including DenseNet, MobileNet, and EfficientNet, obtained $\geq 86.91\%$ ACC, ≥ 0.8693 REC, ≥ 0.8254 κ, ≥ 0.8255 MCC, and ≥ 0.8693 $F1_{mac}$. Among the three backbone networks, EfficientNet consistently outperformed other two backbone networks and MobileNet showed the lowest performance over the five evaluation metrics. To assess the effectiveness of the proposed $\mathcal{L}_{rank}$, we repeated the same experiments without $\mathcal{L}_{rank}$. For each

Table 1. Results of cancer grading.

Network	Loss	ACC (%)	REC	κ	MCC	$F1_{mac}$
DenseNet	$\mathcal{L}_{CE}$	81.50	0.8153	0.7533	0.7577	0.8191
	$\mathcal{L}_{CE}$ & $\mathcal{L}_{tri}$	85.20	0.8522	0.8027	0.8038	0.8554
	$\mathcal{L}_{CE}$ & $\mathcal{L}_{rank}$	**87.00**	**0.8703**	**0.8267**	**0.8275**	**0.8727**
MobileNet	$\mathcal{L}_{CE}$	85.20	0.8523	0.8027	0.8053	0.8579
	$\mathcal{L}_{CE}$ & $\mathcal{L}_{tri}$	86.53	0.8655	0.8204	0.8207	0.8676
	$\mathcal{L}_{CE}$ & $\mathcal{L}_{rank}$	**86.91**	**0.8693**	**0.8254**	**0.8255**	**0.8693**
EfficientNet	$\mathcal{L}_{CE}$	81.88	0.8191	0.7584	0.7668	0.8293
	$\mathcal{L}_{CE}$ & $\mathcal{L}_{tri}$	85.39	0.8541	0.8052	0.8055	0.8547
	$\mathcal{L}_{CE}$ & $\mathcal{L}_{rank}$	**88.80**	**0.8882**	**0.8507**	**0.8508**	**0.8881**

type of backbone networks, the networks were optimized using $\mathcal{L}_{CE}$ only (PlainCNNs) and a combination of $\mathcal{L}_{CE}$ and $\mathcal{L}_{tri}$ (TripletCNNs). Regardless of the type of backbone networks, RankCNNs were substantially superior to both PlainCNNs and TripletCNNs, demonstrating the additive value of the proposed $\mathcal{L}_{rank}$. PlainCNNs, which perform the categorical classification task only, showed the worst performance. TripletCNNs, conducting both categorical ($\mathcal{L}_{CE}$) and (partial) ordinal classification ($\mathcal{L}_{tri}$) tasks, achieved $\leq 86.53\%$ ACC, ≤ 0.8655 REC, ≤ 0.8204 κ, ≤ 0.8207 MCC, and ≤ 0.8676 $F1_{mac}$. These results demonstrate that the ordinal classification could aid in improving the performance of cancer grading and the ranking loss could better exploit the hierarchy of cancer grades. However, the additive value of $\mathcal{L}_{rank}$ was different among the backbone networks. Using $\mathcal{L}_{CE}$ only, MobileNet was better than other two networks, but the performance gain by $\mathcal{L}_{rank}$ and $\mathcal{L}_{tri}$ was lesser for MobileNet. As a result, using $\mathcal{L}_{rank}$, MobileNet was poorer than other two networks. This indicates that the effect of $\mathcal{L}_{rank}$ could vary with the backbone networks.

Moreover, we visualized and quantitatively evaluated the classification results of the proposed approach (Fig. 2 Visual assessment of colorectal cancer grading. Blue, yellow, green, and red colors represent benign, WD, MD, and PD, respectively.). For each tissue image, we slid a rectangular window of size 1024×1024 pixels with a step size of 256 pixels, generating a set of image patches. The image patches were resized by half and used to produce the probabilities for the four classes. Averaging the probabilities over the overlapping patches, we assigned a class label per pixel in the tissue image. For various pathology images, the prediction results are corresponding to the ground truth maps provided by pathologists.

Table 2 inter-class distances among different cancer grades. shows the inter-class distances among different cancer grades where the distance was computed using the features generated by EfficientNet. Numbers represent the average distances and standard deviations in parenthesis. RankCNNs showed substantially higher inter-class distances than other networks (p-value $\ll 0.01$). In comparison to PlainCNNs and TripletCNNs, RankCNNs, on average, exhibited ~3 to 7-fold and ~1 to 3-fold larger distances among different cancer grades, respectively. Moreover, the larger distances we obtained, the more aggressive cancer grades are. For instance, the average distance of BN to WD, MD, and PD was 22.02, 24.51, and 30.80, respectively, i.e., linearly increasing as cancer progresses.

Table 2. Inter-class distances among different cancer grades.

Loss	BN-WD	BN-MD	BN-PD	WD-MD	WD-PD	MD-PD
$\mathcal{L}_{CE}$	4.19	4.22	4.25	1.33	2.98	2.26
	(2.05)	(2.05)	(2.05)	(0.69)	(0.64)	(0.85)
$\mathcal{L}_{CE}$ & $\mathcal{L}_{tri}$	11.30	11.03	12.71	1.79	6.83	5.50
	(4.05)	(4.14)	(4.23)	(1.83)	(1.42)	(2.00)
$\mathcal{L}_{CE}$ & $\mathcal{L}_{rank}$	**22.02**	**24.51**	**30.80**	**5.27**	**10.82**	**6.80**
	(2.64)	(3.03)	(3.13)	(3.12)	(2.98)	(2.49)

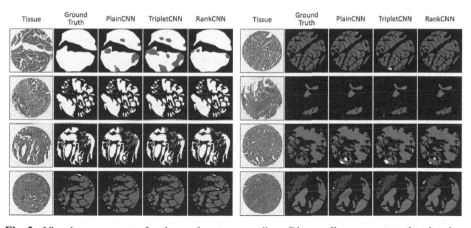

Fig. 2. Visual assessment of colorectal cancer grading. Blue, yellow, green, and red colors represent benign, WD, MD, and PD, respectively.

4 Conclusions

We present a ranking-based deep convolutional neural network that is equipped with the state-of-the-art deep neural network and the ranking loss. The ranking loss attempts to achieve a larger inter-class distance among different pathology classes with respect to the aggressiveness of cancer, leading to the correct ordering of tissue samples with differing cancer grades. The experimental results demonstrate that a substantial performance gain can be obtained without any major modifications of the network architecture, highlighting the effectiveness of the proposed ranking loss.

Acknowledgements. This work was supported by the National Research Foundation of Korea (NRF) grant funded by the Korea government (MSIT) (No.NRF-2021R1A4A1031864).

References

1. Bray, F., Ferlay, J., Soerjomataram, I., Siegel, R.L., Torre, L.A., Jemal, A.: Global cancer statistics 2018: GLOBOCAN estimates of incidence and mortality worldwide for 36 cancers in 185 countries. CA Cancer J. Clin. **68**, 394–424 (2018)
2. Berglund, R.K., Jones, J.S.: A practical guide to prostate cancer diagnosis and management. Clevel. Clin. J. Med. **78**, 321 (2011)
3. Elmore, J.G., et al.: Diagnostic concordance among pathologists interpreting breast biopsy specimens. JAMA **313**, 1122–1132 (2015)
4. Williams, B.J., Bottoms, D., Treanor, D.: Future-proofing pathology: the case for clinical adoption of digital pathology. J. Clin. Pathol. **70**, 1010–1018 (2017)
5. Niazi, M.K.K., Parwani, A.V., Gurcan, M.N.: Digital pathology and artificial intelligence. Lancet Oncol. **20**, e253–e261 (2019)
6. Kwak, J.T., Hewitt, S.M., Sinha, S., Bhargava, R.: Multimodal microscopy for automated histologic analysis of prostate cancer. BMC Cancer **11**, 62 (2011)
7. Doyle, S., Feldman, M.D., Shih, N., Tomaszewski, J., Madabhushi, A.: Cascaded discrimination of normal, abnormal, and confounder classes in histopathology: Gleason grading of prostate cancer. BMC Bioinformatics **13**, 282 (2012)
8. Doyle, S., Feldman, M., Tomaszewski, J., Madabhushi, A.: A boosted Bayesian multiresolution classifier for prostate cancer detection from digitized needle biopsies. IEEE Trans. Biomed. Eng. **59**, 1205–1218 (2010)
9. Kwak, J.T., Hewitt, S.M.: Multiview boosting digital pathology analysis of prostate cancer. Comput. Methods Prog. Biomed. **142**, 91–99 (2017)
10. Wang, X., et al.: Machine learning models for multiparametric glioma grading with quantitative result interpretations. Front. Neurosci. **12**, 1046 (2019)
11. Xu, Y., et al.: Multi-label classification for colon cancer using histopathological images. Microsc. Res. Techniq. **76**, 1266–1277 (2013)
12. Vu, Q.D., Kwak, J.T.: A dense multi-path decoder for tissue segmentation in histopathology images. Comput. Methods Prog. Biomed. **173**, 119–129 (2019)
13. Hou, L., et al.: Sparse autoencoder for unsupervised nucleus detection and representation in histopathology images. Pattern Recogn. **86**, 188–200 (2019)
14. Graham, S., et al.: Hover-net: simultaneous segmentation and classification of nuclei in multi-tissue histology images. Med. Image Anal. **58**, 101563 (2019)
15. Litjens, G., et al.: Deep learning as a tool for increased accuracy and efficiency of histopathological diagnosis. Sci. Rep. **6**, 26286 (2016)
16. Hou, L., Agarwal, A., Samaras, D., Kurc, T.M., Gupta, R.R., Saltz, J.H.: Robust histopathology image analysis: to label or to synthesize? In: Proceedings of the IEEE Conference on Computer Vision and Pattern Recognition, pp. 8533–8542 (2019)
17. Arvaniti, E., et al.: Automated Gleason grading of prostate cancer tissue microarrays via deep learning. Sci. Rep. **8**, 1–11 (2018)
18. Aresta, G., et al.: Bach: Grand challenge on breast cancer histology images. Med. Image Anal. **56**, 122–139 (2019)
19. Ertosun, M.G., Rubin, D.L.: Automated grading of gliomas using deep learning in digital pathology images: a modular approach with ensemble of convolutional neural networks. In: AMIA Annual Symposium Proceedings, p. 1899. American Medical Informatics Association

20. Szegedy, C., et al.: Going deeper with convolutions. In: Proceedings of the IEEE Conference on Computer Vision and Pattern Recognition, pp. 1–9
21. He, K., Zhang, X., Ren, S., Sun, J.: Deep residual learning for image recognition. In: Proceedings of the IEEE Conference on Computer Vision and Pattern Recognition, pp. 770–778
22. Huang, G., Liu, Z., Van Der Maaten, L., Weinberger, K.Q.: Densely connected convolutional networks. In: Proceedings of the IEEE Conference on Computer Vision and Pattern Recognition, pp. 4700–4708
23. Sandler, M., Howard, A., Zhu, M., Zhmoginov, A., Chen, L.-C.: Mobilenetv2: Inverted residuals and linear bottlenecks. In: Proceedings of the IEEE Conference on Computer Vision and Pattern Recognition, pp. 4510–4520
24. Schroff, F., Kalenichenko, D., Philbin, J.: Facenet: A unified embedding for face recognition and clustering. In: Proceedings of the IEEE Conference on Computer Vision and Pattern Recognition, pp. 815–823
25. Hermans, A., Beyer, L., Leibe, B.: In defense of the triplet loss for person re-identification (2017). https://arxiv.org/abs/1703.07737
26. Tan, M., Le, Q.V.: Efficientnet: rethinking model scaling for convolutional neural networks (2019). https://arxiv.org/abs/1905.11946
27. Jurman, G., Riccadonna, S., Furlanello, C.: A comparison of MCC and CEN error measures in multi-class prediction. PLoS One **7**, e41882 (2012)

Spatial Attention-Based Deep Learning System for Breast Cancer Pathological Complete Response Prediction with Serial Histopathology Images in Multiple Stains

Hongyi Duanmu[1], Shristi Bhattarai[2], Hongxiao Li[2], Chia Cheng Cheng[1],
Fusheng Wang[1], George Teodoro[3], Emiel A. M. Janssen[4], Keerthi Gogineni[5],
Preeti Subhedar[5], Ritu Aneja[2], and Jun Kong[2,5(✉)]

[1] Stony Brook University, Stony Brook, NY 11794, USA
[2] Georgia State University, Atlanta, GA 30302, USA
[3] Federal University of Minas Gerais, Belo Horizonte 31270-010, Brazil
[4] Department of Pathology, Stavanger University Hospital, Stavanger, Norway
[5] Emory University, Atlanta, GA 30322, USA

Abstract. In triple negative breast cancer (TNBC) treatment, early prediction of pathological complete response (PCR) from chemotherapy before surgical operations is crucial for optimal treatment planning. We propose a novel deep learning-based system to predict PCR to neoadjuvant chemotherapy for TNBC patients with multi-stained histopathology images of serial tissue sections. By first performing tumor cell detection and recognition in a cell detection module, we produce a set of feature maps that capture cell type, shape, and location information. Next, a newly designed spatial attention module integrates such feature maps with original pathology images in multiple stains for enhanced PCR prediction in a dedicated prediction module. We compare it with baseline models that either use a single-stained slide or have no spatial attention module in place. Our proposed system yields 78.3% and 87.5% of accuracy for patch-, and patient-level PCR prediction, respectively, outperforming all other baseline models. Additionally, the heatmaps generated from the spatial attention module can help pathologists in targeting tissue regions important for disease assessment. Our system presents high efficiency and effectiveness and improves interpretability, making it highly promising for immediate clinical and translational impact.

Keywords: Breast cancer · Convolutional neural network · Pathological complete response · Serial pathology images · Spatial attention

1 Introduction

In triple negative breast cancer (TNBC) treatment, pathological complete response (PCR) to neoadjuvant chemotherapy (NAC) is defined as the lack of

© Springer Nature Switzerland AG 2021
M. de Bruijne et al. (Eds.): MICCAI 2021, LNCS 12908, pp. 550–560, 2021.
https://doi.org/10.1007/978-3-030-87237-3_53

all signs of cancer, especially the absence of cancer cells in pathology images of tissue samples dissected during surgery. It plays an important role in treatment planning and assessment [1,2]. Patients with negative PCR tend to have longer event-free survival and overall survival [1]. Therefore, the accurate prediction of patient PCR to neoadjuvant chemotherapy can significantly help enhance clinical treatment planning by avoiding unnecessary chemotherapy treatment for some patient cohorts. Accurate PCR prediction has a significant clinical impact as it not only reduces adverse chemotherapy effects on patient life quality but also makes it possible to go for other alternative regimes in this treatment window before surgery. However, a precise PCR prediction remains a challenging and unsolved problem.

Early studies have been conducted to predict PCR with ultrasound [3], CT/PET [4], or MRI [5,6]. However, they all have limited accuracy, thus not feasible to be deployed into clinical settings. To our best knowledge, only one study has utilized pathology images for this prediction task, which has limited success [7]. The development of a PCR prediction system using patient histopathology images is indeed conceptually rationale and promising, as histopathology images are the direct imaging source for PCR review. Furthermore, two important biomarkers, Ki-67 and phosphohistone-H3 (PHH3) characterizing tumor cell proliferation circle, are known to have a strong relationship with PCR [8,9]. However, these essential biomarkers from immunohistochemistry (IHC) images have not been jointly studied with spatially aligned tumor phenotypic information from adjacent Hematoxylin and Eosin (H&E) stained slides. Due to the absence of necessary technology development, integrated use of pathophysiological biomarkers with pathology structure features for PCR prediction remains unexplored by far. Recently, deep learning has been rapidly developed in the machine learning research field [10]. This technology has achieved groundbreaking milestones not only in conventional computer science problems [10,11], but also in a large variety of biomedical studies [12–14]. However, deep learning based studies on PCR prediction in breast cancer so far only used radiology images [15,16], limiting the system prediction accuracy and interpretability. Overall, a robust, effective, and interpretable deep learning system for PCR prediction using histopathology images is still in its primitive stage.

To address this unmet clinical need, we have developed a deep learning system that predicts PCR to neoadjuvant chemotherapy in TNBC patients with integrated use of histopathology images of serial tissue sections in multiple stains. The novelty and contribution of this work are threefold. 1) **Biomarkers and pathology features integration**: Instead of using single stained histopathology images, pathology images of serial tissue sections in three PCR relevant stains, including H&E, Ki-67, and PHH3, are jointly utilized in our proposed system, providing complementary molecular and pathology information. 2) **Multi-task**: Our proposed system detects and classifies cells before PCR prediction. Therefore, key information, such as cell type, shape, spatial organization, and the cell proliferation cycle status is provided to the PCR prediction module. This process emulates the reviewing process pathologists follow in clinical settings, making the system more rationale and interpretable. 3) **Spatial attention**

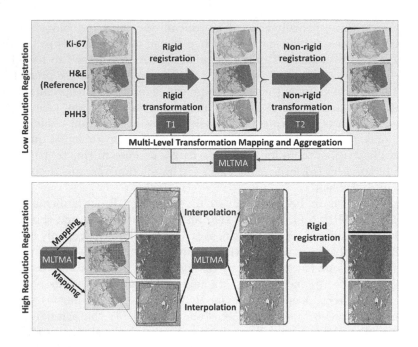

Fig. 1. Schema of registration working pipeline.

mechanism: We have designed a novel spatial attention module that informs the PCR prediction module of tissue spatial importance map. Additionally, the spatial attention module produces heatmaps that make pathologists more informed about the machine-based PCR prediction process, significantly improving the system's interpretability.

2   Methodology

2.1   Image Registration

To enable a joint use of serial histopathology images in multiple stains, we follow a two-step process for pathology image registration [17]. First, the global structure transformations are estimated with low-resolution image representations that can readily fit machine memory for processing. Each whole slide image is scaled down by 16 times. The serial Ki-67 and PHH3 IHC slides are matched to the corresponding reference H&E slide by both rigid and non-rigid registration sequentially. These two registration steps at the low image resolution result in transformations that restore global tissue rotation, translation, scale, and local tissue deformation. Second, low-resolution transformations are mapped to and aggregated at the high image resolution level. Each reference H&E slide is partitioned into a set of $8,000 \times 8,000$ image regions of interest at the high image resolution. The mapped and aggregated transformations are applied to H&E

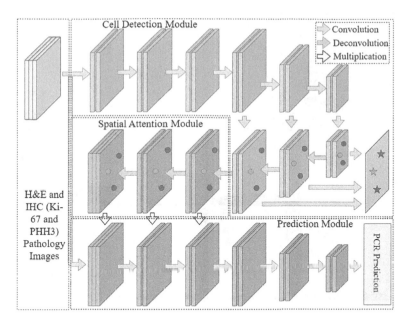

Fig. 2. Architecture schema of our proposed multi-task deep learning system leveraging multi-stained histopathology images of serial tissue sections.

image regions. After mapping and interpolation, the registered image regions are extracted from the serial Ki-67 and PHH3 slides at the high resolution. Additionally, these initial registered Ki-67 and PHH3 images are subject to a second round of rigid registration for final matched image triplets. We present the schema of the registration working pipeline in Fig. 1.

2.2 System Architecture

Presented in Fig. 2, our proposed spatial attention-based deep learning PCR prediction system consists of three primary modules: Cell Detection Module (CDM), Spatial Attention Module (SAM), and Prediction Module (PM).

Cell Detection Module: CDM is designed to recognize cell locations and types in H&E stained histopathology images. The high-level feature maps produced by CDM capture information on cell location, spatial organization, intensity, and types. Such critical information is provided to the next module to form spatial attention. We choose YOLO version 4 as the CDM backbone [18]. YOLO, as the first one-stage detection system, compared with two-stage detection systems, is more efficient in the global feature map generation [19]. With numerous modifications to the architecture, especially the feature-pyramid-like detector header for enhanced spatial feature extractions from different scales, YOLOv4 is improved to accommodate object variations in size [20]. Thus, we use YOLO version 4 for cell detection and classification in CDM.

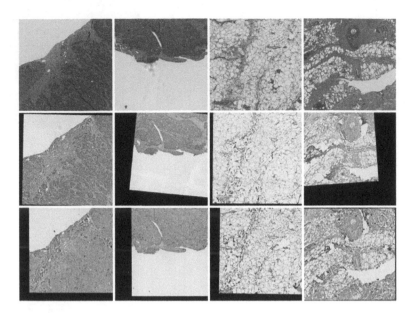

Fig. 3. Four sample cases of registered pathology images in (Top) H&E, (Middle) Ki67, and (Bottom) PHH3 stain.

Spatial Attention Module: SAM consists of three blocks. In each block, there are sequentially two convolutional layers and one deconvolutional layer for upsampling the input feature maps. Informed of such information on cell location, spatial organization, intensity, and class label derived from the detection module, SAM generates spatial attention maps with each pixel value ranging from 0 to 1. These attention maps highlight tissue areas which the system is guided to pay special attention to. SAM includes three blocks, each producing a spatial attention map. The resulting spatial attention maps are respectively multiplied with the original pathology images and the intermediate results from the prediction module in a pixel-wise manner. The essence of the SAM is that it produces a spatial attention map that guides the following prediction module to dynamically emphasize important tissue areas essential to the final PCR prediction.

Prediction Module: PM is used for making the final prediction from spatial attention-guided serial histopathology images in multiple stains. Three different pathology images (H&E, Ki-67, and PHH3) multiplied with spatial attention maps are set as the input of the prediction module. Taking into account the effectiveness and model complexity, we use VGG-16 as the backbone of the prediction module because of its simplicity and efficiency [21]. While the final prediction target in this study is PCR, it is natural to extend this architecture to predict other clinical outcomes, such as residual cancer burden or overall survival.

2.3   Dataset and Training

Our data are pre-NAC biopsies, which were collected before neoadjuvant therapy. We define PCR as having no evidence of residual invasive carcinoma in both the breast tissue and regional lymph nodes with the Residual Cancer Burden (RCB) value being zero. Non-PCR covers varying levels in response with evidence of residual invasive carcinoma. Note that RCB value is calculated based on the lymph nodes and Primary Tumor Bed. A total of 75 NAC treated TNBC cases are collected before neoadjuvant therapy from Dekalb Medical Center in Emory University Healthcare. Of these patients, 43 had PCR and 32 patients had residual disease (i.e. non-PCR). Formalin-fixed paraffin-embedded serial section samples for this study are obtained with information on clinical outcomes. The serial sections are H&E stained and immunohistochemically stained for Ki-67 and PHH3.

Our model training process has two steps. First, we train the Cell Detection Module with 868 40x H&E pathology image regions for tumor cell and TIL (Tumor infiltrating lymphocytes) detection. Bounding boxes for cells of interest (53,314 tumor cells and 20,966 TILs) are labeled and classified by expert pathologists. Non-overlapped 416×416 image patches are cropped from these image regions for training. With the optimizer stochastic gradient descent (SGD) and the loss function for YOLOv4 [18], CDM is trained for 200 epochs with the learning rate of 0.001 using one NVIDIA V100 GPU. When the CDM is fully trained, the CDM is frozen in the later training process to avoid the overwhelming computation burden. For PCR prediction training, we use $1,038$ 40x registered H&E, Ki-67, and PHH3 pathology image regions of size $8,000 \times 8,000$ in pixel. Note this data set is independent from the detection dataset for the CDM training. Typical registered pathology image triplets are presented in Fig. 3. The training set includes 455 regional images from 35 randomly selected patients, while 583 regional images from the remaining 40 patients are allocated for the testing dataset. To facilitate model training, we further partition these registered pathology image regions into non-overlapped image patches of 416×416 in size, generating 41,157 image patches in the training set and 46,029 in the testing set, respectively. With trained CDM fixed, SGD as the optimizer, learning rate as 0.001 for 100 epochs, SAM and PM are further trained with the cross-entropy loss for the PCR prediction.

3   Experiments and Results

Our two main contributions to the PCR prediction system architecture are 1) the integrative use of H&E and IHC biomarker images of adjacent tissue sections and 2) spatial attention-based prediction. To evaluate the effectiveness of these new modules, we have designed three other baseline systems for comparison. The first baseline system only takes H&E histopathology images as input and has only a prediction module. With the first system serving as the building block, the second model upgrades its input and processes the multi-stained input images. By contrast, the third system for comparison takes H&E images, but

Table 1. Comparison of PCR prediction performance of progressively improved deep learning models at the image patch level by metrics of accuracy, AUC, sensitivity, specificity, and balanced accuracy (BA).

	Single stain + Prediction only	Multi-stain + Prediction only	Single stain + SAM prediction	Multi-stain + SAM prediction
Accuracy	0.507	0.635	0.709	0.783
AUC	0.622	0.644	0.762	0.803
Sensitivity	0.726	0.625	0.765	0.701
Specificity	0.467	0.612	0.664	0.829
BA	0.596	0.619	0.715	0.765

Table 2. Prediction performance comparison at patch, region, and patient-level with the number of corrected predictions, total cases, and accuracy.

	Single stain + Prediction only	Multi-stain + Prediction only	Single stain + SAM prediction	Multi-stain + SAM prediction
Patient level	18/40 (45.0%)	27/40 (67.5%)	32/40 (80.0%)	35/40 (87.5%)
Region level	289/583 (49.6%)	387/583 (66.4%)	446/583 (76.5%)	488/583 (83.7%)
Patch level	23325/46029 (50.7%)	29248/46029 (63.5%)	32674/46029 (70.9%)	36059/46029 (78.3%)

it is equipped with the spatial attention mechanism that leverages information from the detection model to guide the prediction module. In other words, "single stain" systems are only provided with H&E stained pathology images without adjacent Ki-67 and PHH3 images. "Prediction only" systems only have a prediction module without the cell detection module and spatial attention module. Finally, "spatial attention" systems retain the same pre-trained detection module for fair comparisons. All models are fully trained to their best performance with the same training and testing configuration.

In Table 1, we present detailed performance comparisons between our proposed system and other baseline models based on prediction accuracy, area under the curve (AUC), sensitivity, specificity, and balanced accuracy (BA). The baseline system taking only H&E stained images and including only the prediction module performs the worst, with 0.507 and 0.622 for accuracy and AUC respectively at the image patch level. Information from images of adjacent tissue sections in multiple stains can improve the prediction performance of the baseline system to 0.635 and 0.644 for accuracy and AUC respectively. When the baseline system includes the spatial attention module integrating the detection with the prediction module, the resulting system performance is significantly improved with accuracy higher than 70%. Our best proposed model, by including both

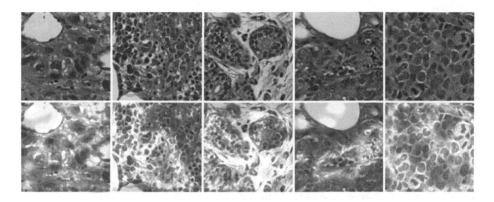

Fig. 4. Typical spatial attention maps from the spatial attention module.

the multi-stain and spatial attention modules, achieves the best accuracy of 0.783 and AUC of 0.803, respectively. Although our proposed model is not the best by sensitivity, it outperforms others by BA. BA is considered as a more general metric as it is the arithmetic average of sensitivity and specificity. With the progressively improved performance demonstrated in Table 1, it is manifested that our proposed two innovative modules help improve the PCR prediction performance significantly.

Additionally, we present in Table 2 PCR prediction performance at different levels. As described in the dataset section, our testing image patches in 416 × 416 pixels are cropped from 583 8,000 × 8,000 image regions of 40 TNBC patients. The PCR prediction at the image region level is determined by the max voting of the patch level results from the region, while the prediction at the patient level is determined by the max voting of the region level results from that patient. As shown in Table 2, the prediction performance of our proposed model is superior to that of other baseline models at all levels, achieving 78.3%, 83.7%, and 87.5% accuracy for patch, region, and patient-level prediction, respectively.

4   Discussion

To our best knowledge, only one study so far aims at predicting PCR to neoadjuvant chemotherapy with histopathology images [7]. By univariate and multivariate analysis with 15 manually designed image features, the best performance achieved by this method was 4.46 by the metric of odds ratio [7]. By comparison, our proposed multi-stain and multi-task deep learning system achieves an odds ratio of 13.3 and 51 at the patch and patient-level, respectively.

Our model is the first work on predicting PCR with multi-stained histopathology images of serial tissue sections. The existing systems use only pathology images of tissue biopsies stained by a single stain, leading to limited accuracy. They also lack full automation for the prediction. As tissue-derived molecular data do not preserve high resolution spatial information in most cases, it has always been a challenge to integrate such information with histopathology features within the same tissue space. As a result, it is ideal to spatially map multiple molecular signatures to the same histology space, enabling multi-modal microscopy integrative analysis for better clinical prediction power. When it comes to PCR prediction, both conventional H&E and IHC biomarker pathology images play an important role. It has been reported that aggressive TNBCs promote cell proliferation with a faster cell cycling kinetics and enhances cell cycle progression [22]. This enhanced cell cycle kinetics can be captured by Ki67 and PHH3 stains in adjacent tissue sections. As a result, we design a PCR prediction system that combines multi-stained serial slides to improve both prediction accuracy and robustness. The superior performance of our novel multi-stain spatial attention system indicates that an integrated analysis of multi-stained serial tissue sections can substantially improve the PCR prediction for NAC TNBC patients.

Our system is also the first work on predicting PCR from pathology images using deep learning techniques. Specifically, we develop the spatial attention module for guided PCR prediction with knowledge from cell detection. Representative spatial attention maps from the spatial attention module are presented in Fig. 4. After the spatial attention module, important areas suggested for spatial attention are highlighted in red. Such attention guidance mechanism effectively directs the following prediction module for enhanced PCR prediction. In the meanwhile, human pathologists may benefit from such interpretable information for treatment planning in clinical practice too.

For future work, first, we will explore incorporating non-imaging features to the PCR prediction system, as several non-imaging clinical variables are proven to be correlated with the PCR. Second, since our current system requires images in three stains to be well registered, we will study improving the reliability of the system for unregistered multi-stained images. Last, besides PCR, we will expand the prediction to additional clinical outcomes such as recurrence and overall survival.

5 Conclusion

In this paper, we present a novel deep learning-based system for the prediction of PCR to neoadjuvant chemotherapy for TNBC patients. By integrating detection and prediction tasks with a new spatial attention mechanism, our proposed system can capture and jointly use information from histopathology images of adjacent tissue sections in three stains (i.e. H&E, Ki-67, and PHH3). Our comparative study with three baseline models demonstrates progressively improved prediction performance of our system. The prediction effectiveness and high interpretability enabled by the spatial attention mechanism suggest its promising clinical potential for enhancing treatment planning in clinical settings.

Funding. This research was supported by National Institute of Health (U01CA 242936), National Science Foundation (ACI 1443054, IIS 1350885), and CNPq.

References

1. Cortazar, P., et al.: Pathological complete response and long-term clinical benefit in breast cancer: the CTNeoBC pooled analysis. Lancet **384**(9938), 164–172 (2014)
2. Ring, A.E., Smith, I.E., Ashley, S., Fulford, L.G., Lakhani, S.R.: Oestrogen receptor status, pathological complete response and prognosis in patients receiving neoadjuvant chemotherapy for early breast cancer. Br. J. Cancer **91**(12), 2012–2017 (2004)
3. Evans, A., et al.: Prediction of pathological complete response to neoadjuvant chemotherapy for primary breast cancer comparing interim ultrasound, shear wave elastography and MRI. Eur. J. Ultrasound **39**(04), 422–431 (2018)
4. van Stiphout, R.G.P.M., et al.: Development and external validation of a predictive model for pathological complete response of rectal cancer patients including sequential PET-CT imaging. Radiother. Oncol. **98**(1), 126–133 (2011)
5. Gollub, M.J., et al.: Dynamic contrast enhanced-MRI for the detection of pathological complete response to neoadjuvant chemotherapy for locally advanced rectal cancer. Eur. Radiol. **22**(4), 821–831 (2012)
6. Yu, N., Leung, V.W.Y., Meterissian, S.: MRI performance in detecting PCR after neoadjuvant chemotherapy by molecular subtype of breast cancer. World J. Surg. **43**(9), 2254–2261 (2019)
7. Raza Ali, H., et al.: Computational pathology of pre-treatment biopsies identifies lymphocyte density as a predictor of response to neoadjuvant chemotherapy in breast cancer. Breast Cancer Res. **18**(1), 1–11 (2016)
8. Tőkés, T., et al.: Expression of cell cycle markers is predictive of the response to primary systemic therapy of locally advanced breast cancer. Virchows Arch. **468**(6), 675–686 (2016). https://doi.org/10.1007/s00428-016-1925-x
9. Penault-Llorca, F., Radosevic-Robin, N.: Ki67 assessment in breast cancer: an update. Pathology **49**(2), 166–171 (2017)
10. LeCun, Y., Bengio, Y., Hinton, G.: Deep learning. Nature **521**(7553), 436–444 (2015)
11. Deng, L., Dong, Yu.: Deep learning: methods and applications. Found. Trends Signal Process. **7**(3–4), 197–387 (2014)
12. Cheplygina, V., de Bruijne, M., Pluim, J.P.W.: Not-so-supervised: a survey of semi-supervised, multi-instance, and transfer learning in medical image analysis. Med. Image Anal. **54**, 280–296 (2019)
13. Shen, D., Guorong, W., Suk, H.-I.: Deep learning in medical image analysis. Annu. Rev. Biomed. Eng. **19**, 221–248 (2017)
14. Litjens, G., et al.: A survey on deep learning in medical image analysis. Med. Image Anal. **42**, 60–88 (2017)
15. Yu-Hong, Q., Zhu, H.-T., Cao, K., Li, X.-T., Ye, M., Sun, Y.-S.: Prediction of pathological complete response to neoadjuvant chemotherapy in breast cancer using a deep learning (DL) method. Thoracic Cancer **11**(3), 651–658 (2020)
16. Cui, Y., et al.: Radiomics analysis of multiparametric MRI for prediction of pathological complete response to neoadjuvant chemoradiotherapy in locally advanced rectal cancer. Eur. Radiol. **29**(3), 1211–1220 (2019)
17. Rossetti, B., Wang, F., Zhang, P., Teodoro, G., Brat, D., Kong, J.: Dynamic registration for gigapixel serial whole slide images. In: IEEE International Symposium on Biomedical Imaging: From Nano to Macro (ISBI), pp. 424–428 (2017)
18. Bochkovskiy, A., Wang, C.-Y., Liao, H.-Y.M.: YOLOv4: optimal speed and accuracy of object detection. arXiv preprint arXiv:2004.10934 (2020)

19. Redmon, J., Divvala, S., Girshick, R., Farhadi, A.: You only look once: unified, real-time object detection. In: Proceedings of the IEEE Conference on Computer Vision and Pattern Recognition (CVPR), June 2016
20. Lin, T.-Y., Dollár, P., Girshick, R., He, K., Hariharan, B., Belongie, S.: Feature pyramid networks for object detection. In: Proceedings of the IEEE Conference on Computer Vision and Pattern Recognition, pp. 2117–2125 (2017)
21. Simonyan, K., Zisserman, A.: Very deep convolutional networks for large-scale image recognition. In: International Conference on Learning Representations (2015)
22. Pannu, V., et al.: HSET overexpression fuels tumor progression via centrosome clustering-independent mechanisms in breast cancer patients. Oncotarget $6(8)$, 6076 (2015)

Integration of Patch Features Through Self-supervised Learning and Transformer for Survival Analysis on Whole Slide Images

Ziwang Huang, Hua Chai, Ruoqi Wang, Haitao Wang, Yuedong Yang[✉], and Hejun Wu[✉]

School of Computer Science and Engineering, Sun Yat-sen University, Guangzhou, China
{yangyd25,wuhejun}@mail.sysu.edu.cn

Abstract. Survival prediction using whole slide images (WSIs) can provide guidance for better treatment of diseases and patient care. Previous methods usually extract and process only image features from patches of WSIs. However, they ignore the significant role of spatial information of patches and the correlation between the patches of WSIs. Furthermore, those methods extract the patch features through the model pre-trained on ImageNet, overlooking the huge gap between WSIs and natural images. Therefore, we propose a new method, called SeTranSurv, for survival prediction. SeTranSurv extracts patch features from WSIs through self-supervised learning and adaptively aggregates these features according to their spatial information and correlation between patches using the Transformer. Experiments on three large cancer datasets indicate the effectiveness of our model. More importantly, SeTranSurv has better interpretability in locating important patterns and features that contribute to accurate cancer survival prediction.

Keywords: WSI · Survival analysis · Transformer · Self-supervised learning

1 Introduction

Survival analysis generally refers to a statistical process that investigates the occurrence time of a certain event. Accurate survival analysis provides invaluable guidance for clinical treatment. For instance, the prognostic models in survival prediction can show the interactions between different prognostic factors

---

Z. Huang and H. Chai contributed equally to this work.
Corresponding authors: Yuedong Yang and Hejun Wu contributed equally to this work.
Corresponding author: Hejun Wu, is with Guangdong Key Laboratory of Big Data Analysis and Processing, Guangzhou 510006, and School of Computer Science and Engineering, Sun Yat-sen University, Guangzhou, China.

© Springer Nature Switzerland AG 2021
M. de Bruijne et al. (Eds.): MICCAI 2021, LNCS 12908, pp. 561–570, 2021.
https://doi.org/10.1007/978-3-030-87237-3_54

in certain diseases. These results from survival prediction would allow clinicians to make early decisions on the treatment of diseases. Such early clinical interventions are crucial for the healthcare of patients.

There have been many computational methods proposed for survival analysis from whole slide images (WSIs) recently. Traditional methods generally select several discriminative patches from manually annotated Region of Interests (RoIs) and then extract features for predictions [16–18,20]. Relatively new methods [11,14,22] choose patches without using RoI annotations, as RoI annotations require heavy manpower. The previous methods that do not need RoI annotations usually adopt the ImageNet [13] pre-trained network to extract patch features from WSIs. For instance, WSISA proposed by Zhu et al. [22] extracts patches from the WSIs and gathers them into clusters of different patterns. WSISA adopts DeepConvSurv [21] to select meaningful patch clusters. These clusters are then aggregated for later prediction. Li et al. [11] propose a survival analysis method that first constructs a topological relationship between features and then learns useful representative and related features from their patches through a graph convolutional network [10] (GCN). However, extracting accurate patch features for survival analysis and integrating patch features to obtain an aggregated set of patient-level features constitute the two significant challenges. As stated, pre-training models overlook the huge gap between WSIs and natural images and no available labels can be used to fine-tune the pre-training models. As a result, the patch features from pre-trained models cannot satisfy the accuracy requirement for survival analysis. Additionally, previous methods do not notice the significant role of patch spatial information and the correlation between patches of WSIs. These methods usually separately process each cluster of patches or every single patch from the WSIs of the patient. This is due to the large scale of WSI, which makes it difficult to integrate spatial information into the model. Therefore, how to integrate patch features to obtain patient-level features is also an open question.

Recent studies have shown that SimCLR [1], a self-supervised learning method, can train a model with excellent feature extraction ability through contrastive learning. The feature extraction ability of this model is comparable to the supervised learning model. Therefore, SimCLR is introduced to train a better model to extract patch features. Otherwise, the Transformer has been widely used for sequence problems recently. The Transformer includes position encodings and self-attention modules. Through certain position encodings, the model can easily restore the WSI spatial information. For each unit in the input sequence, self-attention can get the weight of attention from other units. The weight of attention reflects the correlation between the patches. Since it is impossible to input a whole WSI to fuse the spatial information, we extract patch features selected from the WSI. The features are added with corresponding position encodings to form a sequence to input into the Transformer. The self-attention in Transformer can automatically learn the correlation between patches, and spatial information is also learned through position encodings to obtain patient-level features.

In this paper, we propose a model called SeTranSurv, which adopts **Self-Supervised learning (SSL)** to obtain accurate features from WSIs and employs **Transformer** to aggregate patches according to their correlation and spatial distribution. The contributions are summarized as follows: (1) We adopt Sim-CLR to get a better representation of patch features; (2) We employ the Transformer to aggregate patches according to their correlation and spatial distribution; (3) We use attentional mechanisms to automatically locate features that are highly relevant to survival analysis, which provides better interpretability. Our work attempt to construct the spatial information and correlation between patches and integrates them for accurate survival prediction in WSIs. Extensive experiments on WSI datasets demonstrate that our model outperforms the state-of-the-art models by providing more precise survival risk predictions.

2   Methodology

An overview of the proposed framework is shown in Fig. 1. Motivated by WSISA [22]: Firstly, we select patches from the non-background area of each WSI and use all of them to train the SSL model by SimCLR [1] to train a feature extraction model ResNet18 [7]. Secondly, we re-select 600 patches in the non-background area of each WSI and then use the ResNet18 trained by SimCLR to extract features for every patch. At the third step, a Transformer Encoder takes both each patch feature and the corresponding position embedding information as input. Finally, The fused information from Transformer Encoder is sent to a Muti-Layer Perception (MLP) to get the final risk score.

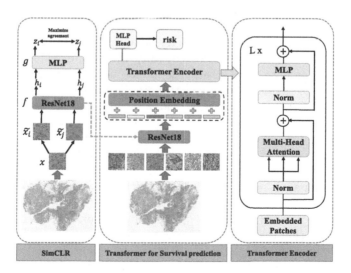

Fig. 1. An overview of the proposed framework. The left part is the advanced SSL method SimCLR [1] for training a feature extraction model ResNet18 [7]. Besides, the middle section is the flow of Transformer Encoder [5] for survival analysis and the right section is the detail of the Transformer Encoder block.

Sampling from WSIs. The primary purpose of this stage is to select some patches from WSIs. A patient often has multiple WSIs, and patch candidates from different WSIs of the patient reflect the survival risk collectively. Therefore, we extract patches from non-background area of each WSI of the same patient and aggregate their WSI results later. The patches with the size of $512 \times 512 \times 3$ are extracted from 20X ($0.5\,\mu$ per pixel) to capture detailed information of the images. While randomly selecting the patches, we also record the corresponding coordinate values of the patches in the original WSI image to facilitate the subsequent position encoding.

Train Feature Extraction Model via Self-supervised Learning. The main goal of this step is to obtain a model that can extract patch features better than the ImageNet pre-trained model. There is a big difference between the ImageNet and WSIs, and we do not have corresponding patch labels to fine-tune the model. SimCLR is a self-supervised learning model proposed by Hinton [1]. SimCLR can train a model with excellent feature extraction ability without the use of labels, and the feature extraction ability of the trained model is comparable to supervised learning. For WSIs, which are significantly different from natural images, we select many unlabeled patches from the WSIs in the training set. These patches are used to train a feature extraction model, ResNet18, through SimCLR. The trained ResNet18 is used to extract the characteristics of patches in the following work.

The specific workflow of SimCLR is shown on the left of Fig. 1. SimCLR learns representations by maximizing consistency between differently augmented views of the same data example. The way to maximizing the consistency is to use the contrastive loss [6] in the potential space. This framework comprises the following four major components: (1) A data augmentation module that transforms any given data example randomly to two correlated views of the same example. The data augmentation followed the same strategies as used in SimCLR for natural images. The image is represented by x. We use two different data augmentation methods to get $\tilde{x}_i$ and $\tilde{x}_j$, which is regarded as a position pair. (2) A neural network based encoder f that extracts representation vectors from augmented data examples. We use ResNet18 [7] to obtain patch features $h_i = f(\tilde{x}_i)$ where h_i is the output after the average pooling layer. (3) A small MLP g maps representations to the space where contrastive loss is applied. We use MLP to obtain $z_i = g(h_i) = W^{(2)}ReLU(W^{(1)}h_i)$. (4) A contrastive loss function defined for a contrastive prediction task. For a given batch size N, the set $\{\tilde{x}_k\}, k \in \{0...N\}$ includes a positive pair of examples $\tilde{x}_i$ and $\tilde{x}_j$. The contrastive prediction task aims to identify $\tilde{x}_j$ in $\{\tilde{x}_k\}_{k \neq i}$ for a given $\tilde{x}_i$.

We randomly sample a minibatch of N examples and define the contrastive prediction task on pairs of augmented examples derived from the minibatch, resulting in $2N$ data points. We do not sample negative examples explicitly. Instead, given a positive pair, similar to [2], we treat the other $2(N-1)$ augmented examples within a minibatch as negative examples. We use NT-Xent loss [12] to optimize the model to enhance feature extraction ability for the

ResNet18. These steps ensure that the views of different images are far apart in the potential space and the views of the same image are close together, thus improving the model's presentation capability. Therefore, we can train a model with excellent feature extraction ability through contrastive learning without labels. The model avoids the inapplicability of features caused by differences of data in different fields compared with the ImageNet pre-trained model.

Feature Fusion via Transformer with Position Encoding. The Transformer includes position encodings and self-attention modules. Through certain position encodings, the model can easily restore the WSI spatial information. For each unit in the input sequence, self-attention can get the weight of attention from other units. The weight of attention reflects the correlation between the patches. Our Transformer Encoder [5] for WSIs follows the architecture design for NLP [5]. For a whole slide image, we sample N (set as 600) patches to get $X \in \mathbf{R}^{N \times H \times W \times C}$ as input into the ResNet18 trained by SimCLR, and the output $h = f(X) \in \mathbf{R}^{N \times 512}$ represents the feature of N patches. $(H \times W \times C)$ is the shape of patches corresponding to $(512 \times 512 \times 3)$.

Position embeddings [5,15] are added to the patch embeddings to retain position information. We use two-dimensional positional embedding [5] in this work. To be specific, consider the inputs as a grid of patches in two dimensions. The corresponding horizontal coordinate and vertical coordinate of each patch in WSI are embedding respectively to obtain the position encodings. The x axis and y axis are represented by X-embedding, and Y-embedding, respectively. The embedding size of x axis and y axis are both 24. The 48-dimensional position vector $p \in \mathbf{R}^{N \times 48}$ is spliced with the corresponding vector h to form a 560-dimensional feature vector, $z_0 = h \oplus p$, where $\oplus$ is the concatenation operator and $z_0 \in \mathbf{R}^{N \times 560}$. We input z_0 into the Transformer Encoder for the integration of features and spatial information.

As shown on the right of Fig. 1, the Transformer Encoder [5] is composed of multiple encoding blocks, and every encoding block has constant widths. The encoding block dimension N is the same as the number of patches sampled from a WSI. Similar to the token of BERT [3], we prepend a learnable embedding to the sequence of embedded patches (z_0^0), whose state at the output of the Transformer encoder (z_L^0) serves as the WSI representation y. The Transformer encoder consists of alternating layers of multiheaded self-attention [3] (MSA) and MLP blocks (Eq. (1), (2)). The self-attention module can calculate the correlation between the features of different patches through attention mechanism. Layernorm (LN) is applied before every block and residual connections [7] after every block. The MLP contains two layers with a GELU non-linearity. Our Transformer Encoder is composed of six encoding blocks, and each encoding block has four heads, among which the hidden size of MLP is 128.

$$t_l = MSA(LN(z_{l-1})) + z_{l-1}, \qquad l = 1...L \qquad (1)$$

$$z_l = MLP(LN(t_l)) + t_l, \qquad l = 1...L \qquad (2)$$

$$L(\boldsymbol{R}) = \sum_{i \in \{i:S_i=1\}} (-R_i + log \sum_{j \in \{j:T_j \leq T_i\}} exp(R_j)) \tag{3}$$

The output $y = LN(\boldsymbol{z}_L^0)$ represents the high-level semantic features fusion by Transformer Encoder. It goes through an MLP Head module [5] $R = W^{(2)}ReLU(W^{(1)}y)$ and directly generates predicted risks (Eq. 3). We integrate the regression of survival risk with high-level feature learning on WSIs. For a patient with multiple WSIs, we average the risk scores of all WSIs for the patient and get the final risk score. The loss function [22] is negative Cox log partial likelihood (Eq. 3) for censored survival data, and S_i, T_i are the censoring status and the survival time of i-th patient, respectively.

3   Experiments

Dataset Description and Baselines. To verify the validity and generalization of SeTranSurv, we apply our methods on three different-sized cancer survival datasets with whole slide pathological images. They are collected from TCGA [8]. The three datasets are Ovarian serous cystadenocarcinoma (OV), Lung squamous cell carcinoma (LUSC), and Breast invasive carcinoma (BRCA). The OV, LUSC and BRCA correspond to small, medium, and large datasets, respectively. The datasets are prepared for multi-omics study, we keep samples with complete multi-omics data. Some statistic facts of WSIs used in the experiments are listed in Table 1. We perform a 5 fold cross-validation on all these datasets.

Table 1. Dataset statistics. Some patients may have multiple WSIs on record.

Cancer subtype	No. patients	No. censored	No. WSIs	No. valid patches
LUSC	329	194	512	117649
OV	298	120	1481	196302
BRCA	609	530	1316	274600

SeTranSurv achieves survival analysis from WSIs without using RoIs annotations, so we compare it with the state of the art methods in survival prediction of WSIs without using RoIs annotations, including WSISA [22], DeepGraphSurv [11], CapSurv [14], DeepAttnMISL [19] and RankSurv [4].

Implementation Details. We use Adam optimizer to optimize all methods, and the learning rate is set to 3e−4 by default. We only changed the batch size to 512 for a balance of performance and running time in SimCLR, and the rest of the parameters are the same as SimCLR. We train the Transformer part with a mini-batch size of 32. All hyperparameters were determined for optimal performance on the validation set. Experiments are conducted on a single NVIDIA GeForce GTX 1080 GPU with 11 GB memory.

Results and Discussions. To assess the performance of SeTranSurv, we use the concordance index (C-index) as the evaluation metric. C-index is a standard evaluation metric in survival prediction [9]. It ranges from 0 to 1. The larger the C-index is, the better the model predicts. The training time of our model increases linearly with the sample size. It takes about 38 h for the SimCLR to train a ResNet18 through WSI patches, and about 6 h to train the final Transformer model for LUSC dataset.

Table 2. Performance comparison of the proposed method and other methods using C-index values on three datasets. The method that using the SimCLR to extract the patch features on the basis of the original method is marked with * in the table. We use OursV1 to indicate that SimCLR and position information are not used in our method, and use OursV2 to indicate that SimCLR is not used in our method.

Model	LUSC	OV	BRCA
WSISA [22]	0.612	0.601	0.637
WSISA *	**0.636**	**0.610**	0.639
DeepGraphSurv [11]	0.647	0.640	0.674
DeepGraphSurv *	**0.675**	**0.659**	**0.685**
CapSurv [14]	0.660	0.641	0.662
CapSurv *	**0.665**	**0.653**	**0.671**
DeepAttnMISL [19]	0.670	0.659	0.675
RankSurv [4]	0.674	0.667	0.687
OursV1	0.662	0.655	0.686
OursV2	0.687	0.673	0.690
SeTranSurv	**0.701**	**0.692**	**0.705**

Table 2 shows the C-index values on three datasets. Our method attains the best C-index values that present the best prediction performance among all methods. Our approach outperforms the previous best approach by an average of 3% on all three datasets. The result illustrates the proposed method is effective and universal.

To explore the effectiveness of SimCLR in extracting features from patches, we conduct a comparative experiment in all methods on whether use the model trained by SimCLR to extract features of patches. As can be seen from Table 2, the features extracted from the SimCLR-trained model can improve the results well in almost methods, which indicates that the model trained with SSL in WSI patches can obtain a better feature extraction ability than the ImageNet pre-trained model. To verify the effectiveness of self-attention and location information in our method, we conduct an ablation experiment. The result of OursV1 shows that self-attention can learn the correlation between patches and obtain good results. The result of OursV2 indicates that position information enables the model to combine the spatial information of entire WSI, which also improves

the results. The above results indicate SeTranSurv has better feature extraction
ability and feature aggregation capability.

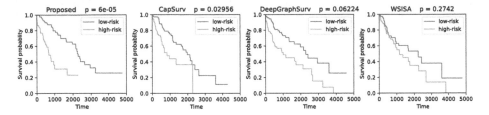

Fig. 2. Kaplan-Meier survival curves of different methods for LUSC datasets in the
test set. High risk (higher than the median) groups are plotted as brown lines, and low
risk (lower than or equal to median) groups are plotted as blue lines. The x-axis shows
the time in days, and the y-axis presents the survival probability. Log-rank p-value is
displayed on each figure. (Color figure online)

Given the trained survival models, we can classify patients into low-risk or
high-risk groups for personalized treatments by the predicted risk scores in the
test set. Two groups are classified by the median of the predicted risk score.
Patients with longer survival time should be divided into the low-risk group,
and with short survival time should be divide into the high-risk group. To measure if those models can correctly divide patients into two groups, we draw
Kaplan-Meier survival curves of LUSC dataset in Fig. 2. The log-rank test is
conducted to test the difference between two curves and evaluate how well the
model will classify testing patients into low and high-risk groups. It is shown
that the proposed method can attain the most significant result of the log-rank
test.

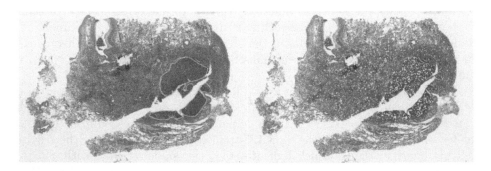

Fig. 3. Left: annotation of RoIs; Right: The blue part represents the parts with larger
weight given by the model in the randomly selected patches. It can be seen that the
patches selected in the RoIs region are generally given a relatively large weight, while
only a small number of patches in the non-RoIs region are given a relatively large
weight. (Color figure online)

SeTranSurv uses the attention mechanism to recognize significant patterns in WSI automatically. As shown in Fig. 3, we draw all the randomly selected patches whose weight assigned by the model exceed the median. We measured the learned attentions patches in Fig. 3, and 20 repeated experiments showed that 85% of selected patches had greater attention values than the average in the ROI regions, significantly higher than the 26% in non-ROI regions. The result indicates that the model can identify the patches that are highly correlated with survival analysis and give these patches a large weight. The patches with large weight correctly highlight most of the RoIs annotated by medical experts, which shows that our method can locate useful features and have good interpretability.

4 Conclusion

We propose SeTranSurv to combine SSL and the Transformer for survival analysis in WSIs. SeTranSurv can extract patch features better and use the correlation and position information between patches to fuse the features that are useful for survival analysis in the entire WSI. Extensive experiments on three large cancer datasets indicate the effectiveness of SeTranSurv.

Acknowledgements. This work was supported by the Meizhou Major Scientific and Technological Innovation Platforms and Projects of Guangdong Provincial Science & Technology Plan Projects under Grant No. 2019A0102005.

References

1. Chen, T., Kornblith, S., Norouzi, M., Hinton, G.: A simple framework for contrastive learning of visual representations. In: ICML 2020: 37th International Conference on Machine Learning, vol. 1, pp. 1597–1607 (2020)
2. Chen, T., Sun, Y., Shi, Y., Hong, L.: On sampling strategies for neural network-based collaborative filtering. In: Proceedings of the 23rd ACM SIGKDD International Conference on Knowledge Discovery and Data Mining, pp. 767–776 (2017)
3. Devlin, J., Chang, M.W., Lee, K., Toutanova, K.N.: BERT: pre-training of deep bidirectional transformers for language understanding. In: Proceedings of the 2019 Conference of the North American Chapter of the Association for Computational Linguistics: Human Language Technologies, vol. 1 (Long and Short Papers), pp. 4171–4186 (2018)
4. Di, D., Li, S., Zhang, J., Gao, Y.: Ranking-based survival prediction on histopathological whole-slide images. In: International Conference on Medical Image Computing and Computer-Assisted Intervention, pp. 428–438 (2020)
5. Dosovitskiy, A., et al.: An image is worth 16x16 words: transformers for image recognition at scale. In: International Conference on Learning Representations (2020)
6. He, K., Fan, H., Wu, Y., Xie, S., Girshick, R.: Momentum contrast for unsupervised visual representation learning. In: 2020 IEEE/CVF Conference on Computer Vision and Pattern Recognition (CVPR), pp. 9729–9738 (2020)
7. He, K., Zhang, X., Ren, S., Sun, J.: Deep residual learning for image recognition. In: 2016 IEEE Conference on Computer Vision and Pattern Recognition (CVPR), pp. 770–778 (2016)

8. Kandoth, C., et al.: Mutational landscape and significance across 12 major cancer types. Nature **502**(7471), 333–339 (2013)
9. Katzman, J.L., Shaham, U., Cloninger, A., Bates, J., Jiang, T., Kluger, Y.: DeepSurv: personalized treatment recommender system using a cox proportional hazards deep neural network. BMC Med. Res. Methodol. **18**(1), 24 (2018)
10. Kipf, T.N., Welling, M.: Semi-supervised classification with graph convolutional networks. In: ICLR (Poster) (2016)
11. Li, R., Yao, J., Zhu, X., Li, Y., Huang, J.: Graph CNN for survival analysis on whole slide pathological images. In: Frangi, A.F., Schnabel, J.A., Davatzikos, C., Alberola-López, C., Fichtinger, G. (eds.) MICCAI 2018. LNCS, vol. 11071, pp. 174–182. Springer, Cham (2018). https://doi.org/10.1007/978-3-030-00934-2_20
12. van den Oord, A., Li, Y., Vinyals, O.: Representation learning with contrastive predictive coding. arXiv preprint arXiv:1807.03748 (2018)
13. Simonyan, K., Zisserman, A.: Very deep convolutional networks for large-scale image recognition. In: ICLR 2015: International Conference on Learning Representations (2015)
14. Tang, B., Li, A., Li, B., Wang, M.: CapSurv: capsule network for survival analysis with whole slide pathological images. IEEE Access **7**, 26022–26030 (2019)
15. Wang, B., Zhao, D., Lioma, C., Li, Q., Zhang, P., Simonsen, J.G.: Encoding word order in complex embeddings. In: ICLR 2020: Eighth International Conference on Learning Representations (2020)
16. Wang, H., Xing, F., Su, H., Stromberg, A.J., Yang, L.: Novel image markers for non-small cell lung cancer classification and survival prediction. BMC Bioinform. **15**(1), 310 (2014)
17. Wang, S., Yao, J., Xu, Z., Huang, J.: Subtype cell detection with an accelerated deep convolution neural network. In: Ourselin, S., Joskowicz, L., Sabuncu, M.R., Unal, G., Wells, W. (eds.) MICCAI 2016. LNCS, vol. 9901, pp. 640–648. Springer, Cham (2016). https://doi.org/10.1007/978-3-319-46723-8_74
18. Yao, J., Wang, S., Zhu, X., Huang, J.: Imaging biomarker discovery for lung cancer survival prediction. In: Ourselin, S., Joskowicz, L., Sabuncu, M.R., Unal, G., Wells, W. (eds.) MICCAI 2016. LNCS, vol. 9901, pp. 649–657. Springer, Cham (2016). https://doi.org/10.1007/978-3-319-46723-8_75
19. Yao, J., Zhu, X., Jonnagaddala, J., Hawkins, N.J., Huang, J.: Whole slide images based cancer survival prediction using attention guided deep multiple instance learning networks. Med. Image Anal. **65**, 101789 (2020)
20. Yu, K.H.: Predicting non-small cell lung cancer prognosis by fully automated microscopic pathology image features. Nat. Commun. **7**(1), 12474 (2016)
21. Zhu, X., Yao, J., Huang, J.: Deep convolutional neural network for survival analysis with pathological images. In: 2016 IEEE International Conference on Bioinformatics and Biomedicine (BIBM), pp. 544–547 (2016)
22. Zhu, X., Yao, J., Zhu, F., Huang, J.: WSISA: making survival prediction from whole slide histopathological images. In: 2017 IEEE Conference on Computer Vision and Pattern Recognition (CVPR), pp. 6855–6863 (2017)

Contrastive Learning Based Stain Normalization Across Multiple Tumor in Histopathology

Jing Ke[1,2,4], Yiqing Shen[3(✉)], Xiaoyao Liang[1], and Dinggang Shen[5,6]

[1] Department of Computer Science and Engineering, Shanghai Jiao Tong University, Shanghai, China
kejing@sjtu.edu.cn
[2] School of Computer Science and Engineering, University of New South Wales, Sydney, Australia
[3] School of Mathematical Sciences, Shanghai Jiao Tong University, Shanghai, China
shenyq@sjtu.edu.cn
[4] BirenTech Research, Shanghai, China
[5] School of Biomedical Engineering, ShanghaiTech University, Shanghai, China
dgshen@shanghaitech.edu.cn
[6] Shanghai United Imaging Intelligence Co., Ltd., Shanghai, China

Abstract. Generative adversarial network (GAN) has been a prevalence in color normalization techniques to assist deep learning analysis in H&E stained histopathology images. The widespread adoption of GAN has effectively released pathologists from the heavy manual workload in the conventional template image selection. However, the transformation might cause significant information loss, or generate undesirable results such as mode collapse in all likelihood, which may affect the performance in the succeeding diagnostic task. To address the issue, we propose a contrastive learning method with a color-variation constraint, which maximally retains the recognizable phenotypic features at the training of a color-normalization GAN. In a self-supervised manner, the discriminative tissue patches across multiple types of tumors are clustered, taken as the salient input to feed the GAN. Empirically, the model is evaluated by public datasets of large cohorts on different cancer diseases from TCGA and Camelyon16. We show better phenotypical recognizability along with an improved performance in the histology image classification.

Keywords: Histopathology · Stain normalization · Self-supervised learning · Contrastive learning · Generative adversarial network

1 Introduction

Histopathology images have been a definitive diagnosis of the cancerous disease through the analysis of tissue specimens since the advent of the Whole-slide Imaging (WSI) scanner. Recently, with the prevalence of convolutional neural

M. de Bruijne et al. (Eds.): MICCAI 2021, LNCS 12908, pp. 571–580, 2021.
https://doi.org/10.1007/978-3-030-87237-3_55

networks (CNNs), stain normalization techniques have been an important pre-processing prior to most computer-aided diagnostic tasks, as slides from different institutions and even slides within the same institution but different batches may vary drastically in stain style [3]. This variability may not bring add recognition difficulty to an experienced pathologist, however, it may significantly reduce the reliability of an AI-assisted system as the latter is possessed slight interpretability [18].

Many successful color normalization techniques have been proposed in the discipline of computational pathology. The very initial approach attempt to subtract the mean of each color channel and then divide by the standard deviation [14]. Conventional algorithms have demonstrated their effectiveness in the past like a non-linear mapping approach employs image-specific color deconvolution [9], or an estimation of the stain vectors using singular value decomposition (SVD) geodesic based stain normalization technique [10], and many others [11,19]. However, due to the reliance on an expertly selected target image, the conventional methods are no more applicable to convolutional neural networks. More recently, generative adversarial networks are widely adopted to reduce color variations between multiple data centers [8]. Specifically, the Cycle-GAN [22] and StainGAN [16], have demonstrated their outstanding experimental results with respect to stain separation and image information preservation. However, these advanced methods may suffer severe information variation due to the universal mode collapse issue (Fig. 1), and generated other unpredictable results. Recently, contrastive learning methods gradually present their capability in domain-specific information extraction in the absence of labels, which assumes that two input image patches should have similar feature representations. And we may leverage this potential in the exploration and preservation of mutual information across two styles in a stain-normalization task.

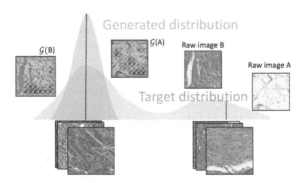

Fig. 1. A few examples of target distribution and generated distribution with mode collapses, the adipose tissue A and stroma tissue B have lost the recognizability in the learning-based style transfer [8] i.e., in $\mathcal{G}(A)$ and $\mathcal{G}(B)$.

In this paper, we address the problem by the proposal of a novel color normalization framework. The contributions are summarized as: 1) We design a self-supervised method to cluster morphologically homogeneous patches across multiple tumors, where the tissue-specific information can be extracted, and the outcome will be taken as latent input in training a GAN. 2) We incorporate a contrastive learning based loss in training a color-transfer GAN with a color-variation constraint, which can well preserve the invariant information in the phenotypical recognition. In contrast with many previous approaches targeting a single organ, this framework tackles multiple types of cancer disease. Empirically, high-quality images with finer phenotypical recognizability can be generated in the color transfer, which is also capable of training a better tissue classifier in the subsequent diagnostic task.

2   Methods

In this section, we introduce the proposed normalization framework, with the overall architecture illustrated in Fig. 2.

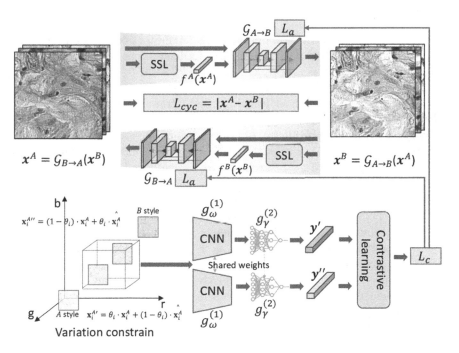

Fig. 2. The overall architecture of the proposed stain normalization framework. A CycleGAN is employed [22] to transfer the stain style with a pre-clustering auxiliary input in a self-supervised learning manner. With a constraint of variation, the images are then fed to a contrastive learning structure for domain-specific feature extraction. The Self-Supervised Learning framework clusters patches prior to the training stage of color normalization, and is also progressively trained together with GAN by loss $\mathcal{L}_p$. Then the clustered output logits, i.e. the input to the final softmax layer in SSL, are concreted with the feature vectors at the bottom layer of the U-Net.

2.1   Self-supervised Clustering to Train a GAN for Normalization

Some color normalization approaches have been proposed in the literature [10,14], yet constrained to classifying tissues from one specific cancer. Some other approaches aim to identify different tissue types across different diseases [5,13] with CNN, yet without an indispensable pre-stage of normalization. In our method, a more generalized GAN is trained towards multiple cancer diseases in a self-supervised learning manner, which learns salient features from raw input images. Innovatively, we group phenotype-homogeneous patches across different tumors to learn mutual features.

We propose a self-supervised pre-clustering model to produce latent input for the target normalization GAN. We first write an input patch as $\mathbf{x}^s \in \mathcal{X}^s$, and the unsupervised soft-clustering model as $f^s : \mathcal{X}^s \to [0,1]^d$, where d is the dimension of the expected clustered categories and the superscript $s \in \mathcal{S}$ writes for stain style s. A soft-clustering model is trained along with the normalization GAN via the pre-clustering loss $\mathcal{L}_p$ i.e.,

$$\mathcal{L}_p = \sum_s \mathbb{E}_{\mathbf{x}^s \in \mathcal{X}^s} H(f^s(\mathbf{x}^s)), \tag{1}$$

where $\mathbb{E}$ denotes the expectation operator, and the function $H(\cdot)$ represents the entropy. The output $f^s(\mathbf{x}^s)$ is taken as an auxiliary input of the normalization GAN as the constraint i.e., $\mathcal{G}_{s_1 \to s_2} : \mathcal{X}^{s_1} \times \mathbb{R}^d \to \mathcal{X}^{s_2}$, where the subscript $s_1 \to s_2$ presents the stain style transformation by the generator $\mathcal{G}$ from $s_1 \in \mathcal{S}$ to $s_2 \in \mathcal{S}$. The self-supervised learning (SSL) framework is trained prior to CycleGAN, the loss $\mathcal{L}_p$ uses the pretrained SSL to improve performance.

Given credit for the prevalence and outstanding performance in the natural-scene images transfer, the CycleGAN [22] is taken in for color transfer in our framework, and the U-Net [15] architecture is employed for the encoder and decoder design. Different from augmented CycleGAN [1], which learns many-to-many mappings by cycling over the original domains augmented with auxiliary latent spaces i.e., map (z_1, x_1) in domain A to (z_2, x_2) in domain B, where z_1, z_2 is the latent inputs, x_1 and x_2 denote images, our framework only does (z_1, x_1) input to x_2 output, without latent label z_2 as output in domain B.

The loss function are composed of three functional terms in this fashion, namely the pre-clustering loss $\mathcal{L}_p$, the GAN loss $\mathcal{L}_g$, and the contrastive loss $\mathcal{L}_c$. The pre-clustering loss $\mathcal{L}_p$ trains the self-supervised model for the pre-text auxiliary input from the morphological features. The GAN loss trains the normalization CycleGAN, which comprises a paired generator $\mathcal{G}_{A \to B}$ and $\mathcal{G}_{B \to A}$ and a paired discriminator $\mathcal{D}_A$ and $\mathcal{D}_B$. And Loss $\mathcal{L}_g$ is composed of two terms of adversarial loss and a cycle loss, depicted as follows:

$$\mathcal{L}_g = \mathcal{L}_a(\mathcal{G}_{A \to B}, \mathcal{D}_A) + \mathcal{L}_a(\mathcal{G}_{B \to A}, \mathcal{D}_B) + \mathcal{L}_{cyc}(\mathcal{G}_{A \to B}, \mathcal{G}_{B \to A}). \tag{2}$$

The prototypical adversarial loss between a paired of generator and discriminator is given as:

$$\mathcal{L}_a(\mathcal{G}s_1 \to s_2, \mathcal{D}_{s_1}) = \mathbb{E}_{\mathbf{x}^{s_1} \in \mathcal{X}^{s_1}} \log \mathcal{D}_{s_1}(\mathbf{x}^{s_1})$$
$$+ \mathbb{E}_{\mathbf{x}^{s_1} \in \mathcal{X}^{s_1}} \log \left(1 - \mathcal{D}_{s^1} \circ \mathcal{G}_{s^1 \to s^2}(\mathbf{x}^{s_1}, f^{s_1}(\mathbf{x}^{s_1}))\right). \tag{3}$$

And the cycle loss will be formulated as:

$$\mathcal{L}_{cyc}(\mathcal{G}_{A \to B}, \mathcal{G}_{B \to A}) = \mathbb{E}_{\mathbf{x}^A \in \mathcal{X}^A} \|x^A - \mathcal{G}_{B \to A} \circ \mathcal{G}_{A \to B}(\mathbf{x}^A, f^A(\mathbf{x}^A))\| \\ + \mathbb{E}_{\mathbf{x}^B \in \mathcal{X}^B} \|x^B - \mathcal{G}_{A \to B} \circ \mathcal{G}_{B \to A}(\mathbf{x}^B, f^B(\mathbf{x}^B))\|. \tag{4}$$

In this scenario, both discriminators are trained to maximize the $\mathcal{L}_g$ while the generators to minimize it. Additionally, the $\mathcal{L}_c$ targets to address the mode collapse issue and also, to preserve the histological structure, which we will further discuss in the following section.

Conclusively, we come to the overall loss function, formulated as

$$\mathcal{L} = \lambda_g \cdot \mathcal{L}_g + \lambda_p \cdot \mathcal{L}_p + \lambda_c \cdot \mathcal{L}_c, \tag{5}$$

where λ_g, λ_p and λ_c are three coefficients to balance each term.

2.2 Contrastive Learning for Feature Preservation

The proposed contrastive learning approach aims to maximize the agreement between the representations of two constrained interporations between the raw image and the generation of the normalization GAN. The designed constrained style transfer with contrastive learning effectively suppresses the outliers in the mutual information extraction. Histological patches $\mathbf{x}_i^A \in \mathcal{X}^A$ in a batch of N images and the associated generated image $\hat{\mathbf{x}}_i = \mathcal{G}_{A \to B}(\mathbf{x}_i, f^A(\mathbf{x}_i^A))$ are fed to the framework to produce adaptively interpolated paired images $\mathbf{x}_i^{A'}$, $\mathbf{x}_i^{A''}$. To stay away from a potential drastic color variation from the original image which may suffer the mode collapse problem or any great information loss, we put a restriction to the neural network training images as a replacement for the pair of a raw image and its generated style. Specifically, an interpolation function with adaptive coefficient to balance the paired image is applied and depicted as follows: $\mathbf{x}_i^{A'} = \theta_i \cdot \mathbf{x}_i^A + (1 - \theta_i) \cdot \widehat{\mathbf{x}_i^A}$ and $\mathbf{x}_i^{A''} = (1 - \theta_i) \cdot \mathbf{x}_i^A + \theta_i \cdot \widehat{\mathbf{x}_i^A}$. The non-linear constraint weights $\theta_i \in (0, 1)$ is determined by the invariant regions:

$$\theta_i = \int_\Omega \mathbb{I}_{<\mu} |\mathbf{x}_i^{A'}(\mathbf{t}) - \mathbf{x}_i^{A''}(\mathbf{t})| d\mathbf{t} / \int_\Omega d\mathbf{t}, \tag{6}$$

where Ω is the valid area in each patch, the coefficient μ is the constraint threshold, and $\mathbb{I}(\cdot)$ is the indicator function.

The interpolated variation-constrained images that share richer morphological features, are then taken as the input of the contrastive self-supervised learning framework to mine latent-space features. In the construction of the framework, we may write the a neural network or a decoder as $g_\omega^{(1)}$ with parameters ω, an auxiliary layer as $g_\gamma^{(2)}$ with parameters γ. Correspondingly, the extracted feature from the paired images will be $\mathbf{y}_i^{A'} = g_\gamma^{(2)} \circ g_\omega^{(1)}(\mathbf{x}_i^{A'})$ and $\mathbf{y}_i^{A''} = g_\gamma^{(2)} \circ g_\omega^{(1)}(\mathbf{x}_i^{A''})$.

Overall, the contrastive loss $\mathcal{L}_c$ is defined as

$$\mathcal{L}_c = \mathbb{E}_{\mathbf{x}^A \in \mathcal{X}^A} l_c(\mathbf{x}^A) + \mathbb{E}_{\mathbf{x}^B \in \mathcal{X}^B} l_c(\mathbf{x}^B), \text{ where} \tag{7}$$

$$l_c(\mathbf{x}_i) = \frac{\exp\left(\cos\left(\mathbf{y}_i^{A\prime}, \mathbf{y}_i^{A\prime\prime}\right)/\tau\right)}{\sum_{1 \leq j \leq N, j \neq i} \left\{ \exp\left(\cos\left(\mathbf{y}_i^{A\prime}, \mathbf{y}_j^{A\prime}\right)/\tau\right) + \exp\left(\cos\left(\mathbf{y}_i^{A\prime\prime}, \mathbf{y}_j^{A\prime\prime}\right)/\tau\right) \right\}},$$
$$\tag{8}$$

where we use the cosine distance to measure the similarity between two feature vectors i.e.,

$$\cos(\mathbf{u}, \mathbf{v}) = \frac{\mathbf{u} \cdot \mathbf{v}}{\|\mathbf{u}\| \cdot \|\mathbf{v}\|}. \tag{9}$$

The temperature coefficient τ helps to weigh different images to achieve hard negative mining.

3   Experiments and Results

3.1   Experimental Setups

Datasets. We use a collection of histopathological datasets with 200 WSIs from 4 different tumors, 1) colon adenocarcinoma from TCGA-COAD, 2) rectum adenocarcinoma from TCGA-READ, 3) stomach adenocarcinoma from TCGA-STAD, and 4) breast cancer metastases from Camelyon16 [2], with a balanced distribution of 50 slides each. All the datasets are publicly available online. WSIs were split into non-overlapped 224×224 patches at the magnitude of $20\times$ to retain the high resolution (0.5 µm/pix).

Settings. We implemented the proposed normalization framework on PyTorch 1.6 with python 3.7 environment. The benchmark test was carried out on an NVIDIA Tesla V100 GPU device with 32 GB memory for performance evaluations. We adopted the ADAM optimizer with a learning rate $= 10^{-4}$ and set the batch size at 16. The maximum epoch number for training the normalization GAN was 100.

We evaluated the proposed model with a couple of state-of-the-art stain normalization approaches proposed by Reinhard et al. [14], Macenko et al. [10], Khan et al. [9], Vahadne et al. [19], StainGAN [16], Harshal et al. [12], and Multimarginal Wasserstein Barycenter [11].

Four datasets are used in our experiment, each containing a variable number of slides from multiple hospitals, and trained by a separate CycleGAN independently. In each dataset, slides from an individual hospital are allocated to either domain A or B, where the distribution criterion is the data balance between the two domains. After the implementation of color normalization to all images, 70% of images are distributed to train a robust classifier and 30% to test in each dataset with the held-out method. The demonstrated results are performed on test sets.

Evaluation Metrics. Two important metrics of the structural similarity index (SSIM) [20] and features similarity index (FSIM) are taken in to evaluate our model [21]. SSIM quantifies the visibility errors and FSIM measures the image quality consistency. A higher value of SSIM and FSIM represents a better performance of the stain normalization. We also train a ResNet-18 [4] classifier to evaluate the normalization performance. We involve NCT-CRC-HE-100K-NORM dataset [6], and another 200 WSIs from CAMELYON16 in our benchmark test to analyze the CNN classification performance after the indispensable pre-processing with the proposed normalization approach. NCT-CRC-HE-100K-NORM contains a number of 100,000 non-normalized 224×224 patches at the magnitude 20× (0.5 μm/pix) [7]. The SSIM and FSIM comparison results are listed in Table 1. Our methods outperform the existing approaches by the higher SSIM and FSIM scores. The empirical results also demonstrate the system's capacity to deal with histology images across multiple cancer tumors.

Table 1. The normalization performance comparison of our methods and current competing approaches, verified by the metrics of SSIM [20] and FSIM [21].

Methods	Camelyon16		TCGA-STAD		TCGA-COAD		TCGA-READ		Aggregrated	
	SSIM	FSIM	SSIM	FSIM	SSIM	FSIM	SSIM	FSIM	SSIM	FSIM
Reinhard et al. [14]	0.631	0.649	0.683	0.653	0.612	0.588	0.532	0.509	0.502	0.492
Macenko et al. [10]	0.621	0.603	0.678	0.654	0.638	0.589	0.691	**0.703**	0.582	0.582
Khan et al. [9]	0.603	0.612	0.647	0.616	0.549	0.533	0.629	0.573	0.512	0.531
Vahadne et al. [19]	0.678	0.632	0.693	0.584	0.674	0.694	0.643	0.612	0.612	0.620
StainGAN [16]	0.701	0.699	0.712	0.659	0.723	0.641	0.687	0.689	0.650	0.661
Harshal et al. [12]	0.712	0.673	0.710	**0.711**	0.693	0.698	0.687	0.683	0.643	0.623
MWB [11]	0.699	0.678	0.689	0.683	0.691	0.692	0.704	0.693	0.645	0.634
Our proposed	**0.743**	**0.732**	**0.713**	0.710	**0.734**	**0.721**	**0.725**	**0.703**	**0.701**	**0.697**

Table 2. A comparison of histology classification accuracy in our proposed method and a couple of competing approaches proposed in the literature, tested with ResNet-18 [4] as a baseline.

Methods	Camelyon16	TCGA-STAD	TCGA-COAD	TCGA-READ	Aggregated
Reinhard et al. [14]	0.893	0.901	0.903	0.883	0.867
Macenko et al. [10]	0.867	0.893	0.912	0.905	0.875
Khan et al. [9]	0.912	0.902	0.893	0.911	0.893
Vahadne et al. [19]	0.908	0.914	0.908	0.906	0.900
StainGAN [16]	0.918	0.921	0.922	0.912	0.882
Harshal et al.[12]	0.913	0.904	0.912	0.907	0.901
MWB [11]	0.878	0.902	0.894	0.889	0.875
Our proposed	**0.923**	**0.927**	**0.921**	**0.925**	**0.910**

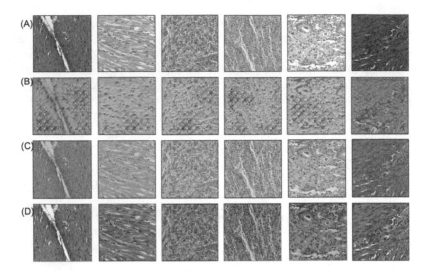

Fig. 3. A few examples of the generated images by a color normalization GAN. (A) The stained raw patches, (B) mode collapse images with a color-transfer GAN [8], (C) the proposed model with $\mu = 0.40$ and (D) with $\mu = 0.20$.

3.2 Experimental Results

As the stain normalization task is widely accepted as an important pre-stage in the histological image analysis, we compare the succeeding classification performance with a couple of state-of-the-art color transfer approaches, with the quantitative comparison results shown in Table 2. On the basis of exactly the same backbone structure, our approach achieves better performance in the downstream tasks of interest, namely the tissue classification. Given the prevalence of ResNet-18 structure [4] in the biomedical imaging domains [17], it is employed in our framework for performance evaluation. As our proposal is structure independent that we can expect a comparable performance rise with other baselines. The experiment results of the ablation study results are shown in Table 3.

Table 3. The ablation results on the aggregated dataset with the proposed normalization method.

Methods	SSIM	FSIM	Accuracy
Without pre-clustering	0.634	0.601	0.877
Without contrastive loss	0.677	0.689	0.902
All settings	**0.701**	**0.697**	**0.910**

We also illustrate our positive results by a few examples in Fig. 3, with a straight parameter of $\mu = 0.4$ and 0.2 in the constrain setting. Phenotypically, the invariant features are well retained. With better interpretability of the framework, we assure the final generalized images of consistency and reliability, which also make the succeeding diagnostic task more accurate and sensible.

4   Conclusions

In this research, we present a novel color-normalization architecture to address the universal color-variation issue across multiple datasets. Within a self-supervised pre-clustering and contrastive learning based loss manner, the phenotypic recognizability is preserved regardless of the potential failure cases from GAN. This approach can also effectively bring down the difficulty in training the network. We demonstrate its advantage in dealing with multiple cancer in one single framework. In the future, we will encompass more cancer types for a more generalized system for the potential unexpected-disease or unseen-organ issue.

References

1. Almahairi, A., Rajeshwar, S., Sordoni, A., Bachman, P., Courville, A.: Augmented cycleGAN: learning many-to-many mappings from unpaired data. In: International Conference on Machine Learning, pp. 195–204. PMLR (2018)
2. Bejnordi, B.E., et al.: Diagnostic assessment of deep learning algorithms for detection of lymph node metastases in women with breast cancer. JAMA **318**(22), 2199–2210 (2017)
3. Ciompi, F., et al.: The importance of stain normalization in colorectal tissue classification with convolutional networks. In: ISBI, pp. 160–163. IEEE (2017)
4. He, K., Zhang, X., Ren, S., Sun, J.: Deep residual learning for image recognition. In: Proceedings of the IEEE Conference on Computer Vision and Pattern Recognition, pp. 770–778 (2016)
5. Hosseini, M.S., et al.: Atlas of digital pathology: a generalized hierarchical histological tissue type-annotated database for deep learning. In: Proceedings of the IEEE/CVF Conference on Computer Vision and Pattern Recognition, pp. 11747–11756 (2019)
6. Kather, J.N., et al.: 100,000 histological images of human colorectal cancer and healthy tissue. In: Zenodo. Zenodo (2018)
7. Kather, J.N., et al.: Deep learning can predict microsatellite instability directly from histology in gastrointestinal cancer. Nat. Med. **25**(7), 1054–1056 (2019)
8. Ke, J., Shen, Y., Jiang, X., Guo, Y., Chen, Y., Liang, X.: Multiple-datasets and multiple-label based color normalization in histopathology with cGAN. In: Medical Imaging 2021: Digital Pathology. vol. 11603, p. 1160310. International Society for Optics and Photonics (2021)
9. Khan, A.M., et al.: A nonlinear mapping approach to stain normalization in digital histopathology images using image-specific color deconvolution. IEEE Trans. Biomed. Eng. **61**(6), 1729–1738 (2014)
10. Macenko, M., et al.: A method for normalizing histology slides for quantitative analysis. In: ISBI: From Nano to Macro, pp. 1107–1110. IEEE (2009)

11. Nadeem, S., Hollmann, T., Tannenbaum, A.: Multimarginal wasserstein barycenter for stain normalization and augmentation. In: Martel, A.L., et al. (eds.) MICCAI 2020. LNCS, vol. 12265, pp. 362–371. Springer, Cham (2020). https://doi.org/10.1007/978-3-030-59722-1_35

12. Nishar, H., Chavanke, N., Singhal, N.: Histopathological stain transfer using style transfer network with adversarial loss. In: Martel, A.L., et al. (eds.) MICCAI 2020. LNCS, vol. 12265, pp. 330–340. Springer, Cham (2020). https://doi.org/10.1007/978-3-030-59722-1_32

13. Park, J., et al.: Aggregation of cohorts for histopathological diagnosis with deep morphological analysis. Sci. Rep. **11**(1), 1–11 (2021)

14. Reinhard, E., et al.: Color transfer between images. IEEE Comput. Graph. Appl. **21**(5), 34–41 (2001)

15. Ronneberger, O., Fischer, P., Brox, T.: U-net: convolutional networks for biomedical image segmentation. In: Navab, N., Hornegger, J., Wells, W.M., Frangi, A.F. (eds.) MICCAI 2015. LNCS, vol. 9351, pp. 234–241. Springer, Cham (2015). https://doi.org/10.1007/978-3-319-24574-4_28

16. Shaban, M.T., et al.: StainGAN: stain style transfer for digital histological images. In: ISBI, pp. 953–956. IEEE (2019)

17. Shen, Y., Ke, J.: A deformable CRF model for histopathology whole-slide image classification. In: Martel, A.L., et al. (eds.) MICCAI 2020. LNCS, vol. 12265, pp. 500–508. Springer, Cham (2020). https://doi.org/10.1007/978-3-030-59722-1_48

18. Tellez, D., et al.: Quantifying the effects of data augmentation and stain color normalization in convolutional neural networks for computational pathology. Med. Image Anal. **58**, 101544 (2019)

19. Vahadane, A., et al.: Structure-preserving color normalization and sparse stain separation for histological images. IEEE Trans. Med. Imaging **35**(8), 1962–1971 (2016)

20. Wang, Z., et al.: Image quality assessment: from error visibility to structural similarity. IEEE Trans. Image Process. **13**(4), 600–612 (2004)

21. Zhang, L., et al.: FSIM: a feature similarity index for image quality assessment. IEEE Trans. Image Process. **20**(8), 2378–2386 (2011)

22. Zhu, J.Y., Park, T., Isola, P., Efros, A.A.: Unpaired image-to-image translation using cycle-consistent adversarial networks. In: Proceedings of the IEEE International Conference on Computer Vision, pp. 2223–2232 (2017)

Semi-supervised Adversarial Learning for Stain Normalisation in Histopathology Images

Cong Cong[1], Sidong Liu[2,3], Antonio Di Ieva[3], Maurice Pagnucco[1], Shlomo Berkovsky[2], and Yang Song[1(✉)]

[1] School of Computer Science and Engineering, University of New South Wales, Sydney, Australia
yang.song1@unsw.edu.au
[2] Centre for Health Informatics, Macquarie University, Sydney, Australia
[3] Computational NeuroSurgery Lab, Macquarie University, Sydney, Australia

Abstract. Hematoxylin and Eosin (H&E) stained histopathology images provide important clues for diagnostic and prognostic assessment of diseases. However, similar tissues can be stained with inconsistent colours which significantly hinder the diagnostic process and training of deep learning models. Various Generative Adversarial Network (GAN) based stain normalisation methods have thus been proposed as a preprocessing step for the downstream classification or detection tasks. However, most of these methods are based on either unsupervised learning which suffers from large discrepancy between domains or supervised learning which requires a target domain and only utilises the target domain images. In this work, we propose to leverage Semi-supervised Learning with GAN to incorporate the source domain images in the learning of stain normalisation without requiring their corresponding ground truth data. Our approach achieves highly effective performance on two classification tasks for brain and breast cancers.

Keywords: Semi-supervised learning · Stain normalisation · Conditional generative adversarial networks

1 Introduction

Tissue staining is used to facilitate effective interpretation of histopathology images. However, the appearance of stained tissue slides can be highly heterogeneous due to the different staining protocols and the subsequent digitisation of the images. This undesired colour variance in histopathology images motivates the study of stain normalisation, which normalises the images to reduce the impact of colour heterogeneity.

Existing studies of stain normalisation normally fall into two main categories, traditional and deep learning-based methods. Specifically, traditional stain normalisation methods use mathematical frameworks to match the colour distribution of an input image with the selected reference images. Examples include the

© Springer Nature Switzerland AG 2021
M. de Bruijne et al. (Eds.): MICCAI 2021, LNCS 12908, pp. 581–591, 2021.
https://doi.org/10.1007/978-3-030-87237-3_56

colour normalisation in the LAB colour space [18], minimisation of the Wasserstein Barycenter between colour distributions [15], and normalisation of stain vectors [12,29]. However, most of these conventional methods rely on a reference image to calculate the stain statistics, therefore the stain normalisation results can be heavily biased by a less representative reference image.

Deep learning-based stain normalisation is used more often these days. Most of these methods leverage the Generative Adversarial Network (GAN) [8] to formulate stain normalisation as an image-to-image translation task. Unsupervised stain normalisation has been widely studied, as it eases the requirement of a reference image. For example, StainGAN [24] utilises the CycleGAN model [31] for unsupervised stain normalisation. SAASN [25] incorporates the self-attention mechanism in CycleGAN to achieve finer details. Another method [13] combines CycleGAN with a pretrained segmentation network to better preserve the cellular structures in the images. While these methods produce satisfactory results in most cases, unsupervised methods still suffer from the large discrepancy between domains in heterogeneous datasets. Thus, supervised stain normalisation, which uses paired images from the target domain, has been developed. A HRNet-based [27] neural style transfer GAN is developed [16], which trains with selected reference images and preserves finer details by including a perceptual loss [9]. Others treat stain normalisation as an image colourisation task, in which they learn a model to repaint the input images with the target domain colour style [23,30]. Compared to unsupervised approaches, these supervised methods produce substantially better normalised images. However, the colourisation task is only performed on the target domain images, without considering the source domain. Such a colourisation formulation does not truly represent the objective of stain normalisation, which is to align the colour distributions between source and target domains.

In this work, we propose to use Semi-Supervised Learning (SSL) with GAN to solve stain normalisation as an image colourisation task. Our model learns to repaint the input images with the target domain colours and we use the image from the source domain to enhance this mapping. Specifically, given the hematoxylin component [21] or grayscale image as input, our GAN-based stain normalisation network learns to repaint it with the target colour styles. In order to incorporate source domain images into the training and explicitly optimise the colourisation for source domain images, a two-decoder generator with a shared encoder is proposed. This design allows us to apply a novel consistency regularisation which enforces the model to produce consistent outputs for the source domain and also minimises their difference from the target domain colour distribution.

Contributions: 1) We design a novel semi-supervised colourisation model for stain normalisation, so that source domain images can be incorporated into the model learning without requiring paired ground truth data for the source domain. 2) Our model adopts a novel two-decoder design with consistency loss to enforce the generator to normalise the unlabelled source images with the desired target domain colour. 3) We conduct extensive experiments on the public

TCGA [6] and BreakHis [26] datasets, and demonstrate that our method leads to large improvement for the downstream classification task on both types of histopathology images.

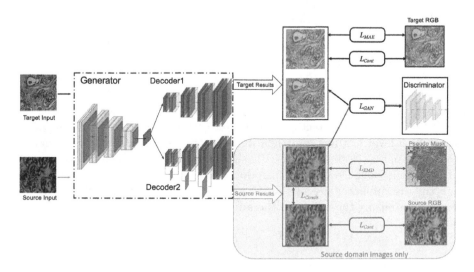

Fig. 1. Our proposed semi-supervised GAN-based stain normalisation model, by incorporating source domain images into the training with pseudo masks in a semi-supervised learning manner.

2   Methods

We design a semi-supervised GAN-based colourisation model for stain normalisation. The objective of this model is to colourise the inputs with the target domain stain colours. For target domain images, we use a supervised learning strategy with paired training data (original H&E stained colour image as ground truth and corresponding grayscale or hematoxylin component as input). Such paired training data are only available in the target domain but not in the source domain. Therefore, to explicitly enhance the colourisation performance for source domain images, we design a semi-supervised learning approach to incorporate the source domain images with pseudo masks into the model training.

Figure 1 shows the overall design of our model. The generator network colourises the input images with target stain style. The PatchGAN [23] discriminator judges whether the generator output is fake or real. The model is trained alternately with batches of labelled target domain images and unlabelled source domain images. For the labelled target domain, our model is trained in a supervised fashion with adversarial loss and content loss [9], whereas on the unlabelled source domain, an additional supervised loss is introduced for consistency regularisation based on the generated RGB images. The average of the two decoder branches' outputs in the generator as the final normalisation results.

2.1 Normalisation via Colourisation

We first describe the stain normalisation process by considering the target domain only. Specifically, the target domain hematoxylin component or grayscale images X and their corresponding RGB images Y are used as labelled paired data to train a Conditional GAN [14] in which the generator learns to colourise the inputs with the target domain colour statistics. The generator, which has an encoder-decoder architecture like U-Net [19] encodes the input images to extract high-level features and then decodes the extracted features to get the colourised images. Note that in Fig. 1, this generator design consists of Encoder and Decoder1, while Decoder2 is introduced for SSL as explained in the Sect. 2.2. Then the discriminator judges the image pairs $(X; Y)$ or $(X; G(X))$, as real or fake by maximising the following the adversarial loss function:

$$\mathcal{L}_{GAN}(X, Y) = \log\left(D(X, Y)\right) + \log\left(1 - D(X, G(X))\right) \tag{1}$$

where, the term $\log\left(D(X, Y)\right)$ will not be calculated for the unlabelled source domain image pairs.

To further regulate the model, such that it not only learns the correct colour mapping but also preserves high-level structural image content, we minimise the content loss L_{Cont} between perceptual features of generated RGB images $\{\hat{Y}\}$ and the original RGB images $\{Y\}$. In our case, the feature presentations of the last four convolutional layers ($n = 4$) in a pretrained VGG16 are used to form the high-level features to derive the content loss:

$$\mathcal{L}_{Cont}(\hat{Y}, Y) = \sum_j^n \omega_j \frac{1}{C_j H_j W_j} ||\phi_j(\hat{Y}) - \phi_j(Y)|| \tag{2}$$

where ϕ_j is the feature map produced from j_{th} convolution layer before the max pooling layer, $C_j H_j W_j$ is the shape of ϕ_j and $\omega_j = 1/n$.

2.2 Semi-supervised Source Domain Normalisation

We then introduce SSL into the model so that the unlabelled source domain images can also be used in learning the correct colourisation mapping. Recent deep learning-based SSL methods normally implement a consistency regularisation that encourages the model to perform consistently with disturbance in the input or model [10,22,28] However, it is likely that such methods could produce consistent but incorrect labels for unlabelled data. Therefore, we propose an additional colour distance-based regularisation which enforces the model output distribution to be closer to the ground truth distribution.

To do this, inspired by [7,10], we force the consistency between the two decoders by minimising the Mean Absolute Distance (L_{MAE}) between their outputs. We further maximise the mutual information [5] by distribution alignment, which is firstly used in [4] by scaling the output to match the label distribution. In our work, we propose to minimise the Earth Mover's Distance [20] (L_{EMD}) between the decoders' outputs and a pseudo mask selected from the target domain images as a form of colour distribution alignment.

We explicitly design **Decoder2** as an improved version of **Decoder1** such that the introduction of **Decoder2** will not degrade the model performance. A simple and effective way of such a modification can be achieved by adding residual blocks which short-circuit the concatenated inputs to the outputs of the convolutional layers. In terms of L_{EMD} calculation, a pseudo mask $\{Y'\}$ with target domain colour statistics is required for the normalised RGB images of unlabelled source domain images to match with. In order to obtain the mask that can best represent the colour statistic of the target domain, we choose the target domain image whose mean and standard deviation of pixel colours are closest to the overall target domain mean and standard deviation as this pseudo mask $\{Y'\}$. This pseudo mask is likely to have a different tissue pattern from the source domain image, but aims to provide a guidance on the colour distribution. Then, for the outputs of the two decoders on unlabelled source domain images $\hat{Y}^s = (\hat{Y}_1^s, \hat{Y}_2^s)$, we apply the following consistency loss:

$$\mathcal{L}_{Consist}(\hat{Y}^s, Y') = L_{MAE}(\hat{Y}_1^s, \hat{Y}_2^s) + L_{EMD}(\hat{Y}_1^s, Y') + L_{EMD}(\hat{Y}_2^s, Y') \quad (3)$$

2.3 Training Pipeline

We evaluate our model with two different inputs, the hematoxylin component of the H&E stained images, which can be extracted from the RGB images using the Beer-Lambert's Law [17], and the grayscale image. They tend to perform differently on different datasets. The generator then colourises the inputs with the target colour style. We use different loss functions based on the input domain. If the inputs are from the target domain, we use adversarial loss, content loss and $L1$ loss to regularise the generator:

$$\mathcal{L}_{target}(X, Y^T) = \mathcal{L}_{GAN}(X, Y^T) + \mathcal{L}_{Cont}(G(X), Y^T) + \mathcal{L}_{MAE}(G(X), Y^T) \quad (4)$$

If the inputs are from the unlabelled source domain, we then incorporate the additional consistency loss in place of the L_{MAE} loss to encourage the network to produce high-quality content-preserved normalised RGB images:

$$\mathcal{L}_{source}(X, Y^S, Y') = \mathcal{L}_{GAN}(X, Y^S) + \mathcal{L}_{Cont}(G(X), Y^S) + \mathcal{L}_{Consist}(G(X), Y') \quad (5)$$

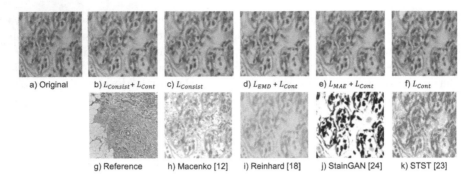

a) Original   b) $L_{Consist} + L_{Cont}$ c) $L_{Consist}$ d) $L_{EMD} + L_{Cont}$ e) $L_{MAE} + L_{Cont}$ f) L_{Cont}

g) Reference   h) Macenko [12]   i) Reinhard [18]   j) StainGAN [24]   k) STST [23]

Fig. 2. Comparison of stain normalised results.

3   Experiments and Results

3.1   Dataset and Implementation

We evaluate our method using two datasets, the TCGA[1] glioma cohort for Isocitrate Dehydrogenase (IDH) prediction [11] and the BreakHis database for breast cancer histopathological image classification [26]. We are grateful to the authors of [11] for providing us the IDH dataset, which is a subset of the public TCGA dataset [6]. It consists of 22,229 images each of 1024×1024 pixels extracted from 921 patients' whole slide images (WSIs) at $10\times$ magnification level. All WSIs have been labelled as either IDH wildtype or mutant confirmed by immunohistochemistry and/or genetic sequencing. The BreakHis dataset contains 7,909 images of 460×700 pixels collected from 82 patients. These images are stored with four magnification levels and are annotated as benign or malignant. In order to train our stain normalisation network, we split the IDH dataset based on the tissue source site (TSS) and choose the largest TSS as the target domain (3,414 images) and the rest as the source domain (18,805 images). The BreakHis dataset does not contain the tissue source site label, thus, we use k-means ($k = 5$) clustering to cluster the images based on the mean and standard deviation of image pixel colours. The largest cluster is used as the target domain (350 images) and the remaining 7,559 images as considered the source domain.

We fine-tune an ImageNet pretrained ResNet50 for the two binary classification tasks using the stain normalised images. For IDH classification, images from 738 randomly selected patients (80% of the cohort) are used for training, those from 91 patients for validation and the remaining 92 patients for testing. For the BreakHis dataset, we follow the 5-fold cross validation setting in [26] with 70% of data for training and 30% for testing in each split, and images of different magnification levels are mixed together during the training and testing. We measure the impact of stain normalisation on the classification performance using F1-score, accuracy and Area Under the Curve (AUC). We also measure the colour consistency of stain normalised images by computing the standard

---

[1] https://portal.gdc.cancer.gov/.

deviation (NMI_{SD}) and coefficient of variation (NMI_{CV}) of Normalised Median Intensity (NMI) [1].

Both the stain normalisation model and ResNet50 classifier are developed using TensorFlow Keras on NVIDIA Tesla P100 GPUs. We reshape the image to 256×256 pixels for both datasets and then train the models with the Adam optimiser with an initial learning rate of 0.0002. We train our stain normalisation model for 200 epochs and fine-tune the ResNet50 classifier for 40 epochs. The weights of loss terms are set to $\lambda_{L1} = 0.25$ and $\lambda_{content} = 0.75$.

3.2 Results

We compare our model with state-of-the-art methods that have experimental results reported on the two datasets. Specifically, for the IDH classification task, we compare with the recent study [11] that collected the IDH dataset. Different from our approach, [11] applies GAN for data augmentation to improve the classification performance without stain normalisation. For BreakHis, many approaches have been reported over the recent years. We choose to compare with the deep learning approaches [2,3] that use the same experimental settings as ours. In particular, [3] has incorporated a traditional stain normalisation method [18] before performing classification. As shown in Table 1, our method (using either the hematoxylin component or grayscale image as input) achieves about 5%–7% performance improvement over [11] and [3]. We find that using the hematoxylin component as inputs is more suitable for images with low magnification levels. Though, using hematoxylin component can enhance the contrast at cell boundaries, it may not always appear in an image patch extracted from high magnification levels.

Table 1. Performance comparison with state-of-the-art on two datasets.

	IDH [11]					BreakHis [26]				
	F1	Acc	Auc	NMI_{SD}	NMI_{CV}	F1	Acc	Auc	NMI_{SD}	NMI_{CV}
w/o normalisation	0.815	0.821	0.90	0.087	0.114	0.823	0.823	0.909	0.072	0.098
IDH study [11]	–	0.870	0.938	–	–	–	–	–	–	–
BreakHis study [3]	–	–	–	–	–	–	0.890	–	–	–
BreakHis study [2]	–	–	–	–	–	–	0.834	–	–	–
Macenko [12]	0.878	0.860	0.914	0.064	0.077	0.899	0.938	0.885	0.025	0.028
Reinhard [18]	0.815	0.833	0.912	0.054	0.052	0.911	0.910	0.918	0.022	0.023
StainGAN [24]	0.878	0.870	0.917	0.044	0.052	0.902	0.898	0.944	0.024	0.028
STST [23]	0.891	0.880	0.918	0.041	0.054	0.937	0.935	0.972	0.018	0.022
Ours-Hematoxylin	**0.937**	**0.934**	**0.984**	0.035	**0.040**	0.948	0.962	0.950	0.020	0.021
Ours-Grayscale	0.878	0.882	0.920	0.060	0.071	**0.980**	**0.980**	**0.996**	**0.017**	**0.019**

We have also trained the same ResNet50 classifier with the stain normalised images using other stain normalisation methods [12,18,23,24]. As shown in Table 1, our method provides better colour consistency (*i.e.* lower NMI_{SD} and NMI_{CV}) and improves the classification performance (*i.e.* 2%–7%). It can also be seen that without (w/o) stain normalisation, the results are consistently lower than using the stain normalised images.

Table 2. Performance comparsion with different pseudo masks.

	IDH [11]			BreakHis [26]		
	P_1	P_2	P_3	P_1	P_2	P_3
Macenko [12]	**0.860**	0.854	0.818	**0.938**	0.922	0.912
Reinhard [18]	**0.833**	0.819	0.780	**0.910**	0.894	0.882
Ours	**0.934**	0.928	0.931	**0.980**	0.978	0.974

We further test the choice of pseudo masks. Besides our pseudo mask design (P_1) described in Sect. 2.2, we evaluated two alternatives: (P_2) a target domain image that is structurally most similar (measured by SSIM) to the source domain, and (P_3) a randomly chosen image from the target domain. The results in Table 2 show that our model has less than 1% accuracy drop when using different masks, whereas other competing methods show 2%–5% drop. This validates our design of the pseudo mask and shows robustness compared to other methods.

Table 3. Performance comparsion with different loss functions.

	$L_{Consist}$	L_{EMD}	L_{Cont}	F1	Accuracy	AUC
IDH [11]			✓	0.878	0.880	0.945
	✓		✓	0.923	0.931	0.972
		✓	✓	0.928	0.929	0.969
	✓	✓		0.860	0.865	0.938
	✓	✓	✓	**0.937**	**0.934**	**0.984**
BreakHis [26]			✓	0.944	0.950	0.956
	✓		✓	0.958	0.968	0.991
		✓	✓	0.969	0.970	0.992
	✓	✓		0.914	0.908	0.964
	✓	✓	✓	**0.980**	**0.980**	**0.997**

Table 3 and Fig. 2 show the results with different loss functions. It can be observed that each term contributes to the performance as removing a single component degrades the model. Visually, using the proposed consistency regularisation alone can already reach a satisfactory result, but adding the content loss brings extra benefits. However, using the content loss alone is not enough to produce satisfactory normalised masks for the unlabelled source domain images.

This can be remitted by adding $L_{Consist}$ or L_{EMD} regularisation which indicates the usefulness of the proposed consistency regularisation. Figure 3 shows the impact of introducing different numbers of source images into training. The number a on the x-axis indicates the ratio of the total number of introduced source domain images relative to the number of target domain images. Generally, the model performs better when more source images are introduced into the training.

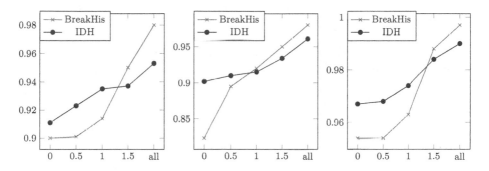

Fig. 3. Performance comparison with different numbers of source image used. Left to right: F1-score, accuracy and AUC.

4   Conclusions

In this paper, we propose a semi-supervised stain normalisation framework. The proposed model learns to colourise input images with the colour style of the target domain using both labelled target domain images and unlabelled source domain images. Our evaluation results show that our model produces higher quality images with high colour consistency with the target domain. We also show performance improvement over the prior art for two different histopathology image classification tasks.

References

1. Basavanhally, A., Madabhushi, A.: EM-based segmentation-driven color standardization of digitized histopathology. In: Medical Imaging 2013: Digital Pathology, vol. 8676, p. 86760G (2013)
2. Bayramoglu, N., Kannala, J., Heikkilä, J.: Deep learning for magnification independent breast cancer histopathology image classification. In: International Conference on Pattern Recognition (ICPR), pp. 2440–2445 (2016)
3. Benhammou, Y., Achchab, B., Herrera, F., Tabik, S.: BreakHis based breast cancer automatic diagnosis using deep learning: taxonomy, survey and insights. Neurocomputing **375**, 9–24 (2020)

4. Berthelot, D., et al.: RemixMatch: semi-supervised learning with distribution align-
    ment and augmentation anchoring. In: International Conference on Learning Rep-
    resentations (ICLR) (2019)
5. Bridle, J.S., Heading, A.J., MacKay, D.J.: Unsupervised classifiers, mutual infor-
    mation and 'phantom targets'. In: Advances in Neural Information Processing
    Systems (NIPS) (1992)
6. Clark, K., et al.: The cancer imaging archive (TCIA): maintaining and operating
    a public information repository. J. Digit. Imaging (JDI) $26(6)$, 1045–1057 (2013)
7. Fang, K., Li, W.-J.: DMNet: difference minimization network for semi-supervised
    segmentation in medical images. In: Martel, A.L., et al. (eds.) MICCAI 2020.
    LNCS, vol. 12261, pp. 532–541. Springer, Cham (2020). https://doi.org/10.1007/
    978-3-030-59710-8_52
8. Goodfellow, I.J., et al.: Generative adversarial networks. In: Conference on Neural
    Information Processing Systems (NIPS) (2014)
9. Johnson, J., Alahi, A., Fei-Fei, L.: Perceptual losses for real-time style transfer
    and super-resolution. In: Leibe, B., Matas, J., Sebe, N., Welling, M. (eds.) ECCV
    2016. LNCS, vol. 9906, pp. 694–711. Springer, Cham (2016). https://doi.org/10.
    1007/978-3-319-46475-6_43
10. Laine, S., Aila, T.: Temporal ensembling for semi-supervised learning. In: Interna-
    tional Conference on Learning Representations (ICLR) (2016)
11. Liu, S., et al.: Isocitrate dehydrogenase (IDH) status prediction in histopathology
    images of gliomas using deep learning. Sci. Rep. $10(1)$, 1–11 (2020)
12. Macenko, M., et al.: A method for normalizing histology slides for quantitative
    analysis. In: IEEE International Symposium on Biomedical Imaging (ISBI), pp.
    1107–1110 (2009)
13. Mahapatra, D., Bozorgtabar, B., Thiran, J.-P., Shao, L.: Structure preserving stain
    normalization of histopathology images using self supervised semantic guidance. In:
    Martel, A.L., et al. (eds.) MICCAI 2020. LNCS, vol. 12265, pp. 309–319. Springer,
    Cham (2020). https://doi.org/10.1007/978-3-030-59722-1_30
14. Mirza, M., Osindero, S.: Conditional generative adversarial nets. arXiv preprint
    arXiv:1411.1784 (2014)
15. Nadeem, S., Hollmann, T., Tannenbaum, A.: Multimarginal Wasserstein barycen-
    ter for stain normalization and augmentation. In: Martel, A.L., et al. (eds.) MIC-
    CAI 2020. LNCS, vol. 12265, pp. 362–371. Springer, Cham (2020). https://doi.
    org/10.1007/978-3-030-59722-1_35
16. Nishar, H., Chavanke, N., Singhal, N.: Histopathological stain transfer using style
    transfer network with adversarial loss. In: Martel, A.L., et al. (eds.) MICCAI 2020.
    LNCS, vol. 12265, pp. 330–340. Springer, Cham (2020). https://doi.org/10.1007/
    978-3-030-59722-1_32
17. Parson, W.W.: Modern Optical Spectroscopy, vol. 2. Springer, Heidelberg (2007)
18. Reinhard, E., Adhikhmin, M., Gooch, B., Shirley, P.: Color transfer between
    images. IEEE Comput. Graph. Appl. (CG&A) $21(5)$, 34–41 (2001)
19. Ronneberger, O., Fischer, P., Brox, T.: U-net: convolutional networks for biomed-
    ical image segmentation. In: Navab, N., Hornegger, J., Wells, W.M., Frangi, A.F.
    (eds.) MICCAI 2015. LNCS, vol. 9351, pp. 234–241. Springer, Cham (2015).
    https://doi.org/10.1007/978-3-319-24574-4_28
20. Rubner, Y., Tomasi, C., Guibas, L.J.: The earth mover's distance as a metric for
    image retrieval. Int. J. Comput. Vis. (IJCV) $40(2)$, 99–121 (2000)
21. Ruifrok, A.C., Johnston, D.A.: Quantification of histochemical staining by color
    deconvolution. Anal. Quantit. Cytol. Histol. (AQCH) $23(4)$, 291–299 (2001)

22. Sajjadi, M., Javanmardi, M., Tasdizen, T.: Regularization with stochastic transformations and perturbations for deep semi-supervised learning. In: Conference on Neural Information Processing Systems (NIPS) (2016)

23. Salehi, P., Chalechale, A.: Pix2pix-based stain-to-stain translation: a solution for robust stain normalization in histopathology images analysis. In: International Conference on Machine Vision and Image Processing (MVIP), pp. 1–7 (2020)

24. Shaban, M.T., Baur, C., Navab, N., Albarqouni, S.: StainGAN: stain style transfer for digital histological images. In: International Symposium on Biomedical Imaging (ISBI), pp. 953–956 (2019)

25. Shrivastava, A., et al.: Self-attentive adversarial stain normalization. In: Del Bimbo, A., et al. (eds.) ICPR 2021. LNCS, vol. 12661, pp. 120–140. Springer, Cham (2021). https://doi.org/10.1007/978-3-030-68763-2_10

26. Spanhol, F.A., Oliveira, L.S., Petitjean, C., Heutte, L.: A dataset for breast cancer histopathological image classification. IEEE Trans. Biomed. Eng. (TBME) **63**(7), 1455–1462 (2015)

27. Sun, K., Xiao, B., Liu, D., Wang, J.: Deep high-resolution representation learning for human pose estimation. In: Proceedings of the IEEE/CVF Conference on Computer Vision and Pattern Recognition (CVPR), pp. 5693–5703 (2019)

28. Tarvainen, A., Valpola, H.: Mean teachers are better role models: Weight-averaged consistency targets improve semi-supervised deep learning results. In: Conferences on Neural Information Processing Systems (NIPS) (2017)

29. Vahadane, A., et al.: Structure-preserving color normalization and sparse stain separation for histological images. IEEE Trans. Med. Imaging **35**(8), 1962–1971 (2016)

30. Yuan, E., Suh, J.: Neural stain normalization and unsupervised classification of cell nuclei in histopathological breast cancer images. arXiv preprint arXiv:1811.03815 (2018)

31. Zhu, J.Y., Park, T., Isola, P., Efros, A.A.: Unpaired image-to-image translation using cycle-consistent adversarial networks. In: Proceedings of the IEEE International Conference on Computer Vision (ICCV), pp. 2223–2232 (2017)

Learning Visual Features by Colorization for Slide-Consistent Survival Prediction from Whole Slide Images

Lei Fan, Arcot Sowmya, Erik Meijering, and Yang Song[(✉)]

School of Computer Science and Engineering, University of New South Wales,
Sydney, NSW 2052, Australia
{lei.fan1,yang.song1}@unsw.edu.au

Abstract. Recent deep learning techniques have shown promising performance on survival prediction from Whole Slide Images (WSIs). These methods are often based on multiple-step frameworks including patch sampling, feature extraction, and feature aggregation. However, feature extraction typically relies on handcrafted features or Convolutional Neural Networks (CNNs) pretrained on ImageNet without fine-tuning, thus leading to suboptimal performance. Besides, to aggregate features, previous studies focus on WSI-level survival prediction but ignore the heterogeneous information that is present in multiple WSIs acquired for the same patient. To address the above challenges, we propose a survival prediction model that exploits heterogeneous features at the patient-level. Specifically, we introduce colorization as the pretext task to train the CNNs which are tailored for extracting features from patches of WSIs. In addition, we develop a patient-level framework integrating multiple WSIs for survival prediction with consistency and ranking losses. Extensive experiments show that our model achieves state-of-the-art performance on two large-scale public datasets.

Keywords: Survival prediction · Histopathology · Colorization · Whole Slide Images · Deep learning

1 Introduction

Survival prediction is aimed at estimating the expected time at which an event of interest occurs (*e.g.* death). Among the various data modalities, histopathological Whole Slide Images (WSIs) are one of the most crucial for survival prediction, since WSIs have extremely high resolution (*i.e.* giga-pixels) and capture detailed multi-level pathological information of tumor and tissues.

Recent deep learning techniques [1,3,11,12,17,19,20,22–24,28,29] have shown promising performance in survival prediction from WSIs. Due to their giga-pixel resolution, WSIs cannot be fed into a CNN directly to implement end-to-end training on raw WSIs for survival prediction. Therefore, most methods have focused on obtaining high-quality representations of WSIs. Zhu *et al.* [28]

© Springer Nature Switzerland AG 2021
M. de Bruijne et al. (Eds.): MICCAI 2021, LNCS 12908, pp. 592–601, 2021.
https://doi.org/10.1007/978-3-030-87237-3_57

proposed DeepConvSurv where a CNN is used for survival prediction on patches selected from WSIs by pathologists. After that, SCNNs [12] and CDOR [20] were trained by using selected patches and achieved high performance on glioma cancer. However, obtaining representative patches of WSIs is expensive and time-consuming, and a small set of patches may not completely and properly reflect the patients' tumor morphology [23]. Therefore, recent studies [1,3,11,22,23,29] have adopted a sampling strategy to represent WSIs by cropping a number of patches from WSIs, and patch-level information is then aggregated for the WSI-level prediction. Among these approaches, WSISA [29] is one of the most well-known models. More advanced models such as the DeepGraphConv [11] and RankSurv [3] employ graph neural networks (GNNs) and hypergraph structure to obtain hierarchical representations of WSIs respectively. In the above studies, patch-level feature extraction typically relies on handcrafted features [29] or CNNs pretrained on ImageNet [3,11,22,23] without any fine-tuning due to the lack of patch-level annotations. These pretrained CNN models are not tailored for WSIs, and hence could lead to suboptimal performance. In addition, existing studies [3,11] often focus on WSI-level survival prediction, whereas generally a patient has several WSIs acquired from different parts of the tissue that are heterogeneous. There are other methods [22,23,29] that make patient-level prediction by adopting a clustering strategy on all WSIs belonging to a single patient, but the clustering performance would be largely affected by the varying imaging quality of different WSIs.

To address the above challenges, we propose a survival prediction model that exploits heterogeneous features at the patient-level. The contributions of this paper are summarized as follows: (1) We introduce colorization as a pretext task for self-supervised feature learning, so that the CNN-based feature extraction is customized for WSI patches without requiring patch-level annotations. (2) We develop a framework for patient-level survival prediction by incorporating multiple WSIs with consistency loss for regularizing the high-level features and ranking loss for comparison among different patients. (3) We conduct extensive experiments on two large-scale datasets: TCGA-GBM and TCGA-LUSC [6]. The ablation study shows the effectiveness of our patient-level prediction framework and our feature learning component customized via colorization. Our proposed model achieves state-of-the-art performance on both datasets.

2   Methodology

Figure 1 illustrates our proposed framework that consists of three main steps: patch sampling, colorization for extracting features, and patient-level survival prediction. Firstly, a number of patches are automatically selected from WSIs. Then, the colorization task is employed for training CNN-based feature extraction with self-supervised learning. After that, the final survival prediction is obtained by integrating multiple WSIs of the same patient.

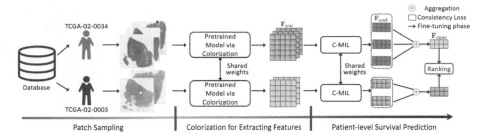

Fig. 1. Overall architecture of our proposed framework. In the first and second steps, WSIs are processed to generate feature maps ($\mathbf{F}_{wsi}$) separately. Then, $\mathbf{F}_{wsi}$ is fed into C-MIL to obtain embedding feature ($\mathbf{F}_{emb}$), and several $\mathbf{F}_{emb}$ are used for generating case-level feature ($\mathbf{F}_{case}$) by the aggregation module.

2.1 Patch Sampling

Considering a set of N patients, each patient x_i ($i \in \{1, \ldots, N\}$) has survival information ($\mathbf{W}_i^k, t_i, \delta_i$). $\mathbf{W} = (W_1, \ldots, W_k)$ and $k \in \{1, \ldots, K_i\}$ denote the WSI set and WSI number of the patient x_i with K_i WSIs. The observation time t_i means the censored or survival time when the survival indicator δ_i is 0 (censored) or 1 (uncensored) respectively.

Previous studies [1,3,22,23,29] have demonstrated that sampled patches from a WSI can represent the WSI-level information. In our implementation, WSIs are firstly processed to coarsely localize the region of tissue by using filters based on Otsu's thresholding [14]. Then, patches of size 256×256 pixels are cropped from the localized region, and patches belonging to the background, blood capillary, hole of tissues, or covered by marker pens are removed. Patches that are out of focus are also removed by filtering according to the variance of the second-order derivative of patches calculated by the Laplacian operator [16]. Finally, M (*i.e.* 1000) patches I_j ($j \in \{1, \ldots, M\}$) are selected from each WSI.

2.2 Colorization for Extracting Features

Recently, self-supervised learning (SSL) techniques have shown remarkable results on several standard computer vision tasks [8]. By designing pretext tasks related to the downstream task, SSL creates surrogate supervision for training pretext tasks where the inputs and labels are derived from the raw data without human annotations. In survival prediction from WSIs, designing CNN-based feature extraction can be treated as the pretext task, and survival prediction is the downstream task. Hence, the main challenge is how to design an appropriate pretext task associated with survival prediction. Previous studies [1,13] for WSIs have employed image reconstruction as the pretext task where autoencoder models are trained for recovering original images from input images.

Different from these methods, we introduce the colorization task as the pretext task. Colorization requires the model to colorize images based on the lightness of raw images. The learned features of the colorization model can then

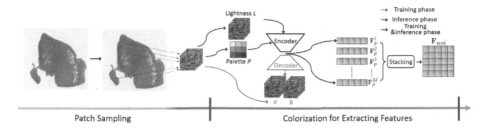

Fig. 2. Pipeline of patch sampling and colorization for extracting features.

be used for downstream tasks [9, 10, 26]. The effectiveness of colorization-based learning has been attributed to the fact that if the model can colorize arbitrary images, the model will be able to capture some semantic information and localize various objects in the images [9]. This representation capability of high-level information thus motivates us to choose the colorization model instead of the more commonly used reconstruction-based feature learning.

Specifically, for a WSI with M patches, each patch can be split into the lightness channel $L \in \mathbb{R}^{256 \times 256}$ as the input and color channels $ab \in \mathbb{R}^{256 \times 256 \times 2}$ as labels in the CIE Lab color space. We adopt the Encoder-Decoder architecture [26] as our baseline model where the encoder follows a standard CNN model (e.g. VGG [18], ResNet [4]), and the decoder consists of two transposed convolutional blocks with batch normalization and the ReLU activation function.

Furthermore, considering that different WSIs can have varying color distributions, similar structures of nuclei and tissue may have been stained with disparate color distributions among these WSIs. However, due to the absence of color information, the colorization model will eventually learn the average color distributions among all WSIs as shown in Fig. 3. Hence, we introduce a color palette as an input to explicitly guide the model with the color distributions of the corresponding WSI. The color palette P is generated by K-means clustering of all pixels RGB values in the corresponding WSI and provides guided signals for the colorization model (Fig. 2). We empirically set the cluster number to 9.

Training Model via Colorization: All patches are used for training the colorization model with a loss function L_{color}, which is defined as:

$$L_{color} = L_{ce}(\hat{\mathbf{C}}, \mathbf{C}) = -\sum_q^Q \sum_x^H \sum_y^W \mathbf{C}_{x,y,q} \log(\hat{\mathbf{C}}_{x,y,q}) \tag{1}$$

where $L_{ce}(\cdot, \cdot)$ denotes the cross entropy loss. $\hat{\mathbf{C}}$ and $\mathbf{C}$ are the model's output and labels respectively. Here H and W are the patch's height and width respectively. ab channels are jointly quantized into Q (following [26], Q is 313) color bins and then $\mathbf{C} \in [0, 1]^{H \times W \times Q}$ is the quantized color distribution of labels.

Inference for Extracting Features: At test time, a patch $I_m \in \mathbb{R}^{256 \times 256}$ ($m \in \{1, \dots, M\}$) is fed into the model, and then the output of the encoder is obtained and reshaped into a feature vector $\mathbf{F}_p^m \in \mathbb{R}^{1 \times 512}$ as the patch feature. Therefore, a WSI has M feature vectors, and all $\mathbf{F}_p^m$ are stacked into a feature map $\mathbf{F}_{wsi} \in \mathbb{R}^{1000 \times 512}$.

2.3   Patient-Level Survival Prediction

Previous methods [3,11] often perform survival prediction by treating each WSI individually, or by adopting a clustering strategy [22,23,29] where patches are selected from all WSIs altogether. However, we conjecture that the relation between WSIs and patients can be summarized in three aspects: (1) the qualities of different WSIs acquired from the same patient vary and should be processed separately; (2) under the same supervision of survival information, high-level features of several WSIs of the same patient should exhibit some consistency; and (3) high-level features from different patients should be distinguishable.

Based on the above assumptions, we propose a patient-level survival prediction model as illustrated in Fig. 1. The model mainly consists of two modules: Convolutional Multiple Instance Learning (C-MIL) [21] and the aggregation module. For a patient x_i with K_i WSIs, C-MIL is used to further reduce the dimension of each feature map $\mathbf{F}_{wsi}^k$ of WSIs, generating discriminative embedding feature $\mathbf{F}_{emb}^k \in \mathbb{R}^{1000 \times L}$ (L is 64 and $k \in \{1, \ldots, K_i\}$). Then the aggregation module is used to combine the embedding features $\mathbf{F}_{emb}^1, \ldots, \mathbf{F}_{emb}^{K_i}$ into the case-level feature $\mathbf{F}_{case}^i$, which is formulated as:

$$\mathbf{F}_{case}^i = \mathbf{F}_{out}^i * \tanh(\mathcal{A}(\mathbf{F}_{out}^i))) \tag{2}$$

where $\mathbf{F}_{case}^i \in \mathbb{R}^{64 \times 1}$ and $*$ means the matrix multiplication. $\mathbf{F}_{out}^i \in \mathbb{R}^{64 \times K_i}$ is stacked by $Conv(\mathcal{T}(\mathbf{F}_{emb}^1)), \ldots, Conv(\mathcal{T}(\mathbf{F}_{emb}^{K_i}))$ where $\mathcal{T}$ is transpose operation, $Conv$ is the convolutional block with 1×1 size and $Conv(\mathcal{T}(\mathbf{F}_{emb}^k)) \in \mathbb{R}^{64 \times 1}$. $\mathcal{A}(\mathbf{F}_{out}) \in \mathbb{R}^{K_i \times 1}$ denotes that $\mathbf{F}_{out}^i$ is transformed into a vector by passing through the Adaptive Average Pooling operation $\mathcal{A}$ in PyTorch [15].

We employ a two-phase approach to train the survival prediction model from the coarse-fine strategy. During the first phase, we train the model with the negative log-likelihood loss to learn the coarse mapping from the patient to risk based on patient-wise information, where $\mathbf{F}_{case}^i$ is processed to generate the final risk R_i for survival prediction [2]. We also design the consistency loss L_{cons} as an auxiliary loss, which is formulated as:

$$L_{cons} = \frac{1}{H} \sum_{(i,j)}^{H} |\mathbf{F}_{emb}^i - \mathbf{F}_{emb}^j| \tag{3}$$

where H is the number of WSI pairs of the patient x_i. The consistency loss L_{cons} is used for explicitly regularizing embedding features, which encourages consistency of $\mathbf{F}_{emb}^1, \ldots, \mathbf{F}_{emb}^{K_i}$ features of the same patient x_i.

At the second phase, we train the model based on pairs of patients, and we use the ranking loss L_{rank} [3] to fine-tune the model by comparing pairs of patients. L_{rank} is formulated as:

$$L_{rank} = \frac{1}{T} \sum_{i,j}^{T} (\frac{1}{2}(1 - \mathbb{I}_{t_i,t_j})\sigma(R_i - R_j) + \log(1 + e^{-\sigma(R_i - R_j)})) \tag{4}$$

where T is the number of patient pairs and T is $\frac{N(N-1)}{2}$. σ is the sigmoid function, and t_i means the survival time of patient x_i. $\mathbb{I}_{t_i,t_j}$ is the indicator function, and $\mathbb{I}_{t_i,t_j}$ is $[1, 0, -1]$ if $t_i > t_j$, $t_i = t_j$, and $t_i < t_j$ respectively.

3   Experiment

3.1   Dataset and Implementation Details

We conduct our experiments on two large-scale datasets: glioblastoma multiforme (GBM) and lung squamous cell carcinoma (LUSC), obtained from The Cancer Genome Atlas (TCGA) [6][1]. Following previous work [22,24,29], we adopt a core sample set from UT MD Anderson Cancer Center [25], which is called the *Core Dataset*. In addition, we build a more comprehensive set: *Whole Dataset* containing more patient cases, and the WSIs include both high-quality formalin-fixed paraffin-embedded (FFPE) slides and low-quality frozen specimens slides. The dataset information is summarized in Table 1.

Table 1. Dataset statistics.

Datasets	Core dataset		Whole dataset		Avg. size
	No. patient	No. WSI	No. patient	No. WSI	
TCGA-GBM	126	255	617	2053	0.50 GB
TCGA-LUSC	121	485	504	1612	0.72 GB

We apply 5-fold cross validation with the Concordance index (C-Index) [5] as our evaluation metric. C-Index is a common evaluation metric for survival prediction with the value ranging from 0 to 1. A larger value of C-Index means better prediction performance of the model, and a value of 0.5 means random guess. Since we employ a two-phase training approach, during the first phase, we train the model with the negative log-likelihood loss and use Adam optimization [7] with weight decay 5×10^{-4}. We employ the step learning rate schedule and set the training epochs to 60, where the learning rate is set to 1×10^{-3} initially and halved after 20 and 40 epochs. At the second stage, we fine-tune the model with the ranking loss, where the epoch and learning rate are set to 15 and 1×10^{-4} respectively.

---

[1] https://portal.gdc.cancer.gov/.

Table 2. Comparison results with state-of-the-art methods. (§ denotes $p < 0.005$).

Methods	C-Index			
	Core dataset		Whole dataset	
	TCGA-GBM	TCGA-LUSC	TCGA-GBM	TCGA-LUSC
WSISA [29]	0.6450	0.6380	0.5789	0.6076
DeepCorrSurv [24]	0.6452	0.6287	–	–
DeepGraphSurv [11]	–	–	0.5877	0.5964
MILSurv [22]	0.6570	–	0.6165	0.6235
RankSurv [3]	0.6686	0.6713	0.6627	0.6608
Our model	**0.6892**§	**0.7039**§	**0.6654**§	**0.6772**§

3.2   Results

Table 2 reports the performance of our proposed model and state-of-the-art methods including WSISA [29], DeepCorrSurv [24], DeepGraphSurv [11], MIL-Surv [22] and RankSurv [3]. The original papers of WSISA, DeepCorrSurv, and MILSurv have reported their performance on the Core Dataset. For the Whole Dataset, we obtain the experimental results reported by RankSurv in [3]. In addition, the authors of RankSurv did not report the results on the Core Dataset, but they kindly provided these upon our request[2]. Overall, our proposed model achieves better performance than the compared approaches on both GBM and LUSC datasets. The advantage of our proposed model is mainly attributed to the fact that we use the colorization-based feature extraction to generate high-quality features and develop our patient-level survival prediction framework incorporating the consistency and ranking losses. DeepGraphSurv and RankSurv attempted to obtain the representation of each WSI by employing the more complex Graph Neural Networks, which takes advantage of topological information of patches in WSIs. DeepCorrSurv builds a model integrating WSIs and molecular information, but patches are selected by pathologists.

Table 3. Ablation study of feature extraction on the core dataset.

Datasets	C-Index					
	ResNet18⁻	ResNet18*	ResNet18⁺	ResNet34⁻	ResNet34*	ResNet34⁺
TCGA-GBM	0.5995	0.6271	0.6390	0.5970	0.6211	**0.6415**
TCGA-LUSC	0.6311	0.6485	0.6509	0.6274	0.6520	**0.6627**

Evaluation of Feature Extraction via Colorization: Table 3 shows the comparison results of different CNN-based feature extraction approaches on the Core Dataset. Here $^-$ and * denote the model pretrained on ImageNet without fine-tuning and via colorization respectively, and $^+$ denotes that the color palette is

---

[2] We gratefully acknowledge the help and suggestions from the authors of RankSurv.

introduced. In order to have direct comparison, only C-MIL and the aggregation module are employed without L_{cons} and L_{rank}. All experiments follow the same training settings. Compared with models pretrained on ImageNet, both pretrained ResNet18* and ResNet34* via colorization achieve better performance on both datasets. By introducing the color palette, ResNet18+ and ResNet34+ with the color palette obtain higher performance. In addition, in order to have a visual understanding of the colorization task, we also employ Class Activation Mapping (CAM) [27] to generate a set of visualization images, as shown in Fig. 3. It can be seen that different from models pretrained on ImageNet, pretrained models via colorization can highlight larger areas covering the overall structure of nuclei and tissue, which is more suitable for extracting features.

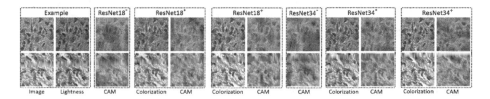

Fig. 3. CAM-based visualization and colorization of different CNN models.

Evaluation of Patient-Level Survival Prediction Framework: The effectiveness of each component in our patient-level survival prediction framework is illustrated in Table 4. All experiments are based on ResNet34+ with the color palette. *Agg* means that the aggregation module is used to aggregate all embedding features into case-level features. *Avg* means that each embedding feature is processed to generate a survival risk separately, and the average of these risks is the final survival prediction. L_{cons} and L_{rank} mean that the consistency loss and ranking loss are used respectively. Compared with (1) which uses *Avg*, (2) achieves better performance by using the aggregation module. By adding the consistency loss, (3) and (4) gain about 0.02 improvement over (1) and (2) respectively, which demonstrates the effectiveness of the consistency loss. When all components are used in the survival prediction framework, our model (5) obtains the highest performance on both GBM and LUSC datasets.

Table 4. Ablation study of patient-level survival prediction on the Core Dataset.

Methods		Settings			C-Index	
		Agg	L_{cons}	L_{rank}	TCGA-GBM	TCGA-LUSC
(1)	*Avg*				0.6372	0.6504
(2)	*Agg*	✓			0.6415	0.6627
(3)	*Avg*+L_{cons}		✓		0.6639	0.6619
(4)	*Agg*+L_{cons}	✓	✓		0.6684	0.6876
(5)	Our model	✓	✓	✓	**0.6892**	**0.7039**

4 Conclusion

In this paper, we propose a survival prediction model that exploits heterogeneous features at the patient-level. We introduce the colorization task as a pretext task to train the CNN-based feature extraction. Moreover, we develop a framework to implement patient-level survival prediction. Specifically, we propose the consistency loss to regularize several high-level features of WSIs acquired from the same patient, and incorporate the ranking loss to fine-tune the model by making comparisons among different patients. Extensive experiments show the effectiveness of our colorization-based feature extraction and our proposed survival prediction framework, and our model achieves state-of-the-art results on both GBM and LUSC datasets.

References

1. Abbet, C., Zlobec, I., Bozorgtabar, B., Thiran, J.-P.: Divide-and-rule: self-supervised learning for survival analysis in colorectal cancer. In: Martel, A.L., et al. (eds.) MICCAI 2020. LNCS, vol. 12265, pp. 480–489. Springer, Cham (2020). https://doi.org/10.1007/978-3-030-59722-1_46
2. Davidson-Pilon, C.: lifelines: survival analysis in python. J. Open Sour. Softw. **4**(40), 1317 (2019)
3. Di, D., Li, S., Zhang, J., Gao, Y.: Ranking-based survival prediction on histopathological whole-slide images. In: Martel, A.L., et al. (eds.) MICCAI 2020. LNCS, vol. 12265, pp. 428–438. Springer, Cham (2020). https://doi.org/10.1007/978-3-030-59722-1_41
4. He, K., Zhang, X., Ren, S., Sun, J.: Deep residual learning for image recognition. In: CVPR (2016)
5. Heagerty, P.J., Zheng, Y.: Survival model predictive accuracy and ROC curves. Biometrics **61**(1), 92–105 (2005). https://doi.org/10.1111/j.0006-341X.2005.030814.x
6. Kandoth, C., et al.: Mutational landscape and significance across 12 major cancer types. Nature **502**(7471), 333–339 (2013)
7. Kingma, D.P., Ba, J.: Adam: a method for stochastic optimization. arXiv preprint arXiv:1412.6980 (2014)
8. Kolesnikov, A., Zhai, X., Beyer, L.: Revisiting self-supervised visual representation learning. In: CVPR, pp. 1920–1929 (2019)
9. Larsson, G., Maire, M., Shakhnarovich, G.: Learning representations for automatic colorization. In: Leibe, B., Matas, J., Sebe, N., Welling, M. (eds.) ECCV 2016. LNCS, vol. 9908, pp. 577–593. Springer, Cham (2016). https://doi.org/10.1007/978-3-319-46493-0_35
10. Larsson, G., Maire, M., Shakhnarovich, G.: Colorization as a proxy task for visual understanding. In: CVPR, pp. 6874–6883 (2017)
11. Li, R., Yao, J., Zhu, X., Li, Y., Huang, J.: Graph CNN for survival analysis on whole slide pathological images. In: Frangi, A.F., Schnabel, J.A., Davatzikos, C., Alberola-López, C., Fichtinger, G. (eds.) MICCAI 2018. LNCS, vol. 11071, pp. 174–182. Springer, Cham (2018). https://doi.org/10.1007/978-3-030-00934-2_20
12. Mobadersany, P., et al.: Predicting cancer outcomes from histology and genomics using convolutional networks. PNAS **115**(13), E2970–E2979 (2018). https://doi.org/10.1073/pnas.1717139115

13. Muhammad, H., et al.: Unsupervised subtyping of cholangiocarcinoma using a deep clustering convolutional autoencoder. In: Shen, D., et al. (eds.) MICCAI 2019. LNCS, vol. 11764, pp. 604–612. Springer, Cham (2019). https://doi.org/10.1007/978-3-030-32239-7_67

14. Otsu, N.: A threshold selection method from gray-level histograms. IEEE Trans. Syst. Man Cybern. **9**(1), 62–66 (1979)

15. Paszke, A., et al.: PyTorch: an imperative style, high-performance deep learning library. In: Wallach, H., Larochelle, H., Beygelzimer, A., d'Alché-Buc, F., Fox, E., Garnett, R. (eds.) NeurIPS, pp. 8024–8035. Curran Associates, Inc. (2019)

16. Pech-Pacheco, J.L., Cristobal, G., Chamorro-Martinez, J., Fernandez-Valdivia, J.: Diatom autofocusing in brightfield microscopy: a comparative study. In: ICPR 2000, vol. 3, pp. 314–317 (2000). https://doi.org/10.1109/ICPR.2000.903548

17. Shao, W., et al.: Diagnosis-guided multi-modal feature selection for prognosis prediction of lung squamous cell carcinoma. In: Shen, D., et al. (eds.) MICCAI 2019. LNCS, vol. 11767, pp. 113–121. Springer, Cham (2019). https://doi.org/10.1007/978-3-030-32251-9_13

18. Simonyan, K., Zisserman, A.: Very deep convolutional networks for large-scale image recognition (2015)

19. Wulczyn, E., et al.: Deep learning-based survival prediction for multiple cancer types using histopathology images. PLoS One **15**(6), e0233678 (2020)

20. Xiao, L., et al.: Censoring-aware deep ordinal regression for survival prediction from pathological images. In: Martel, A.L., et al. (eds.) MICCAI 2020. LNCS, vol. 12265, pp. 449–458. Springer, Cham (2020). https://doi.org/10.1007/978-3-030-59722-1_43

21. Yang, H., Tianyi Zhou, J., Cai, J., Soon Ong, Y.: MIML-FCN+: multi-instance multi-label learning via fully convolutional networks with privileged information. In: CVPR (2017)

22. Yao, J., Zhu, X., Huang, J.: Deep multi-instance learning for survival prediction from whole slide images. In: Shen, D., et al. (eds.) MICCAI 2019. LNCS, vol. 11764, pp. 496–504. Springer, Cham (2019). https://doi.org/10.1007/978-3-030-32239-7_55

23. Yao, J., Zhu, X., Jonnagaddala, J., Hawkins, N., Huang, J.: Whole slide images based cancer survival prediction using attention guided deep multiple instance learning networks. Med. Image Anal. **65**, 101789 (2020)

24. Yao, J., Zhu, X., Zhu, F., Huang, J.: Deep correlational learning for survival prediction from multi-modality data. In: Descoteaux, M., Maier-Hein, L., Franz, A., Jannin, P., Collins, D.L., Duchesne, S. (eds.) MICCAI 2017. LNCS, vol. 10434, pp. 406–414. Springer, Cham (2017). https://doi.org/10.1007/978-3-319-66185-8_46

25. Yuan, Y., et al.: Assessing the clinical utility of cancer genomic and proteomic data across tumor types. Nat. Biotechnol. **32**(7), 644–652 (2014)

26. Zhang, R., Isola, P., Efros, A.A.: Colorful image colorization. In: Leibe, B., Matas, J., Sebe, N., Welling, M. (eds.) ECCV 2016. LNCS, vol. 9907, pp. 649–666. Springer, Cham (2016). https://doi.org/10.1007/978-3-319-46487-9_40

27. Zhou, B., Khosla, A., Lapedriza, A., Oliva, A., Torralba, A.: Learning deep features for discriminative localization. In: CVPR (2016)

28. Zhu, X., Yao, J., Huang, J.: Deep convolutional neural network for survival analysis with pathological images. In: BIBM, pp. 544–547. IEEE, December 2016. https://doi.org/10.1109/BIBM.2016.7822579

29. Zhu, X., Yao, J., Zhu, F., Huang, J.: WSISA: making survival prediction from whole slide histopathological images. In: CVPR (2017)

Adversarial Learning of Cancer Tissue Representations

Adalberto Claudio Quiros[1]([⊠]), Nicolas Coudray[2], Anna Yeaton[2],
Wisuwat Sunhem[1], Roderick Murray-Smith[1], Aristotelis Tsirigos[2],
and Ke Yuan[1]([⊠])

[1] University of Glasgow School of Computing Science, Scotland, UK
{a.claudio-quiros.1,w.sunhem.1}@research.gla.ac.uk,
{roderick.murray-smith,ke.yuan}@glasgow.ac.uk
[2] New York University School of Medicine, New York, NY, USA
{nicolas.coudray,anna.yeaton,aristotelis.tsirigos}@nyulangone.org

Abstract. Deep learning based analysis of histopathology images shows promise in advancing the understanding of tumor progression, tumor micro-environment, and their underpinning biological processes. So far, these approaches have focused on extracting information associated with annotations. In this work, we ask how much information can be learned from the tissue architecture itself.

We present an adversarial learning model to extract feature representations of cancer tissue, without the need for manual annotations. We show that these representations are able to identify a variety of morphological characteristics across three cancer types: Breast, colon, and lung. This is supported by 1) the separation of morphologic characteristics in the latent space; 2) the ability to classify tissue type with logistic regression using latent representations, with an AUC of 0.97 and 85% accuracy, comparable to supervised deep models; 3) the ability to predict the presence of tumor in Whole Slide Images (WSIs) using multiple instance learning (MIL), achieving an AUC of 0.98 and 94% accuracy.

Our results show that our model captures distinct phenotypic characteristics of real tissue samples, paving the way for further understanding of tumor progression and tumor micro-environment, and ultimately refining histopathological classification for diagnosis and treatment (The code and pretrained models are available at: https://github.com/AdalbertoCq/Adversarial-learning-of-cancer-tissue-representations).

Keywords: Generative adversarial networks · Histology

Electronic supplementary material The online version of this chapter (https://doi.org/10.1007/978-3-030-87237-3_58) contains supplementary material, which is available to authorized users.

M. de Bruijne et al. (Eds.): MICCAI 2021, LNCS 12908, pp. 602–612, 2021.
https://doi.org/10.1007/978-3-030-87237-3_58

1   Introduction

Histological images, such as hematoxylin and eosin (H&E) stained tissue microarrays (TMAs) and whole slide images (WSIs), are an imaging technology routinely used in clinical practice, that relay information about tumor progression and tumor microenvironment to pathologists. Recently, there has been advances in relating tissue phenotypes from histological images to genomic mutations [2–4,10], molecular subtypes [18,19], and prognosis [3,4]. While these previous works have contributed greatly to the field, and have highlighted the richness of information in H&E slides, they are limited by the frequently unavailable labels required to train supervised methods.

Unsupervised learning offers the opportunity to build phenotype representations based on tissue architectures and cellular attributes, without expensive labels or representations that are only correlated with a selected predicted outcome as discriminative models.

Within unsupervised models, Generative Adversarial Networks (GANs) have been widely used in digital pathology, from nuclei segmentation [13], stain transformation and normalization [17,21], to high-quality tissue samples [12]. In addition, there has been some initial work on building representations of cells [5] or larger tissue patches [15].

In particular, PathologyGAN [15] offers a Generative Adversarial Network (GAN) that captures tissue features and uses these characteristics to give structure to its latent space (e.g. colour, texture, spatial features of cancer and normal cells, or tissue type). The generator has representation learning properties where distinct regions of the latent space are directly related to tissue characteristics. However, it does not offer the ability to project real tissue images to its latent space, only offering latent representations for synthesized tissue. Such representations are crucial if we want to relate morphological and cellular features of tissue with genetic, molecular, or survival patient information.

Contributions. We propose an adversarial learning model to extract feature representations of cancer tissue, we show that our tissue representations are built on morphological and cellular characteristics found on real tissue images. We present a Generative Adversarial Network with representation learning properties that includes an encoder, allowing us to project real tissue onto the model's latent space. In addition, we show evidence that these representations capture meaningful information related to tissue, illustrating their applicability in three different scenarios:

1) We visualize the representations of real tissue and show how distinct regions of the latent space enfold different characteristics, and reconstructed tissue from latent representations follow the same characteristics as the original real image; 2) We quantify how informative these representation are by training a linear classifier to predict tissue types; 3) We demonstrate the suitability of the tissue representations on a multiple instance learning (MIL) task, predicting presence of tumor on WSIs.

2   Method

We build upon PathologyGAN [15], and introduce an encoder E that maps back generated tissue to the GAN's latent space. Effectively learning to interpret tissue morphologies and acting as the inverse of the generator G. After training, the encoder can be used independently to map real tissue samples to their representations in the latent space. Figure 1 captures the high level architecture of our model.

The loss functions for the discriminator L_{Dis} and the generator L_{Gen} are defined as the Relativistic Average Discriminator [7], where the discriminator's goal is to estimate the probability of the real data being more realistic than the fake (Eqs. 1 and 2). P_{data} is the distribution of real data, $G(w)$ is the distribution of synthetic data produced by the Generator G, $C(x)$ is the non-transformed discriminator output or critic, W the transformed latent space with representation learning properties, and $P_z = \mathbb{N}(0, I)$ the original latent space:

$$L_{Dis} = -\mathbb{E}_{x_r \sim P_{data}} \left[\log \left(\tilde{D}\left(x_r \right) \right) \right] - \mathbb{E}_{x_f \sim G(w)} \left[\log \left(1 - \tilde{D}\left(x_f \right) \right) \right], \quad (1)$$

$$L_{Gen} = -\mathbb{E}_{x_f \sim G(w)} \left[\log \left(\tilde{D}\left(x_f \right) \right) \right] - \mathbb{E}_{x_r \sim P_{data}} \left[\log \left(1 - \tilde{D}\left(x_r \right) \right) \right], \quad (2)$$

$$\tilde{D}\left(x_r \right) = \text{sigmoid}\left(C\left(x_r \right) - \mathbb{E}_{x_f \sim G(w)} C\left(x_f \right) \right),$$

$$\tilde{D}\left(x_f \right) = \text{sigmoid}\left(C\left(x_f \right) - \mathbb{E}_{x_r \sim P_{data}} C\left(x_r \right) \right),$$

$$w = M(z), \; z \sim P_z.$$

We use the mean square error between latent vectors w and their reconstruction from generated images $w' = E(G(w))$ as the encoder loss function, L_{Enc} (Eq. 3):

$$L_{Enc} = \mathbb{E}_{z \sim P_z} \left[\frac{1}{n} \sum_{i=1}^{n} (w_i - w'_i)^2 \right] \; where \; w' = E(G(w)), \; w = M(z). \quad (3)$$

Although the encoder E is simultaneously trained with the GAN model, we can separate the model training into two parts: The mapping network M, generator G, and discriminator D that are trained as a GAN, and the encoder E, which is trained to project back the generated cancer tissue images onto the latent space. In practice, the encoder E learns with the Generator G. We

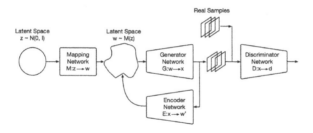

Fig. 1. High level architecture of our GAN model.

trained our encoder based on the assumption that the generator is successful in reproducing cancer tissue. Therefore the encoder will learn to project real tissue images if it is able to do so with generated ones. Based on this logic, we use only generated images to train the encoder.

Additionally, the encoder is only updated when the generator is not trained with style mixing regularization [8]. Style mixing regularization is a technique that promotes disentanglement where the generator G generates an image from two different latent vectors w_1 and w_2, these vector are feed at different layers of the generator G. However, it becomes impractical to train the encoder in these steps because these images have no clear assignation in the latent space W. Therefore, The style mixing regularization is only preformed 50% of times in the generator training, so our encoder is updated every two steps per the generator.

Datasets. We trained our model with three different cancer types: Breast, colon, and lung. We provide a detailed description on these datasets and how they were built in the supplementary material.

The breast H&E cancer dataset is composed by the Netherlands Cancer Institute (NKI, Netherlands) and Vancouver General Hospital (VGH, Canada) cohorts [1] with 248 and 328 patients, each patient with associated Tissue Micro-Arrays (TMAs). Each TMA is divided into 224×224 tiles and labeled subject to density of cancer cells in the tile using CRImage [20], we use 9 different classes with class 8 accounting for tiles with the largest count of cancer cells. This dataset is composed by a training set of 249K tiles and 460 patients, and a test set of 13K tiles and 116 patients, with no overlapping patients between sets.

The colorectal H&E cancer dataset from National Center for Tumor diseases (NCT, Germany) [9] provides tissue images of 224×224 resolution with an associated type of tissue label: Adipose, background, debris, lymphocytes, mucus, smooth muscle, normal colon mucosa, cancer-associated stroma, and colorectal adenocarcinoma epithelium (tumor). The dataset is divided into a training set of 100K tissue tiles and 86 patients, and a test set of 7K tissue tiles and 50 patients, there is no overlapping patients between train and test sets. Finally, in order to compare our model to supervised methods on tissue type classification, we combine the classes stroma and smooth muscle into a class 'simple stroma' as in reference publications [11, 16].

The lung H&E cancer dataset contains samples with adenocarcinoma (LUAD), squamous cell carcinoma (LUSC), and normal tissue, composed by 1807 Whole Slide Images (WSIs) of 1184 patients from the Cancer Genome Atlas (TCGA). Each WSI is labeled as tumor and non-tumor depending on the presence of lung cancer in the tissue and divided into 224×224 tiles. In addition, we split the dataset into a training set of 916K tissue tiles and 666 patients, and a test set of 569K tissue tiles and 518 patients, with no overlapping patients between both sets.

3   Results

Since our tissue representations are built in an unsupervised manner and from tissue features alone, we studied how meaningful real tissue representations are.

We show results quantifying the tissue morphology and cellular information contained in the representations, and provide examples of how they can be exploited: Latent space visualization and tissue reconstruction, tissue type classification, and tumor prediction in a multiple instance learning setting.

3.1   Visualizations of Tissue Representations and Reconstructions

We first aim to test how interpretable the latent representations of real tissue are, and if they capture enough information to recreate tissue with the same characteristics. We do so by visualizing the latent representations along with the corresponding real images and by reconstructing images from real tissue projections.

We used the breast cancer and colorectal cancer datasets for these results. As covered in Sect. 2, the breast tissue patches have an associated label with the density of cancer cells in the image and the colorectal tissue patches have an associated label with the corresponding tissue type. In both cases, we used the training set to train our GAN model and later used the encoder E to project images from test sets, obtaining representations of real tissue samples.

In Fig. 2 we used UMAP [14] to reduce the dimensionality of latent representations from 200 to 2 and plot each latent vector with its associated real tissue image and label. In the breast cancer case, tissue with the highest density of cancer cells is distributed outwards while no presence of them concentrates inwards. Colorectal cancer samples are located in different regions of the space depending of their tissue types. In both examples, tissue characteristics of real images, whether if it is tissue type or cancer cell density, determines the location of the representation in the latent space.

In addition, we wanted to compare real images with the synthetic images reconstructed by the generator at the specific position in the latent space where each real image was projected, $X_{recon} = G(E(X_{real}))$. Figure 3 shows real images and their associated reconstructions, we used latent representations of real images (a) to synthesize their reconstructions (b) with the GAN's generator. We provide examples of the colorectal cancer tissue types (1–5) and different cancer cell densities in breast cancer tissue (6–10). We can see that the reconstructions follow the characteristics of the real tissue images.

We conclude that tissue representations are not only interpretable but also hold the relevant information needed to synthesize tissue with the same characteristics.

3.2   Tissue Type Classification over Latent Representations

In this task, we aim to quantify how informative latent representation are, verifying that the model is able to learn tissue patterns that define tissue type. We train a linear classifier to predict tissue type over latent representations.

We used the colorectal cancer dataset with each tissue sample and its associated tissue type. We trained our GAN with the training set and again used the Encoder E to project the training and test sets onto the GAN's latent space, obtaining representations for each tissue image. Consecutively, we used the latent representations for the training set to train a logistic regression (one-versus-rest) and evaluate performance using test set projections.

Table 1 shows the performance of the logistic regression, reaching an average AUC (one-vs-rest) of 0.976 and multi-class accuracy of 85.43% just from latent

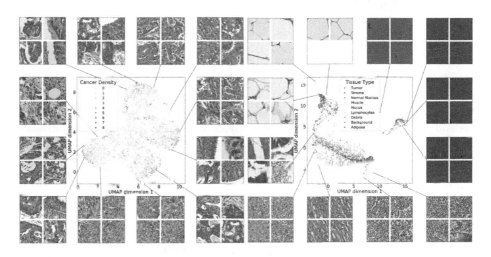

Fig. 2. Uniform Manifold Approximation and Projection (UMAP) vectors of PathologyGAN's latent representations, we present breast cancer tissue from NKI and VGH (left image) and colorectal cancer tissue from NCT (right image). Breast cancer tissue images are labeled using cancer cell counts, class 8 accounting for the largest cell number. Colorectal cancer tissue images are labeled based on their tissue type. In both cases, we observe that real tissue projected to the latent space retain cellular information and tissue morphology.

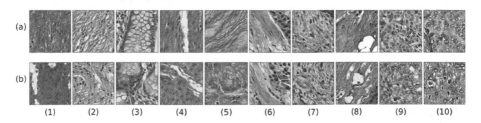

Fig. 3. Real tissue images and their reconstructions. We take real tissue images and map them to the latent space with our encoder, then we use the generator with the latent vector representations to generate the image reconstructions. (a) correspond to the real tissue images X_{real} and (b) to the reconstructions $X_{recon} = G(E(X_{real}))$, the images are paired in columns. We present samples of colorectal cancer tissue from NCT (1–5) and breast cancer tissue from VGH and NKI (5–10). We show different examples of tumor(1, 9, 10), stromal (2, 8), normal mucosa (3), muscle (3), and lymphocytes (6, 7), the reconstructions follow the real image attributes.

Table 1. Logistic regression Accuracy and AUC on tissue type classification. We used the colorectal cancer tissue images from NCT to train a classifier over latent representations. A logistic regression (one-vs-rest) is able to reliably find information in tissue representations to predict tissue types.

Total AUC: 0.976							
Tumor	Simple stroma	Mucosa	Mucus	Lymph.	Debris	Back.	Adipose
0.974	0.929	0.964	0.997	0.994	0.959	1.0	0.998
Total Accuracy: 85.43%							
Tumor	Simple Stroma	Mucosa	Mucus	Lymph.	Debris	Back.	Adipose
89%	71%	68%	91%	83%	63%	100%	96%

Table 2. Performance comparison on tissue type classification between existing methods and our tissue latent representations. These results reflect baseline performance of supervised deep learning and non-deep learning approaches. Our representations on logistic regression without any transformation or projection, and the fact that they are comparable with supervised performance, demonstrate the applicability and information hold in them.

Model	AUC	Accuracy
Ours	0.976	85.43%
Bayesian DNN [16]	**0.995**	**99.2%**
RBF-SVM [11]	0.976	87.4%

representations. Table 2 provides a comparison between other existing supervised methods, such as Raczkowski et al. [16] where a Bayesian deep neural network is trained for the purpose of tissue classification achieving an AUC of 0.992 and 92.44% accuracy, in addition, Kather et al. [11] provides another performance reference using an RNF-SVM with an AUC of 0.995 and 92.44% accuracy. We provide further details on ROC and confusion matrices in the supplementary material.

Phenotype representations from our model provide robust information such that a linear classifier is able to predict tissue types with high accuracy. Despite a small loss of performance when compared to the best supervised method, our fully unsupervised representations could be an effective solution when extensive and precise manual annotations cannot be obtained.

3.3   Multiple Instance Learning on Latent Representations

Finally, we tested the reliability of the tissue phenotype representations in a weakly supervised setting. We used tissue representations in a multiple instance learning (MIL) task for tumor presence prediction in Whole Slide Images (WSIs), where each WSI has an average, minimum, and maximum of 974, 175, and 14K, tiles, respectively.

We used the lung cancer dataset where each WSI has an associated label tumor or normal subject to presence of tumor tissue. We divided each WSI into 224×224 patches to train our GAN model and obtain tissue representations, and we later used all tissue representations of the WSI.

In the case of the MIL problem, we have a bag of instances $X = \{x_1, ..., x_n\}$ with an individual label $Y \in \{0, 1\}$. We further assume that each instance of the bag has an associated label $y_i \in \{0, 1\}$ to which we have no access:

$$Y = \begin{cases} 0, & \text{iff } \sum_k y_k = 0 \\ 1, & \text{otherwise} \end{cases}$$

In our case, we have tissue tiles that we translated into tissue representations $W = \{w_1, ..., w_n\}$, and use them to determine the presence of lung tumor $Y = 1$ in the WSI. We used the attention-based deep MIL [6] as it assigns a weight to each instance of the bag x_k, allowing us to measure which representations are relevant for the prediction.

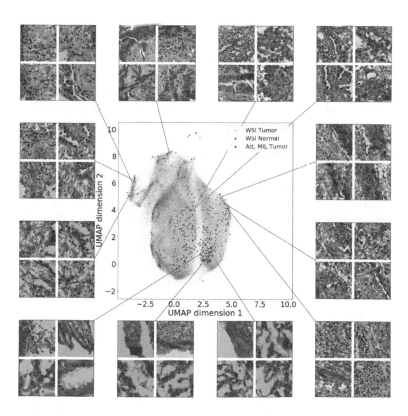

Fig. 4. Uniform Manifold Approximation and Projection (UMAP) vectors of lung cancer tissue representations. We labeled each patch of the WSI with the corresponding label subject to presence of tumor in the WSI, and highlight images and representations where the attention-based deep MIL focuses to predict the outcome. We can see that the MIL framework emphasizes on regions where there is only the presence of tumor patches, relying on the information contained in the latent representations.

The attention-based deep MIL over latent representations achieves an AUC of 0.98 and accuracy of 94%. These results are comparable to Coudray et al. [2], where an Inception-V3 network was tested on the same dataset and purpose achieving an AUC of 0.993 and accuracy of 97.5%.

Figure 4 shows UMAP reductions of tissue patches representations for the test set, we labeled each patch representation with the WSI label, tumor or normal depending on the presence of tumor. In addition we highlighted images and representations of the top 0.1% most weighted representations for the tumor outcome prediction. We can see that the MIL model focuses on regions of the latent space where there is no presence of normal tissue.

Given the accurate prediction of lung tumor presence in the WSIs and the focus of the MIL framework on representations solely present in tumor tissue, we conclude that the phenotype representations are reliable enough to capture tissue characteristics such as tumor tissue at scale.

4   Conclusion

We presented an adversarial learning model that builds phenotype representations of cancer tissue. Our model overcomes previous limitations [15] by introducing an Encoder, enabling a direct mapping between real tissue images and phenotype representations. We have illustrated the applicability of its representations in three different scenarios, providing evidence of the morphological and cellular information enfold on the real tissue representations. Furthermore, we found that these latent representations learn such stable and relevant features of histopathology images that they can be used as interpretable visualizations, as feature space of a linear classifier, or as input in a weakly supervised setting such as MIL. We envision our model to be used as a tool to characterize phenotype patterns. These learned features of histopathology images can be used to find associations between tissue and matched clinical and biological data such as genomic, transcriptomic, or survival information, contributing to a further characterize tumor micro-environment and improved patient stratification.

Acknowledgements. We will like to acknowledge funding support from University of Glasgow on A.C.Q scholarship, K.Y from EPSRC grant EP/R018634/1., and R.M-S. from EPSRC grants EP/T00097X/1 and EP/R018634/1. This work has used computing resources at the NYU School of Medicine High Performance Computing Facility.

References

1. Beck, A.H., et al.: Systematic analysis of breast cancer morphology uncovers stromal features associated with survival. Sci. Transl. Med. **3**(108), 108ra113 (2011). https://doi.org/10.1126/scitranslmed.3002564
2. Coudray, N., et al.: Classification and mutation prediction from non-small cell lung cancer histopathology images using deep learning. Nat. Med. **24**(10), 1559–1567 (2018). https://doi.org/10.1038/s41591-018-0177-5

3. Coudray, N., Tsirigos, A.: Deep learning links histology, molecular signatures and prognosis in cancer. Nature Cancer **1**(8), 755–757 (2020). https://doi.org/10.1038/s43018-020-0099-2
4. Fu, Y., et al.: Pan-cancer computational histopathology reveals mutations, tumor composition and prognosis. Nature Cancer **1**(8), 800–810 (2020). https://doi.org/10.1038/s43018-020-0085-8
5. Hu, B., Tang, Y., Chang, E.I.C., Fan, Y., Lai, M., Xu, Y.: Unsupervised learning for cell-level visual representation in histopathology images with generative adversarial networks. IEEE J. Biomed. Health Inform. **23**(3), 1316–1328 (2019). https://doi.org/10.1109/jbhi.2018.2852639
6. Ilse, M., Tomczak, J., Welling, M.: Attention-based deep multiple instance learning. In: Dy, J., Krause, A. (eds.) Proceedings of the 35th International Conference on Machine Learning. Proceedings of Machine Learning Research, vol. 80, pp. 2127–2136 (2018)
7. Jolicoeur-Martineau, A.: The relativistic discriminator: a key element missing from standard GAN. In: International Conference on Learning Representations (2019)
8. Karras, T., Laine, S., Aila, T.: A style-based generator architecture for generative adversarial networks. 2019 IEEE/CVF Conference on Computer Vision and Pattern Recognition (CVPR), June 2019. https://doi.org/10.1109/cvpr.2019.00453
9. Kather, J.N., Halama, N., Marx, A.: 100,000 histological images of human colorectal cancer and healthy tissue, April 2018. https://doi.org/10.5281/zenodo.1214456
10. Kather, J.N., Heij, L.R., Grabsch, H.I., et al.: Pan-cancer image-based detection of clinically actionable genetic alterations. Nature Cancer **1**(8), 789–799 (2020). https://doi.org/10.1038/s43018-020-0087-6
11. Kather, J.N., et al.: Multi-class texture analysis in colorectal cancer histology. Sci. Rep. **6**(1), 27988 (2016)
12. Krause, J., et al.: Deep learning detects genetic alterations in cancer histology generated by adversarial networks. J. Pathol. **254**(1), 70–79 (2021)
13. Mahmood, F., et al.: Deep adversarial training for multi-organ nuclei segmentation in histopathology images. IEEE Trans. Med. Imaging 1 (2020). https://doi.org/10.1109/tmi.2019.2927182
14. McInnes, L., Healy, J., Saul, N., Großberger, L.: UMAP: uniform manifold approximation and projection. J. Open Source Softw. **3**(29) (2018)
15. Quiros, A.C., Murray-Smith, R., Yuan, K.: PathologyGAN: learning deep representations of cancer tissue. In: Medical Imaging with Deep Learning (2020)
16. Raczkowski, L., Mozejko, M., Zambonelli, J., Szczurek, E.: Ara: accurate, reliable and active histopathological image classification framework with Bayesian deep learning. Sci. Rep. **9**(1), 14347 (2019)
17. Rana, A., Yauney, G., Lowe, A., Shah, P.: Computational histological staining and destaining of prostate core biopsy RGB images with Generative Adversarial Neural Networks. In: 2018 17th IEEE International Conference on Machine Learning and Applications (ICMLA), December 2018. https://doi.org/10.1109/icmla.2018.00133
18. Schmauch, B., et al.: A deep learning model to predict RNA-seq expression of tumours from whole slide images. Nat. Commun. **11**(1), 3877 (2020). https://doi.org/10.1038/s41467-020-17678-4
19. Woerl, A.C., et al.: Deep learning predicts molecular subtype of muscle-invasive bladder cancer from conventional histopathological slides. Eur. Urol. **78**(2), 256–264 (2020)

20. Yuan, Y., et al.: Quantitative image analysis of cellular heterogeneity in breast tumors complements genomic profiling. Sci. Transl. Med. 4(157), 157ra143 (2012). https://doi.org/10.1126/scitranslmed.3004330
21. Zanjani, F.G., Zinger, S., Bejnordi, B.E., van der Laak, J.A.W.M., de With, P.H.N.: Stain normalization of histopathology images using generative adversarial networks. In: 2018 IEEE 15th International Symposium on Biomedical Imaging (ISBI 2018), pp. 573–577 (2018)

A Multi-attribute Controllable Generative Model for Histopathology Image Synthesis

Jiarong Ye[1], Yuan Xue[1], Peter Liu[2], Richard Zaino[3], Keith C. Cheng[3], and Xiaolei Huang[1(✉)]

[1] College of Information Sciences and Technology, The Pennsylvania State University, University Park, PA, USA
suh972@psu.edu
[2] Upper Dublin High School, Fort Washington, PA, USA
[3] College of Medicine, The Pennsylvania State University, Hershey, PA, USA

Abstract. Generative models have been applied in the medical imaging domain for various image recognition and synthesis tasks. However, a more controllable and interpretable image synthesis model is still lacking yet necessary for important applications such as assisting in medical training. In this work, we leverage the efficient self-attention and contrastive learning modules and build upon state-of-the-art generative adversarial networks (GANs) to achieve an attribute-aware image synthesis model, termed AttributeGAN, which can generate high-quality histopathology images based on multi-attribute inputs. In comparison to existing single-attribute conditional generative models, our proposed model better reflects input attributes and enables smoother interpolation among attribute values. We conduct experiments on a histopathology dataset containing stained H&E images of urothelial carcinoma and demonstrate the effectiveness of our proposed model via comprehensive quantitative and qualitative comparisons with state-of-the-art models as well as different variants of our model.

Keywords: Histopathology image synthesis · Attribute-aware conditional generative model · Conditional contrastive learning

1 Introduction

Discriminative models, especially those based on deep learning, have been proven effective in various medical image analysis tasks [15]. However, such models

---

J. Ye and Y. Xue—These authors contributed equally to this work.
P. Liu—Independent Researcher.

Electronic supplementary material The online version of this chapter (https://doi.org/10.1007/978-3-030-87237-3_59) contains supplementary material, which is available to authorized users.

M. de Bruijne et al. (Eds.): MICCAI 2021, LNCS 12908, pp. 613–623, 2021.
https://doi.org/10.1007/978-3-030-87237-3_59

primarily focus on discovering distinguishable patterns and features existing in medical images for down-stream analysis tasks, thus may neglect patterns that are characteristic of the images but not distinct enough for discriminative tasks. Meanwhile, generative models provide a complementary way of learning all image patterns by modeling the entire data distribution. Towards a better comprehension of medical image attributes, we propose an attribute-guided generative adversarial network, termed AttributeGAN, to model the data distribution conditioned on different attributes and link the attribute values with image patterns and characteristics. Different from existing generative models proposed in the medical image domain for applications such as cross-modality translation [1], synthetic augmentation [21] and image reconstruction [13], we investigate the problem of synthesizing histopathology images conditioned on different image attributes to build a more controllable and interpretable medical image generative model.

Existing literature on controllable and interpretable image synthesis models [16,18] focus on noticeable attributes such as human body pose, hair color, age of human face, among others. However, attributes of medical images are more nuanced and harder to model and thus the problem of generating medical images based on controllable attributes is more challenging to solve. For conditional image synthesis, conditional GANs (cGANs) [11,12] have utilized various types of discriminator networks to help the models capture the relationships between input conditions and image features. However, few of them work on multiple attribute inputs or are studied for medical image applications.

In this work, our goal is to develop an attribute-guided medical image synthesis model which can generate high-resolution and realistic images as well as make sure the generated images accurately reflect the attributes given to the model. We build upon a successful unsupervised generative model, leverage a carefully designed attribute-attention model, and employ a conditional contrastive learning strategy to efficiently model the conditional data distribution. Multiple attributes are one-hot encoded and concatenated with the noise vector and fed into different stages of the proposed model. Our proposed model generates photo-realistic histopathology images while being more controllable and interpretable than unconditional generative models. We conduct experiments on a histopathology dataset containing stained H&E images of urothelial carcinoma and compare our proposed AttributeGAN with the state-of-the-art cGAN as well as different variants of our model. We summarize our contributions in this work as follows:

* We propose a multi-attribute controllable generative model for high quality histopathology image synthesis. To the best of our knowledge, our work is the first to develop an attribute-aware GAN model with the capability to precisely control cellular features while preserving photo-realism for synthesized images.
* We incorporate efficient attention modules and conditional contrastive learning in both the generator and the discriminator to significantly improve quality as well as achieve better attribute-awareness of the generated images. Experiments on a histopathology dataset show better image quality using our proposed AttributeGAN than the state-of-the-art conditional GAN model.

2   Methodology

To guarantee the quality of synthesized images, we build our model upon a recent unsupervised backbone generative model introduced by [10]. For attribute-aware and controllable generation, we incorporate multi-attribute annotations of each image as the additional condition information to explicitly control the generation process. With attribute conditions inserted, the synthesized results are expected to maintain sufficiently photo-realistic while accurately capturing the distinguishable image feature patterns within attributes. To fulfill the first goal, we adopt a skip-layer channel-wise excitation (SLE) module and include additional reconstruction loss in discriminator as in [10]. SLE leverages learned feature patterns from a lower abstract level to further re-calibrate the channel-wise features map of higher scale. As demonstrated in the architecture of our proposed controllable cellular attribute-aware generative model in Fig. 1, in addition to the basic structure of SLE, we further improve the backbone by incorporating a global attention pooling for context modeling [3] at earlier stages of upsampling before the transformation through the bottleneck blocks to capture channel-wise dependencies.

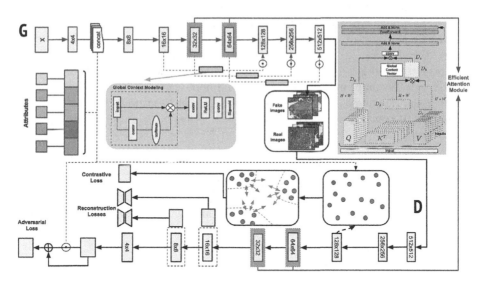

Fig. 1. The architecture of our proposed controllable cellular attribute-aware generative model. Each color block of the attribute vector input represents a corresponding cellular attribute feature: cell crowding, cell polarity, mitosis, prominence of nucleoli and state of nuclear pleomorphism. Different colors in the feature space for contrastive learning refers to the label constructed by combination of 5 cellular attribute levels (*e.g. (cell-crowding-severe, cell-polarity-completely-lacking, mitosis-frequent, nucleoli-prominent, pleomorphism-moderate)*)

For the second goal of attribute learning, while existing conditional GANs (cGANs) [11] concatenate noise vectors with the conditional vectors and leverage projection discriminator for condition correctness, such models may not be able to capture the nuanced changes in attribute levels of medical images. In addition to input concatenation and projection discriminator, we integrate conditional contrastive losses [6] to both discriminator and generator to exploit the relation between images and the attributes they contain. Integrating a self-supervised learning based module to exploit data-to-data and data-to-attribute relations within a mini-batch of proper size comes with two merits. First, with known attributes available for reference, the performance no longer heavily relies on the hard negative and positive samples mining. We consider the anchor image itself together with real images with the same attribute combination as positive samples, while real images with different attribute combinations in the same mini-batch as negative samples. Second, the performance of capturing the explicitly distinguishable feature representations in a fine-grained manner is substantially enhanced. Theoretically, this is achieved by minimizing the feature-level distances between positive samples while maximizing the distances between positive and negative samples. During training, the knowledge of attribute-dependent feature distinction learned by the discriminator is then passed to the generator for synthesizing images that are more sensitive to inter/intra-attribute characteristics. The effectiveness is further proven empirically in the qualitative ablation study of model architecture with and without the contrastive learning objective as demonstrated in Fig. 3. To elaborate, first we denote $X = \{x_1, x_2, ..., x_n\}$ as extracted features from the intermediate stage of discriminator, and $Y = \{y_1, y_2, ..., y_n\}$ as the combination of multiple attributes. Intuitively, after mapping data to the hypersphere via feature and attribute projectors f and l, our goal is to push the inter-attribute samples further and pull intra-attribute ones closer at the feature level. Thus, our conditional contrastive loss is formulated as:

$$\mathcal{L}(x_i, y_i; t) = -\log\left(\frac{\exp(\frac{f(x_i)^\top l(y_i)}{t}) + \sum_{k=1}^n \mathbb{1}_{y_k=y_i} \cdot \exp(\frac{f(x_i)^\top f(x_k)}{t})}{\exp(\frac{f(x_i)^\top l(y_i)}{t}) + \sum_{k=1}^n \mathbb{1}_{k\neq i} \cdot \exp(\frac{f(x_i)^\top f(x_k)}{t})}\right), \quad (1)$$

where $\mathbb{1}$ is the indicator function and the scalar value t plays the role as the regularizer to balance the push and pull force among samples across different and within the same group of attributes.

Recent GAN models [22] for image synthesis have adopted the self-attention module [20] to capture long-range dependencies within the image. However, the dot-product based self-attention can quadratically increase computational complexity and constrain the number of images inside each batch. Meanwhile, the aforementioned contrastive learning efficiency heavily relies on a relatively large batch size as both data-to-data and data-to-attribute relation learning would be seriously compromised with a small batch size and insufficient number of positive/negative pairs. Hence, in order to free up more space to accommodate a larger volume of data in each batch and train with lower computational complexity, we apply a more efficient equivalence [17] of self-attention. As illustrated in the efficient attention module in Fig. 1, feature vectors at intermediate stages in both generator and discriminator are projected onto three latent spaces through convolution operations termed as query, key and value as in the original self-attention [20], and denoted as Q, K, V, respectively. Here, $Q \in \mathbb{R}^{(H*W) \times d_q}$, $K \in \mathbb{R}^{(H*W) \times d_k}$, $V \in \mathbb{R}^{(H*W) \times d_v}$, $d_q = d_k$ and H, W refer to the height and width of the image. Leveraging the associative property of matrix multiplication, rather than start with the multiplication of QK^T as formulated in [20] to measure the pair-wise similarity exhaustively, instead we begin with the multiplication between K^T and V. It is feasible because $(\frac{QK^T}{n})V = \frac{Q}{\sqrt{n}}(\frac{K^T}{\sqrt{n}}V)$. Following this procedure, we obtain a matrix $g \in \mathbb{R}^{d_k \times d_v}$, representing the intermediate global context vector with dimension of d_v in d_k channels after aggregating from $H * W$ positions through weighted summation. At the next step, the context vector is acquired by having each pixel gathering positional features from all d_k channels for d_v dimensions, by multiplying Q and the result of $(K^T V)$. With the efficient attention, the memory complexity is reduced to $\mathcal{O}(d_k * d_v)$ from the original $\mathcal{O}(n^2)$, escalating convergence speed and freeing up more space, making it possible for conditional contrastive learning to deliver its performance to the fullest.

More specifically, for conditional attributes, we encode the input condition into a one-hot vector with attribute level labels for all five cellular features. The attribute vector is later concatenated with the input noise vector after the initial stage of upsampling both vectors using transposed convolution operators. For synthesizing images with resolution 512×512, efficient attention modules are applied in two intermediate upsampling stages at 32×32 and 64×64 resolutions as shown in Fig. 1. For each upsampling block without attention module, input images first go through an upsampling layer with scale factor set as 2, immediately followed by a gaussian blurring kernel for antialiasing. Next, to enlarge the feature learning space channel-wise, a basic block including a convolutional layer, a batch normalization layer and an activation layer is added as another major component in each individual upsampling block. Gated Linear Units (GLU) is utilized for every activation layer in the AttributeGAN architecture, as it has shown quality-improving potential over the commonly used ReLU or GELU activations [14]. Additionally, three skip-layer connections are applied at the resolutions of 16×16, 32×32, and 64×64 to 128×128, 256×256 and 512×512 in order to strengthen the gradient signals between layers.

For the discriminator, the conditional attributes are required together with either synthesized or real images to be further utilized in a projection based discrimination. Attribute vectors are fed into a feed-forward layer before being incorporated into the output of discriminator. As shown in Fig. 1, at the resolution of 128×128 the feature vectors and the attribute level information are projected to an embedded space for contrastive learning, which is later included in the losses for the discriminator. To further refine the discriminator's capability of capturing a more comprehensive feature map to be differentiated from the fakes, two auxiliary reconstruction losses are added. We utilize two additional simple decoders trained within the discriminator for the 8×8 and 16×16 feature vectors, and calculate the mean squared error (MSE) for both in the reconstruction loss.

3   Experiments and Results

Dataset. We conduct comprehensive experiments on a histopathology dataset representing patients with bladder cancer collected by [23]. The dataset contains 4, 253 histopathology image patches with 512×512 resolution. Each patch is accompanied with a paragraph of pathology report descriptions provided by multiple experienced pathologists. Each report follows a template format that describes 5 types of key morphological visual cellular features essential for classifying urothelial carcinoma, including cell crowding, cell polarity, mitosis, prominence of nucleoli and state of nuclear pleomorphism.

To achieve a more concise representation of attributes and their levels, we extract feature-describing keywords in the report as annotations (see Table 1, 2, 3, 4 and 5 in Supplementary Materials). Converting raw reports to categorical levels for each cellular attribute facilitates the manipulation of semantic editing in our experiments, as demonstrated in Fig. 2. There are 4, 3, 3, 2, 4 levels assigned to describe different degrees of cell crowding, cell polarity, mitosis, nucleoli and pleomorphism, respectively. Following this procedure, each patch is paired with a combination of levels from all 5 cellular attributes. To accelerate the learning of attribute-relevant patterns, we discard the combinations with frequency less than the 20th percentile since most of those merely appear in the dataset once or twice.

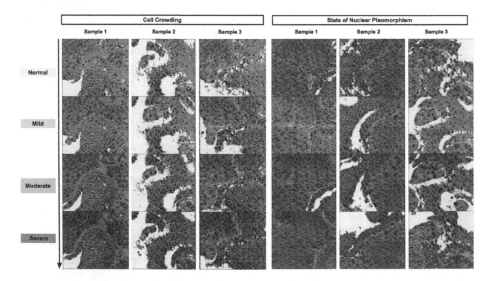

Fig. 2. The AttributeGAN generated histopathology patches based on different levels of cell crowding and the state of nuclear pleomorphism. The input noise vector is set to be identical for each sample, which explains the resemblance of general shape and texture shared within each column and rich diversity across columns. Zoom in for better view.

Implementation Details. AttributeGAN is trained on two NVIDIA Quadro RTX 6000 GPUs each with 24 GB RAM in parallel by applying the PyTorch DistributedDataParallel module together with SyncBatchNorm. The GPU space freed up from the attention module efficiency enables a larger batch size. In our experiments, the batch size is set as 64, and each device processes half of the inputs from the current batch. The learning rate is fixed to be $2e - 4$ throughout the entire 50000 steps of training.

We present example images generated by our AttributeGAN in Fig. 2. To demonstrate the smooth progression through different attribute levels and showcase disentanglement among attributes, the input attribute is framed as a 5-dimensional vector where we only alter one attribute at a time inside each result batch. Other than the attribute whose level is being varied, the remaining dimensions are fixed to be a combination of the other four attributes that frequently appear in the dataset. With attribute conditions given in such manner, the generated images show clear progressions in cellular pattern in accordance with the changes in input attribute condition.

To examine the effectiveness of our proposed AttributeGAN and its components, we compare images generated by different models as well as the real images in Fig. 3. Various well-developed and extensively-used models are relevant

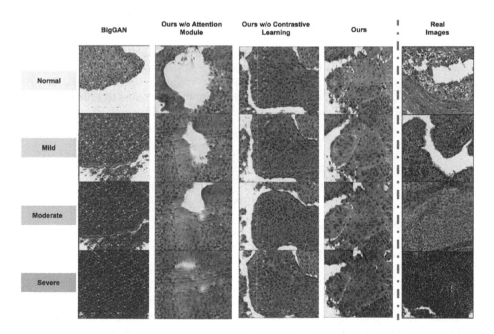

Fig. 3. Generated images from ablation study. The selected attribute for ablation study is cell crowding. We present the comparison among images synthesized using our baseline model BigGAN, our proposed AttributeGAN w/o the efficient attention module, our proposed AttributeGAN w/o the conditional contrastive loss, and real images for 4 levels of cell crowding: normal, mild, moderate and severe. Zoom in for better view.

to attribute-controlling, such as Fader Networks [9], StyleGAN [7] and StyleGAN v2 [8]. Although the aforementioned models present state-of-the-art results on photo-realism and attribute accuracy, they are not suitable to be directly compared with our approach for the conditional histopathology image synthesis task, because they are designed for slightly different goals such as semantic editing of assigned attributes (e.g. the Fader Networks), or unconditional image synthesis (e.g. StyleGAN, StyleGAN v2). Hence we consider the state-of-the-art conditional GAN model, BigGAN [2], as the most appropriate baseline model. Since BigGAN can only handle single-dimensional condition, we train 5 different Big-GAN models for different attributes. Considering that BigGAN consumes larger memory and requires longer time to converge, we train all baseline BigGAN models with image resolution 256×256. During comparison, we resize all images to the same size for fair comparison. One can observe that images generated by our models show superb realism. Compared with the BigGAN model, different variants of AttributeGAN model keep the global shape and texture well inside each column. On the contrary, the global image pattern changes for BigGAN given different attribute level inputs. For variants of our AttributeGAN, our proposed model without the attention module generates less realistic images, and the model without the conditional contrastive learning reacts less responsively to the changes in attribute level. The full AttributeGAN model respects the changes in attribute level and retains the global patterns well.

Table 1. Quantitative evaluation results of different methods. Real images are from a holdout validation set during fine-tuning of the pre-trained classifier. Note that we report BigGAN results from five independently trained BigGAN models for five attributes as it can only work with single attribute inputs. EA refers to Efficient Attention module and CCL refers to the Conditional Contrastive Loss.

Methods	FID↓	Attribute Error↓				
		Cell Crowding	Cell polarity	Mitosis	Nucleoli	Pleomorphism
Real Images*	–	.011	.034	.037	.018	.014
BigGAN [2]	158.39	.112	.080	.104	**.049**	.065
AttributeGAN (Ours) w/o EA	142.015	.035	**.078**	.208	.056	**.023**
AttributeGAN (Ours) w/o CCL	55.772	.094	.112	.111	.056	.070
AttributeGAN (Ours)	**53.689**	.021	.098	**.088**	.081	.063

In Table 1, we show quantitative comparison results between different models. Following conventions in image synthesis works [2,22], we adopt Fréchet Inception Distance (FID) [5] score which has shown to correlate well with human perception of realism. FID measures the Fréchet distance between two multivariate Gaussians fit to features of generated and real images extracted by the pre-trained Inception V3 [19] model. Compared with BigGAN whose FID score is averaged from five BigGAN models, all AttributeGAN variants achieve better

FID score indicating better realism. After including the attention module, the FID score improved significantly for the AttributeGAN model. To better evaluate the correctness of represented attributes, we further calculate an Attribute Error to measure the discrepancy between attribute levels predicted by an ImageNet pre-trained ResNet18 [4] model fine-tuned on the histopathology dataset and the groundtruth attribute levels. Images generated by all models are first normalized to same resolution 224×224 for fair comparison. All attribute levels are normalized to the range $[0, 1]$ and the MSE of the predicted attributes and the groundtruth attributes are computed as the attribute error value. During fine-tuning of the ResNet18 model, we keep a holdout validation set and the corresponding attribute error evaluated on the holdout real images are also reported in Table 1. For BigGAN and our proposed AttributeGAN without attention, although they achieve small attribute errors for certain attributes, the quality of generated images are lower which makes them differ more from real images, thus the attribute prediction model trained on real images may not be able to correctly predict the attribute level for such images. Compared to AttributeGAN without contrastive learning, the full AttributeGAN generally gets lower attribute error, especially on cell crowding. Based on both the qualitative and quantitative comparisons, we prove the necessity of the attention module and the conditional contrastive loss, and show that one multi-attribute AttributeGAN model can generate images with better quality than multiple BigGAN models for conditional histopathology image synthesis.

4 Discussion

To assess the quality of the generated images and how well the images correspond to the input attribute levels, we presented five sets of images that were generated based on different cellular attribute levels to two expert pathologists. Both pathologists commented that the synthetic images are remarkably good in resembling routinely stained H&E images of urothelial carcinoma. In the set of images generated according to different levels of cell crowding (see examples in Fig. 2-Left), the crowding of nuclei occurs appropriately overall at each of the described levels, and the degree of crowding remains within the realm of reality, although for a few images, the increase in crowding seems to be by increasing the epithelial/stromal ratio, rather than increasing the density of cells within the same amount of epithelium. For the set of images generated according to different levels of pleomorphism (see examples in Fig. 2-Right), an increase in nuclear pleomorphism was observed as the images progress through the pleomorphism prominence levels. For the other three sets of images generated based on different levels of cell polarity, mitosis, and prominence of nucleoli (see Figs. 1–3 in Supplementary Materials), the pathologists commented that no obvious progression was observed through those sequences of images. We plan to further investigate these three attributes in our future work, study whether the attributes are correlated in some fashion in real images and learn how to improve the responsiveness of generated images to varying input conditions.

5 Conclusion

In this work, we present a multi-attribute guided generative model, Attribute-GAN, for synthesizing highly realistic histopathology images. Images generated by the proposed model show smooth progression through different input attribute levels and contain photo-realistic patterns. With the quality of synthesized images, AttributeGAN can be potentially used for medical education or training and support various medical imaging applications.

References

1. Armanious, K., et al.: MedGAN: medical image translation using GANs. Comput. Med. Imaging Graph. **79**, 101684 (2020)
2. Brock, A., Donahue, J., Simonyan, K.: Large scale GAN training for high fidelity natural image synthesis. In: International Conference on Learning Representations (2018)
3. Cao, Y., Xu, J., Lin, S., Wei, F., Hu, H.: Global context networks. IEEE Trans. Pattern Anal. Mach. Intell. (2020)
4. He, K., Zhang, X., Ren, S., Sun, J.: Deep residual learning for image recognition. In: Proceedings of the IEEE Conference on Computer Vision and Pattern Recognition, pp. 770–778 (2016)
5. Heusel, M., Ramsauer, H., Unterthiner, T., Nessler, B., Hochreiter, S.: GANs trained by a two time-scale update rule converge to a local Nash equilibrium. In: Advances in Neural Information Processing Systems, pp. 6626–6637 (2017)
6. Kang, M., Park, J.: ContraGAN: contrastive learning for conditional image generation. In: NeurIPS 2020, Neural Information Processing Systems (2020)
7. Karras, T., Laine, S., Aila, T.: A style-based generator architecture for generative adversarial networks. In: Proceedings of the IEEE/CVF Conference on Computer Vision and Pattern Recognition, pp. 4401–4410 (2019)
8. Karras, T., Laine, S., Aittala, M., Hellsten, J., Lehtinen, J., Aila, T.: Analyzing and improving the image quality of styleGAN. In: Proceedings of the IEEE/CVF Conference on Computer Vision and Pattern Recognition, pp. 8110–8119 (2020)
9. Lample, G., Zeghidour, N., Usunier, N., Bordes, A., Denoyer, L., Ranzato, M.: Fader networks: generating image variations by sliding attribute values. In: Advances in Neural Information Processing Systems, pp. 5963–5972 (2017)
10. Liu, B., Zhu, Y., Song, K., Elgammal, A.: Towards faster and stabilized GAN training for high-fidelity few-shot image synthesis. ArXiv abs/2101.04775 (2021)
11. Miyato, T., Koyama, M.: cGANs with projection discriminator. In: International Conference on Learning Representations (2018)
12. Odena, A., Olah, C., Shlens, J.: Conditional image synthesis with auxiliary classifier gans. In: International Conference on Machine Learning, pp. 2642–2651. PMLR (2017)
13. Quan, T.M., Nguyen-Duc, T., Jeong, W.K.: Compressed sensing MRI reconstruction using a generative adversarial network with a cyclic loss. IEEE Trans. Med. Imaging **37**(6), 1488–1497 (2018)
14. Shazeer, N.: GLU variants improve transformer. arXiv preprint arXiv:2002.05202 (2020)
15. Shen, D., Wu, G., Suk, H.I.: Deep learning in medical image analysis. Annu. Rev. Biomed. Eng. **19**, 221–248 (2017)

16. Shen, Y., Gu, J., Tang, X., Zhou, B.: Interpreting the latent space of GANs for semantic face editing. In: Proceedings of the IEEE/CVF Conference on Computer Vision and Pattern Recognition, pp. 9243–9252 (2020)
17. Shen, Z., Zhang, M., Zhao, H., Yi, S., Li, H.: Efficient attention: attention with linear complexities. In: Proceedings of the IEEE/CVF Winter Conference on Applications of Computer Vision, pp. 3531–3539 (2021)
18. Shoshan, A., Bhonker, N., Kviatkovsky, I., Medioni, G.: Gan-control: explicitly controllable GANs. arXiv preprint arXiv:2101.02477 (2021)
19. Szegedy, C., Vanhoucke, V., Ioffe, S., Shlens, J., Wojna, Z.: Rethinking the inception architecture for computer vision. In: Proceedings of the IEEE Conference on Computer Vision and Pattern Recognition, pp. 2818–2826 (2016)
20. Vaswani, A., et al.: Attention is all you need. In: Proceedings of the 31st International Conference on Neural Information Processing Systems, pp. 6000–6010 (2017)
21. Xue, Y., et al.: Selective synthetic augmentation with HistoGAN for improved histopathology image classification. Med. Image Anal. 67, 101816 (2021)
22. Zhang, H., Goodfellow, I., Metaxas, D., Odena, A.: Self-attention generative adversarial networks. In: International Conference on Machine Learning, pp. 7354–7363. PMLR (2019)
23. Zhang, Z., et al.: Pathologist-level interpretable whole-slide cancer diagnosis with deep learning. Nat. Mach. Intell. 1(5), 236–245 (2019)

Modalities - Ultrasound

USCL: Pretraining Deep Ultrasound Image Diagnosis Model Through Video Contrastive Representation Learning

Yixiong Chen[1,4], Chunhui Zhang[2], Li Liu[3,4(✉)], Cheng Feng[5,6], Changfeng Dong[5,6], Yongfang Luo[5,6], and Xiang Wan[3,4]

[1] School of Data Science, Fudan university, Shanghai, China
[2] Institute of Information Engineering, Chinese Academy of Sciences, Beijing, China
[3] Shenzhen Research Institute of Big Data, Shenzhen, China
liuli@cuhk.edu.cn
[4] The Chinese University of Hong Kong Shenzhen, Shenzhen, China
[5] Shenzhen Third People's Hospital, Shenzhen, China
[6] Southern University of Science and Technology, Shenzhen, China

Abstract. Most deep neural networks (DNNs) based ultrasound (US) medical image analysis models use pretrained backbones (*e.g.*, ImageNet) for better model generalization. However, the domain gap between natural and medical images causes an inevitable performance bottleneck. To alleviate this problem, an US dataset named US-4 is constructed for direct pretraining on the same domain. It contains over 23,000 images from four US video sub-datasets. To learn robust features from US-4, we propose an US semi-supervised contrastive learning method, named USCL, for pretraining. In order to avoid high similarities between negative pairs as well as mine abundant visual features from limited US videos, USCL adopts a sample pair generation method to enrich the feature involved in a single step of contrastive optimization. Extensive experiments on several downstream tasks show the superiority of USCL pretraining against ImageNet pretraining and other state-of-the-art (SOTA) pretraining approaches. In particular, USCL pretrained backbone achieves fine-tuning accuracy of over 94% on POCUS dataset, which is 10% higher than 84% of the ImageNet pretrained model. The source codes of this work are available at https://github.com/983632847/USCL.

Keywords: Ultrasound · Pretrained model · Contrastive learning

---

Y. Chen and C. Zhang—Contributed equally. This work was done at Shenzhen Research Institute of Big Data (SRIBD).

Electronic supplementary material The online version of this chapter (https://doi.org/10.1007/978-3-030-87237-3_60) contains supplementary material, which is available to authorized users.

© Springer Nature Switzerland AG 2021
M. de Bruijne et al. (Eds.): MICCAI 2021, LNCS 12908, pp. 627–637, 2021.
https://doi.org/10.1007/978-3-030-87237-3_60

1   Introduction

Due to the low cost and portability, ultrasound (US) is a widely used medical imaging technique, leading to the common application of US images [2,24] for clinical diagnosis. To date, deep neural networks (DNNs) [9] are one of the most popular automatic US image analysis techniques. When training DNN on US images, a big challenge is the data scarcity, which is often dealt with parameters transferred from pretrained backbones (*e.g.*, ImageNet [19] pretrained VGG or ResNet). But model performance on downstream tasks suffers severely from the domain gap between *natural* and *medical* images [12]. There is a lack of public well-pretrained models specifically for US images due to the insufficient labeled pretraining US data caused by the high cost of specialized annotations, inconsistent labeling criterion and data privacy issue.

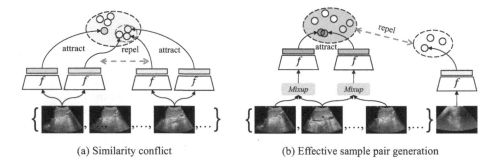

(a) Similarity conflict   (b) Effective sample pair generation

Fig. 1. Motivation of USCL. SPG tackles the harmful similarity conflict of traditional contrastive learning. (a) Similarity conflict: if a negative sample pair comes from different frames of the same video, they might be more similar than positive samples augmented from a frame, which confuses the training. (b) SPG ensures negative pairs coming from different videos, thus are dissimilar. The sample interpolation process also helps the positive pairs to have appropriate similarities, and enriches the feature involved in comparison. Representations are learned by gathering positive pairs close in representation space and pushing negative pairs apart.

Recently, more and more literature tend to utilize unsupervised methods [3,7] to avoid medical data limitation for pretraining. The common practice is to pretrain models with pretext tasks and evaluate the representations on specific downstream tasks. Yet most existing methods can only outperform ImageNet pretraining with high-cost multi-modal data [11,14]. To get powerful pretrained models from US videos, we first build an US video dataset to alleviate data shortage. Secondly, contrastive learning[4,7,25] is also exploited to reduce the dependence on accurate annotations due to its good potential ability to learn robust visual representations without labels. However, given the fact that most US data are in video format, normal contrastive learning paradigm (*i.e.*, Sim-CLR [4] and MoCo [7], which considers two samples augmented from each image as a positive pair, and samples from different images as negative pairs) will cause high similarities between negative pairs sampled from the same video and mislead the training. This problem is called *similarity conflict* (Fig. 1 (a)) in this work. *Thus, is there a method which can avoid similarity conflict of contrastive learning and train a robust DNN backbone with US videos?*

Table 1. Statistics of the US-4 dataset containing 4 video-based sub-datasets. The total number of images is 23,231, uniformly sampled from 1051 videos. Most videos contain 10–50 similar images, which ensures the good property of semantic clusters.

Sub-dataset	Organ	Image size	Depth	Frame rate	Classes	Videos	Images
Butterfly [1]	Lung	658 × 738	–	23 Hz	2	22	1533
CLUST [24]	Liver	434 × 530	–	19 Hz	5	63	3150
Liver Fibrosis	Liver	600 × 807	∼8 cm	28 Hz	5	296	11714
COVID19-LUSMS	Lung	747 × 747	∼10 cm	17 Hz	4	670	6834

To answer this question, we find that image features from the same US video can be seen as a cluster in semantic space, while features from different videos come from different clusters. We design a sample pair generation (SPG) scheme to make contrastive learning fit the natural clustering characteristics of US video (Fig. 1 (b)). Two samples from the same video act as a positive pair and two samples from different videos are regarded as a negative pair. In this process, two positive samples can naturally be seen as close feature points in the representation space, while negative samples have enough semantic differences to avoid similarity conflict. In addition, SPG does not simply choose frames as samples (*e.g.*, key frame extraction [18]), we put forward sample interpolation contrast to enrich features. Samples are generated from multiple-frame random interpolation so that richer features can be involved in positive-negative comparison. This method makes the semantic cohesion appear at the volume level of the ultrasound representation space [13] instead of the instance level. Combined with SPG, our work develops a semi-supervised contrastive learning method to train a generic model with US videos for downstream US image analysis. Here, the whole framework is called *ultrasound contrastive learning (USCL)*, which combines supervised learning to learn category-level discriminative ability, and contrastive learning to enhance instance-level discriminative ability.

2   US-4 Dataset

In this work, we construct a new US dataset named US-4, which is collected from four different convex probe [2] US datasets, involving two scan regions (*i.e.*, lung and liver). Among the four sub-datasets of US-4, *Liver Fibrosis* and *COVID19-LUSMS* datasets are collected by local sonographers [6,17], *Butter-fly* [1] and *CLUST* [24] are two public sub-datasets. The first two sub-datasets are collected with *Resona 7T* ultrasound system, the frequency is FH 5.0 and the pixel size is $0.101\,\text{mm}$–$0.127\,\text{mm}$. All sub-datasets contain labeled images captured from videos for classification task. In order to generate a diverse and sufficiently large dataset, images are selected from original videos with a suitable sampling interval. For each video with frame rate T, we extract $n = 3$ samples per second with sampling interval $I = \frac{T}{n}$, which ensures that US-4 contains sufficient but not redundant information of videos. This results in 1051 videos and 23,231 images. The different attributes (*e.g.*, depth and frame rate) of dataset are described in Table 1. The US-4 dataset is relatively balanced in terms of images in each video, where most videos contain tens of US images. Some frame examples are shown in Fig. 2.

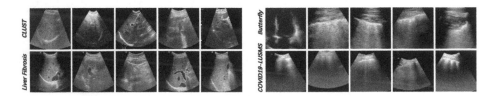

Fig. 2. Examples of US image in US-4.

3   Methodology

This section first formulates the proposed USCL framework (Fig. 3), then describes the details of sample pair generation. Finally, the proposed USCL will be introduced.

3.1   Problem Formulation

Given a video V_i from the US-4 dataset, USCL first extracts images to obtain a balanced distributed frame set $\mathbb{F}_i^K = \{\mathbf{f}_i^{(k)}\}_{k=1}^K$, where K is the number of extracted images. Next, a *sampler* Θ is applied to randomly sample M images, denoted as $\mathbb{F}_i^M = \{\mathbf{f}_i^{(m)}\}_{m=1}^M$ with $2 \leq M \ll K$. A following *mixed frame generator* $G : \mathbb{F}_i^M \rightarrow \mathbb{S}_i^2$ obtains two images, where $\mathbb{S}_i^2 = \{\mathbf{x}_i^{(1)}, \mathbf{x}_i^{(2)}\}$ is a positive pair followed by two data augmentation operations $Aug = \{Aug_i, Aug'_i\}$. These augmentations including random cropping, flipping, rotation and color jittering are used for perturbing positive pairs, making the trained backbones invariant to scale, rotation, and color style.

The objective of USCL is to train a backbone f from training samples $\{(\mathbf{x}_i^{(1)}, \mathbf{x}_i^{(2)}), \mathbf{y}_i\}_{i=1}^N$ by combining self-supervised contrastive learning loss $\mathcal{L}_{con}$ and supervised cross-entropy (CE) loss $\mathcal{L}_{sup}$, where N is the number of videos in a training batch. Therefore, the USCL framework formulation aims to minimize following loss $\mathcal{L}$:

$$\mathcal{L} = \mathcal{L}_{con}(g(f(Aug(G(\mathbf{f})); \mathbf{w}_f); \mathbf{w}_g)) + \lambda \mathcal{L}_{sup}(h(f(Aug(G(\mathbf{f})); \mathbf{w}_f); \mathbf{w}_h); \mathbf{y}), \tag{1}$$

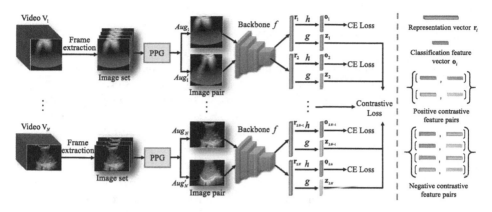

Fig. 3. System framework of the proposed USCL, which consists of sample pair generation and semi-supervised contrastive learning. (i) USCL extracts evenly distributed image sets from every US video as image dataset. (ii) The positive pair generation (PPG) module consists of a *sampler* Θ random sampling several images from an image set, and a *mixed frame generator* G obtaining two images. A generated positive pair is processed by two separate data augmentation operations. (iii) A backbone f, a projection head g and a classifier h are trained simultaneously by minimizing the self-supervised contrastive learning loss and supervised CE loss.

where λ is a hyper-parameter, $\mathbf{f} = \{\{\mathbf{f}_i^{(m)}\}_{m=1}^M\}_{i=1}^N$ are frames sampled from a batch of videos for training, $G(\mathbf{f}) = \{\mathbf{x}_i^{(1)}, \mathbf{x}_i^{(2)}\}_{i=1}^N$ are positive pairs, and $\mathbf{y} = \{\mathbf{y}_i\}_{i=1}^N$ are corresponding class labels. f, g and h denote backbone, projection head (two-layer MLP) and linear classifier, respectively. Different from most existing contrastive learning methods, USCL treats contrastive loss in Eq. (1) as a consistency regularization (CR) term, which improves the performance of pretraining backbone by combining supervised loss in a mutually reinforcing way. Here, label information instructs the model to recognize samples with different labels to be negative pairs, and contrastive process learns how US images can be semantically similar or different to assist better classification.

3.2 Sample Pair Generation

Most of the existing contrastive learning approaches construct positive pairs by applying two random data augmentations image by image. When directly applying them to the US frames, the contrastive learning fails to work normally due to the similarity conflict problem (*i.e.*, two samples coming from the same video are too similar to be a negative pair). To solve this problem, a sample pair generation (SPG) scheme is designed: it generates positive pairs with the positive pair generation (PPG) module[7], and any two samples from different positive pairs are regarded as a negative pair.

---

[7] For more details of PPG module, see the Supplementary Material Sect. 2.

The PPG module regards an evenly distributed image set extracted from a video as a semantic cluster, and different videos belong to different clusters. This kind of organization fits the purpose of contrastive learning properly. We expect the model can map the semantic clusters to feature clusters. Then PPG generates two images as a positive sample pair from each cluster. Note that only one positive pair is generated from a video, which can prevent the aforementioned similarity conflict problem.

In detail, firstly, a *sampler* Θ is applied to randomly sample three images $\widehat{\mathbf{x}}_i^{(1)}, \widehat{\mathbf{x}}_i^{(2)}$, and $\widehat{\mathbf{x}}_i^{(3)}$ in chronological order from an image set $\{\mathbf{f}_i^{(m)}\}_{m=1}^{M}$. Secondly, a delicate *mixed frame generator* G is performed to generate a positive sample pair. The image $\widehat{\mathbf{x}}_i^{(2)}$ is set as the anchor image, while $\widehat{\mathbf{x}}_i^{(1)}$ and $\widehat{\mathbf{x}}_i^{(3)}$ are perturbation images. In a mini-batch, G constructs positive sample pairs in interpolation manner via the mixup operation between anchor image and two perturbation images as follows.

$$\begin{cases} (\mathbf{x}_i^{(1)}, \mathbf{y}_i^{(1)}) = \xi_1(\widehat{\mathbf{x}}_i^{(2)}, \widehat{\mathbf{y}}_i^{(2)}) + (1 - \xi_1)(\widehat{\mathbf{x}}_i^{(1)}, \widehat{\mathbf{y}}_i^{(1)}), \\ (\mathbf{x}_i^{(2)}, \mathbf{y}_i^{(2)}) = \xi_2(\widehat{\mathbf{x}}_i^{(2)}, \widehat{\mathbf{y}}_i^{(2)}) + (1 - \xi_2)(\widehat{\mathbf{x}}_i^{(3)}, \widehat{\mathbf{y}}_i^{(3)}) \end{cases}, \tag{2}$$

where $\{\widehat{\mathbf{y}}_i^{(k)}\}_{k=1}^{3}$ are corresponding labels. $\xi_1, \xi_2 \sim Beta(\alpha, \beta)$, where α, β are parameters of *Beta* distribution.

In our contrastive learning process, sample pairs are then fed to the backbone followed by the projection head for contrastive learning task. The proposed PPG module has several benefits: 1) Interpolation makes every point in the feature convex hull enclosed by the cluster boundary possible to be sampled, making the cluster cohesive as a whole; 2) Positive pairs generated with Eq. (2) have appropriate mutual information. On the one hand, positive pairs are random offsets from the anchor image to the perturbation images, which ensures that they share the mutual information from the anchor image. On the other hand, the sampling interval $I \geq 5$ frames in US-4, resulting in low probability for SPG to sample temporarily close $\{\widehat{\mathbf{x}}_i^{(k)}\}_{k=1}^{3}$ which are too similar.

3.3   Ultrasound Contrastive Learning

The proposed USCL method learns representations not only by the supervision of category labels, but also by maximizing/minimizing agreement between positive/negative pairs as CR. Here, assorted DNNs can be used as backbone f to encode images, where the output representation vectors $\mathbf{r}_{2i-1} = f(\mathbf{x}_i^{(1)})$ and $\mathbf{r}_{2i} = f(\mathbf{x}_i^{(2)})$ are then fed to the following projection head and classifier.

Contrastive Branch. The contrastive branch consists of a projection head g and corresponding contrastive loss. The g is a two layer MLP which nonlinearly maps representations to other feature space for calculating contrastive regularization loss. The mapped vector $\mathbf{z}_i = g(\mathbf{r}_i) = \mathbf{w}_g^{(2)} \sigma(\mathbf{w}_g^{(1)} \mathbf{r}_i)$ is specialized for a contrast, where σ is ReLU activation function and $\mathbf{w}_g = \{\mathbf{w}_g^{(1)}, \mathbf{w}_g^{(2)}\}$ are the weights of g. The contrastive loss is proposed by Sohn [22], which aims at minimizing the distance between positive pairs $\{\mathbf{x}_i^{(1)}, \mathbf{x}_i^{(2)}\}_{i=1}^N$ and maximizing the distance between any negative pair $\{\mathbf{x}_i^{(1/2)}, \mathbf{x}_j^{(1/2)}\}$, $i \neq j$ for CR:

$$\mathcal{L}_{con} = \frac{1}{2N} \sum_{i=1}^N (l(2i-1, 2i) + l(2i, 2i-1)), \tag{3}$$

where

$$l(i,j) = -\log \frac{\exp(s_{i,j}/\tau)}{\sum_{k=1}^{2N} \mathbb{1}_{i \neq k} \cdot exp(s_{i,k}/\tau)}, \tag{4}$$

and

$$s_{i,j} = \mathbf{z}_i \cdot \mathbf{z}_j / (\|\mathbf{z}_i\| \|\mathbf{z}_j\|), \tag{5}$$

where τ is a tuning temperature parameter.

Classification Branch. We use a linear classifier h with weights $\mathbf{w}_c$ to separate sample features linearly in the representation space similar to [9,10]. The classification loss with corresponding one-hot label $\mathbf{y}_i$ is

$$\mathcal{L}_{sup} = \frac{1}{2N} \sum_{i=1}^N (CE(\mathbf{o}_{2i-1}, \mathbf{y}_i) + CE(\mathbf{o}_{2i}, \mathbf{y}_i)), \tag{6}$$

where $\mathbf{o}_i = h(\mathbf{r}_i) = softmax(\mathbf{w}_c \mathbf{r}_i)$.

Note that USCL is a semi-supervised training method, only contrastive branch works when the framework receives unlabeled data. This semi-supervised design is intuitively simple but effective, which makes it easy to be implemented and has great potential to be applied to various pretraining scenarios.

4 Experiment

4.1 Experimental Settings

Pretraining Details. ResNet18 is chosen as a representative backbone. We use US-4 dataset (the ratio of training set to validation set is 8 to 2) with 1% labels for pretraining, and fine-tune pretrained models for various downstream tasks. During pretraining, US images are randomly cropped and resized to 224×224 pixels as the input, followed by random flipping and color jittering. We use Adam optimizer with learning rate 3×10^{-4} and weight decay rate 10^{-4} to optimize network parameters. The backbones are pretrained on US-4 for 300 epochs with batch size $N = 32$. The pretraining loss is the sum of contrastive loss and standard cross-entropy loss for classification. Like SimCLR, the backbones are used for fine-tuning on target tasks, projection head g and classifier h are discarded when the pretraining is completed. The λ in Eq. (1) is 0.2, parameters α and β in Eq. (2) are 0.5 and 0.5, respectively. The temperature parameter τ in Eq. (4) is 0.5. The experiments are implemented using PyTorch with an Intel Xeon Silver 4210R CPU@2.4 GHz and a single Nvidia Tesla V100 GPU.

Fine-Tuning Datasets. We fine-tuned the last 3 layers of pretrained backbones on POCUS [2] and UDIAT-B [26] datasets to testify the performance of our USCL. On POCUS and UDIAT-B datasets, the learning rates are 0.01 and 0.005, respectively. The POCUS is a widely used lung convex probe US dataset for COVID-19 consisting of 140 videos, 2116 images from three classes (*i.e.*, COVID-19, bacterial pneumonia and healthy controls). The UDIAT-B consists of 163 linear probe US breast images from different women with the mean image size of 760×570 pixels, where each of the images presents one or more lesions. Within the 163 lesion images, 53 of them are cancerous masses and other 110 are benign lesions. In this work, we use UDIAT-B dataset to perform the lesion detection and segmentation comparison experiments. 50 of 163 images are used for validation and the rest are used for training.

Table 2. Ablation study of two contrastive ingredients during pretraining: assigning a negative pair from samples of different videos to overcome similarity conflict (I_1) and using mixup operation to enrich the features of positive pairs (I_2). They both improve the model transfer ability significantly, and the classification brunch is also beneficial. All results are reported as POCUS fine-tuning accuracy.

Method	ImageNet	USCL	I_1		✓		✓	✓
			I_2			✓	✓	✓
			CE loss					✓
Accuracy (%)	84.2			87.5	90.8	92.3	93.2	94.2

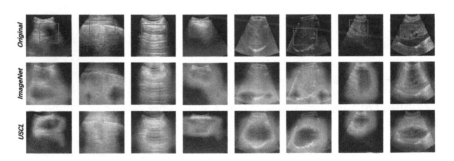

Fig. 4. The visualization results of the last Conv layer in ImageNet pretrained model and USCL model with Grad-CAM [21]. The first 4 columns are lung US images, models trained with USCL on US-4 can focus on the regions of A-line and pleural lesion instead of concentrating on regions without valid information like the ImageNet counterpart. The last 4 columns are liver US images, models trained with USCL accurately attend to the liver regions.

4.2 Ablation Studies

Here, we report the last 3 layers fine-tuning results on POCUS of US-4 pretrained backbones (ResNet18) to validate different components of USCL.

SPG *and* **CE Loss.** We implement five pretraining methods considering the influence of different contrastive ingredients and the classification brunch with CE loss (Table 2). Compared with ImageNet, vanilla contrastive learning improves the accuracy by 3.3% due to a smaller domain gap. It is regarded as the method baseline. The negative pair assigning scheme and positive pair generation method further improves the fine-tuning performance by 3.3% and 4.8%. They can be combined to reach higher performance. In addition, CE loss improves fine-tuning accuracy by 1.0%. This indicates that extra label information is able to enhance the power of contrastive representation learning.

Visualization of Feature Representation. To illustrate the robust feature representation of pretrained backbone, we visualize the last Conv feature map of some randomly selected images produced by USCL pretrained model and ImageNet pretrained model with Grad-CAM [21] (Fig. 4). Compared with ImageNet pretrained backbone, attention regions given by the USCL backbone are much more centralized and more consistent with clinical observation.

Table 3. Comparison of fine-tuning accuracy (%) on POCUS classification dataset and average precision (AP [16]) on UDIAT-B detection (Det), segmentation (Seg) with SOTA methods. (AP is calculated as the area under the precision-recall curve drawn with different Intersection over Union (IoU) thresholds.)

Method	Classification					Det	Seg
	COVID-19	Pneumonia	Regular	Total Acc	F1	AP	AP
ImageNet [9]	79.5	78.6	88.6	84.2	81.8	40.6	48.2
US-4 supervised	83.7	82.1	86.5	85.0	82.8	38.3	42.6
TE [20]	75.7	70.0	89.4	81.7	79.0	38.7	46.6
Π Model [20]	77.6	76.4	88.7	83.2	80.6	36.1	45.5
FixMatch [23]	83.0	77.5	85.7	83.6	81.6	39.6	46.9
MoCo v2 [5]	79.7	81.4	88.9	84.8	82.8	38.7	47.1
SimCLR [4]	83.2	89.4	87.1	86.4	86.3	43.8	51.3
USCL	**90.8**	**97.0**	**95.4**	**94.2**	**94.0**	**45.4**	**52.8**

4.3 Comparison with SOTA

We compare USCL with ImageNet pretrained ResNet18 [9] and other backbones pretrained on US-4 dataset with supervised method (*i.e.*, plain supervised), semi-supervised methods (*i.e.*, Temporal Ensembling (TE) [20], Π Model [20], Fix-Match [23]), and self-supervised methods (*i.e.*, MoCo v2 [5], SimCLR [4]).

Results on Classification Task. On POCUS dataset, we fine-tune the last three layers to testify the representation capability of backbones on classification task (Table 3). USCL has consistent best performance on classification of all classes, and its total accuracy of 94.2% is also significantly better than all 7 counterparts. Compared with ImageNet pretrained backbone, USCL reaches a much higher F1 score of 94.0%, which is 12.2% higher.

Results on Detection and Segmentation Tasks. Table 3 shows the comparison results of detection and segmentation on UDIAT-B dataset. Mask R-CNN [8] with ResNet18-FPNs [15], whose backbones are pretrained, is used to implement this experiment. USCL generates better backbones than ImageNet and US-4 supervised learning. For detection and segmentation, it outperforms ImageNet pretraining by 4.8% and 4.6%, respectively. Importantly, the UDIAT-B images are collected with linear probe instead of convex probe like US-4, showing a superior texture encoding ability of USCL.

5 Conclusion

This work constructs a new US video-based image dataset US-4 and proposes a simple but efficient contrastive semi-supervised learning algorithm USCL for US analysis model pretraining. USCL achieves significantly superior performance than ImageNet pretraining by learning compact semantic clusters from US videos. Future works include adding more scan regions of US videos to US-4 dataset for a better generalization on more diseases.

Acknowledgement. This work is supported by the Key-Area Research and Development Program of Guangdong Province (2020B0101350001); the GuangDong Basic and Applied Basic Research Foundation (No. 2020A1515110376); Guangdong Provincial Key Laboratory of Big Data Computation Theories and Methods, The Chinese University of Hong Kong (Shenzhen).

References

1. Butterfly videos. https://www.butterflynetwork.com/index.html. Accessed 20 Sept 2020
2. Born, J., et al.: Accelerating detection of lung pathologies with explainable ultrasound image analysis. Appl. Sci. **11**(2), 672 (2021)
3. Celebi, M. Emre., Aydin, Kemal (eds.): Unsupervised Learning Algorithms. Springer, Cham (2016). https://doi.org/10.1007/978-3-319-24211-8
4. Chen, T., Kornblith, S., Norouzi, M., Hinton, G.: A simple framework for contrastive learning of visual representations. arXiv:2002.05709 (2020)
5. Chen, X., Fan, H., Girshick, R., He, K.: Improved baselines with momentum contrastive learning. arXiv:2003.04297 (2020)
6. Gao, L., et al.: Multi-modal active learning for automatic liver fibrosis diagnosis based on ultrasound shear wave elastography. In: 2021 IEEE 18th International Symposium on Biomedical Imaging (ISBI), pp. 410–414. IEEE (2021)
7. He, K., Fan, H., Wu, Y., Xie, S., Girshick, R.: Momentum contrast for unsupervised visual representation learning. In: CVPR, pp. 9729–9738 (2020)

8. He, K., Gkioxari, G., Dollar, P., Girshick, R.: Mask R-CNN. IEEE TPAMI **42**(2), 386–397 (2020)
9. He, K., Zhang, X., Ren, S., Sun, J.: Deep residual learning for image recognition. In: CVPR, pp. 770–778 (2016)
10. Huang, G., Liu, Z., Van Der Maaten, L., Weinberger, K.Q.: Densely connected convolutional networks. In: CVPR, pp. 4700–4708 (2017)
11. Jiao, Jianbo, Cai, Yifan, Alsharid, Mohammad, Drukker, Lior, Papageorghiou, Aris T., Noble, J. Alison.: Self-supervised contrastive video-speech representation learning for ultrasound. In: Martel, Anne L., et al. (eds.) MICCAI 2020. LNCS, vol. 12263, pp. 534–543. Springer, Cham (2020). https://doi.org/10.1007/978-3-030-59716-0_51
12. Ke, A., Ellsworth, W., Banerjee, O., Ng, A.Y., Rajpurkar, P.: Chextransfer: Performance and parameter efficiency of ImageNet models for chest X-ray interpretation. arXiv:2101.06871 (2021)
13. Kwitt, R., Vasconcelos, N., Razzaque, S., Aylward, S.: Localizing target structures in ultrasound video-a phantom study. Med. Image Anal. **17**(7), 712–722 (2013)
14. Li, X., Jia, M., Islam, M.T., Yu, L., Xing, L.: Self-supervised feature learning via exploiting multi-modal data for retinal disease diagnosis. IEEE TMI **39**(12), 4023–4033 (2020)
15. Lin, T.Y., Dollár, P., Girshick, R., He, K., Hariharan, B., Belongie, S.: Feature pyramid networks for object detection. In: CVPR, pp. 2117–2125 (2017)
16. Lin, Tsung-Yi., et al.: Microsoft COCO: common objects in context. In: Fleet, David, Pajdla, Tomas, Schiele, Bernt, Tuytelaars, Tinne (eds.) ECCV 2014. LNCS, vol. 8693, pp. 740–755. Springer, Cham (2014). https://doi.org/10.1007/978-3-319-10602-1_48
17. Liu, L., Lei, W., Wan, X., Liu, L., Luo, Y., Feng, C.: Semi-supervised active learning for Covid-19 lung ultrasound multi-symptom classification. In: 2020 IEEE 32nd International Conference on Tools with Artificial Intelligence (ICTAI), pp. 1268–1273. IEEE (2020)
18. Liu, T., Zhang, H.J., Qi, F.: A novel video key-frame-extraction algorithm based on perceived motion energy model. IEEE TCSVT **13**(10), 1006–1013 (2003)
19. Russakovsky, O., et al.: ImageNet large scale visual recognition challenge. IJCV **115**(3), 211–252 (2015)
20. Samuli, L., Timo, A.: Temporal ensembling for semi-supervised learning. In: International Conference on Learning Representations (ICLR), vol. 4, p. 6 (2017)
21. Selvaraju, R.R., Cogswell, M., Das, A., Vedantam, R., Parikh, D., Batra, D.: Grad-CAM: visual explanations from deep networks via gradient-based localization. In: ICCV, pp. 618–626 (2017)
22. Sohn, K.: Improved deep metric learning with multi-class N-pair loss objective. In: NeurIPS, pp. 1857–1865 (2016)
23. Sohn, K., et al.: FixMatch: simplifying semi-supervised learning with consistency and confidence. arXiv:2001.07685 (2020)
24. Somphone, O., Allaire, S., Mory, B., Dufour, C.: Live feature tracking in ultrasound liver sequences with sparse demons. In: MICCAI Workshop, pp. 53–60 (2014)
25. Vu, Y.N.T., Wang, R., Balachandar, N., Liu, C., Ng, A.Y., Rajpurkar, P.: MedAug: contrastive learning leveraging patient metadata improves representations for chest X-ray interpretation. arXiv:2102.10663 (2021)
26. Yap, M.H., et al.: Automated breast ultrasound lesions detection using convolutional neural networks. IEEE J. Biomed. Health Inform. **22**(4), 1218–1226 (2017)

Identifying Quantitative and Explanatory Tumor Indexes from Dynamic Contrast Enhanced Ultrasound

Peng Wan[1], Chunrui Liu[2], Fang Chen[1], Jing Qin[3], and Daoqiang Zhang[1(✉)]

[1] College of Computer Science and Technology, Nanjing University of Aeronautics and Astronautics, Nanjing, China
dqzhang@nuaa.edu.cn
[2] Department of Ultrasound, Affiliated Drum Tower Hospital, Medical School of Nanjing University, Nanjing, China
[3] School of Nursing, The Hong Kong Polytechnic University,Hung Hom, Hong Kong

Abstract. Contrast-enhanced ultrasound (CEUS) has been one of the most promising imaging techniques in tumor differential diagnosis since the real-time view of intra-tumor blood microcirculation. Existing studies primarily focus on extracting those discriminative imaging features whereas lack medical explanations. However, accurate quantitation of some clinical experience-driven indexes regarding intra-tumor vascularity, such as tumor infiltration and heterogeneity, still faces significant limitations. To tackle this problem, we present a novel scheme to identify quantitative and explanatory tumor indexes from dynamic CEUS sequences. Specifically, our method mainly comprises three steps: 1) extracting the stable pixel-level perfusion pattern from dynamic CEUS imaging using an improved stable principal component pursuit (SPCP) algorithm; 2) performing local perfusion variation comparison by the proposed Phase-constrained Wasserstein (PCW) distance; 3) estimating three clinical knowledge-induced tumor indexes, i.e. infiltration, regularity, and heterogeneity. The effectiveness of this method was evaluated on our collected CEUS dataset of thyroid nodules, and the resulting infiltration and heterogeneity index with $p < 0.05$ between different pathological types validated the efficacy of this quantitation scheme in thyroid nodule diagnosis.

Keywords: Contrast enhanced ultrasound · Perfusion analysis · Quantitative parameters estimation

1 Introduction

As a 'hallmark of cancer', tumor-induced angiogenesis acts as one of the most important biological behaviors by which tumors adapt to the change of nutrient requirement. Since the use of micro-bubble contrast agent, contrast-enhanced

---

P. Wan and C. Liu—These authors contributed equally to this work.

© Springer Nature Switzerland AG 2021
M. de Bruijne et al. (Eds.): MICCAI 2021, LNCS 12908, pp. 638–647, 2021.
https://doi.org/10.1007/978-3-030-87237-3_61

ultrasound (CEUS) provides a real-time visualization of dynamic tissue perfusion around lesion regions, and thus widely applied in differential diagnosis of various types of tumors [1].

Computer-aided analysis of dynamic CEUS imaging is quite challenging due to the following three aspects: Firstly, owing to irregular microbubble destruction during the acquisition of CEUS imaging, the inconsistency of intensity changes at each pixel is inevitable among adjacent temporal points; Secondly, there exists local temporal distortions when comparing pixel-wise perfusion patterns; Thirdly, existing tumor characteristics concluded by clinical experiences are especially qualitative and subjective, lack of precise numerical values for tumor quantitation [2].

Recently, existing studies mainly concentrate on the automated extraction of image features with the 'Black Box' characteristic. For example, traditional quantitative assessments of CEUS imaging rely on regional averaged Time Intensity Curves (TICs) by extracting a number of kinetics parameters. However, these features have no direct link to biological behaviors over tumor progression and lose spatial information. In addition, most machine learning or deep learning-based methods attempt to extract high-dimensional imaging features and learn latent representations, which is hard to be interpreted from a clinical point [3].

Different from previous studies, our study aims at quantifying some clinical experience-driven indexes to aid clinical tumor diagnosis. From the clinical point of view, professional radiologists concluded a few experienced characteristics of dynamic CEUS imaging that are commonly used in daily practices. These non-quantifiable indexes mainly include, lesion infiltration [4], regularity and homogeneity [5]. To the best of our knowledge, quantifying these experience-driven and explanatory tumor indexes from dynamic CEUS imaging has not yet been well studied.

To address these issues, we proposed a novel scheme to identify these quantitative and explanatory tumor indexes from CEUS imaging. The main innovations of this scheme include: 1) an improved Stable Principal Component Pursuit (SPCP) technique is adopted to extract stable pixel-wise perfusion patterns; 2) a novel Phase-constrained Wasserstein Distance (PCW) is proposed for pixel-level perfusion patterns analysis; 3) clinical experience-driven indexes of tumors are quantified based on the derived Area under the curve (AUC) and PCW view.

2   Method

Figure 1 presents a graphical overview of the proposed scheme. Our method consists of three main steps: 1) stable pixel-wise perfusion pattern extraction by the Stable Principal Component Pursuit (SPCP) (Sect. 2.1); 2) pixel-wise perfusion pattern analysis using Phase-constrained Wasserstein Distance (PCW) (Sect. 2.2); and 3) explanatory tumor indexes quantification based on the Area under the curve (AUC) and PCW views (Sect. 2.3).

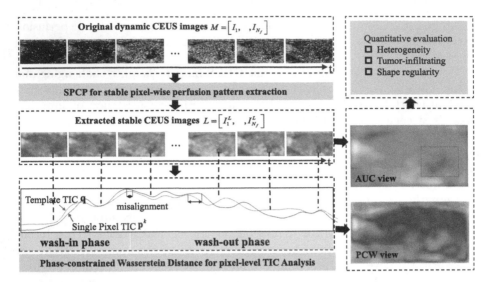

Fig. 1. Graphical overview of the proposed scheme. The input is sequential dynamic CEUS frames M and the output is the quantified tumor indexes which simultaneously preserve the spatial information and have clinical explanation. The overall quantitation process consists of three stages, 1) stable pixel-wise perfusion pattern extraction by the Stable Principal Component Pursuit (SPCP); 2) pixel-wise TIC analysis using Phase-constrained Wasserstein Distance (PCW); 3) explanatory tumor indexes quantification based on the Area under the curve (AUC) and PCW views.

2.1 SPCP for Stable Pixel-Wise Perfusion Pattern Extraction

Pixel-Wise Perfusion Pattern. Given one CEUS sequence $M = [I_1, \ldots, I_{N_f}]$, where I_t is the vectorization of the t_{th} 2D CEUS frame and N_f is the length of the whole perfusion sequence. The k_{th} row of CEUS matrix $\mathbf{p}^k = [p_1^k, \ldots, p_{N_f}^k]$ denotes the Time Intensity Curve (TIC) at the k_{th} pixel ($k = 1, \ldots, N_j$, N_j is the number of pixels in each frame), also called pixel-wise perfusion pattern in this work.

Stable Pixel-Wise Perfusion Pattern Extraction. Although pixel-level TICs provide us an opportunity to evaluate perfusion pattern at the maximal spatial resolution compared with regional TICs, irregular microbubble oscillation or destruction might lead to inconsistent intensity fluctuation among adjacent frames at the pixel level. That is, apparent intensity change is a mixture of inherent microbubble concentration variations caused by intra-tumor blood supply and irregular fluctuations incurred by microbubble disruption. Therefore, an accurate evaluation of pixel-wise perfusion patterns depends on an effective recovery of fluctuation-free pixel-level TICs.

To extract the stable pixel-wise perfusion pattern, we attempt to decompose the original CEUS sequence M into a low rank component $L = [I_1^L, \ldots, I_{N_f}^L]$

(i.e. the slow and smoothing intensity changes) and a sparse component $S = \left[I_1^S, \ldots, I_{N_f}^S\right]$ (i.e. the rapid and irregular intensity fluctuations). In addition, for general CEUS imaging, an additional noise component ($\varepsilon > 0$) also needs to be considered. To accomplish this matrix decomposition, we apply an improved Stable Principal Component Pursuit (SPCP) algorithm [7], which is formulated as,

$$\min_{L,S} \max \left(\|L\|_*, \alpha\|S\|_1\right)$$
$$s.t. \|L + S - M\|_2 \leq \varepsilon \tag{1}$$

where $\|\cdot\|_1$, $\|\cdot\|_2$, and $\|\cdot\|_*$ denote l_1-norm, l_2-norm, and nuclear norm respectively, α is the trade-off parameter which is fine-tuned according to the coefficient of determination R^2 in [6]. Equation(1) is a typical convex optimalization problem which is solved by quasi-Newton method [7]. Accordingly, each row of the solution L is regarded as the stable perfusion pattern at one pixel position.

2.2 Phase-Constrained Wasserstein Distance for Porfuslon Pattern Analysis

Tcmplate Perfusion Pattern. To refine tumor edge extraction and quantify internal heterogeneity, we resort to find a template perfusion pattern $\mathbf{q} = \left[q_1, \ldots, q_{N_f}\right]$, which satisfies that distances between $\mathbf{q}$ and $\mathbf{p}_b^k$ (pixel-wise perfusion patterns from boundary) are nearly to zero as possible, while distances between $\mathbf{q}$ and $\mathbf{p}_t^k$ (those from intratumor) are large enough to quantify the local perfusion variations. Hence, we utilize the average of TICs from the coarse boundary outlined manually as the template $\mathbf{q}$.

Difference of Pixel-Level Perfusion Pattern. The next step is to define an effective distance metric for pixel-wise perfusion pattern comparison, such that local blood supply variation could be highlighted. Ideally, the resulting parametric map based on the new distances between $\mathbf{p}^k$ and $\mathbf{q}$ is able to delineate tumor boundary and reveal internal vascularity distinction. As shown in Fig. 1, local temporal alignment is essential for enhancement degree (i.e., blood supply) comparison since there exist temporal misalignments between pixel-wise TIC, i.e., instances of different sequences in the same temporal position may correspond to different enhancement phases.

Phase-Constrained Wasserstein Distance. Wasserstein distance provides a flexible way to match instances of two sets based on their pair-wise similarity [8]. As for dynamic CEUS sequence comparison, we propose a novel Phase-constrained Wasserstein distance (PCW), where a phase-related temporal regularization is added to ensure that matched intensities are temporally adjacent. Additionally, clinical diagnosis experiences tell us that the phase of contrast agent uptake generally contains more biological behavior information than that of wash-out phase, which suggests that different phases should have different matching flexibilities.

Given $\mathbf{p}^k = \left[p_1^k, \ldots, p_{N_f}^k\right]$ and $\mathbf{q} = [q_1, \ldots, q_{N_f}]$, by viewing intensity p_t^k and q_t as samples drawn from discrete distributions f and g respectively, Wasserstein distance is taken as the metric between TICs. The objective of Wasserstein distance is to find an optimal coupling matrix T (which belongs to $U = \left\{T \in R_+^{N_f \times N_f} | T1_{N_f} = f, T^T 1_{N_f} = g\right\}$) that transport the distribution f to g with the minimal cost. For simplicity, f and g are both viewed as uniform discrete distribution, and $d_{ij} = \left(p_i^k - q_j\right)^2$ is the squared distance between p_i^k and q_i. Thus, Wasserstein distance between TICs is formulated as,

$$d_{wd}\left(\mathbf{p}^k, \mathbf{q}\right) = \sum_{i=1}^{N_f} \sum_{j=1}^{N_f} T_{ij} d_{ij} \tag{2}$$

To encourage temporally adjacent elements to be matched, we introduce the phase-constrained temporal regularization $w\left(T\right)$, where $w\left(T\right) = KL\left(T||Q\right) = \sum_{i=1}^{N} \sum_{j=1}^{N} T_{ij} \log \frac{T_{ij}}{Q_{ij}}$ is the Kullback-Leibler divergence between two coupling matrices. The matrix Q represents the prior distribution of matching weights in T,

$$Q_{ij} = \frac{1}{\sqrt{2\pi\sigma^2}} e^{-\frac{(i-j)^2}{2\sigma^2}} \tag{3}$$

where σ controls the size of nonzero area around the diagonal of Q, and higher value indicates larger local matching flexibility. In order to control matching flexibility for different phases, we partition Q into two submatrices Q_{in} and Q_{out}, $Q = \begin{bmatrix} Q_{in} & 0 \\ 0 & Q_{out} \end{bmatrix}$, where $Q_{in} \in R_+^{N_p \times N_p}$, $Q_{out} \in R_+^{(N_f-N_p) \times (N_f-N_p)}$. N_p denotes Time to Peak (TTP) of template TIC, and interval $[0, N_p]$ and $[N_p, N_f]$ represent the wash-in and wash-out phase, respectively. In this work, we set $\sigma_{in} < \sigma_{out}$ to ensure temporal alignments stricter in wash-in phase. Hence, the proposed Phase-constrained Wasserstein Distance (PCW) is formulated as,

$$PCW\left(\mathbf{p}^k, \mathbf{q}\right) = \min_{T \in U(f,g)} \sum_{i=1}^{N_f} \sum_{j=1}^{N_f} T_{ij} d_{ij} + \lambda KL(T||Q) \tag{4}$$

where λ is the trade-off parameter. The Lagrangian function $L\left(T, f, g\right)$ is written as $L\left(T, \theta, v\right) = \sum_{i=1}^{N} \sum_{j=1}^{N} T_{ij} d_{ij} + \lambda T_{ij} \log \frac{T_{ij}}{Q_{ij}} + \theta^T \left(T1_N - f\right) + v^T \left(T^T 1_N - g\right)$. By setting the derivative $\frac{\partial L}{\partial t_{ij}}$ to zero, we can obtain $T^\lambda = e^{diag\left(-\frac{1}{2} - \frac{\theta}{\lambda}\right)} K e^{diag\left(-\frac{1}{2} - \frac{v}{\lambda}\right)}$, $k_{ij} = e^{-\frac{d'_{ij}}{\lambda}}, d'_{ij} = d_{ij} + \frac{\lambda}{2} \frac{(i-j)^2}{\sigma_{in(out)}^2}$. Motivated by the Sinkhorn distance, the solution of Eq. 4 can be efficiently obtained by matrix scaling algorithm [9].

2.3   PCW and AUC View for Quantifying the Explanatory Tumor Indexes

Tumor Infiltration. First we define the outer-edge of tumor $s(i), i = 1, 2...n_1$, a slightly expanded contour compared with original edge $c(j), j = 1, 2...n_2$, $n_1 \geq n_2$, and then the degree of tumor infiltration is defined as the Dynamic time warping (DTW) divergence of sequences based on AUC view [10], $TI = dtw(s, c)$. The smaller TI means more similar vascular properties around the tumor edge, that is, more evident tumor invasion.

Shape Regularity. Fractal dimension (FD) is widely used to quantify the complexity of geometric forms [11]. In our work, we take the ratio of FD to tumor size S as the degree of shape regularity (SR), $SR = \frac{1}{S} \frac{\log(N_r)}{\log(1/r)}$, where N_r is the number of self-similar shapes and r is the corresponding scaling factor. Apparently, higher SR value represents less shape regularity.

Perfusion Heterogeneity. We utilize the image entropy of tumor region based on AUC or PCW view to measure internal perfusion heterogeneity [12]. Similarly, the value of entropy is normalized by the size of tumor S, $PH = -\frac{1}{S} \sum_i w_i \log w_i$, where w_i is the statistical frequency of tumor area. By the definition, larger PH value indicates that vascularity distributions within tumor region are more heterogeneous.

3   Experimental Setup and Evaluation

Dataset. Our dataset is a collection of 55 consecutive patients (Gender, F/M = 35/20; Age, 45.8 ± 12.3 years) attending Affiliated Drum Tower Hospital, Medical School of Nanjing University for thyroid nodules examination from September 2016 to July 2018. Only solitary nodules are included in this study. Three pathological types of nodules were incorporated, i.e., 17 Nodular Goiter, 19 Adenoma, and 19 Papillary Thyroid Carcinoma. The average maximum diameter of nodules is 19.5 ± 7.1 mm. All patients were examined by an expert radiologist with over 10-year clinical experience. Examinations were performed on a Logiq E9 ultrasound scanner (GE Healthcare, Milwaukee, WI, USA) with the second-generation microbubble contrast SonoVue at a low mechanical index (0.05–0.08). Pathologies results of all cases were confirmed by biopsy or surgical specimens. Each video lasts around 3 min with a frame rate of 15 fps and the spatial resolution of dual-view imaging is 600 × 800 pixels, where conventional gray-level view and contrast-specific view are displayed side by side. Approval was obtained by the ethics review board of local hospital and the informed consent was obtained from patients before this study.

Experimental Setup. In order to obtain a reliable quantitative analysis results, standard pre-processing steps were performed on raw video data, including motion correction, co-registration, and speckle noise reduction [13], etc. In our experiments, part of the beginning frames (the uptake of contrast agent has not yet started) and ending frames (the concentration of contrast agents no longer declines) were removed from raw videos. For pixel-wise perfusion pattern extraction using Stable Principal Component Pursuit, the balancing parameter α was set around $\frac{1}{\sqrt{m \times n}}$ (where m and n are the width and height of CEUS view). The optimal α value was chosen based on the coefficient of determination R^2 in [6]. ε was fixed to 0.05 for noise component. For Phase-constrained Wasserstein Distance, σ_{in} and σ_{out} control the expected bandwidth of warping for wash-in and wash-out phase, respectively. We set σ_{in} and σ_{out} to 0.75 and 1.5 in this study, which were fine-tuned ranging from 0.25 to 5 with the gap of 0.25. The optimal values are determined when the mean distance between $\mathbf{q}$ and $\mathbf{p}_b^k$ is nearly to zero as possible. As for temporal regularization, we chose $\lambda = 5$ to balance the matching flexibility and the temporal constraint.

3.1 Evaluation of the Quantified Tumor Indexes

To evaluate the validity of our proposed quantitative clinical experience-driven indexes in tumor differential diagnosis, we compared tumor infiltration(TI), shape regularity(SR) and perfusion heterogeneity(PH) from the perspective of benign and malignancy nodules and three pathological subtypes.

Table 1. Quantitative parameters. Except for SR, the other two indexes TI and PH (heterogeneity based on AUC and PCW parametric map respectively) show significant difference between benign and malignant nodules (p $\leq$ 0.05)

Indexes	Benign	Malignant	p-value
Infiltration (TI)	3.09 ± 1.59	2.41 ± 0.81	0.04
Shape regularity (SR)	1.18 ± 0.73	1.33 ± 0.78	>0.05
Heterogeneity (PH from AUC)	3.84 ± 2.03	5.95 ± 3.68	0.03
Heterogeneity (PH from PCW)	3.56 ± 1.79	6.46 ± 4.21	0.01

First, Student t-test was performed to check for a significant difference between benign and malignant nodules, and the results are listed in Table 1. As can be observed, heterogeneity derived from PCW parametric map shows stronger discrimination than that estimated from AUC view, which confirms that PCW has the ability to characterize the pixel-level perfusion difference, leading to an effective perfusion index for differentiating benign and malignant nodules. Second, we further assess the quantitative indexes among three pathological types, Fig. 2 shows the boxplot of the three parameters, among which, degree of perfusion heterogeneity is calculated both on AUC and PCW maps.

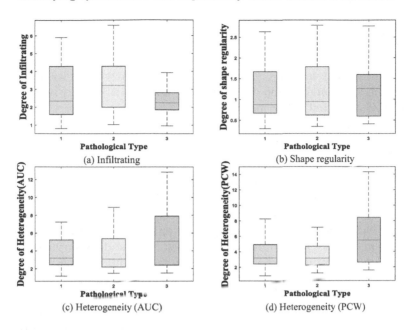

Fig. 2. Boxplots for values of three quantitative indexes among 1-Nodular Goiter, 2-Thyroid Adenoma, and 3-Papillary Thyroid Carcinoma.

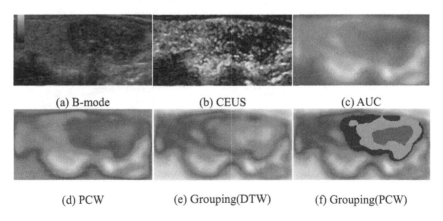

Fig. 3. A visualization of CEUS data and parametric maps, red line marks the manually outlined boundary. (a) B-mode gray-scale image I_{gs}; (b) Contrast-enhanced imaging I_t; (c–e) Parametric maps based on various estimated parameters; (f) Grouping result based on PCW view;

As for TI, the value of Papillary Thyroid Carcinoma is significantly smaller than Nodular Goiter and Thyroid Adenoma. Regarding benign nodules, Nodular Goiter has slightly stronger invasion than Thyroid Adenoma. Comparatively, shape of regularity is less discriminative among different pathological types.

Finally, Fig. 3 provides a visualization of tumor infiltration, shape regularity, heterogeneity and grouping results with the same spatial resolution as original CEUS. Apparently, PCW based map improved the enhancement along the boundary of nodule, meanwhile, in terms of internal heterogeneity, more abundant details on hemodynamic distribution of nodules is marked in PCW view than that of AUC and DTW maps.

4   Conclusion

We presented a novel scheme for the quantitative evaluation of dynamic CEUS imaging. In this framework, we first apply stable principal component pursuit to extract stable and smoothing perfusion pattern at each pixel, then utilize the proposed Phase-constrained Wasserstein distance to refine tumor delineation extraction and derive the parametric map (i.e., AUC and PCW view) with the same spatial resolution, and finally introduces three clinical experience-induced indexes for quantitative perfusion analysis. Currently, template TIC is determined by pixel-wise TICs from initial manually outlined boundary, which might degrade the eventual quantitation performance. It could be a promising direction to unify tumor boundary and internal heterogeneity information into template TIC selection in the future work.

Acknowledgement. This work was supported by the National Natural Science Foundation of China (Nos. 62136004, 61876082, 61732006, 61901214, U20A20389), the General Research Fund from Hong Kong Research Grants Council (Nos. 15205919), the National Key R&D Program of China (Grant Nos. 2018YFC2001600, 2018YF C2001602), the Nanjing Medical Science and Technique Development Foundation (Nos. YKK19054), and also by the CAAI-Huawei MindSpore Open Fund.

References

1. Jiang, Y., Zhou, Q., Zhu, C.: Contrast-enhanced ultrasound in the diagnosis of benign and malignant hepatic tumors. J. Cent. South Univ. Med. Sci. **37**(1), 53–60 (2012)
2. Balleyguier, C., et al.: New potential and applications of contrast-enhanced ultrasound of the breast: Own investigations and review of the literature. Eur. J. Radiol. **69**(1), 14–23 (2009)
3. Moon, W.K., Chen, I.L., Chang, J., Shin, S., Lo, C., Chang, R.: The adaptive computer-aided diagnosis system based on tumor sizes for the classification of breast tumors detected at screening ultrasound. Ultrasonics **76**, 70–77 (2017)
4. Wang, Y.M., Fan, W., Zhao, S., Zhang, K., Zhang, L., Zhang, P., et al.: Qualitative quantitative and combination score systems in differential diagnosis of breast lesions by contrast-enhanced ultrasound. Eur. J. Radiol. **85**(1), 48–54 (2016)
5. Hocke, M., Schulze, E., Gottschalk, P., Topalidis, T., Dietrich, C.F.: Contrast-enhanced endoscopic ultrasound in discrimination between focal pancreatitis and pancreatic cancer. World J. Gastroenterol. **12**(2), 246–50 (2006)

6. Christofides, D., Leen, E., Averkiou, M.A.: Automatic respiratory gating for contrast ultrasound evaluation of liver lesions. IEEE Trans. Ultrason. Ferroelectr. Freq. Control **61**(1), 25–32 (2014)
7. Aravkin, A., Becker, S., Cevher, V., Olsen, P.: A variational approach to stable principal component pursuit. In: Proceedings of the Thirtieth Conference on Uncertainty in Artificial Intelligence, UAI, vol. 2014, pp. 32–41 (2014)
8. Bing, S., Hua, G.: Order-preserving Wasserstein distance for sequence matching. In: Proceedings of the IEEE Conference on Computer Vision and Pattern Recognition, CVPR, vol. 2017, pp. 1049–1057 (2017)
9. Cuturi, M.: Sinkhorn distances: lightspeed computation of optimal transport. In: Proceedings of the 27th Annual Conference on Neural Information Processing Systems, NIPS 2013, pp. 2292–2300 (2013)
10. Keogh, E.J., Ratanamahatana, C.: Exact indexing of dynamic time warping. Knowl. Inf. Syst. **7**(3), 358–386 (2003)
11. Balankin, A.S., Ochoa, D.S., Miguel, I.A., Ortiz, J.: Fractal topology of hand-crumpled paper. Phys. Rev. E **81**(6), 11–26 (2010)
12. Yanai, K., Barnard, K.: Image region entropy: a measure of visualness of web images associated with one concept. In: Proceedings of the 13th ACM International Conference on Multimedia, ACM 2005, pp. 419–422 (2005)
13. Coupé, P., Hellier, P., Kervrann, C., Barillot, C.: Nonlocal means-based speckle filtering for ultrasound images. IEEE Trans. Image Process. **18**(10), 2221–2229 (2009)

Weakly-Supervised Ultrasound Video Segmentation with Minimal Annotations

Ruiheng Chang[1,5], Dong Wang[2], Haiyan Guo[4], Jia Ding[3], and Liwei Wang[1,2(✉)]

[1] Center for Data Science, Peking University, Beijing, China
{changrh,wanglw}@pku.edu.cn
[2] Key Laboratory of Machine Perception, MOE, School of EECS, Peking University, Beijing, China
wangdongcis@pku.edu.cn
[3] Yizhun Medical AI Co., Ltd, Beijing, China
jia.ding@yizhun-ai.com
[4] The First Affiliated Hospital of Zhengzhou University, Zhengzhou, China
fccguohy@zzu.edu.cn
[5] Zhejiang Lab, Zhejiang, China

Abstract. Ultrasound segmentation models provide powerful tools for the diagnosis process of ultrasound examinations. However, developing such models for ultrasound videos requires densely annotated segmentation masks of all frames in a dataset, which is unpractical and unaffordable. Therefore, we propose a weakly-supervised learning (WSL) approach to accomplish the goal of video-based ultrasound segmentation. By only annotating the location of the start and end frames of the lesions, we obtain frame-level binary labels for WSL. We design Video Co-Attention Network to learn the correspondence between frames, where CAM and co-CAM will be obtained to perform lesion localization. Moreover, we find that the essential factor to the success of extracting video-level information is applying our proposed consistency regularization between CAM and co-CAM. Our method achieves an mIoU score of 45.43% in the breast ultrasound dataset, which significantly outperforms the baseline methods. The codes of our models will be released.

Keywords: Ultrasound · Weakly-supervised · Segmentation

1 Introduction

Ultrasound is an imaging method that uses high-frequency sound waves to generate images reflecting the body's condition. It has a wide range of applications,

---

R. Chang, D. Wang and H. Guo—Equal contribution.

Electronic supplementary material The online version of this chapter (https://doi.org/10.1007/978-3-030-87237-3_62) contains supplementary material, which is available to authorized users.

such as examining breast lesions, evaluating blood flow, diagnosing gallbladder disease, and prenatal screening [12,17]. Finding and analyzing lesions is one of the primary purposes of ultrasound examination.

In order to obtain a deep model for video lesion segmentation, the regular pipeline (Fig. 2(a)) includes two steps: a) Annotating pixel-level lesion masks of all frames in a collected ultrasound video dataset. b) Training a model for video-based lesion segmentation. Whereas the difficulties lie in the labeling step. Ultrasound can only be labeled by qualified experts and it is also unpractical and unaffordable to annotate a dataset in detail which is large enough for each kind of the examinations. Consequently, most literature about ultrasound analysis work on processing static ultrasound image [6], and that of ultrasound video is absent.

In this paper, we propose a weakly-supervised learning (WSL) approach to accomplish the goal of automatic video-based ultrasound segmentation.

Firstly, we propose an efficient labeling strategy that accommodates WSL for ultrasound video data. In our method, annotators are only required to label the start and end frame of each lesion (Fig. 2(b)), then we can

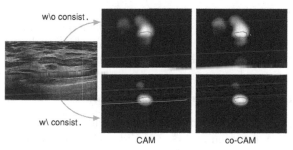

Fig. 1. Visualization of CAM and co-CAM. Above: without consistency loss; Below: with consistency loss. The red contours are ground-truth segmentations (Color figure online).

obtain the information about whether each frame contains a lesion.

Then, we propose to leverage video-level information to conduct WSL for ultrasound segmentation. We propose Video Co-Attention Network to learn the correspondences across frames. In addition to classifying each frame separately (to generate CAM), the network also learns to identify the co-existing lesions across different frames in a video and thereby generates co-attentive CAM (co-CAM). However, the visualization results show that the masks of CAM and co-CAM are obviously larger than the ground-truth (Fig. 1). By analyzing the properties of CAM and co-CAM, we conclude that co-CAM tends to make aggressive predictions on regions with correspondences across frames while CAM usually makes conservative predictions. Therefore, we apply pixel-wise consistency regularization across CAM and co-CAM. Benefiting from the consistency regularization, unnecessary correlations in co-CAM are suppressed by the supervision of CAM, and the improved co-CAM leads to higher quality features for CAM through co-attention module. In consequence, CAM and co-CAM improve jointly (see Fig. 1).

Experimental results validate the effectiveness of our proposed method. We collect an ultrasound dataset with 1565 video fragments to evaluate our method.

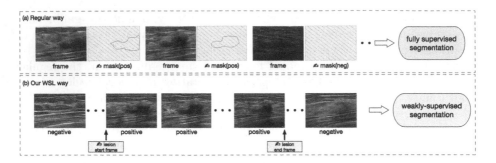

Fig. 2. Process of annotating data to train the segmentation model.

Our method achieves 45.43% mIoU in the test set, which significantly outperforms the single-image baselines. We also conduct several ablation studies and the results prove that the consistency regularization plays an essential role in the network.

Our contributions can be summarized as follows:

- We propose a novel labeling method for weakly-supervised ultrasound video segmentation and design Video Co-Attention Network for this task.
- By analyzing the behaviors of CAM and co-CAM, we propose consistency regularization between them, which brings significant improvement.

2   Related Work

2.1   Weakly Supervised Semantic Segmentation

Labeling segmentation masks is an expensive process, so weakly-supervised semantic segmentation (WSSS) is proposed to reduce the labeling cost. Currently, most image-level WSSS methods are based on Class Activation Maps (CAM) [28]. CAM identifies the most informative regions for the classification task. However, CAM tends to be incomplete for large-scale objects and imprecise for small-scale objects [1]. Numerous attempts have been made to improve the performance of CAM such as "seed and expand" strategy [7,9,21,28], "erasing" method [5,8,19] and saliency models [7,11,21–23]. There are also two other methods related to our approach. Araslanov and Roth [1] propose normalised Global Weighted Pooling (nGWP). Sun *et al.* [20] address the importance of cross-image semantic relation.

2.2   Automatic Ultrasound Analysis

Ultrasound is a medical examination with huge demand, where the computer-aided diagnosis system is expected to assist the analysis process. Recently, deep learning methods for ultrasound analysis are applied to various types of anatomical structures, such as breast [3,26], liver [2], thyroid [15] and kidney [27]. To conduct lesion segmentation, typical methods employ 2D segmentation network (*e.g.* U-Net [18]), which deals with static ultrasound images [6]. The disadvantage is that 2D network is not designed for video data and only works in controlled settings with high-quality images [24].

While in this paper, we provide a solution to the online ultrasound analysis for ultrasound video streams, where only limited annotation effort is required. Therefore, our setting is more meaningful for clinical usage.

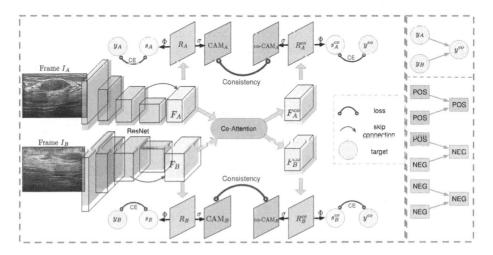

Fig. 3. Overview of our proposed Video Co-attention Network. The right part shows the strategy of label assignment for y^{co}.

3   Methodology

The general pipeline of WSSS includes three steps: *1) Training a classification network that can discover the most discriminative foreground regions (e.g. CAM). 2) Generating pseudo masks on the training set. 3) Training a segmentation model supervised by the pseudo masks.*

Our method follows the same pipeline while improving each step for our ultrasound task. We will introduce our method in the following sections.

3.1   Correspondence Reasoning for WSSS

Compared with common WSSS datasets with natural images, there are two obstacles existing in ultrasound dataset, which increase the difficulties of WSSS:

- Objects (*i.e.* lesions) in ultrasound are much smaller than those in natural images and have more ambiguous boundaries.
- Image-level class labels can only provide extremely limited information in ultrasound since there's only one category (the lesion) in ultrasound data.

To overcome these problems, we introduce Video Co-Attention Network. Figure 3 illustrates an overview of the network.

Video Co-attention Network. Co-attention module is a powerful tool for building correlations of different images [13,14,20,25]. We adopt the co-attention module to enable the network to find the co-existing image patterns of the frames (lesion regions), while suppressing the activations of the regions without correlation findings (*i.e.* background regions).

Specifically, as shown in Fig. 3, for frame I_A and I_B from the same video with binary labels $y_A, y_B \in \{0, 1\}$, they are processed by backbone network and output feature maps $F_A, F_B \in \mathbb{R}^{C \times H \times W}$. Then, we use a convolution layer to squeeze the channel of F_A and F_B to 1 and get R_A and R_B, which represent the responses of the foreground class. Then, an aggregation function Φ is applied to R_A and R_B and outputs the class score scalars s_A and s_B, respectively. The form of Φ will be introduced in Sect. 3.2. Then, the sigmoid cross entropy (CE) loss is applied to supervise the class scores:

$$L_{\mathrm{CAM}}(I_A, I_B) = CE(s_A, y_A) + CE(s_B, y_B) \tag{1}$$

To obtain the CAMs, we apply *Sigmoid* activation function $\sigma(x) = \frac{1}{1+e^{-x}}$ to the response feature maps R_A and R_B.

Besides the regular CAM branch, our model also learns to predict whether there is a lesion co-exists in the two frames I_A and I_B. In order to do this, we first apply co-attention module to F_A and F_B. The co-attention module obtains the affinity matrix P by

$$P = F_A^\top W_P F_B \in \mathbb{R}^{HW \times HW} \tag{2}$$

where F_A and F_B are flattened with shape $C \times HW$, and W_P is learnable. Each element in the affinity matrix P represent the relation between a location pair in F_A and F_B. Then, we apply row-wise and column-wise softmax operations to P and multiply the outputs with F_B and F_A respectively to get the co-attentive features F_A^{co} and F_B^{co}. Then the co-attentive response feature maps R_A^{co} and R_B^{co} can be obtained after a convolution layer. Then we can calculate the co-attentive class score s_A^{co} and s_B^{co} using the same manner of s_A and s_B. The supervision of co-attentive class score is by *and* operation, *i.e.*, $y^{\mathrm{co}} = y_A \wedge y_B$. Hence, the loss function of co-attentive branch is

$$L_{\mathrm{co\text{-}CAM}}(I_A, I_B) = CE(s_A^{\mathrm{co}}, y^{\mathrm{co}}) + CE(s_B^{\mathrm{co}}, y^{\mathrm{co}}) \tag{3}$$

Here, we name the CAM generated after co-attention operation as co-CAM, which can be extracted using a similar way with CAM.

The overall training loss is the summation of L_{CAM} and $L_{\mathrm{co\text{-}CAM}}$.

Consistency of CAM and co-CAM. CAM and co-CAM are introduced to locate discriminate regions of ultrasound frames. However, the design of co-CAM barely brings an improvement (See Table 2 for detail). By visualizing the results (Fig. 1), we find that both CAM and co-CAM frequently predict larger masks than the ground-truth masks, which leads to lower precision.

To tackle this problem, we first analyze the properties of CAM and co-CAM intuitively. CAM and co-CAM have different behaviors. CAM identifies the trustable regions only from the information of individual frames, hence tends to make relatively conservative predictions only on the regions with high confidence. On the contrary, co-CAM extracts information using relevant frames, which means co-CAM can recognize not only the most discriminative areas but also regions with correspondences across different frames, and finally makes relatively aggressive predictions. Above viewpoint is supported by the experimental results that the CAM has higher precision but lower recall than co-CAM (The first line in Table 2).

To obtain tight masks with higher precision, we apply pixel-wise consistency regularization across CAM and co-CAM. Consistency loss is defined as following:

$$
\begin{aligned}
L_{\text{consist}} = {} & \mathbb{I}(\boldsymbol{y}^{\text{co}} = 1) \cdot MSE(\text{CAM}_A, \text{co-CAM}_A) \\
& + \mathbb{I}(\boldsymbol{y}^{\text{co}} = 1) \cdot MSE(\text{CAM}_B, \text{co-CAM}_B)
\end{aligned}
\tag{4}
$$

where MSE is the mean square loss and $\mathbb{I}$ is the identity function. Note that we only apply consistency loss on positive frame pairs (*i.e.* $\boldsymbol{y}^{\text{co}} = 1$) since the target co-CAMs for negative ones are empty.

Benefiting from the consistency regularization, the unnecessary correlations in co-CAM are suppressed by the supervision of CAM. Meanwhile, since the features of co-CAM are extracted by co-attention module from the features of CAM, the improved co-CAM also encourages the CAM to predict masks with higher precision. In consequence, CAM and co-CAM promote each other and improve in a joint manner. After adding the consistency loss, the loss function can be summarized as: (λ is the weight of consistency loss.)

$$
L_{\text{total}} = L_{\text{CAM}} + L_{\text{co-CAM}} + \lambda \cdot L_{\text{consist}}
\tag{5}
$$

3.2 Structure of Classification Network

In ultrasound data, lesions usually occupy only a small proportion of the image. Therefore, we adopt several practical designs for better performance of small objects on our network such as smaller down-sample rate and *normalised Global Weighted Pooling* (nGWP) [1]

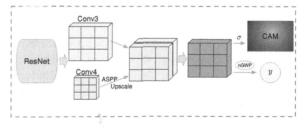

Fig. 4. Structure of the classification network.

aggregation function Φ to enable size-invariant masks predictions. The network structure is illustrated in Fig. 4.

$$
\Phi(\boldsymbol{R}) = \frac{\sum_{h,w} \boldsymbol{R}_{h,w} \cdot \sigma(\boldsymbol{R}_{h,w})}{\epsilon + \sum_{h,w} \sigma(\boldsymbol{R}_{h,w})}
\tag{6}
$$

3.3   Lesion Segmentation

In our WSSS pipeline, once the video co-attention network is trained, we generate pseudo masks for the train set and train the video segmentation network.

Pseudo Mask Generation. We use co-CAM to generate pseudo masks since co-CAM takes advantage of video-level information and achieves higher localization performance than CAM. For each frame I with positive annotation, we first uniformly sample N positive frames $\{I_i\}_{i=1}^{N}$ from the frames that contain the same lesion, and then compute $L_{\text{co-CAM}}(I, I_i)$ for all N frames. $L_{\text{co-CAM}}(I, I_i)$ reflects the strength of correlation between I and I_i. As the loss becomes smaller, the correlation become stronger. Hence, we select top K frames and ensemble the co-CAMs between I and the K frames for final pseudo masks. Here we use pixel-wise max operation for the ensemble procedure.

Table 1. Compare with baselines. The metric is mIoU (%).

Method	Pseudo masks (Val)	Seg (Test)
CAM [28]	10.91	18.90
Improved CAM	35.27	39.36
Video Co-Attention Network(ours)	**44.82**	**45.43**

Video Segmentation Network. The last step is training a video segmentation network with the supervision of generated pseudo masks. We adopt 3DC-SEG [16] for this task, which is state-of-the-art model for video object segmentation. 3D ResNet-34 is used as the backbone.

4   Experiments

4.1   Dataset and Metric

Dataset Description. We collect an in-house breast ultrasound dataset with 1565 videos. The average duration of these videos is 96.40 s, with 30 frames per second. More details are shown in the supplementary material. For the train and validation set, the start frames and end frames for the appearances of lesions are annotated by experts. We annotate segmentation masks for one frame within each lesion in the validation and test set to evaluate the performance. We report the performance of pseudo masks on the validation set, while the final segmentation performance is evaluated on the test set.

Evaluation Metric. We adopt the mean Intersection over Union (mIoU) criterion to evaluate the segmentation performance. If not specified, we report the performance of co-CAM on the validation set. We also report Precision and Recall in the ablation studies to analyze the behaviors of CAM and co-CAM.

4.2   Implementation Details

We adopt ResNet-34 [4] as the backbone network. We train the model on 8 TITAN RTX GPU cards for 30k iterations with 64 frame pairs per batch. We adopt ADAM optimizer [10] with $\beta_1 = 0.9$, $\beta_2 = 0.999$, and the learning rate starts from 1e−4, which is reduced by a factor of 0.1 after 20k iterations. If not specified, the weight of consistency loss is set to $\lambda = 10.0$, and the hyper-parameters of pseudo mask generation are set to $N = 10$ and $K = 3$.

4.3   Comparisons with Baselines

Considering that there is no existing work studying the problem of weakly-supervised video segmentation in our setting, we compare our method with two single image baselines:

- **CAM.** We directly use the method in [28] to generate pseudo masks and train the segmentation network (*i e* 3DC SEC).
- **Improved CAM.** We add the method we discussed in Sect. 3.2 to improve the performance of CAM baseline. This baseline is actually a degeneration of our method by removing the co-attention module and co-CAM.

Table 2. Ablation study: weight (λ).

λ	CAM			co-CAM		
	mIoU	Prec.	Recall.	mIoU	Prec.	Recall.
0	35.91	53.34	70.56	35.03	48.40	76.92
0.5	36.34	53.47	71.55	36.03	47.69	79.74
1.0	39.12	58.53	70.75	36.50	49.66	77.15
5.0	41.67	62.69	71.81	41.47	55.15	79.40
10.0	**43.45**	64.38	70.85	**44.52**	64.69	70.79
20.0	36.96	74.49	50.88	38.45	71.75	55.99
50.0	36.73	78.95	47.55	37.36	76.45	50.37

Table 3. Ablation study: downsample rates.

Conv2	Conv3	Conv4	Downsample	mIoU
		✓	16×	41.32
	✓		8×	39.63
	✓	✓	8×	**44.82**
✓	✓		4×	30.23
✓		✓	4×	31.45

The results are shown in Table 1. The performance of the CAM baseline is 10.91 for pseudo masks and 18.90 for segmentation, which is unsatisfying for practical usage. The improved CAM baseline outperforms CAM baseline by a large margin, which may be contributed by the enhanced expressive power of small objects. However, these two baselines only use single image information and ignore the correspondence between frames. By leveraging video-level information, our method achieves significant improvement compared to the baselines and reaches an mIoU score of 45.43 on the test set. We show the qualitative results in the supplementary material.

4.4   Ablation Study

In this section, we study the contributions of each component in our design. We compare the performance of pseudo masks generation on the validation set. More results can be found in the supplementary material.

Consistency Loss. The consistency regularization is an essential component to the success of extracting visual correspondence across frames. We study the behaviors of CAM and co-CAM with different weights of consistency loss (λ) in Table 2. Without consistency loss (*i.e.* $\lambda = 0$), the mIoUs of CAM and co-CAM are similar to the improved CAM baseline in Table 1. Meanwhile, the precision of co-CAM is slightly lower than that of CAM, which shows that the co-CAM has more aggressive predictions than CAM and confirms our conjecture in Sect. 3.1.

The non-consistent CAM and co-CAM are with low precision. By increasing the value of λ, the precision of both CAM and co-CAM grow in unison. The results are in line with our intuition that the consistency regularization promotes both CAM and co-CAM with tighter masks and higher precision. In our experiments, we achieve a trade-off between precision and recall when $\lambda = 10.0$, and obtain the highest mIoU score 44.52, which is an improvement of 9.49 mIoU score compared with non-consistent co-CAM.

Downsample Scales. In Sect. 3.2, we use a lower downsample rate to enlarge the resolution of outputs feature maps, which aims at more accurate segmentation for small lesions. We evaluate the performance of different downsample scales in Table 3. In the experiments, the 8x downsample rate implemented by combining Conv3 and Conv4 achieves the best performance.

5   Conclusion

In this paper, we discuss the problem of weakly-supervised learning for ultrasound video segmentation. We propose Video Co-Attention Network for this task and apply consistency regularization for more precise predictions. Our work is a successful attempt. Future work could include:

- Refining the boundaries of lesions masks.
- Exploring to leverage annotations with richer information (*e.g.* boxes).

Acknowledgement. This work was supported by National Key R&D Program of China (2018YFB1402600), Key-Area Research and Development Program of Guangdong Province (No. 2019B121204008), BJNSF (L172037), Beijing Academy of Artificial Intelligence, Project 2020BD006 supported by PKU-Baidu Fund.

References

1. Araslanov, N., Roth, S.: Single-stage semantic segmentation from image labels. In: Proceedings of the IEEE/CVF Conference on Computer Vision and Pattern Recognition, pp. 4253–4262 (2020)

2. Biswas, M., et al.: Symtosis: a liver ultrasound tissue characterization and risk stratification in optimized deep learning paradigm. Comput. Meth. Prog. Biomed. **155**, 165–177 (2018)
3. Han, S., et al.: A deep learning framework for supporting the classification of breast lesions in ultrasound images. Phys. Med. Biol. **62**(19), 7714 (2017)
4. He, K., Zhang, X., Ren, S., Sun, J.: Deep residual learning for image recognition. In: Proceedings of the IEEE Conference on Computer Vision and Pattern Recognition, pp. 770–778 (2016)
5. Hou, Q., Jiang, P., Wei, Y., Cheng, M.M.: Self-erasing network for integral object attention. In: Advances in Neural Information Processing Systems, pp. 549–559 (2018)
6. Huang, Q., Huang, Y., Luo, Y., Yuan, F., Li, X.: Segmentation of breast ultrasound image with semantic classification of superpixels. Med. Image Anal. **61**, 101657 (2020)
7. Huang, Z., Wang, X., Wang, J., Liu, W., Wang, J.: Weakly-supervised semantic segmentation network with deep seeded region growing. In: Proceedings of the IEEE Conference on Computer Vision and Pattern Recognition, pp. 7014–7023 (2018)
8. Jing, L., Chen, Y., Tian, Y.: Coarse-to-fine semantic segmentation from image-level labels. IEEE Trans. Image Process. **29**, 225–236 (2019)
9. Khoreva, A., Benenson, R., Hosang, J., Hein, M., Schiele, B.: Simple does it: weakly supervised instance and semantic segmentation. In: Proceedings of the IEEE Conference on Computer Vision and Pattern Recognition, pp. 876–885 (2017)
10. Kingma, D.P., Ba, J.: Adam: a method for stochastic optimization. arXiv preprint arXiv:1412.6980 (2014)
11. Lee, J., Kim, E., Lee, S., Lee, J., Yoon, S.: FickleNet: weakly and semi-supervised semantic image segmentation using stochastic inference. In: Proceedings of the IEEE Conference on Computer Vision and Pattern Recognition, pp. 5267–5276 (2019)
12. Liu, S., et al.: Deep learning in medical ultrasound analysis: a review. Engineering **5**(2), 261–275 (2019)
13. Lu, J., Yang, J., Batra, D., Parikh, D.: Hierarchical question-image co-attention for visual question answering. In: Advances in Neural Information Processing Systems, pp. 289–297 (2016)
14. Lu, X., Wang, W., Ma, C., Shen, J., Shao, L., Porikli, F.: See more, know more: unsupervised video object segmentation with co-attention Siamese networks. In: Proceedings of the IEEE Conference on Computer Vision and Pattern Recognition, pp. 3623–3632 (2019)
15. Ma, J., Wu, F., Jiang, T., Zhu, J., Kong, D.: Cascade convolutional neural networks for automatic detection of thyroid nodules in ultrasound images. Med. Phys. **44**(5), 1678–1691 (2017)
16. Mahadevan, S., Athar, A., Ošep, A., Hennen, S., Leal-Taixé, L., Leibe, B.: Making a case for 3D convolutions for object segmentation in videos. arXiv preprint arXiv:2008.11516 (2020)
17. Reddy, U.M., Filly, R.A., Copel, J.A.: Prenatal imaging: ultrasonography and magnetic resonance imaging. Obstet. Gynecol. **112**(1), 145 (2008)
18. Ronneberger, O., Fischer, P., Brox, T.: U-Net: convolutional networks for biomedical image segmentation. In: Navab, N., Hornegger, J., Wells, W.M., Frangi, A.F. (eds.) MICCAI 2015. LNCS, vol. 9351, pp. 234–241. Springer, Cham (2015). https://doi.org/10.1007/978-3-319-24574-4_28

19. Singh, K.K., Lee, Y.J.: Hide-and-seek: forcing a network to be meticulous for weakly-supervised object and action localization. In: 2017 IEEE International Conference on Computer Vision (ICCV), pp. 3544–3553. IEEE (2017)
20. Sun, G., Wang, W., Dai, J., Van Gool, L.: Mining cross-image semantics for weakly supervised semantic segmentation. arXiv preprint arXiv:2007.01947 (2020)
21. Wang, X., You, S., Li, X., Ma, H.: Weakly-supervised semantic segmentation by iteratively mining common object features. In: Proceedings of the IEEE Conference on Computer Vision and Pattern Recognition, pp. 1354–1362 (2018)
22. Wei, Y., Feng, J., Liang, X., Cheng, M.M., Zhao, Y., Yan, S.: Object region mining with adversarial erasing: a simple classification to semantic segmentation approach. In: Proceedings of the IEEE Conference on Computer Vision and Pattern Recognition, pp. 1568–1576 (2017)
23. Wei, Y., Xiao, H., Shi, H., Jie, Z., Feng, J., Huang, T.S.: Revisiting dilated convolution: a simple approach for weakly-and semi-supervised semantic segmentation. In: Proceedings of the IEEE Conference on Computer Vision and Pattern Recognition, pp. 7268–7277 (2018)
24. Xian, M., Zhang, Y., Cheng, H.D., Xu, F., Zhang, B., Ding, J.: Automatic breast ultrasound image segmentation: a survey. Pattern Recogn. **79**, 340–355 (2018)
25. Xiong, C., Zhong, V., Socher, R.: Dynamic coattention networks for question answering. arXiv preprint arXiv:1611.01604 (2016)
26. Yap, M.H., et al.: Automated breast ultrasound lesions detection using convolutional neural networks. IEEE J. Biomed. Health Inform. **22**(4), 1218–1226 (2017)
27. Yin, S., et al.: Multi-instance deep learning with graph convolutional neural networks for diagnosis of kidney diseases using ultrasound imaging. In: Greenspan, H., et al. (eds.) CLIP/UNSURE -2019. LNCS, vol. 11840, pp. 146–154. Springer, Cham (2019). https://doi.org/10.1007/978-3-030-32689-0_15
28. Zhou, B., Khosla, A., Lapedriza, A., Oliva, A., Torralba, A.: Learning deep features for discriminative localization. In: Proceedings of the IEEE Conference on Computer Vision and Pattern Recognition, pp. 2921–2929 (2016)

Content-Preserving Unpaired Translation from Simulated to Realistic Ultrasound Images

Devavrat Tomar[1], Lin Zhang[1(✉)], Tiziano Portenier[1], and Orcun Goksel[1,2]

[1] Computer-Assisted Applications in Medicine, ETH Zurich, Zurich, Switzerland
lin.zhang@vision.ee.ethz.ch
[2] Department of Information Technology, Uppsala University, Uppsala, Sweden

Abstract. Interactive simulation of ultrasound imaging greatly facilitates sonography training. Although ray-tracing based methods have shown promising results, obtaining realistic images requires substantial modeling effort and manual parameter tuning. In addition, current techniques still result in a significant appearance gap between simulated images and real clinical scans. Herein we introduce a novel *content-preserving* image translation framework (ConPres) to bridge this appearance gap, while maintaining the simulated anatomical layout. We achieve this goal by leveraging both simulated images with semantic segmentations and unpaired in-vivo ultrasound scans. Our framework is based on recent contrastive unpaired translation techniques and we propose a regularization approach by learning an auxiliary segmentation-to-real image translation task, which encourages the disentanglement of content and style. In addition, we extend the generator to be class-conditional, which enables the incorporation of additional losses, in particular a cyclic consistency loss, to further improve the translation quality. Qualitative and quantitative comparisons against state-of-the-art unpaired translation methods demonstrate the superiority of our proposed framework.

Keywords: Image translation · US simulation · Contrastive learning

1 Introduction

Ultrasound (US) is a commonly used medical imaging modality that supports real-time and safe clinical diagnosis, in particular in gynecology and obstetrics. However, the limited image quality and the hand-eye coordination required for probe manipulation necessitate extensive training of sonographers in image interpretation and navigation. Volunteer access and realism of phantoms being limited

---

D. Tomar and L. Zhang—Both authors contributed equally to this manuscript.

Electronic supplementary material The online version of this chapter (https://doi.org/10.1007/978-3-030-87237-3_63) contains supplementary material, which is available to authorized users.

M. de Bruijne et al. (Eds.): MICCAI 2021, LNCS 12908, pp. 659–669, 2021.
https://doi.org/10.1007/978-3-030-87237-3_63

for training, especially of rare diseases, computational methods become essential as simulation-based training tools. To that end, interpolation of pre-acquired US volumes [6] provide only limited image diversity. Nevertheless, ray-tracing based methods have been demonstrated to successfully simulate images with realistic view-dependent ultrasonic artifacts, *e.g.* refraction and reflection [4]. Monte-Carlo ray-tracing [14] has further enabled realistic soft shadows and fuzzy reflections, while animated models and fusion of partial-frame simulations were also presented [20]. However, the simulation realism depends highly on the underlying anatomical models and the parametrization of tissue properties. Especially the noisy appearance of ultrasound images with typical speckle patterns are nontrivial to parameterize. Despite several approaches proposed to that end [13,21,27], images simulated from anatomical models still lack realism, with the generated images appearing synthetic compared to real US scans.

Learning-based image translation techniques have received increasing interest in solving ultrasound imaging tasks, *e.g.* cross-modality translation [11], image enhancement [10,25,26], and semantic image synthesis [2,22]. The aim of these techniques is to map images from a source domain to target domain, e.g. mapping low- to high-quality images. Generative adversarial networks (GANs) [7] have been widely used in image translation due to their superior performance in generating realistic images compared to supervised losses. In the paired setting, where images in the source domain have a corresponding ground truth image in the target domain, a combination of supervised per-pixel losses and a conditional GAN loss [15] has shown great success on various translation tasks [9]. In the absence of paired training samples, the translation problem becomes underconstrained and additional constraints are required to learn a successful translation. To tackle this issue, a cyclic consistency loss (cycleGAN) was proposed [28], where an inverse mapping from target to source domain is learned simultaneously, while a cycle consistency is ensured by minimizing a reconstruction loss between the output of the inverse mapping and the source image itself. Recent works have extended and applied cycle consistency on multi-domain translation [1,5,29]. Cycle consistency assumes a strong bijective relation between the domains. To relax the bijectivity assumption and reduce the training burden, Park et al. [17] proposed an alternative with a single-sided unpaired translation technique with contrastive learning. For US simulation, the standard cycleGAN was used in [24] to improve the realism of simulated US image frames, however, this method is prone to generate unrealistic deformations and hallucinated features.

In this work, we aim to improve the realism of computationally-simulated US images by converting their appearance to that of real in-vivo US scans, while preserving their anatomical content and view-dependent artefacts originating from the preceeding computational simulation. We build our framework on a recent contrastive unpaired translation framework [17] and introduce several contributions to improve translation quality. In particular, to encourage content preservation, we propose to (i) constrain the generator with the accompanying semantic labels of simulated images by learning an auxiliary segmentation-to-real image translation task; and (ii) apply a class-conditional generator, which in turn enables the incorporation of a cyclic loss.

2   Method

Given unpaired source images $X = \{x \in \mathbb{X}\}$ and target images $Y = \{y \in \mathbb{Y}\}$, we aim to learn a generator function $G : \mathbb{X} \mapsto \mathbb{Y}$, such that mapped images $G(x)$ have similar appearance (style) as images in Y, while preserving the structural content of the input image x. To achieve this goal, we divide G into an encoder G_{enc} and a decoder G_{dec}. G_{enc} is restricted to extract content-related features only, while G_{dec} learns to generate a desired target appearance using a patch contrastive loss. Combined with both cyclic and semantic regularizations, we design a multi-domain translation framework consisting of a single generator and discriminator (Fig. 1).

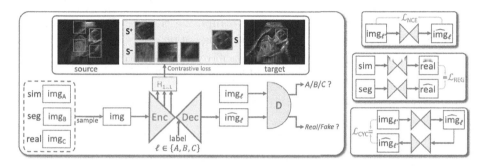

Fig. 1. (Left) Overview of our proposed framework. (Right) Illustrations of some of the loss functions used to train our model.

Adversarial Loss. We adopt the patchGAN discriminator [17] that discriminates real and fake images using a least squares GAN loss:

$$\mathcal{L}_{\mathrm{GAN}}(X, Y) = \mathbb{E}_y \log[(D(y) - 1)^2] + \mathbb{E}_x \log[D(G(x))^2] . \tag{1}$$

Contrastive Loss. An unpaired contrastive translation framework (CUT) is presented in [17] that maximizes mutual information between image patches in the source and target domain to maintain the content of source images. The core of this approach is to enforce each translated patch to be (i) similar to the corresponding input patch, while (ii) different from any other input patches. For the similarity assessment, image patches are represented by hidden features of G_{enc}. A multi-layer perceptron (MLP) H_l with two hidden layers is then used to map the chosen encoder features h_l to an embedded representation $z_l = H_l(h_l) \in \mathbb{R}^{S_l \times C_l}$ with S_l spatial locations and C_l channels, where $h_l = G_{\mathrm{enc}}^l(x)$ is the l-th hidden layer of G_{enc}. For each spatial location s in z_l, the corresponding patch feature vector $z_l^{s+} \in \mathbb{R}^{C_l}$ is then the positive sample and the features at any other locations are the negatives $z_l^{s-} \in \mathbb{R}^{(S_l - 1) \times C_l}$. The corresponding patch feature $\hat{z}_l^s = h_l(G_{enc}^l(\hat{y})) \in \mathbb{R}^{C_l}$ of the output image $\hat{y}$ acts as the query. The contrastive loss is defined as the cross-entropy loss

$$l(\hat{z}_l^s, z_l^{s+}, z_l^{s-}) = -\log \left[\frac{\exp(\hat{z}_l^s \cdot z_l^{s+}/\tau)}{\exp(\hat{z}_l^s \cdot z_l^{s+}/\tau) + \sum_{k=1}^{S_l-1} \exp(\hat{z}_l^s \cdot z_{l,k}^{s-}/\tau)} \right], \quad (2)$$

with the temperature parameter τ set to 0.07, following [17]. Using features from multiple encoder depths allows us to enforce patch similarity on multiple scales, leading to the following noise contrastive estimation (NCE) loss

$$\mathcal{L}_{\mathrm{NCE}}(X) = \mathbb{E}_x \sum_{l=1}^{L} \sum_{s=1}^{S_l} l(\hat{z}_l^s, z_l^{s+}, z_l^{s-}), \quad (3)$$

where L is the number of layers used for computing the loss. To encourage the generator to translate the domain-specific image appearance only, $\mathcal{L}_{\mathrm{NCE}}$ is also evaluated on the target domain $\mathbb{Y}$, which acts as an identity loss, similarly to the cyclic consistency loss in [28]. The final objective in CUT [17] is defined as

$$\mathcal{L}_{\mathrm{CUT}}(X, Y) = \mathcal{L}_{\mathrm{GAN}}(X, Y) + \mathcal{L}_{\mathrm{NCE}}(X) + \mathcal{L}_{\mathrm{NCE}}(Y). \quad (4)$$

Semantic-Consistent Regularization. To encourage the disentanglement of content and style, we leverage available surrogate segmentation maps $S = \{s \in \mathbb{S}\}$ of the simulated images (sim). In addition to sim-to-real translation, our generator then learns to also synthesize real images from segmentation maps (seg), *i.e.* seg-to-real translation. Since segmentation maps contain only content and no style, it is ensured that, after passing G_{enc}, there is no style left in the features, therefore G_{dec} has to introduce styles entirely from scratch. Learning this auxiliary task thus helps to prevent style leakage from G_{enc}, enforcing G_{enc} to extract only content-relevant features. In this modified CUT framework with semantic input (CUT+S), we minimize

$$\mathcal{L}_{\mathrm{CUT+S}} = \mathcal{L}_{\mathrm{CUT}}(X, Y) + \mathcal{L}_{\mathrm{GAN}}(S, Y) + \mathcal{L}_{\mathrm{NCE}}(S). \quad (5)$$

In addition, we regularize G to generate the same output for paired seg and sim, thus explicitly incorporating the semantic information of simulated images into the generator. We achieve this by minimizing the following semantic-consistent regularization loss: $\mathcal{L}_{\mathrm{REG}}(X, S) = \mathbb{E}_{x,s}||G(x) - G(s)||_1$. Our consistency-based training objective then becomes:

$$\mathcal{L}_{\mathrm{CUT+SC}} = \mathcal{L}_{\mathrm{CUT+S}} + \lambda_{\mathrm{REG}}\mathcal{L}_{\mathrm{REG}}(X, S). \quad (6)$$

Multi-Domain Translation. In preliminary experiments, we observed that despite the identity contrastive loss and semantic inputs, the generator still alters the image content, since the above losses do not explicitly enforce the structural consistency between input and translated images. To mitigate this issue, we require a cyclic consistency loss similar to [28]. For this purpose, we extend the so-far single-direction translation to a multi-domain translation framework, while keeping a unified (now conditional) generator and discriminator, inspired by StarGAN [5]. Here, G_{dec} is trained to transfer the target appearance, conditioned by the target class label $\ell \in \{\mathbb{A}, \mathbb{B}, \mathbb{S}\}$ given the classes $\mathbb{A}$ simulated image, $\mathbb{B}$ real image, and $\mathbb{S}$ semantic map. The class label is encoded as a one-hot vector and concatenated to the input of the decoder. The cyclic consistency loss is then defined as

$$\mathcal{L}_{\text{CYC}}(X) = \mathbb{E}_{x,\ell,\ell'}||x - G(G(x,\ell),\ell')||_1, \tag{7}$$

where ℓ' is the class label of the input image and ℓ is label of the target class.

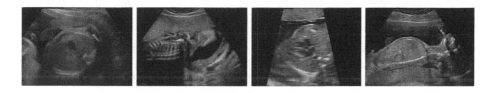

Fig. 2. Examples of in-vivo images used to train our model.

Classification Loss. To enable class-dependent classification (CLS) with the discriminator [5], D tries to predict the correct domain class label ℓ' for a given *real* image x as an auxiliary task, *i.e.*

$$\mathcal{L}_{\text{CLS,r}}(X) = \mathbb{E}_{x,\ell'}[-\log D(\ell'|x)], \tag{8}$$

while G tries to fool D with *fake* images to be classified as target domain ℓ by minimizing

$$\mathcal{L}_{\text{CLS,f}}(X) = \mathbb{E}_{x,\ell}[-\log D(\ell|G(x,\ell))]. \tag{9}$$

Final Objective. For our final model (ConPres), the training objective is evaluated by randomly sampling two pairs of domains $(X_i, Y_i) \in \{(\mathbb{A}, \mathbb{B}, \mathbb{S}) \backslash X_i \neq Y_i\}$ for $i = [1, 2]$, given the following discriminator and generator losses

$$\mathcal{L}_{\text{ConPres}}^{\text{D}} = \sum_{i=1}^{2} -\mathcal{L}_{\text{GAN}}(X_i, Y_i) + \lambda_{\text{CLS,r}} \mathcal{L}_{\text{CLS,r}}(X_i), \tag{10}$$

$$\mathcal{L}_{\text{ConPres}}^{\text{G}} = \sum_{i=1}^{2} \mathcal{L}_{\text{CUT}}(X_i, Y_i) + \lambda_{\text{CLS,f}} \mathcal{L}_{\text{CLS,f}}(X_i) + \lambda_{\text{CYC}} \mathcal{L}_{\text{CYC}}(X_i)$$
$$+ \mathbb{1}_{[(X_1=\mathbb{A} \wedge X_2=\mathbb{S}) \vee (X_1=\mathbb{S} \wedge X_2=\mathbb{A})]} \lambda_{\text{REG}} \mathcal{L}_{\text{REG}}(X_1, X_2) \tag{11}$$

with the indicator function $\mathbb{1}_{[.]}$ and the hyperparameters $\lambda_{\{.\}}$ for weighting loss components. We set $\lambda_{\text{REG}} = 0$ when the two source domains are not $\mathbb{A}$ and $\mathbb{S}$.

3   Experiments and Results

Real In-vivo Images. 22 ultrasound sequences were collected using a GE Voluson E8 machine during standard fetal screening exams of 8 patients. Each sequence is several seconds long. We extracted all 4427 frames and resize them to 256×354, see Fig. 2 for some examples. The resulting image set was randomly split into training-validation-test sets by a 80–10–10% ratio.

US Simulation. We used a ray-tracing framework to render B-mode images from a geometric fetal model, by simulating a convex probe placed at multiple locations and orientations on the abdominal surface, with imaging settings listed in the supplement. At each location, simply rasterizing a cross-section through the triangulated anatomical surfaces at the ultrasound center imaging plane provided corresponding semantic maps. Figure 3 shows example B-mode images with corresponding semantic maps. A total of 6669 simulated frames were resized to 256×354 and randomly split into training-validation-test sets by 80–10–10%.

Metrics. We use the following metrics to quantitatively evaluate our method:

- **Structural similarity index** (SSIM) measures the structural similarity between simulated and translated images, quantifying content preservation. We evaluate SSIM within regions having content in simulated images.
- **Fréchet inception distance** (FID) [8] measures the feature distribution difference between two sets of images, herein real and translated, using feature vectors of Inception network. Since a large number of samples is required to reduce estimation bias, we use the *pre-aux* layer features, which has a smaller dimensionality than the default pooling layer features.
- **Kernel inception distance** (KID) [3] is an alternative unbiased metric to evaluate GAN performance. KID is computed as the squared maximum mean-discrepancy between the features of Inception network. We use the default pooling layer features of Inception, to compute this score.

Implementation Details. We use a least-squares GAN loss with patchGAN discriminator as in [5]. The generator follows an encoder-decoder architecture, where the encoder consists of two stride-2 convolution layers followed by 4 residual blocks, while the decoder consists of 4 residual blocks followed by two convolution layers with bilinear upsampling. For architectural details, please see the supplementary material. To compute the contrastive loss, we extract features from the input layer, the stride-2 convolution layers, and the outputs of the first three residual blocks of the encoder. For CUT and its variants CUT+S and CUT+SC, we used the default layers in [17]. To compute λ_{REG}, the sampled simulated and segmentation images in each batch are paired. We used Adam [12] optimizer to train our model for 100 epochs with an l_2 regularization of 10^{-4} on model parameters with gradient clipping and $\beta = (0.5, 0.999)$. We set $\lambda_{CLS,*} = 0.1$, $\lambda_{REG} = 1$ and $\lambda_{CYC} = 10$. We set the hyper-parameters based on similar losses in the compared implementations, for comparability; while we grid-searched the others, *e.g.* λ_{REG}, for stable GAN training. We implemented our model in PyTorch [19]. For KID and FID computations, we used the implementation of [16].

Comparative Study. We compare our proposed ConPres to several state-of-the-art unpaired image translation methods:

- **CycleGAN** [28]: A conventional approach with cyclic consistency loss.
- **SASAN** [23]: CycleGAN extension with self-attentive spatial adaptive normalization, leveraging semantic information to retain anatomical structures, while translating using spatial attention modules and SPADE layers [18].
- **CUT** [17]: Unpaired contrastive framework for image translation.
- **StarGAN** [5]: A unified GAN framework for multi-domain translation.

We used the official implementations and default hyperparameters for training all the baselines. To assess the effectiveness of the proposed architecture and losses, we also compare with the models CUT+S (CUT plus the seg-to-real translation) and CUT+SC (CUT+S plus $\mathcal{L}_{REG}$).

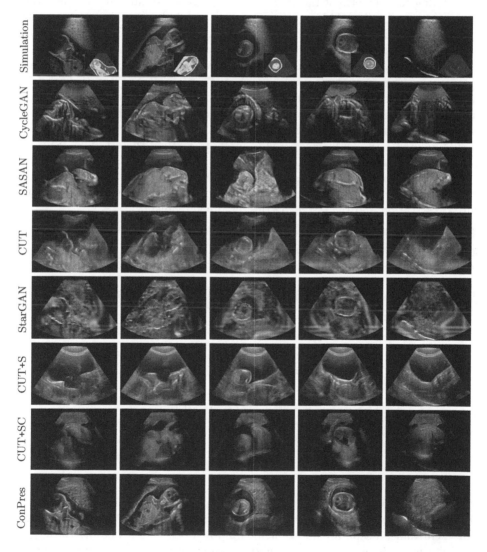

Fig. 3. Qualitative results, with images masked by foreground in segmentations.

In Fig. 3 we show that only learning an auxiliary seg-to-real translation, i.e. CUT+S, cannot guide the network to learn the semantics of simulated images.

CUT+SC with the loss term $\mathcal{L}_{REG}$ largely reduces hallucinated image content, although it still fails to generate fine anatomical details. With the multi-domain conditional generator and additional losses of ConPres, translated images preserve content and feature a realistic appearance. Training without $\mathcal{L}_{NCE}$ leads to training instability.

Comparison to State-of-the-Art. As seen qualitatively from the examples in Fig. 3, our method substantially outperforms the alternatives in terms of content preservation, while translating realistic US appearance. CycleGAN, SASAN, and CUT hallucinate inexistent tissue regions fail to generate fine anatomical structures, e.g. the ribs. StarGAN fails to generate faithful ultrasound speckle appearance, which leads to highly unrealistic images. Our method ConPres preserves anatomical structures, while enhancing the images with a realistic appearance. It further faithfully preserves acoustic shadows, even without explicit enforcement. However, as seen from the last column, the refraction artefact appears artificial in the images translated by all the methods. Note that although the imaging field-of-view (FoV) and probe opening in the simulation is significantly different from the real in-vivo images (Fig. 2) used for training, our ConPres maintains the input FoV closely compared to previous state-of-the-art. The results in Table 1 quantitatively confirm the superiority of our method. Note that SSIM and FID/KID are used to measure translation performance from two different and sometimes competing aspects, with the former metric for quantifying structure preservation and the latter metrics for image realism.

Table 1. Quantitative metrics and ranking from the user study (mean ±std). Best results are marked bold. "Seg" gives if semantic maps are used as network input.

	Seg	Method	SSIM ↑	FID ↓	KID ↓	Ranking $\in [1,6]$↓
	—	Simulation	—	2.37	0.41	3.98 ± 1.35
Others	✗	CycleGAN [28]	71.73 ± 5.18	1.78	0.32	2.86 ± 1.27
	✓	SASAN [23]	68.20 ± 4.00	2.36	0.39	3.59 ± 1.55
	✗	CUT [17]	67.28 ± 4.62	1.77	0.31	2.92 ± 1.20
	✓	StarGAN [5]	63.62 ± 4.82	1.93	0.47	5.76 ± 0.61
Ours	✓	CUT+S	68.88 ± 4.63	2.25	0.41	
	✓	CUT+SC	$\mathbf{80.56 \pm 2.11}$	1.87	0.38	
	✓	ConPres	72.13 ± 4.58	**1.51**	**0.24**	**1.89±1.07**

A user study was performed with 18 participants (14 technical and 4 clinical ultrasound experts) to evaluate the realism of translated images for 20 US frames. For each frame, a separate questionnaire window opened in a web interface, presenting the participants with six candidate images including the input simulated famre and its translated versions using CUT, CycleGAN, SASAN, StarGAN, and ConPres. As a reference for the given ultrasound machine appearance, we also showed a fixed set of 10 real in-vivo images. The participants were asked to rank the candidate images based on "their likelihood for being an image from this machine". The average rank score is reported in Table 1. Based on a paired Wilcoxon signed rank test, our method is significantly superior to any competing method (all p-values $< 10^{-18}$).

Discussion. Note that, despite both being fetal images, the simulated and the real images have substantially different anatomical contents, which makes the translation task extremely challenging. Nevertheless, our proposed framework is able to generate images with appearance strikingly close to real images, with far superior realism than its competitors. Besides sim-to-real translation, given its multi-domain conditional nature, our proposed framework without any further training can also translate images between the other domains, *e.g.* seg-to-real or seg-to-sim, with examples presented in the supplementary material.

4   Conclusions

We have introduced a contrastive unpaired translation framework with a class-conditional generator, for improving ultrasound simulation realism. By applying cyclic and semantic consistency constraints, our proposed method can translate domain-specific appearance, while preserving the original content. This is shown to outperform state-of-the-art unpaired translation methods. With the proposed methods, we largely close the appearance gap between simulated and real images. Future works may include an evaluation of the effects of translated images on US training as well as an investigation of seg-to-real image translation, which can enable to completely dispense with any expensive rendering.

Acknowledgements. Funding was provided by the Swiss Innovation Agency Innosuisse.

References

1. Almahairi, A., Rajeshwar, S., Sordoni, A., Bachman, P., Courville, A.: Augmented CycleGAN: learning many-to-many mappings from unpaired data. In: International Conference on Machine Learning (ICML), pp. 195–204 (2018)
2. Bargsten, L., Schlaefer, A.: SpeckleGAN: a generative adversarial network with an adaptive speckle layer to augment limited training data for ultrasound image processing. Int. J. Comp. Asst. Radiol. Surg. **15**(9), 1427–1436 (2020)
3. Bińkowski, M., Sutherland, D.J., Arbel, M., Gretton, A.: Demystifying MMD GANs. preprint arXiv:1801.01401 (2018)
4. Burger, B., Bettinghausen, S., Radle, M., Hesser, J.: Real-time GPU-based ultrasound simulation using deformable mesh models. IEEE Trans. Med. Imaging **32**(3), 609–618 (2013)

5. Choi, Y., Choi, M., Kim, M., Ha, J.W., Kim, S., Choo, J.: StarGAN: unified generative adversarial networks for multi-domain image-to-image translation. In: Proceedings of the IEEE Conference on Computer Vision and Pattern Recognition (CVPR), pp. 8789–8797 (2018)
6. Goksel, O., Salcudean, S.E.: B-Mode ultrasound image simulation in deformable 3-D medium. IEEE Trans. Med. Imaging **28**(11), 1657–1669 (2009)
7. Goodfellow, I., et al.: Generative adversarial nets. In: Advances in Neural Information Processing Systems (NeurIPS), pp. 2672–2680 (2014)
8. Heusel, M., Ramsauer, H., Unterthiner, T., Nessler, B., Hochreiter, S.: GANs trained by a two time-scale update rule converge to a local nash equilibrium. In: Advances in Neural Information Processing Systems (NeurIPS), pp. 6626–6637 (2017)
9. Isola, P., Zhu, J.Y., Zhou, T., Efros, A.A.: Image-to-image translation with conditional adversarial networks. In: IEEE Conference on Computer Vision and Pattern Recognition (CVPR), pp. 1125–1134 (2017)
10. Jafari, M.H., et al.: Cardiac point-of-care to cart-based ultrasound translation using constrained CycleGAN. Int. J. Comp. Asst. Radiol. Surg. **15**, 1–10 (2020)
11. Jiao, J., Namburete, A.I., Papageorghiou, A.T., Noble, J.A.: Self-supervised ultrasound to MRI fetal brain image synthesis. IEEE Trans. Med. Imaging **39**(12), 4413–4424 (2020)
12. Kingma, D.P., Ba, J.: Adam: a method for stochastic optimization. In: ICLR (2015)
13. Mattausch, O., Goksel, O.: Image-based reconstruction of tissue scatterers using beam steering for ultrasound simulation. IEEE Trans. Med. Imaging **37**(3), 767–780 (2017)
14. Mattausch, O., Makhinya, M., Goksel, O.: Realistic ultrasound simulation of complex surface models using interactive Monte-Carlo path tracing. Comput. Graph. Forum **37**, 202–213 (2018)
15. Mirza, M., Osindero, S.: Conditional generative adversarial nets. preprint arXiv:1411.1784 (2014)
16. Obukhov, A., Seitzer, M., Wu, P.W., Zhydenko, S., Kyl, J., Lin, E.Y.J.: High-fidelity performance metrics for generative models in pytorch (2020). https://github.com/toshas/torch-fidelity. Accessed 26 Feb 2021
17. Park, T., Efros, A.A., Zhang, R., Zhu, J.-Y.: Contrastive learning for unpaired image-to-image translation. In: Vedaldi, A., Bischof, H., Brox, T., Frahm, J.-M. (eds.) ECCV 2020. LNCS, vol. 12354, pp. 319–345. Springer, Cham (2020). https://doi.org/10.1007/978-3-030-58545-7_19
18. Park, T., Liu, M.Y., Wang, T.C., Zhu, J.Y.: Semantic image synthesis with spatially-adaptive normalization. In: Proceedings of the IEEE Conference on Computer Vision and Pattern Recognition (CVPR), pp. 2337–2346 (2019)
19. Paszke, A., et al.: Pytorch: an imperative style, high-performance deep learning library. preprint arXiv:1912.01703 (2019)
20. Starkov, R., Tanner, C., Bajka, M., Goksel, O.: Ultrasound simulation with animated anatomical models and on-the-fly fusion with real images via path-tracing. Comput. Graph. **82**, 44–52 (2019)
21. Starkov, R., Zhang, L., Bajka, M., Tanner, C., Goksel, O.: Ultrasound simulation with deformable and patient-specific scatterer maps. Int. J. Comp. Asst. Radiol. Surg. **14**(9), 1589–1599 (2019)
22. Tom, F., Sheet, D.: Simulating patho-realistic ultrasound images using deep generative networks with adversarial learning. In: IEEE International Symposium on Biomedical Imaging (ISBI), pp. 1174–1177 (2018)

23. Tomar, D., Lortkipanidze, M., Vray, G., Bozorgtabar, B., Thiran, J.P.: Self-attentive spatial adaptive normalization for cross-modality domain adaptation. IEEE Trans. Med. Imaging (2021)
24. Vitale, S., Orlando, J.I., Iarussi, E., Larrabide, I.: Improving realism in patient-specific abdominal ultrasound simulation using CycleGANs. Int. J. Comp. Asst. Radiol. Surg. **15**, 1–10 (2019)
25. Zhang, L., Portenier, T., Goksel, O.: Learning ultrasound rendering from cross-sectional model slices for simulated training. Int. J. Comp. Asst. Radiol. Surg. **16**(5), 721–730 (2021)
26. Zhang, L., Portenier, T., Paulus, C., Goksel, O.: Deep image translation for enhancing simulated ultrasound images. In: Hu, Y., et al. (eds.) ASMUS/PIPPI -2020. LNCS, vol. 12437, pp. 85–94. Springer, Cham (2020). https://doi.org/10.1007/978-3-030-60334-2_9
27. Zhang, L., Vishnevskiy, V., Goksel, O.: Deep network for scatterer distribution estimation for ultrasound image simulation. IEEE Trans. Ultrason. Ferroelectr. Freq. Control (TUFFC) **67**(12), 2553–2564 (2020)
28. Zhu, J.Y., Park, T., Isola, P., Efros, A.A.: Unpaired image-to-image translation using cycle-consistent adversarial networks. In: IEEE International Conference on Computer Vision (CVPR), pp. 2223–2232 (2017)
29. Zhu, J.Y., et al.: Toward multimodal image-to-image translation. In: Advances in Neural Information Processing Systems (NeurIPS) (2017)

Visual-Assisted Probe Movement Guidance for Obstetric Ultrasound Scanning Using Landmark Retrieval

Cheng Zhao[1]([✉]), Richard Droste[1], Lior Drukker[2], Aris T. Papageorghiou[2], and J. Alison Noble[1]

[1] Institute of Biomedical Engineering, University of Oxford, Oxford, UK
cheng.zhao@eng.ox.ac.uk
[2] Nuffield Department of Women's and Reproductive Health, University of Oxford, Oxford, UK

Abstract. Automated ultrasound (US)-probe movement guidance is desirable to assist inexperienced human operators during obstetric US scanning. In this paper, we present a new visual-assisted probe movement technique using automated landmark retrieval for assistive obstetric US scanning. In a first step, a set of landmarks is constructed uniformly around a virtual 3D fetal model. Then, during obstetric scanning, a deep neural network (DNN) model locates the nearest landmark through descriptor search between the current observation and landmarks. The global position cues are visualised in real-time on a monitor to assist the human operator in probe movement. A Transformer-VLAD network is proposed to learn a global descriptor to represent each US image. This method abandons the need for deep parameter regression to enhance the generalization ability of the network. To avoid prohibitively expensive human annotation, anchor-positive-negative US image-pairs are automatically constructed through a KD-tree search of 3D probe positions. This leads to an end-to-end network trained in a self-supervised way through contrastive learning.

Keywords: Obstetric US · Probe guidance · Landmark retrieval

1 Introduction

Motivation: Obstetric US scanning is known to be highly experienced-operator dependent. Simplifying US to be more accessible to non-expert operators is a recognized priority for wider deployment of US in clinical practice. Automatic probe movement guidance may assist less-experienced operators to perform scanning

Electronic supplementary material The online version of this chapter (https://doi.org/10.1007/978-3-030-87237-3_64) contains supplementary material, which is available to authorized users.

more confidently, and widen the use of US in existing and new areas of clinical medicine. Our target is to develop automated machine learning (ML)-based visual interventions to provide helpful visualization cues for guiding an inexperienced operator using US scanning as an exemplar. In this case the target end-user might be a sonographer trainee, midwife, emergency medicine doctors, or primary care practitioners for instance.

Automatic ML-based probe movement guidance to assist a human operator (rather than a robot) is currently an open research problem. Two recent methods [3,6] propose to predict control parameters of probe movement such as translation distance and rotation degree. Li *et al.* [6] propose an Iterative Transformation Network (ITN) to automatically detect 2D standard planes from a prescanned 3D US volume. The CNN-based ITN learns to predict the parameters of the geometric transformation required to move the current plane towards the position/orientation of the 2D standard plane in the 3D volume. Droste *et al.* [3] develop a real-time probe rotation guidance algorithm using US images with Inertial Measurement Unit (IMU) signals for obstetric scanning. The proposed deep multi-modality model predicts both the rotation towards the standard plane position, and the next rotation that an expert operator might perform.

These control parameter prediction style methods are best suited for guiding a robot agent rather than a human. There is a parallel here with the self-driving vehicle literature where, for example, the most efficient way to assist a person driving is via real-time GPS localization visualization, while control parameter (steering wheel and accelerator) prediction is more useful for a self-driving car. We are therefore interested in discovering whether a similar visual intervention such as [12] can assist obstetric US scanning.

Grimwood *et al.* [5] formulate the probe guidance problem as a high-level command classification problem during prostate external beam radiotherapy using US images and transducer pose signals. The proposed CNN-RNN based classification network predicts 6 different high-level guidance cues i.e. outside prostate, prostate periphery, prostate centre for position and move left, move right, stop for direction to recommend probe adjustments. However, training this classification network requires a large number of expensive ground-truth annotated by physicists and radiotherapy practitioners.

From a technical viewpoint, deep regression-based methods such as [3,6] take advantage of the powerful non-linearity of a DNN to regress the control parameters from the collected data. These methods leverage the DNN to learn to overfit on the training data of some specific users, so these methods naturally lack generalization ability, as mentioned in [8], for real clinical applications.

Contribution: In this paper we propose a landmark retrieval-based method as a visual-assisted intervention to guide US-probe movement as shown in Fig. 1. The goal is to provide global position visualization cues to the operator during US scanning. To be specific, we firstly construct a set of landmarks uniformly around a virtual fetal model. Each landmark stores a data-pair of information: the 3D position relative to the virtual fetal model, and the global descriptor of the US

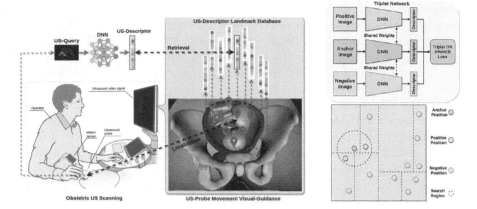

Fig. 1. Overview of landmark retrieval-based US-probe movement guidance.

Fig. 2. (Up) The triplet network architecture; (Down) The probe position KD-tree based anchor-positive-negative triplet data construction.

image captured at this position. During US scanning, the network transforms the current observed US image to a global descriptor, and then retrieves the landmark dataset to locate the nearest landmark through descriptor search. The nearest landmark provides the relative 3D position between the probe and the virtual fetal model in 3D space. This global position visualization is displayed on the monitor in real-time as visual guidance to assist the operator.

This descriptor learning-based landmark retrieval method abandons any need for deep parameter regression, which can avoid the degeneration of network generalization ability. The proposed method is trained end-to-end in a self-supervised way without any expensive human expert annotation. The main contributions are: 1) we formulate US-probe movement guidance as a landmark retrieval problem through learned descriptor search; 2) a Transformer-VLAD network is proposed to learn a generalized descriptor for automatic landmark retrieval; 3) the descriptor learning is achieved by contrastive learning using self-constructed anchor-positive-negative US image-pairs.

2   Methodology

Overview: Building on the representation ability of DNN, we cast US-probe movement guidance as landmark retrieval. The query, i.e. current observed US image, at an unknown position is used to visually search a landmark dataset. The positions of top-ranked landmarks are used as suggestions for the query position. It is achieved by designing a DNN, i.e. Transformer-VLAD, to extract a global descriptor given an US image for visual search. During inference, only the descriptor of the query US image is computed online, while the other descriptors of the landmarks are computed once offline and stored in memory, thus enabling a real-time performance (0.01 s on NVIDIA TITAN RTX). The visual search is

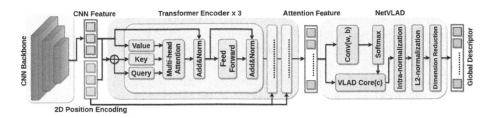

Fig. 3. The Transformer-VLAD network architecture.

performed by finding the nearest landmarks to the query. This can be achieved through fast approximate nearest neighbour search by sorting landmarks according to the Euclidean distance between the learned descriptors.

The proposed Transformer-VLAD network is a typical triplet network which is a variation of a Siamese network, as shown in Fig. 2 up. It utilizes a triplet of images, including anchor, positive and negative US images in network training. The triplet network simultaneously minimizes the feature distance between the anchor and positive US image-pair, and maximizes the feature distance between the anchor and negative US image-pair through contrastive learning. The anchor-positive-negative triplet data is automatically constructed according to the KD-tree based probe 3D position without use of human annotation. Hence, the whole network is trained end-to-end in a self-supervised way.

The more detailed architecture inside the Transformer-VLAD network is illustrated in Fig. 3. It consists of three components: feature extraction (left), Transformer (middle) and NetVLAD (right). The feature extraction is composed of a series of convolution stacks to extract the local feature representation from the US image. The Transformer includes three transformer encoder stacks in series with 2D position encoding, enabling co-contextual information extraction from a set of feature representations. The NetVLAD is a differentiable version of the vector of locally aggregated descriptors (VLAD), which aggregates a set of local descriptors and generate one global descriptor.

Local Feature Extraction: We employ VGG-16 [9] per-trained on the ImageNet dataset as a backbone to extract local features. This CNN-backbone transforms the initial US image $\mathcal{I}_{US} \in \mathbb{R}^{1 \times H_0 \times W_0}$ to a lower-resolution feature map $\mathcal{F}_0 \in \mathbb{R}^{D \times H \times W}$, where $H_0 = 400$, $W_0 = 274$, $D = 512$ and $H, W = H_0/32, W_0/32$. So each pixel feature representation in the final feature map represents a 32×32 US patch in the original US image. Finally, we collapse the feature map $\mathcal{F}_0$ into a one-dimensional sentence-like feature vector $\mathcal{F} \in \mathbb{R}^{D \times H \cdot W}$ as input to the Transformer.

Contextual Feature Extraction: Given the feature vector $\mathcal{F} \in \mathbb{R}^{D \times H \cdot W}$, the Transformer [10] extracts the contextual cues within the CNN feature representations to generate a new feature vector $\mathcal{A} \in \mathbb{R}^{D \times H \cdot W}$. The Transformer consists of three encoders, and each of which is composed of a series of modules, i.e. multi-head self-attention (MHSA), feed-forward network (FFN) and layer normalization (LN). Each encoder can be stacked on top of each other multiple times.

Because the Transformer architecture is permutation-invariant, we supplement it with fixed positional encodings $\mathcal{P} \in \mathbb{R}^{D \times H \cdot W}$ that are added to each encoder. Specifically, $\mathcal{P}$ is a sinusoidal positional encoding following [7]. We add $\mathcal{P}$ to the query Q and key K without value V in each MHSA to maintain the position information of the feature representation,

$$Q = K = \mathcal{F} + \mathcal{P}, V = \mathcal{F}. \tag{1}$$

Then the Transformer encoder can learn a co-contextual message $Attn$ captured by the MHSA mechanism,

$$Attn([Q_i, K_i, V_i]) = \text{concat}([\text{softmax}(\frac{Q_i \cdot K_i^T}{\sqrt{d_i}})V_i]), \tag{2}$$

where Q_i, K_i, V_i stand for ith head of queries, keys, values of the feature representation respectively, and d_i refers to the dimension of queries. In this implementation, an eight head attention (i.e. $i = 1, 2, ..., 8$) is adopted to enhance the discriminativeness of the feature attributes. The MSHA mechanism automatically builds the connections between the current representation and the other salient representations within the sentence-like feature vector.

Finally, the attentional representation $\mathcal{A}$ can be obtained as,

$$\mathcal{A}_0 = LN(\mathcal{F} + Attn), \quad \mathcal{A} = LN(FFN(\mathcal{A}_0) + \mathcal{A}_0), \tag{3}$$

where FFN contains two fully connected layers. This procedure is performed three times in the three encoders, and the position encoding is inputted to the MHSA in each encoder.

Feature Aggregation: In order to improve permutation invariance of the feature representation $\mathcal{A} \in \mathbb{R}^{D \times H \cdot W}$, we adopt NetVLAD [1] rather than a bag-of-visual-words or max-pooling operation. It is designed to aggregate a set of local descriptors $\mathcal{A} = \{\mathbf{x_i}\}$ to generate one global descriptor $\mathcal{V}_0 \in \mathbb{R}^{D \times K}$, where $K = 64$ denotes the number of cluster centers $\{c_k\}$,

$$\mathcal{V}_0(d, k) = \sum_{i=1}^{H \cdot W} \alpha_k(\mathbf{x_i})(x_i(d) - c_k(d)), \quad \alpha_k(\mathbf{x_i}) = \frac{e^{\mathbf{w}_k \mathbf{x}_i + b_k}}{\sum_{k'} e^{\mathbf{w}_{k'} \mathbf{x}_i + b_{k'}}}. \tag{4}$$

Here $x_i(d)$ denotes the dth dimension of the ith descriptor, and $c_k(d)$ denotes dth dimension of the kth cluster center. $\{\mathbf{w}_k\}$, $\{b_k\}$ and $\{c_k\}$ are the trainable parameters of the kth cluster. In contrast to conventional VLAD, the parameters of NetVLAD, especially the assignment score $\alpha_k(\mathbf{x_i})$ of the descriptor $\mathbf{x_i}$ to kth cluster center, are learned through an end-to-end training.

NetVLAD records statistical information with respect to local signatures and sums the differences between these signatures and their respective cluster. To avoid computationally expensive descriptor search, we use a fully connected layer to compress the high-dimensional descriptor $V_0 \in \mathbb{R}^{D \times K}$ into a compact descriptor $V \in \mathbb{R}^{4096}$.

Loss Function: After getting the query, positive, negative global descriptors V_q, V_{pos}, V_{neg} of the triplet data from the Transformer-VLAD network, we explore both Triplet loss and InfoNCE loss to train the network through contrastive learning. The contrastive learning aims to push representations of positive pairs closer together, while representations of negative pairs are pushed farther with each other. Triplet loss requires the positive pairs to be closer than the negative pairs by a fixed margin δ given the same anchor,

$$\mathcal{L}_{Trip}(V_q, V_{pos}, V_{neg}) = \max\{0, dis(V_q, V_{pos}) - dis(V_q, V_{neg}) + \delta\}, \qquad (5)$$

where $\delta = 0.3$ and $dis(\cdot, \cdot)$ denotes the Euclidean distance. InfoNCE loss formulates it as a dictionary look-up task using cross-entropy to measure the descriptor similarity from the similar/dissimilar date-pairs,

$$\mathcal{L}_{InN}(V_q, V_{pos}, \{V_{neg}\}) = -\log \frac{\exp(V_q \cdot V_{pos}/\tau)}{\exp(V_q \cdot V_{pos}/\tau) + \sum \exp(V_q \cdot V_{neg}/\tau)}, \qquad (6)$$

where $\tau = 0.5$ is a temperature hyper-parameter.

3   Experiments

Data Acquisition and Processing: Data acquired in this work came from a ScanTrainer Simulator[1] (Intelligent Ultrasound Ltd). This realistic simulator is based on real clinical 3D US volumes and allows a user to learn how to acquire 2D images for a virtual patient. In this case, we captured the 2D US image with the corresponding 6DoF probe pose during virtual obstetric scanning from the simulator. We collected a large number of obstetric US images of 2nd (20 weeks) and 3rd trimester (28 weeks) scans from different subjects in the simulator library of examples. We acquired 535,775 US images with the corresponding 6DoF probe pose captured to construct the anchor-positive-negative triple data for the network training. We constructed 5 landmark-query testing cases for the 2nd trimester scanning, and also 5 landmark-query testing cases for the 3rd trimester scanning. For the landmark setting, we firstly collected a very large number of US images with probe poses. Then, a spatially distributed sampling was used to generate 400 evenly distributed landmarks in 3D space, which can not only transform an arbitrary size position to a fixed number of positions, but also simultaneously preserve structural information within the original positions. The query number of 5 test cases in the 2nd trimester are 1471, 927, 1295,

---

[1] https://www.intelligentultrasound.com/scantrainer/.

934, 1031 respectively, and that of the 3rd trimester are 1027, 936, 813, 830, 818 respectively. Note the training and testing data are collected from different cases/women of 2nd and 3rd trimester scans.

Self-supervised Network Training: To avoid expensive human annotation, we construct anchor-positive-negative triple data using KD-tree searching according to the 3D probe position, as shown in Fig. 3 down. To be specific, we extract the 3D probe position from the US-probe data-pair to build a KD-tree. Each node in the KD-tree stores the corresponding US image. Given an anchor US image, we set the search radius to 15mm for the KD-tree search region. The US images located inside the search region are assigned as positive US images related to the anchor image, while those outside US images are assigned as negative US images. In this case, the anchor-positive-negative triple data is

Table 1. Performance comparison on different test cases with different losses.

Test cases	Trans-VLAD$_{Trip}$			Trans-VLAD$_{InN}$		
	r@1	r@5	r@10	r@1	r@5	r@10
case 1_{Sec}	85.3	92.3	93.4	82.6	92.9	94.5
case 2_{Sec}	87.9	94.4	95.7	84.3	**95.7**	**98.0**
case 3_{Sec}	77.2	87.2	90.7	73.3	85.5	90.4
case 4_{Sec}	**90.3**	**96.8**	**98.1**	**88.6**	95.6	97.8
case 5_{Sec}	83.0	92.8	94.4	77.1	93.4	95.7
case 1_{Thi}	81.7	92.2	94.1	78.0	91.2	94.6
case 2_{Thi}	89.3	96.4	97.9	86.5	94.4	97.2
case 3_{Thi}	80.6	91.4	94.8	76.2	90.2	94.8
case 4_{Thi}	75.5	87.3	89.7	72.1	86.3	91.1
case 5_{Thi}	82.8	94.4	95.3	77.8	90.3	94.1
Average	83.4	92.5	94.4	79.7	91.6	94.8

Trans signifies Transformer. r@N signifies recall@number(%). Trip and InN signify Triplet and InfoNCE loss. Sec and Thi signify 2nd and 3rd Trimester.

Table 2. Performance comparison with baselines using ablation analysis.

Method	r@1	r@5	r@10
Trans-VLAD	**83.4**	**92.5**	**94.4**
NetVLAD [1]	80.2	90.9	93.5
ViT [2,4]-VLAD	81.8	91.8	93.8
Trans-Max	77.2	87.8	92.1
Trans-TEN [11]	82.5	91.5	94.0

Trans signifies Transformer. Max signifies Max-pooling operation.

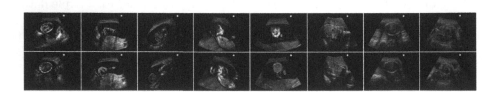

Fig. 4. Selected examples of query US images (first row) and successfully retrieved top1 US landmarks (second row). The images in the first 5 columns are captured from 2nd trimester, and the last 3 columns are captured from 3rd trimester.

constructed automatically from data itself without human annotation so that the network is trained end-to-end in a self-supervised way. The hyper-parameter 15mm is empirically set according to the number of landmarks and 3D volume i.e. density of landmarks. It can be adjusted according to specific clinical tasks.

Performance Evaluation: A standard evaluation procedure of image retrieval is employed for performance evaluation. Specifically, the query image is deemed correctly retrieved if at least one of the topN retrieved landmarks is within 15mm from the probe position of the query. The percentage of correctly retrieved queries (recall) is calculated for different values of N, i.e. recall@topN number(%). Some selected examples of query US images and successfully retrieved top1 US landmarks are shown in the Fig. 4. We can see the successfully retrieved top1 landmark has very similar appearance to the query US image.

The recall@number(%) of each test case for the 2nd and 3rd trimester cases are given in the Table 1. We can see that the contrastive learning with Triplet loss achieves better performance than with InfoNCE loss. Performance for the 2nd trimester cases is slightly better than that for the 3rd trimester cases. A performance comparison with baselines using ablation analysis is provided in the Table 2. Compared with Transformer-VLAD, there is no Transformer sub-network in the baseline NetVLAD [1]. The baselines Transformer-Max and Transformer-TEN replace differentiable VLAD with Max-pooling and DeepTEN [11] respectively for the local feature aggregation. The baseline ViT [2,4]-VLAD uses a pure Transformer encoder instead of a CNN backbone operated on a sequence of 16×16 image patches. Note the latest research [4] achieves SOAT

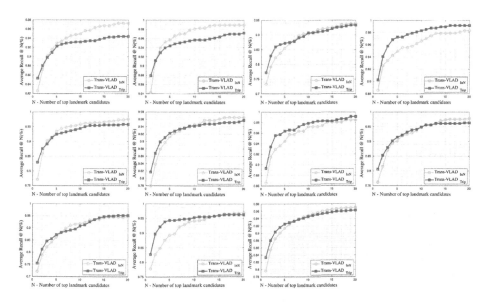

Fig. 5. The average recall curves from top1 to top20 landmark candidates for all 2nd and 3rd trimester test cases.

performance on the public benchmarks of natural image retrieval and we replaces its Max-pooling with VLAD to get better results in our dataset. We can see the that performance difference between the compared methods decreases as the number N increases. The Transformer sub-network improves performance compared with its absence. The VLAD-pooling outperforms Max-pooling significantly when the dataset does not achieve the large-scale level as public benchmark dataset. The VLAD-pooling provides slightly performance improvement comparing with DeepTEN-pooling due to their similar mechanism. We also find that the CNN backbone achieves better performance than a patch-style Transformer for US image retrieval although ViT [2,4] has attained excellent results compared to CNN on some public benchmarks. We also report the average recall curves from top1 to top20 landmark candidates for all 2nd and 3rd trimester test cases in the Fig. 5. The sub-figures from left to right, top to bottom refer to the recall curves of case 1, 2, 3, 4, 5 for 2nd trimester, and case 1, 2, 3, 4, 5 for 3rd trimester, and the average recall curve of all 10 test cases (last sub-figure).

4   Conclusions

In this paper, we present a novel visual-assisted US-probe movement guidance method using landmark retrieval aimed at assisting inexperienced operators to scan. In contrast to conventional control parameter prediction methods, we design a global position visualization intervention which is more intuitive and suitable for the human operator. We also proposed a Transformer-VLAD network to learn a generalized descriptor of each US image to achieve automated landmark retrieval. To avoid the need for expensive human annotation, we take advantage of the 3D probe position to construct anchor-positive-negative US image-pairs automatically for contrastive learning. The experiments demonstrate the potential of the proposed method to simulate realistic imaging acquisitions.

Acknowledgement. This paper is funded by the ERC (ERC-ADG-2015 694581, project PULSE), the EPSRC (EP/MO13774/1, EP/R013853/1), and the NIHR Biomedical Research Centre funding scheme.

References

1. Arandjelovic, R., Gronat, P., Torii, A., et al.: NetVLAD: CNN architecture for weakly supervised place recognition. In: CVPR, pp. 5297–5307. IEEE (2016)
2. Dosovitskiy, A., Beyer, L., Kolesnikov, A., et al.: An image is worth 16×16 words: Transformers for image recognition at scale. In: ICLR (2021)
3. Droste, R., Drukker, L., Papageorghiou, A.T., Noble, J.A.: Automatic probe movement guidance for freehand obstetric ultrasound. In: Martel, A.L., et al. (eds.) MICCAI 2020. LNCS, vol. 12263, pp. 583–592. Springer, Cham (2020). https://doi.org/10.1007/978-3-030-59716-0_56
4. El-Nouby, A., Neverova, N., Laptev, I., Jégou, H.: Training vision transformers for image retrieval. arXiv preprint arXiv:2102.05644 (2021)

5. Grimwood, A., McNair, H., Hu, Y., Bonmati, E., Barratt, D., Harris, E.J.: Assisted probe positioning for ultrasound guided radiotherapy using image sequence classification. In: Martel, A.L., et al. (eds.) MICCAI 2020. LNCS, vol. 12263, pp. 544–552. Springer, Cham (2020). https://doi.org/10.1007/978-3-030-59716-0_52

6. Li, Y., et al.: Standard plane detection in 3D fetal ultrasound using an iterative transformation network. In: Frangi, A.F., Schnabel, J.A., Davatzikos, C., Alberola-López, C., Fichtinger, G. (eds.) MICCAI 2018. LNCS, vol. 11070, pp. 392–400. Springer, Cham (2018). https://doi.org/10.1007/978-3-030-00928-1_45

7. Parmar, N., Vaswani, A., Uszkoreit, J., et al.: Image transformer. In: ICML, pp. 4055–4064. PMLR (2018)

8. Sattler, T., Zhou, Q., Pollefeys, M., Leal-Taixe, L.: Understanding the limitations of CNN-based absolute camera pose regression. In: CVPR, pp. 3302–3312. IEEE (2019)

9. Simonyan, K., Zisserman, A.: Very deep convolutional networks for large-scale image recognition. arXiv preprint arXiv:1409.1556 (2014)

10. Vaswani, A., Shazeer, N., Parmar, N., et al.: Attention is all you need. In: NeurIPS, pp. 5998–6008. Curran Associates, Inc. (2017)

11. Zhang, H., Xue, J., Dana, K.: Deep TEN: texture encoding network. In: CVPR, pp. 708–717. IEEE (2017)

12. Zhao, C., Shen, M., Sun, L., Yang, G.Z.: Generative localization with uncertainty estimation through video-CT data for bronchoscopic biopsy. IEEE Robot. Autom. Lett. 5(1), 258–265 (2019)

Training Deep Networks for Prostate Cancer Diagnosis Using Coarse Histopathological Labels

Golara Javadi[1]([✉]), Samareh Samadi[1], Sharareh Bayat[1], Samira Sojoudi[1],
Antonio Hurtado[3], Silvia Chang[3], Peter Black[3], Parvin Mousavi[2],
and Purang Abolmaesumi[1]

[1] Department of Electrical and Computer Engineering, University of British
Columbia, Vancouver, BC, Canada
[2] Vancouver General Hospital, Vancouver, BC, Canada
[3] School of Computing, Queen's University, Kingston, ON, Canada

Abstract. Motivation: Accurate detection of prostate cancer using ultrasound data is a challenging yet highly relevant clinical question. A significant roadblock for training accurate models for cancer detection is the lack of histopathology labels with high resolution that correspond to the presence of cancer in the entire imaging or biopsy planes. Histopathology reports only provide a coarse, representation of cancer distribution in an image region; the distribution of cancer in itself is only approximately reported, making labels generated from these reports very noisy. Method: We propose a multi-constraint optimization method in a co-teaching framework with two deep neural networks. These networks are simultaneously and jointly trained, where each network uses data identified by its peer network as less noisy, to update itself. We propose two additional constraints based on the statistics of cancer distribution and noisy nature of labels to the conventional co-teaching framework. Results: We demonstrate the effectiveness of the proposed learning methodology using a challenging ultrasound dataset with 380 biopsy cores obtained from 89 patients during systematic prostate biopsy. Our results show that our proposed multi-constraint optimization method leads to a significant improvements in terms of area under the curve and balanced accuracy over baseline co-teaching method for detection of prostate cancer.

Keywords: Noisy label · Histopathology coarse label · Prostate cancer · Ultrasound

This work is funded in part by the Natural Sciences and Engineering Research Council of Canada (NSERC), the Canadian Institutes of Health Research (CIHR), and Borealis AI through the Borealis AI Global Fellowship Award.
G. Javadi and S. Samadi—Joint first authors, the order is selected randomly.
P. Black, P. Mousavi and P. Abolmaesumi—Joint senior authors.

M. de Bruijne et al. (Eds.): MICCAI 2021, LNCS 12908, pp. 680–689, 2021.
https://doi.org/10.1007/978-3-030-87237-3_65

1   Introduction

Histopathology analysis of biopsy samples is an indispensable tool in cancer diagnosis that provides gold-standard assessment of tissues for abnormality. In recent years with evolution of deep learning in medical imaging, several deep learning approaches have been proposed for Prostate Cancer (PCa) diagnosis with ultrasound (US) imaging [7,8,11,14,15,17], where histopathology of biopsy cores is the basis for labeling of tissue structure and its characteristics. Histopathology reports of PCa cores include information on the presence of cancer, its grade, and the extent of cancer involvement in a core (in percentage or length). Measurements of cancer involvement are usually performed by visual estimation using a regular ruler or the side graticule available on most microscopes [2]. Given the absence of detailed information about the spatial distribution of cancer in core, using pathology reports as ground truth leads to weak and noisy labels for training deep networks. These networks tend to over fit to such noisy labels [20].

Several groups have tackled the problem of training deep networks with weak and noisy labels in the machine learning literature [3,5,9,13], and for medical imaging, where small numbers of samples are available [10]. In one category of solutions a weighted loss is used to mitigate label noise [4,6,18]. In these methods, an estimation of the label noise is used as a weight for samples. Samples that have a higher likelihood of label error are down-weighted, and sometimes completely ignored, during model training. Estimating label noise is usually challenging, in practice. Meta-Weight-Net (MW-Net) [19] uses a small number of "clean" samples to learn a weighting function. Obtaining such a set of clean samples, in itself, is not always feasible either. Wei et al. use co-teaching [6] and remedy the problem by training two deep neural networks simultaneously. Each network selects a set of clean data, using the samples that perform well, for its peer's training.

In this paper, we reformulate the weakly supervised problem of prostate cancer detection as a multi-constraint optimization problem. We combine the co-teaching framework and an adaptive weighted loss to analyze a sequence of ultrasound images (Fig. 1). Using data from 89 patients undergoing systematic biopsy, we leverage the reported "involvement of cancer" within each biopsy core to estimate label noise. We use these estimates to down-weight samples from cancerous cores that have low involvement. To reflect the uncertainty associated with the reported cancer involvement values and to calculate them, we compute a distribution via data augmentation. We demonstrate that by using the involvement information while considering its uncertainty as an adaptive loss, we can improve the performance of PCa classification. Furthermore, since the core labels are reliable, we consider an additional constraint to assure that the network learn core labels. To the best of our knowledge, this paper is the first study which uses noisy labels along with cancer involvement in core as prior information to train deep neural networks for PCa detection.

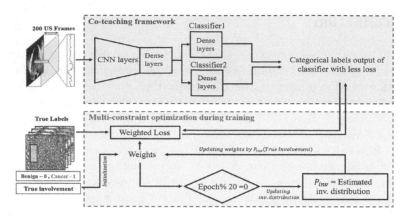

Fig. 1. An overview of proposed framework for training deep neural networks for PCa detection with noisy labels. The training consists of two steps to address noisy labels: first, in a co-teaching framework, two classifiers are trained simultaneously. Then, an adaptive loss function is used to decrease the contribution of none-cancerous regions in each biopsy core. The input data are sequences of ultrasound images from systematic biopsy. The labels for training and initial weights for the loss function are driven from histopathology reports.

2   Materials and Methods

2.1   Data

Our data consist of 380 biopsy cores obtained from 89 subjects during systematic prostate biopsy. The participants provided informed consent to be a part of this study, and the Institutional Research Ethics Board approved the investigation. Based on the prostate volume, 8 to 12 samples are taken from a patient during sextant biopsy. We use the data acquisition protocol suggested by [7]. For each biopsy core, 200 frames of radio-frequency (RF) ultrasound data are captured by holding the transducer still for approximately 5 s. We use a BK3500 ultrasound machine in conjunction with a software development kit (SDK) to connect our in-house data collection software to ultrasound machine for collecting RF signals. The biopsy gun is then fired to collect the tissue sample.

Preprocessing: As the first step in processing the data, we exclude the data with artifacts due to patient and hand motion or significant shadowing. To match the pathology results to the biopsied tissue on ultrasound images, we analyze RF data in the area around the needle. Therefore, we first localize the needle tip in US frames manually. Subsequently, a region of interest (ROI) of size 2×18 mm starting 2 mm from the tip of needle is selected. As a result, each data sample is a sequence of 200 frames of cropped ultrasound images associated with a biopsy core. A review of the literature shows that temporal ultrasound data is promising for detection of prostate cancer [7,8,16] compared to methods that only use a single ultrasound image. As a result, we use this protocol as a base for our data analysis. The data are then labeled as cancer or benign, based on the histopathology results for each core.

2.2 Method

Let each data sample be a bag of signals $\mathbf{X}_i = \{\mathbf{x}_1, \ldots \mathbf{x}_{n_i}\}$, where n_i, is the number of signals in each biopsy core $(\mathbf{X}_i)$ and $\mathbf{x}_j$ is a sequence of 200 time points. Pathology reports provide us with two labels for each core (i): 1) label $(\tilde{y}_i)$, which is zero or one for benign or cancer, respectively, and 2) involvement (C_i), that varies between zero and one with zero representing benign and any other value representing the proportion of cancer in the biopsied sample. The ground truth for each signal in a bag, which is defined by $\mathbf{y} = \{y_j | j = 1, \ldots, n\}$, is unknown, but is related to the core labels by $\max(\mathbf{y}) = \tilde{y}$, we ignore the core index (i) for simplicity. Consequently, PCa classification would be considered in the form of weakly supervised learning approach. We propose to use "involvement" as auxiliary information and define our problem as a multi-constraint optimization. For each core i, we solve the following set of equations:

$$\min_{\Theta, \mathbf{y}_i} \quad loss_{Main}(\hat{\mathbf{y}}_i, \mathbf{y}_i) \quad (Main);$$

$$\text{s.t.} \quad \max(\hat{\mathbf{y}}_i) = \tilde{y}_i \quad (Max); \tag{1}$$

$$\frac{|\hat{\mathbf{y}}_i|}{n_i} = C_i \quad (Involvement),$$

where C is the reported involvement value, and $loss_{Main}$ can be any loss function in general.

Main Objective: To solve the Main optimization problem, the signal level true labels $(\mathbf{y})$ are required. The only histopathology labels available are those for an entire biopsy core. Therefore, we label all signals in a core with the core labels, making the labels inherently noisy. We use a state-of-the-art approach called co-teaching [6] to tackle label noise. In this method, two different networks with the same structure but distinct initializations are used for classification. Each classifier's easy inputs (inputs with lower classification error) are used to update the other classifier. The idea behind using two networks is to prevent biased prediction from one network to directly back propagate in the same network and this is up to their peer network to select what data should be used for training. As a result, we expect this framework can deal with label noise better than the self-evolving one. To select the easy inputs we select a number of samples that has the lower loss value. In a batch D which has $|D|$ number of samples, $R(e)|D|$ will be selected to minimize $loss_{Main}(\hat{\mathbf{y}}, \mathbf{y}|D')$, where D' is the sub batch and $R(e)$ is the ratio of a batch that would be selected in each epoch and decreases gradually to a fixed value $1 - \tau$ as:

$$R(e) = 1 - min(\frac{e}{e_{max}}, \tau), \tag{2}$$

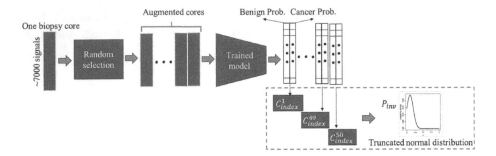

Fig. 2. Estimating the probability distribution function of involvement. We calculate the involvement of outputs across augmented versions of one biopsy core and compute mean (μ) and standard deviation (σ) of calculated involvements to estimate a Gaussian distribution for involvement.

where e and e_{max} are the current epoch, and the maximum number of epochs, respectively and τ is a constant variable in the range of $[0, 1]$.

The input to the co-teaching network is a batch of signals selected randomly from all signals of all cores and patients in the training set. Although the optimization problem (Eq. 1) is defined on core level, due to the limited number of training samples, signal level training is performed. This approach also sees a wider range of patients in every training batch, which leads to a more generalized model that can capture patients' variations more accurately in the future. The connection between signal level and core level labels is explained in the following.

Max Constraint: To apply the Max constraint, a shared memory is considered to reserve the maximum value of the predicted labels ($\max(\hat{\mathbf{y}})$) for each core. $\max(\hat{\mathbf{y}})$ is the core level label estimation. During the training, whenever we detect a cancerous signal the core level estimation of the related core will be equal to one. By defining a new loss $loss_{Max} = |\max(\hat{\mathbf{y}}) - \tilde{y}|$ and using the standard Lagrangian-dual optimization method, the total loss is defined as:

$$loss_{Total} = loss_{Main} + \lambda\, loss_{Max}. \tag{3}$$

Involvement Constraint: As described previously, involvement (C_i) is a rough estimate of the cancer ratio in a core. Therefore, mathematically, we can consider it as a random variable. Generally, the expected value of a random variable is used to constrain the optimization objective. However, in our case, each batch of training data contains signals from multiple cores, and accurate estimation of the involvement of individual cores in that batch is challenging. Therefore, the Involvement constraint cannot be added as a loss term to $loss_{Total}$. Moreover, there are uncertainties associated with the involvement values, that will be ignored by using a fixed value. We empirically show that considering the variation improves the classification performance.

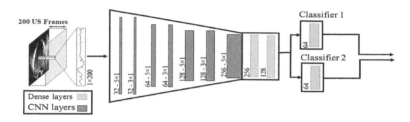

Fig. 3. Network structure and details of convolutional and dense layers.

To account for the uncertainty of the involvement values we propose to estimate the probability distribution of the predicted involvement and use the probability of the involvement as sample weight. Estimation of the involvement probability requires considerable computational resources and it is not a trivial task to
be performed per epoch. Therefore, we estimate $Pr(\frac{|\hat{\mathbf{y}}_i|}{n_i} = C_i)$ every 20 epochs,
and reward the signals in each core with their related probability values.

Estimating Probability Distribution: To estimate the probability distribution, an augmentation method to compute mean (μ) and standard deviation (σ)
of predicted involvement value is considered (Fig. 2). 50 augmented cores are
generated from every core by selecting 80% of its signals randomly. For each
of the augmented cores, C_i is computed by dividing the number of cancerous
signals by the total number of signals in the core. We assume C_i is a truncated
Gaussian variable, $0 < C_i < 1$. Therefore, its probability distribution can be
written as:

$$P_{inv}(c) = \frac{1}{\sigma} \frac{\Phi(\frac{c-\mu}{\sigma})}{\Phi(\frac{1-\mu}{\sigma}) - \Phi(\frac{-\mu}{\sigma})}, \tag{4}$$

$$\Phi(x) = \frac{1}{2\pi} \exp(-\frac{1}{2}x^2). \tag{5}$$

3   Experiments and Results

We divide our patients into mutually exclusive training (182 cores from 42
patients), validation (92 cores from 34 patients) and test (106 cores from 13
patients) sets. We design a network of seven 1D convolutional layers followed
by batch normalization and dropout and two dense layers as a feature generator
model. The two classifiers each have a dense layer. Figure 3 shows the details of
convolutional and dense layers of the network. The output of classifiers are cate-
gorical labels; $\hat{\mathbf{y}}_c = f(\mathbf{X}, \Theta)$, and $\hat{\mathbf{y}} = argmax(\hat{\mathbf{y}}_c)$, where $\hat{\mathbf{y}} = \{\hat{y}_j | j = 1, \ldots, n\}$
is a vector of labels for all the signals in the batch. $loss_{Main}$ is set to cross
entropy. Adam is used as the optimizer with a constant learning rate of $1e - 3$
and the batch size is set to 2024.

Table 1. The two top rows show model performance for classification of cores in the test data. The two bottom rows show the performance by two different strategies. Easy refers to a model that learns from cores that have high P_{inv}, and Hard refers to a model that learns from cores with low P_{inv}.

Method	AUC	Balanced accuracy	Sensitivity	Specificity
Co-teaching [6]	61	58	65	57
Proposed method	70	67	78	57
Easy	77	53	91	42
Hard	63	60	61	60

The clinical standard for evaluation of the performance of an imaging technology for prostate cancer detection is set by the PROMIS study (740 patients, 11 clinical sites) [1] comparing mp-MRI with ultrasound-guided sextant biopsy. In that study, the reported sensitivity and specificity of mp-MRI for detection of aggressive cancer was 88% and 45%, respectively, vs. those of 48% and 99% for the sextant biopsy, respectively. We compare our method with co-teaching as the baseline [6]. Table 1 shows a promising improvement in terms of area under the curve (AUC), balanced accuracy, sensitivity, and specificity.

The prediction of the biopsy region is shown in Fig. 4 with heat maps of the biopsy cores depicted in the corner of each US image. The colormaps reflect cancer likelihood as predicted by our model. The red and blue colors refer to cancer and benign predictions, respectively. As seen from these images, the proportion of the red regions on each colormap is correlated with the involvement value for that core. In case of benign cores, a significant portion of the heat map is blue.

3.1 Ablation Study

The main optimization technique proposed in our work is a combination of two constraints: a) max constraint that limits the detected cancer ratio in benign cores, which is crucial in our optimization problem because it helps increase the specificity of the model. Low specificity is also a well-known issue in detection of prostate cancer with other imaging modalities such as multi-parametric MRI [1] and b) involvement, as reported by pathology which constrains the fraction of detected cancer in each biopsy core. In an ablation study (Fig. 5), we show the effect of each of these constraints. Starting with a baseline AUC of 61% with co-teaching, the results improved to 64% by incorporating the max constraint (Fig. 5b). The results further improved to 70% by applying the involvement constraint, which further shrinks the search space for the max constraint.

We perform two experiments to study the effect of adaptive weighted loss on prostate cancer diagnosis: 1) using the involvement reported in histopathology reports as a fixed value to weigh the loss while this weight does not change during training; 2) using an adaptive weighted loss, where the weights are updated every 20 epochs with a new estimate of the probability of involvement. Figure 5a shows the receiver operating characteristic (ROC) curve for both weighting methods.

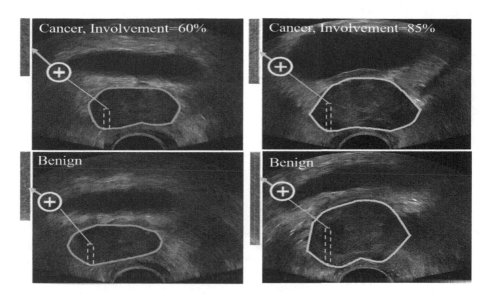

Fig. 4. Cancer likelihood of biopsy cores (dashed box). The red and blue colors refer to cancer and benign predictions, respectively. Involvement shows the proportion of cancer in cores that are labeled as cancer by histopathology. (Color figure online)

Focal loss, a dynamic weighted loss approach, has been proposed in [12]. Here, the weights are modified during training such that a network learns more from cores with higher loss values. Although the idea works well when labels are mostly clean, in our data with noisy labels implementing such an approach will result in higher loss values. We perform an experiment to show that in our data with noisy labels, training from easy cores (i.e. high involvement and low loss values) will lead to higher AUC than learning from hard cores (i.e. low involvement and high loss values). To encourage the network to learn from easy cores, we use P_{inv} as a weight in the loss, and to learn from hard cores we use $1 - P_{inv}$ as such. Results in Table 1 show that when the models focus on easy samples, specificity is lower while the overall performance (represented by AUC) is better. The prostate has a wide range of tissue patterns, which makes learning benign cores difficult. Any deviation from majority benign signals would be considered as cancer. Therefore, in our framework benign cores are counted as hard cores and when the network is encouraged to learn from easy cores, it would not learn benign cores well. Interestingly, this observation from ultrasound data corroborates with findings from multi-parametric MRI, which also suffers from low specificity [1]. However, sensitivity is often more significant in a cancer classification problem. By adding the Max constraint, the network is forced strongly to predict higher probability of benign than cancer for all benign signals. This fact is proven by the result of our proposed method in Table 1, which shows that using the Max constraint simultaneously with the Involvement constraint improves the specificity.

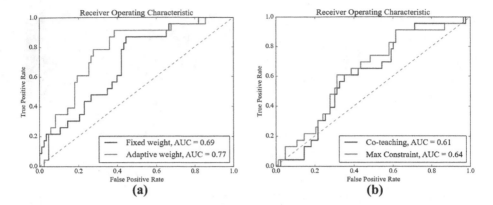

Fig. 5. The effect of each constraint in ROC is compared with a reference method. (a) ROC curve is compared between fixed weight and our proposed adaptive weight approach. (b) ROC curve is shows the effect of adding the Max constraint to co-teaching [6] method.

4   Conclusion

In this paper, we address the prostate cancer classification as a weakly supervised problem and provide a solution that involves dual-constraint optimization: 1) Max constraint, where in addition to the main classification objective a constraint is applied to the maximum prediction of all signals in a core to encourage its equality with the core label; 2) Involvement constraint, where we apply a constraint to adjust the proportion of cancer prediction in a core to the involvement value reported in histopathology. To account for the uncertainty of involvement measurements, we propose to use the probability of involvement as a sample weight. Each signal in a core is weighted with the probability of its involvement using its probability distribution function.

References

1. Ahmed, H.U., et al.: Diagnostic accuracy of multi-parametric MRI and TRUS biopsy in prostate cancer PROMIS: a paired validating confirmatory study. Lancet **389**(10071), 815–822 (2017)
2. Amin, M.B., et al.: The critical role of the pathologist in determining eligibility for active surveillance as a management option in patients with prostate cancer. Arch. Pathol. Lab. Med. **138**(10), 1387–1405 (2014)
3. Feng, L., An, B.: Partial label learning with self-guided retraining. In: Proceedings of the AAAI Conference on Artificial Intelligence, vol. 33, pp. 3542–3549 (2019)
4. Ghosh, A., Lan, A.: Do we really need gold samples for sample weighting under label noise? In: Proceedings of the IEEE/CVF Winter Conference on Applications of Computer Vision (WACV), pp. 3922–3931, January 2021
5. Gong, C., Zhang, H., Yang, J., Tao, D.: Learning with inadequate and incorrect supervision. In: 2017 IEEE International Conference on Data Mining (ICDM), pp. 889–894. IEEE (2017)

6. Han, B., et al.: Co-teaching: robust training of deep neural networks with extremely noisy labels. In: Advances in Neural Information Processing Systems 2018, pp. 8527–8537, 4 December 2018
7. Javadi, G., et al.: Multiple instance learning combined with label invariant synthetic data for guiding systematic prostate biopsy: a feasibility study. Int. J. Comput. Assist. Radiol. Surg. (2020)
8. Javadi, G., et al.: Complex cancer detector: complex neural networks on nonstationary time series for guiding systematic prostate biopsy. In: Martel, A.L., et al. (eds.) MICCAI 2020. LNCS, vol. 12263, pp. 524–533. Springer, Cham (2020). https://doi.org/10.1007/978-3-030-59716-0_50
9. Jiang, L., Zhou, Z., Leung, T., Li, L.J., Fei-Fei, L.: MentorNet: learning data-driven curriculum for very deep neural networks on corrupted labels. In: International Conference on Machine Learning, pp. 2304–2313. PMLR (2018)
10. Karimi, D., Dou, H., Warfield, S.K., Gholipour, A.: Deep learning with noisy labels: exploring techniques and remedies in medical image analysis. Med. Image Anal. **65**, 101759 (2020)
11. Klotz, L., et al.: Comparison of micro-ultrasound and multiparametric magnetic resonance imaging for prostate cancer: a multicenter, prospective analysis. Can. Urol. Assoc. J. **15**(1), E11 (2021)
12. Lin, T.Y., Goyal, P., Girshick, R., He, K., Dollár, P.: Focal loss for dense object detection. In: Proceedings of the IEEE International Conference on Computer Vision, pp. 2980–2988 (2017)
13. Ren, M., Zeng, W., Yang, B., Urtasun, R.: Learning to reweight examples for robust deep learning. In: International Conference on Machine Learning, pp. 4334–4343. PMLR (2018)
14. Rohrbach, D., Wodlinger, B., Wen, J., Mamou, J., Feleppa, E.: High-frequency quantitative ultrasound for imaging prostate cancer using a novel micro-ultrasound scanner. Ultrasound Med. Biol. **44**(7), 1341–1354 (2018)
15. Sedghi, A., et al.: Improving detection of prostate cancer foci via information fusion of MRI and temporal enhanced ultrasound. Int. J. Comput. Assist. Radiol. Surg. (2020)
16. Sedghi, A., et al.: Deep neural maps for unsupervised visualization of high-grade cancer in prostate biopsies. Int. J. Comput. Assist. Radiol. Surg. **14**, 1009–1016 (2019)
17. Shao, Y., Wang, J., Wodlinger, B., Salcudean, S.E.: Improving prostate cancer (PCa) classification performance by using three-player minimax game to reduce data source heterogeneity. IEEE Trans. Med. Imaging **39**(10), 3148–3158 (2020)
18. Shu, J., Zhao, Q., Chen, K., Xu, Z., Meng, D.: Learning adaptive loss for robust learning with noisy labels. arXiv preprint arXiv:2002.06482 (2020)
19. Shu, Q.X., Lixuan, Y., Qian, Z., Sanping, Z., Zongben, X., Deyu, M.: Meta-weight-net: learning an explicit mapping for sample weighting. In: NeurIPS, pp. 1919–1930 (2019)
20. Zhang, C., Bengio, S., Hardt, M., Recht, B., Vinyals, O.: Understanding deep learning requires rethinking generalization. arXiv preprint arXiv:1611.03530 (2017)

Rethinking Ultrasound Augmentation: A Physics-Inspired Approach

Maria Tirindelli[1], Christine Eilers[1(✉)], Walter Simson[1], Magdalini Paschali[1],
Mohammad Farid Azampour[1,2], and Nassir Navab[1,3]

[1] Computer Aided Medical Procedures, Technical University of Munich,
Munich, Germany
christine.eilers@tum.de
[2] Department of Electrical Engineering, Sharif University of Technology, Tehran, Iran
[3] Computer Aided Medical Procedures, John Hopkins University,
Baltimore, MD, USA

Abstract. Medical Ultrasound (US), despite its wide use, is characterized by artefacts and operator dependency. Those attributes hinder the gathering and utilization of US datasets for the training of deep neural networks used for computer-assisted intervention systems. Data augmentation is commonly used to enhance model generalization and performance. However, common data augmentation techniques, such as affine transformations do not align with the physics of US and, when used carelessly can lead to unrealistic US images. To this end, we propose a set of physics-inspired transformations, including deformation, reverb and signal-to-noise ratio, that we apply on US B-mode images for data augmentation. We evaluate our method on a new spine US dataset for the tasks of bone segmentation and classification.

Keywords: Ultrasound · Computer-assisted interventions · Data augmentation · Classification · Segmentation

1 Introduction

Ultrasound (US) is a radiation-free, low-cost, and flexible imaging technique. However, US is characterized by low signal-to-noise ratio (SNR), artefacts, such as phase aberration, reverberation or scattering and an increased operator dependency. These attributes account for high variability in US images. Due to these shortcomings, interpreting US scans is an especially challenging task.

With the rise of machine learning in medical imaging, Deep Neural Networks (DNN) are applied to US imaging to facilitate their interpretation [1]. Applications for these methods include bone segmentation and bone registration [10,21–23]. Successful execution of these tasks can enable the development of innovative applications with an increased degree of autonomy, including robotic scans and

---

M. Tirindelli and C. Eilers—The authors contributed equally.

© Springer Nature Switzerland AG 2021
M. de Bruijne et al. (Eds.): MICCAI 2021, LNCS 12908, pp. 690–700, 2021.
https://doi.org/10.1007/978-3-030-87237-3_66

diagnostic support [18–20]. However, training DNNs requires large and diverse datasets. For medical US such datasets are limited due to the strenuous acquisition and annotation process.

Moreover, US datasets that can be used for training DNNs should cover a wide range of variability, induced by operator dependency, US machines, acquisition parameters, and subject-anatomies. Such diverse US datasets could ensure the generalization of DNNs to an unseen test subject during a computer-aided intervention.

In many computer vision tasks, data augmentation is applied to overcome the lack of training data [2]. For DNNs trained with natural images, datasets are artificially increased by applying different transformation techniques. Augmentation methods could broadly be divided into two categories, namely synthetic data generation and image modification. In the first category, generative adversarial networks (GANs) [3] are used to create synthetic data based on the limited available dataset. Such models have been applied by Zaman et al. [4] on US images for different time gain compensations, different depths and different roll and pitch motions of the US probe. Synthetic augmentations, however, require a rather large amount of data to train the GAN and are, therefore, not suited for every scenario.

In the second category, classical image modifications, such as random scaling, translations, rotations, and Gaussian noise additions, are applied to a dataset. In US this approach has been used in different works. Baka et al. [5] performed data augmentation through mirroring and small free-form deformations in US spine images for bone segmentation. Other works applied random shifting [6,11,14], random flipping [6–9,11,13,14], different translations [8,12], rotation transformations [9,10,12–14] and varying brightness [7,9] as an approach for data augmentation.

However, these classical augmentations are based on the mechanisms behind optical cameras which strongly differ from the principles of US. Applying these transformations to US scans could create unrealistic US images inconsistent with the real variability in US acquisitions. A horizontal flipping (Fig. 2 a)) of the US image is still consistent with a 180-degree rotation of the US transducer. A vertical flipping, however, would result in a shadowing region between a strong reflector and the transducer, as shown in Fig. 2 b) which does not reflect the physical model of attenuation. Rotations and translations of the image (shown in Fig. 2 c), d)) result in displacement between the location of the transducer at the top of the image and the image content, therefore creating a gap between the wave source and reflective tissue.

To this end, we propose a novel augmentation technique for US imaging that is inspired by the physical behavior of US. In this paper our contributions are:

- We propose a novel data augmentation method, using a set of US image modifications that take into account realistic sources of variability in US (Fig. 1). Our method can expand the size of US datasets and provide anatomically and physically consistent variability.
- We comprehensively evaluate our method on the challenging tasks of bone segmentation and classification regarding the occurrence of bone per frame

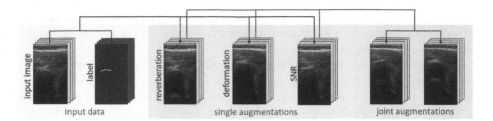

Fig. 1. Our proposed data augmentation pipeline: from US images and corresponding bone masks (yellow), different augmentations are generated (green) and can be merged in the same image (blue). (Color figure online)

to showcase its suitability for a variety of crucial tasks for computer-assisted interventions.

• We provide a new spine US dataset, that can be used for tasks such as automated robotic US scanning and intelligent localization of regions of interest.

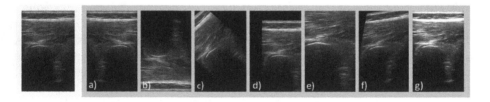

Fig. 2. Classical augmentations applied to an US image: a) horizontal flip, b) vertical flip, c) rotation, d) translation, e) scaling, f) shearing, g) brightness adaption.

2   Methods

The proposed augmentations are inspired by the physical model of wave propagation in medical US. These augmentations use the identification of regions of high-echogenicity or attenuation in order to model and augment the wave propagation and resulting B-mode image. We propose augmenting training data based on deformation due to probe pressure, reverberation artifacts and signal-to-noise-ratio, which have been tailored to linear US imaging (1).

2.1   Deformation

In this section, we propose a deformation model, seen in Fig. 3 that simulates deformations from variations in the contact pressure of the US probe on interrogated tissues. Assuming a transducer displacement d_{probe} for a given augmentation, we derive its respective Displacement Field (DF) for the deformed medium.

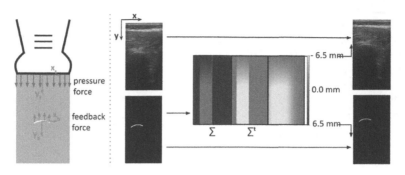

Fig. 3. Deformation Pipeline: Left: The forces applied by the US probe (red arrows) and bones (green arrows), and the coordinate systems centered in the bone (x_b, y_b) and the probe centroids (x_p, y_p), respectively. Right: The original B-mode image and label. The label is used to compute the DF (Σ) induced by the probe pressure. To avoid unrealistic gap above the skin layer, the DF is expressed in the probe coordinate system (Σ^t) and blurred. Σ^t is finally applied to both image and label. (Color figure online)

This DF is then applied to the input B-mode image resulting in our proposed augmentation. The DF is generated from a simplified physical model of the interactions of soft tissues, bones and the transducer. Specifically, we assume that soft-tissues are isotropic and homogeneous, that the probe pressure is applied along the axial direction and that the bone is a static body without deformation or transformation. Furthermore, we assume that only tissues between the probe and bone undergo compression and lateral tissue deformation is negligible. In lateral tissues there is no deformation, thus the DF is constant and equal to d_{probe}. In tissues laying between bone and probe, we can derive the deformation components as $\epsilon_{yy} = F/EA$, where A is the transducer area and F is the force applied by the probe and E is the Young's Modulus. This can be rewritten as $F = d_{\text{probe}}EA/y_{\text{probe}}$, where y_{probe} is the position of the probe in the bone coordinate system. Hence, we have:

$$\Sigma(x, y) = \int \epsilon_{yy} dy \bigg|_{\Sigma(x,0)=0} = -H(-y)\frac{F}{EA}y = -H(-y)\frac{d_{\text{probe}}}{y_{\text{probe}}}y \qquad (1)$$

where $\Sigma(x, y)$ is the DF.

In order to avoid unrealistic gaps between skin and transducer, we rewrite the displacements in the transducer coordinate system. In this coordinate system y_{bone} is the position of the bone with respect to the probe. This corresponds to applying an offset of d_{probe} to the DF equation. To ensure smooth transitions between regions with large and small displacements, we add lateral gaussian smoothing. The transducer translation d_{probe} is randomly sampled in our US augmentation. Pseudo-code is shown in Algorithm 1.

Algorithm 1. Computation of Σ^t given d_{probe}

---

for $i, j = 1 :$ Width, Height **do**

   $\Sigma(i,j)^t = -d_{\text{probe}}$ **if** (i,j) is bone or below bone

   $\Sigma(i,j)^t = -d_{\text{probe}}/y_{\text{bone}} \cdot j$ **if** (i,j) is above bone

   $\Sigma(i,j)^t = 0$ **else**

end for

smooth($\Sigma^t(i,j)$)

2.2   Reverberation

In this section we propose a method to simulate reverberation artifacts on US data as can be seen in Fig. 4. Our model uses a ray-based approximation and assumes constant a speed of sound c in tissues. Following these assumptions, a highly reflective structure at depth Δ in the interrogated tissue will generate an echo at $\Delta = \dfrac{ct_1}{2}$. If the echo intensity is sufficiently high, the signal is again reflected at the tissue-transducer interface back once more at the tissue-interface level. This generates an additional echo in the recorded signal, located at Δ_r:

$$\Delta_r = 2\Delta = t_1 c = \frac{t_2 c}{2} \tag{2}$$

Multiple reflections, commonly known as reverberation, can occur several times, generating reverberation artifacts located at multiples of Δ in the B-mode image.

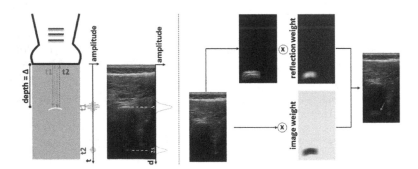

Fig. 4. Reverberation Pipeline. Left: The transmitted signal and the echos generated by a bone at depth Δ. In the time-amplitude plot the signals generated by the first echo (green arrow) and reverberation echo (red arrow) are reported. The first echo generates a bright area in the B-mode image at Δ, while the reverberation echo generates an artifact at 2Δ. Right: The generation of reverberation artifacts on B-mode data. The patch containing the bone is extracted and replicated at multiples of Δ. The replicated patch is weighted and summed up to the original image. (Color figure online)

In the proposed method we simulate reverberation artifacts, by first computing the bone centroid (x_c, y_c) on the label image. Secondly, we shift the image patch containing the bone along the axially by $2y_c$. Finally, we compute the resulting image as the weighted sum of the shifted patch and the original image. The multiplication weights for the reverberation region w_r are defined as the shifted label filtered with a Gaussian filter (kernel size=45 px, sigma=20 px) and scaled by a factor r_i, which we call reverberation intensity. The multiplication weights for the original image are defined as $1 - w_r$. The factor r_i defines the intensity of the reverberation artifact and is randomly sampled during the augmentation.

2.3 Signal-to-Noise Ratio

Signal-to-Noise Ratio (SNR) provides information on the relation between the amount of desired signal and the background noise. For bone segmentation, the signal is given by coherent structures such as bone, and the noise consists of the background speckle. In our method we propose to tune the SNR in B-Mode data by first extracting and scaling the signal in the image to enhance or reduce the SNR, e.g. the visibility of bones compared to the background. The proposed pipeline is shown in Fig. 5. To extract signal from the B-mode, we use the method proposed by [15] to compute local energy (LE) maps from B-Mode data. LE provides pixel-wise information on the signal energy at each location in space and is defined as:

$$LE(x) = f_e(x)^2 + f_{o1}(x)^2 + f_{o2}(x)^2 \tag{3}$$

where $f_e(x)$, $f_{o1}(x)$ and $f_{o2}(x)$ are the components of the monogenic signal extracted from the US data. To tune the SNR in the US data, we first normalize the images by the LE. Afterwards, we tune the LE maps by multiplying bone and non-bone pixels by different scaling factors, i_b and i_{bg}. These factors define the scaling between signal and background energies. For $i_b > i_{bg}$ the bone structure is enhanced, while for $i_b < i_{bg}$ the background is intensified, making the bone less visible. Both factors are randomly sampled during the augmentation. Finally, we re-scale the B-mode image by the tuned LE map, thus obtaining a new image with an enhanced or reduced SNR.

3 Experiments and Results

We evaluated the proposed US augmentations on the tasks of bone segmentation and bone classification.

Model Architecture: For the segmentation task we used a U-Net architecture [16], while for classification we use DenseNet121 [17]. For training we used learning rate of 0.01, Adam optimizer and Binary Cross Entropy loss function.

Dataset Acquisition: Our models were trained on an US dataset consisting of 10.656 US images (size 272 × 503) of 24 healthy volunteers with a BMI ranging from 20 to 25. The US scans were acquired with a Zonare z.one ultra

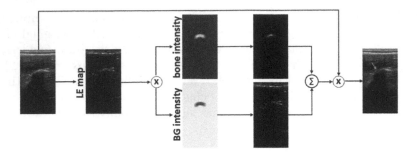

Fig. 5. SNR augmentation pipeline. The local energy (LE) map is computed based on the input image. This image is then multiplied with the label or its inverse and the intensity values to obtain tuned local energy maps for bone and background (BG) regions. The overall tuned local energy is computed by adding the bone and background parts and the augmented image is obtained by multiplication of the input image with the tuned local energy.

Table 1. Value ranges for the classical and proposed augmentation parameters selection during training. For each algorithm, the parameter is uniformly sampled from the value range.

Augmentation	Parameter	Value range
Classical	Rotation in degree	−10–10
	Translation (horizontal and vertical)	0.2, 0.2
	Scaling in both axis	1, 1
	Shearing in both axis	1, 1
	Brightness	0.2
Proposed	Deformation - d_{probe}	30–100
	Reverb - r_i	0.50–0.9
	SNR - i_b, i_{bg}	0.70–1.40

sp Convertible Ultrasound System (Zonare Medical Systems Inc.) with a L8-3 linear probe. We set the image depth to 7 cm, the gain to 92%, the frequency to 10 MHz and the sampling rate 13 Hz.

Segmentation. For the bone segmentation task, we used 5.284 frames containing bones. On each of these frames, bones were annotated pixel-wise. The dataset was split subject-level to training (3972 frames from 17 subjects), validation (782 frames from 5 subjects) and testing (500 frames from 2 subjects).

Classification. For the bone classification task, we leveraged 5.692 US frames from 22 subjects. We split the dataset into two classes: one containing at least one bone per frame, the other containing no bone in each frame. The dataset was split subject-level to training (3821 frames from 16 subjects), validation (1037 from 4 subjects) and testing (834 frames from 2 subjects).

Table 2. Baseline comparisons for bone segmentation with UNet and bone classification with DenseNet. We report the average metrics over 5-fold cross validation along with their respective standard deviation ($\pm$).

	Segmentation		Classification	
	DSC	HDF	ACC	F1
None	0.589 ± 0.07	20.72 ± 3.84	0.876 ± 0.06	0.770 ± 0.15
Classical	0.625 ± 0.03	17.76 ± 3.17	$\mathbf{0.883 \pm 0.04}$	0.780 ± 0.09
Reverb	0.604 ± 0.03	19.71 ± 2.20	$\mathbf{0.883 \pm 0.03}$	$\mathbf{0.802 \pm 0.04}$
Deformation	$\mathbf{0.626 \pm 0.01}$	19.06 ± 3.63	0.865 ± 0.04	0.759 ± 0.11
SNR	$\mathbf{0.626 + 0.02}$	$\mathbf{17.24 \pm 1.83}$	0.877 ± 0.06	0.764 ± 0.16
All	0.600 ± 0.02	17.32 ± 2.97	0.834 ± 0.02	0.742 ± 0.04

Implementation. Our method was implemented in PyTorch 1.7.1 and the DNNs were trained on a NVIDIA Titan V 12 GB HBM2 using Polyaxon[1]. The source code for our method and our dataset are publicly available[2]. For each task we evaluated the network performance using different augmentation techniques, that are shown in detail in Table 1. The value ranges were chosen empirically. Augmentations were only applied in training for both segmentation and classification tasks and were generated on the fly during training with a probability of 30%.

Evaluation Metrics. All our models were trained using 5-fold cross validation. For the segmentation model we report the average Dice Score (DSC) and Hausdorff Distance (HDF) with standard deviation. Regarding classification, we evaluate average accuracy (ACC) and F1-score (F1) with standard deviation.

4   Results and Discussion

Table 2 showcases the results for the segmentation and classification networks for different augmentations. "All" denotes models trained with all three proposed augmentations. For the segmentation task, it can be seen that augmentation substantially improves the network performance both in terms of DSC by 2–4% and HDF. This signifies the fact that data augmentation for the challenging task of bone segmentation is crucial and has a positive effect. The proposed transformations of Deformation and SNR show a marginal improvement of 1% for DSC compared to the classical augmentations, while SNR achieves the lowest HDF for all techniques. Additionally, the models trained with the proposed transformations had the lowest standard deviation among folds, highlighting their consistency. Combining all proposed transformations, the performance slightly drops by 2%, which could be attributed to the fact that the resulting combination of transformations is not present on our unseen test set.

---

[1] https://polyaxon.com/.
[2] https://github.com/mariatirindelli/UltrasoundAugmentation.

For the task of bone classification, the model trained with Reverb augmentation outperforms the other methods in terms of F1-Score by 2–7%, highlighting the potential of this transformation. Consistent with our segmentation findings, combining all transformations did not provide an additional benefit. Overall, the results indicated that Deformation and SNR transformations were beneficial for bone segmentation and Reverb for classification.

5   Conclusion

In this conference paper we introduced a novel, physics-inspired augmentation method for US B-mode images. We proposed augmentations that tune the SNR, deformations and reverberations. Our augmentations were evaluated on a new US spine dataset for the tasks of bone segmentation and bone classification. The results showcased the impact of data augmentation on training DNNs for medical US. US augmentation with deformations and reverberation marginally outperformed the classical augmentation baseline, highlighting the potential of these transformation approaches. Future work includes investigating further realistic and anatomically-consistent US augmentations that contribute towards training generalizable CNNs that can be leveraged for robotic US computer-assisted interventions.

Acknowledgements. This paper was partially funded by the Bayerische Forschungsstiftung, under Grant DOK-180-19, as well as the H2020 EU grant 688279 (EDEN2020) and the German Central Innovation Program for Small and Medium-sized Enterprises under grant agreement ZF4190502CR8 (PUMBA). We would also like to thank NVIDIA for the GPU donation.

References

1. Van Sloun, R.J.G., Cohen, R., Eldar, Y.C.: Deep learning in ultrasound imaging. Proc. IEEE **108**(1), 11–29 (2019)
2. Shorten, C., Khoshgoftaar, T.M.: A survey on image data augmentation for deep learning. J. Big Data **6**(1), 1–48 (2019)
3. Goodfellow, I.J., et al.: Generative adversarial networks. arXiv preprint arXiv:1406.2661 (2014)
4. Zaman, A., Park, S.H., Bang, H., Park, C., Park, I., Joung, S.: Generative approach for data augmentation for deep learning-based bone surface segmentation from ultrasound images. Int J. Cars 15, 931–941 (2020). https://doi.org/10.1007/s11548-020-02192-1
5. Baka, N., Leenstra, S., van Walsum, T.: Ultrasound aided vertebral level localization for lumbar surgery. IEEE Trans. Med. Imaging **36**(10), 2138–2147 (2017). https://doi.org/10.1109/TMI.2017.2738612
6. Duong, D.Q., et al.: Fully automated segmentation of alveolar bone using deep convolutional neural networks from intraoral ultrasound images. In: 41st Annual International Conference of the IEEE Engineering in Medicine and Biology Society (EMBC), Berlin, Germany, pp. 6632–6635 (2019). https://doi.org/10.1109/EMBC.2019.8857060

7. Hohlmann, B., Glanz, J., Radermacher, K.: Segmentation of the distal femur in ultrasound images. Curr. Dir. Biomed. Eng. **6**(1), 20200034 (2020)
8. Qi, X., Voar, N., Riera, L., Sarangi, A., Youssef, G., Vives, M., Hacihaliloglu, I.: Automatic Scan Plane Identification from 2D Ultrasound for Pedicle Screw Guidance. In: CAOS 2018 (EPiC Series in Health Sciences, vol. 2), pp. 168–174 (2018)
9. Benjdira, B., Ouni, K., Al Rahhal, M.M., Albakr, A., Al-Habib, A., Mahrous, E.: Spinal cord segmentation in ultrasound medical imagery. Appl. Sci. **10**(4), 1370 (2020)
10. Alsinan, A. Z., Vives, M., Patel, V., Hacihaliloglu, I.: Spine surface segmentation from ultrasound using multi-feature guided CNN. In: CAOS 2019 (EPiC Series in Health Sciences), vol. 3, pp. 6–10 (2019)
11. Nguyen, K.C.T., et al.: Alveolar bone segmentation in intraoral ultrasonographs with machine learning. J. Dental Res. **99**(9), 1054–1061 (2020). https://doi.org/10.1177/0022034520920593
12. Patel, H., Hacihaliloglu, I.: Improved automatic bone segmentation using large-scale simulated ultrasound data to segment real ultrasound bone surface data. In: IEEE 20th International Conference on Bioinformatics and Bioengineering (BIBE), Cincinnati, OH, USA, pp. 288–294 (2020). https://doi.org/10.1109/BIBE50027.2020.00054
13. Luan, K., Li, Z., Li, J.: An efficient end-to-end CNN for segmentation of bone surfaces from ultrasound. In: Computerized Medical Imaging and Graphics, vol. 84, p. 101766 (2020), ISSN 0895–6111. https://doi.org/10.1016/j.compmedimag.2020.101766
14. Ungi, T., et al.: Automatic spine ultrasound segmentation for scoliosis visualization and measurement. IEEE Trans. Biomed. Eng. **67**(11), 3234–3241 (2020). https://doi.org/10.1109/TBME.2020.2980540
15. Bridge, C.P., Noble, J.A.: Object localisation in fetal ultrasound images using invariant features. In: 2015 IEEE 12th International Symposium on Biomedical Imaging (ISBI), pp. 156–159. IEEE (2015)
16. Ronneberger, O., Fischer, P., Brox, T.: U-Net: convolutional networks for biomedical image segmentation. In: Navab, N., Hornegger, J., Wells, W.M., Frangi, A.F. (eds.) MICCAI 2015. LNCS, vol. 9351, pp. 234–241. Springer, Cham (2015). https://doi.org/10.1007/978-3-319-24574-4_28
17. Huang, G., Liu, Z., Van Der Maaten, L., Weinberger, K.Q.: Densely connected convolutional networks. In: Proceedings of the IEEE Conference on Computer Vision and Pattern Recognition, pp. 4700–4708 (2017)
18. Tirindelli, M., et al.: Force-ultrasound fusion: bringing spine robotic-us to the next "level." IEEE Robot. Autom. Lett. **5**(4), 5661–5668 (2020)
19. Esteban, J., et al.: Robotic ultrasound-guided facet joint insertion. Int. J. Comput. Assist. Radiol. Surg. **13**(6), 895–904 (2018)
20. Hase, H., et al.: Ultrasound-guided robotic navigation with deep reinforcement learning. In: IEEE/RSJ International Conference on Intelligent Robots and Systems (IROS) (2020)
21. Wang, P., Vives, M., Patel, V.M., Hacihaliloglu, I.: Robust real-time bone surfaces segmentation from ultrasound using a local phase tensor-guided CNN. Int. J. Comput. Assist. Radiol. Surg. **15**, 1127–1135 (2020)

22. Wang, P., Patel, V.M., Hacihaliloglu, I.: Simultaneous segmentation and classification of bone surfaces from ultrasound using a multi-feature guided CNN. In: Frangi, A.F., Schnabel, J.A., Davatzikos, C., Alberola-López, C., Fichtinger, G. (eds.) MICCAI 2018. LNCS, vol. 11073, pp. 134–142. Springer, Cham (2018). https://doi.org/10.1007/978-3-030-00937-3_16
23. Hetherington, J., Lessoway, V., Gunka, V., Abolmaesumi, P., Rohling, R.: SLIDE: automatic spine level identification system using a deep convolutional neural network. Int. J. Comput. Assist. Radiol. Surg. **12**(7), 1189–1198 (2017)

Author Index

Printed in the United States
by Baker & Taylor Publisher Services